A CENSUS OF GREEK MEDICAL MANUSCRIPTS

Manuscripts containing Greek medical texts were inventoried by author and work at the beginning of the 20th century by a group of philologists under the direction of Hermann Diels. Useful as it was—and will continue to be—Diels' catalogue omitted authors and works, misidentified manuscripts, and overlooked codices. Furthermore, since the publication of the catalogue, some libraries have adopted a new system of classification, manuscripts have been destroyed, items have changed location, and new ones have come to light.

The present *Census* is a checklist of the Greek medical manuscripts currently known in collections worldwide. It is both an amended and updated index of Diels' catalogue, and a list of the items missed or overlooked in Diels, or located since. Although it does not supersede Diels' catalogue, it is the indispensable instrument for a New Diels, and will be the reference for years to come for any new critical edition and medico-historical research based on manuscripts, besides providing the basis for a broad range of other historical inquiries, from codicology to the history of medicine and science, including Byzantine intellectual history, Renaissance studies and humanism, history of the book and early printing, and the history of medical philology and learning.

Alain Touwaide, Institute for the Preservation of Medical Traditions, Washington, DC, USA

Medicine in the Medieval Mediterranean

Medicine in the Medieval Mediterranean is a series devoted to all aspects of medicine in the Mediterranean area during the Middle Ages, from the 3rd/4th centuries to the 16th. Though with a focus on Greek medicine, diffused through the whole Mediterranean world and especially developed in Byzantium, it also includes the contributions of the cultures that were present or emerged in the area during the Middle Ages and after, and which interacted with Byzantium: the Latin West and early vernacular languages, the Syrian and Arabic worlds, Armenian, Georgian and Coptic groups, Jewish and Slavic cultures and Turkish peoples, particularly the Ottomans.

Medicine is understood in a broad sense: not only medical theory, but also the health conditions of people, nosology and epidemiology, diet and therapy, practice and teaching, doctors and hospitals, the economy of health, and the non-conventional forms of medicine from faith to magic, that is, all the spectrum of activities dealing with human health.

The series includes texts and studies. It will bring to light previously unknown, overlooked or poorly known documents interpreted with the most appropriate methods, and publish the results of cutting-edge research, so providing a wide range of scholarly and scientific fields with new data for further explorations.

A Census of Greek Medical Manuscripts

From Byzantium to the Renaissance

ALAIN TOUWAIDE

Institute for the Preservation of Medical Traditions,
Washington, DC, USA

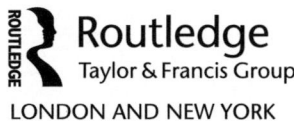

Routledge
Taylor & Francis Group

LONDON AND NEW YORK

First published 2016
by Routledge

2 Park Square, Milton Park, Abingdon, Oxfordshire OX14 4RN
52 Vanderbilt Avenue, New York, NY 10017

Routledge is an imprint of the Taylor & Francis Group, an informa business

First issued in paperback 2019

The Library of Congress has cataloged the printed edition as follows:
Library of Congress Control Number: 2015951326

ISBN: 978-1-4094-0656-3 (hbk)
ISBN: 978-0-367-87893-1 (pbk)

Typeset in Garamond Premier Pro
by Swales & Willis

Contents

Foreword by Paul Canart   *vii*

Introduction   *ix*

Notes for consultation   *xiii*

Acknowledgements   *xvii*

Census of Byzantine and Renaissance Manuscripts   1

Bibliography   *375*

Index   *423*

Foreword

As many other catalogers of ancient manuscripts—this has been my profession for more than 40 years—I sometimes need to describe Greek codices containing medical or related treatises. To this end, I have regularly consulted the well-known catalogue compiled by Hermann Diels and his collaborators, which has, and will continue to be, extremely useful. However, as Alain Touwaide appropriately reminds us in the *Introduction* to the present work, its limits, its shortcomings and its mistakes have long made it desirable to have, if not a completely revised edition of Diels' catalogue, at least a list of the many corrections and complements made possible thanks to the scholarly research over the past 60 years. The author of the present *Census* provides such a list.

Having followed for several decades—though episodically—Alain Touwaide's painstaking and time-consuming investigation, I can bear witness to the perseverance with which he has performed and completed his endeavor. Now having carefully and patiently read his impressive volume, I can attest to the extreme accuracy, as well as to the sheer magnitude, of his accomplishment. His work is the result of long and difficult research in the catalogues of manuscript collections and scholarly literature, completed by personal *in-situ* inspection of many codices. With the present volume, all the data resulting from this quest are made available to the scholarly community.

The present *Census* is not a *New Diels*, but the indispensable foundation for such a new catalogue. To compile such a work, all the Greek treatises, compilations and medical fragments contained in all the manuscripts that can be traced through history or that have been preserved through present day should be identified and described precisely enough to be distinguished from any other (be it in their original form or in later rearrangements). Then, their presence in all the manuscripts in which they are said to be found should be verified or negated on the basis of a direct analysis of the codices. Alain Touwaide's *Census* provides two major instruments toward such a new catalogue: first, his *Census* is an index that makes it possible to trace all the mentions of all the manuscripts listed in Diels. This index goes further, however, as it provides verification of the identification of all the manuscripts listed in Diels' catalogue (location and shelfmark), and also of their contents. His work does not supersede Diels' catalogue, however, as it does not repeat Diels' data once it has established their accuracy. Second, Touwaide's work lists a great number of manuscripts omitted by or unknown to Diels, together with a short, yet precise, description of the medical texts they contain.

The most significant contribution of the *Census*—one that I cannot stress enough—is that, in the many cases where Diels' catalogue provides incorrect information, Touwaide goes from one clue to another like a detective, and succeeds not only in catching the culprits of manuscript misidentifications in literature, sometimes going as far back as the Renaissance, but also—if not above all—in rescuing their victims and establishing the correct identity of the manuscripts misidentified in the scholarly tradition up to Diels and his collaborators. Those who work in the field know how much talent, flair, intuition, and patience such inquiries require.

I will not expand on the astute presentation of data in the *Census*, which deftly combines and clearly distinguishes between Diels' material reproduced *ad litteram* and Touwaide's own corrections and additions. I stress instead some of his strategic choices, aimed to make consultation of the work straightforward. For the many manuscripts incorrectly cited several times in Diels' lists, correct data are provided only for the first occurrence, instead of using cross-references which, in the footnotes of some publications, force readers through annoying gymnastics. Also, abandoning

19th- and even 20th-century scholarly usage, Touwaide provides an English translation for all the library and collection names originally in other languages, although one might regret that nowadays this is useful, if not necessary. For the identification of the contents of the manuscripts, however, Touwaide maintains the traditional usage of authors' names and titles in Latin, something that will be particularly useful in the future for catalographic purposes. In the bibliography, he deliberately applied the adage *quod abundat non vitiat* which, by way of consequence, causes pleasure when reading the endless titles cherished by 16th-, 17th- and 18th-century classical scholars.

Working from Touwaide's *Census*, it will be interesting to evaluate Diels' data and to make some statistic approximations. This could be done, for example, with the number of apparently different manuscripts listed in Diels which refer, in fact, to the same codices or are simply incorrect. One could also do similar evaluations about wrong or inaccurate locations of manuscripts, erroneous shelfmarks, or inexact identification of contents. Similar quantitative evaluation could be applied to the number of manuscripts added to those listed in Diels' catalogue by Touwaide.

As an example, and limiting myself to the first 250 manuscripts mentioned in Diels, I have calculated the number of codices newly introduced and analyzed by Touwaide: they total 194, that is, a number equivalent to 78 per cent of the sample of 250. Bearing in mind that the 250 items do not correspond by any means to 250 actual manuscripts, but to a smaller number because of inexact, inaccurate or redundant information in Diels' catalogue, it becomes immediately clear that Touwaide's *Census* richly increases the number of Greek codices with medical contents currently known.

If we add to this all the supplementary data and corrections provided by the *Census*, we can only acknowledge the magnitude and the accuracy of Alain Touwaide's achievement, congratulate him for his contribution to scholarship, and thank him for such a *magnum opus*.

Mgr. Paul Canart
Biblioteca Apostolica Vaticana
June 2015

Introduction[1]

In the study of ancient Greek medicine, manuscripts are of fundamental importance as they provide the primary sources without which no documented history can be written. In spite of centuries of activity,[2] no comprehensive inventory is available. The present volume aims to compensate for this lacuna and offers a world census of currently known Greek manuscripts with medical content.

This census is not entirely unprecedented as lists of Greek medical manuscripts have already been compiled in scholarship, from the *Bibliotheca botanica* and the *Bibliotheca medicinae practicae* by the Swiss physician, naturalist and encyclopedist Albrecht von Haller (1707–1777), published in 1771–1772 and 1776–1788, respectively, to *Die Handschriften der antiken Ärzte, Griechische Abteilung*, edited by the German historian of ancient Greek philosophy and science Hermann Diels (1848–1922) and published in 1905–1908 by the Berlin Academy of Sciences. However, these and similar compilations list only the manuscripts containing the treatises of a select number of ancient physicians. In addition, they do not offer in all cases exhaustive lists of manuscripts for the works under consideration, and even the most recent, Diels' *Handschriften der antiken Ärzte*, is now obsolete because new manuscripts have come to light since its publication, others have changed location, and further still, others were destroyed during the two World Wars of the 20th century.[3]

An attempt toward a systematic inventory of manuscripts was made in mid-19th century by the French librarian and historian of medicine Charles Daremberg (1817–1872). In order to compile a *Catalogue raisonné des manuscrits médicaux*,[4] Daremberg traveled extensively so as to personally inspect entire manuscript collections and identify all relevant items.[5] In spite of his efforts, however, he could not complete his project.

The present census departs from previous work in two ways: not only does it list the manuscripts of all currently identified Greek medical texts—authored or anonymous—produced in the Greek world from Hippocrates to the fall of Constantinople, but also it aims to be up-to-date and to reflect as closely as possible current knowledge of Greek medical literature and manuscripts. It is not a New Diels as the time has not yet come for such a new catalogue in spite of substantial

---

[1]   Bibliographical references in the footnotes provide the last name of the author(s), the year of publication of the work and the exact pages referred to. Full identification of works is provided in the Bibliography on pages 375–421 where abbreviated references are listed in alphabetical order of author's last name and, for each author, in chronological order of publication.

[2]   For a history of the search of Greek medical manuscripts in scholarship, see Touwaide 2009.

[3]   On these limitations of Diels' catalogue, see Touwaide 2009: 509–524. The conclusions presented in this article are based on an analysis of the manuscripts that were either listed by Diels as being preserved in libraries of the United Kingdom and Ireland, or are presently located in those libraries. As further study has revealed, these conclusions can be extended to the whole work.

[4]   On this project, see Touwaide 2009: 500–503.

[5]   For reports on these travels, see Daremberg 1845 and 1845/2, 1848, 1851 and 1852, with a re-edition of the latter two in the form of a monograph in Daremberg 1853.

progress in the inventory and description of ancient manuscripts worldwide, and the introduction of computerization in the humanities.

Building on available literature, the census presented here is largely an index of the manuscripts listed in Diels' *Handschriften der antiken Ärzte*. This index includes a full discussion of the not-infrequent manuscript citations that are incorrect in Diels (be it *in toto* or *in parte*). Examination of the contents, history or cataloguing of such items does not aim to replace Diels, even though the results provide data towards a *New Diels*. The aim is only to allow for proper identification of these manuscripts by providing correct shelfmark, collection, library or location according to the cases. The census goes beyond this corrected index of Diels: besides providing the current name of the cities and libraries mentioned in Diels in the original language and according to current English usage, it introduces many new items as a result of an expansion of the field in two directions: medical topics and chronology.

Medicine is understood here in a broad sense that encompasses many components during the period of the texts contained in preserved manuscripts: not only the canonical works of the so-called "Founding Fathers" Hippocrates and Galen, but also treatises of Christian anthropology,[6] analytical medicine,[7] psychology including oniromancy[8] and physiognomy, lists of *materia medica* and illustrated botanical reference compilations,[9] pharmaceutical formularies and hospital pharmacopeias, and literary works medical in nature.[10] Translations into Greek have also been taken into consideration, mostly from Arabic and Persian, but also from Latin. Lexica (mostly botanical) are included as a corollary of the translations, since they were tools for the practice of medicine in a multilingual and multicultural society. Manuscripts are also included for forms of medicine that may be deemed non-scientific by present standards, but were a part of contemporary medicine, medicinal practice, or world of medicine, health and disease. This is the case for iatromathematics, for example, the *Cyranides*, and the different forms of what is called the *Physiologus*.

Timewise, Diels is limited to the period spanning Hippocrates to Paul of Aegina, from the 5th century BCE to the 7th century CE. Although a few later physicians are present in the 1906 issue and the 1908 supplement, they are not numerous.[11] Many major and minor authors and works of the mid- or late-Byzantine periods are omitted, such as Theophanes Chrysobalantes, the *Efodia*, Symeon Seth, Nicephorus Gregoras, Nicephorus Blemmydes, Demetrius Pepagomenus, the many translations from Arabic or Persian, hospital manuals, or Johannes Argyropoulus to note just a few. I have tried to include as many post-7th-century CE physicians as identifications of authors and

---

6   Gregorius Nyssenus, Gregorius Nazianzenus, Nemesius and Meletius, for example.

7   The Aristotelian *Problemata*.

8   From Aristoteles, *De insomniis*, to Nicephorus Gregoras' commentary on Synesius' treatise.

9   Actually copies of Dioscorides, *De materia medica*, with plant representations.

10   The poems of Nicander, for instance.

11   Among the authors who can be ascribed with some plausibility to the period after Paul of Aegina listed in the 1906 issue (= II) and in the supplement (= N), are Abraham (I.3; N.42), Antonius Pyropulus (II.15; N.45), Beniaminus (II.22; N.46), Cassius iatrosophista (II.22; N.46), Chariton (II.23), Constantinus Meliteniota (II.24; N.47), Damascenus (II.25), Eleutherus (II.35), Esdras propheta (II.37–38; N.50–51), Euphemius Siculus (II.38; N.51), Iacobus Psychrestus (II.50), Ioannes Chumnos (II.52), Ioannes Esdra (II.53), Ioannes episcopus Prisdyanensis (II.54; N.55), Ioannes Staphidaces (II.55; N.55), Leo (II.57; N.56), Manuel Comnenus (N.57), Maximus (Planudes?) (II.62; N.57), Neophytus Prodromenus (II.68; N.60), Nicolaus Myrepsus (II.69; N.60), Nicomedes iatrosophista (II.69), Paulus Nicaeensis (II.81; N.63), Perzoe (II.81), Philippus Xerus (N.63), Photius monachus (II.85), Taronitus (II.100; N.67), Theophilus (II.101–106; N.68), Theophylactus Simocata (II.106; N.68), and Ioannes Zacharias Actuarius (II.108–111; N.69).

descriptions of texts in catalogues, relevant publications or personal inspection of collections *in situ* made possible.

For economy's sake, Diels' and new data are merged in a unique list. Several devices have been created to facilitate consultation: cross-referencing where appropriate, running titles on top of the pages, graphic presentation and organization of data on the pages, and also an index. All such finding aids are explained in the *Notes for consultation* that follow this introduction.

———————

This census is the result of three decades of research *in persona* in libraries all over the world, of constant and repeated travels (including to remote locations), of innumerable contacts started in a time when neither the Internet nor email existed, of long hours spent over catalogues in search for information that could not be found at first glance, of patient scrutiny of ancient and more recent lists of manuscripts, of tenacity and sometimes also of serendipity, and of active collaboration, the admirable erudition of many of my contacts, and most generous sharing of information.

I have been fortunate to receive help from many colleagues, curators, experts in auction houses, antiquarian book dealers, and specialists across the globe whose names appear in the *Acknowledgements* that follow the *Notes for consultation*. The length of the list is an eloquent witness to the generosity with which all of them have replied to my many questions. Also, I have benefitted from the services of the often-anonymous personnel in reading rooms of libraries worldwide who made it possible for me to consult the many manuscripts I requested. Without all of them—known or anonymous, named in the *Acknowledgements* or not—I would not have been able to collect the information presented here. All are in a certain way the co-authors of this volume, though they do not share the responsibility for its imperfections, imprecision or mistakes, all of which are mine.

———————

For the preparation of this census, I have collected information from available bibliographies, indexed relevant literature, made or acquired images of manuscripts, and, with the development of computerization, increasingly stored relevant information on digital media, and generated computerized databases allowing for multi-criteria retrieval. All this material is held and curated by the Institute for the Preservation of Medical Traditions in Washington, DC, where it is available for consultation by any scholar interested in Greek medical manuscripts and the history of ancient and Byzantine medicine. Likewise, scholars working on specific manuscripts, texts, or ancient physicians are invited to share their discoveries and communicate the results of their investigations—published or not—so that the inventory and description of manuscripts, together with the identification of their texts, will improve, making it possible to shorten the time until a complete *New Diels* is compiled. In the meantime, all material received by the Institute for the Preservation of Medical Traditions will be deposited in its library and will be made available for study to the scholarly community.

Notes for consultation

1. Identification of manuscripts

Throughout this volume manuscripts are designated by means of four identifiers according to standard codicological practice:

- name of the city where they are preserved;
- name of the library;
- name of a collection when applicable;
- shelfmark.

City names are followed by the two-letter code of their country.[1] They are cited in the original language and script, followed by their English form. Similarly, library names are in the original language and script, and translated into English. All such additional elements appear between parentheses.

The graphic presentation of data reflects the four-level system of identification of manuscripts with four levels of indentation. For example:

> Wrocław (PL)
>> Biblioteka Uniwersytecka we Wrocławiu (University Library Wrocław)
>>> Rehd.
>>>> 34

2. Special scripts

City and library names that are not originally in the Latin alphabet are cited in their original writing (Greek, Cyrillic, and Armenian), followed for the latter two by a transcription into the Latin alphabet according to standard tables of conversion, and in all cases the commonly accepted English form or translation, respectively.[2]

The spelling of Greek terms, author's names and publication titles reflects both the evolution of Greek language (especially the 1982 legislation sanctioning the passage from poly- to monotonic spelling) and the use of single authors, even though such use may contradict contemporary legislation.[3]

---

[1] This is the ISO 3166-1 alpha-2 code defined in ISO 3166-1, as a part of the ISO 3166 standard published by the International Organization for Standardization (ISO).

[2] For the Greek alphabet, ISO 843: 1997; for the Cyrillic alphabet, ISO 9: 1995; for the Armenian alphabet, ISO 9985: 1996.

[3] On these questions, see Adrados 2005: 296–297.

3. Index of Diels

For the manuscripts cited in Diels, city and library names exactly reproduce the form provided in Diels. Since it is in German in most cases, I provide the original name and its current English form. For the sake of accuracy, incorrect locations, possible mistaken identifiers, and misspellings exactly reproduce Diels' data. Abbreviated library and collection names have been spelled out.

An index at the end of the volume lists all the library names in the form they have in Diels, in the original language, and in their English form.

Shelfmarks have been treated in the same way and thus reflect all peculiarities present in Diels. As a consequence, shelfmarks possibly differing by minor variants (including Roman numerals instead of Arabic, for instance) have been considered as different items.

All elements of manuscript identification reproduced from Diels are printed in boldface to be easily distinguished from any other information provided in this volume.

All mentions of manuscripts cited in Diels are followed by references to their occurrences. References are made of two elements: a Roman number I or II indicating the volumes of Diels (I for the 1905 issue and II for the 1906 one), or an N for the supplement (Nachtrag, published in 1908). This first element is followed by one or more Arabic numbers corresponding to the page or pages where the manuscripts are mentioned. When manuscripts appear several times on the same page, references are followed by an Arabic number between parentheses indicating the number of citations. A reference as I.90 (3), for example, indicates that a manuscript cited in volume I (1905, on Hippocrates and Galen), page 90, appears three times on that page.

Lists of occurrences are followed by reference to the catalogues where the manuscripts are listed and/or described. In most cases, these catalogues are those consulted by Diels' collaborators.

Manuscripts that are *iatrosofia* (medical manuals of the Greek-speaking populations in the Ottoman Empire) or humanist/scholarly copies (such as extracts, anthologies or indexes by post-16th-century scholars) are identified as such, possibly with an indication of their period of copy and/or copyist/author.

If manuscripts have changed location, current ones are provided. No such indication is provided for *iatrosofia* or recent humanist/scholarly copies, as special catalogues for these manuscripts will be published in the future.

4. Census

The census lists manuscripts on the basis of their current location. However, for those cited in Diels, it also cross-references the index.

For the many newly introduced manuscripts, a brief summary of their content is provided with the identification of the folios in which the texts appear. Both identification of texts and references to folios reproduce data provided in available catalogues or relevant publications. References of these works follow the summary.

For the manuscripts that have not been previously described and are listed on the basis of a personal inspection, Latin author's names and titles have been created according to standard cataloguing practice.

5. Cross-referencing

To facilitate cross-referencing between Diels' index and the census the following elements have been introduced:

- all manuscripts listed in Diels are identified by means of a number from 0001 to 1859 between brackets;
- these numbers are placed in the lefthand margin of each page so as to be easily distinguished;
- the numbers attributed to the manuscripts listed on each double page appear in the running titles of the pages on the right side (odd numbers);
- similarly, the names of the cities for which manuscripts are listed on each double page are mentioned in the running titles of the pages on the left side (even numbers).

6. Bibliography

All references to catalogues and relevant publications in the body of the volume are abbreviated. Only the name of the author(s), the year of publication, and the page numbers on which the references are found are provided. In the case of a reference to notes, the page number is immediately followed by the number of the note preceded by the letter n (without space) (e.g. 127n3). Full identification of publications is provided in the bibliography that follows the list of manuscripts. Abbreviated references are listed in alphabetical order of authors' last names and, for each author, in chronological order of publication.

7. General index

The index lists all the names of libraries mentioned in the volume, including the German names provided in Diels and the current names as per the census (in both cases with their original form and their English equivalent).

Acknowledgements[1]

Research for this census started in a structured form as early as 1986 and benefitted at that time of the advice of Charles Astruc, Bibliothèque nationale, Paris; Paul Canart, Biblioteca Apostolica Vaticana; Dieter Harlfinger, Freie Universität Berlin; Jean Irigoin, then at the Ecole Pratique des Hautes Etudes Paris; Joseph Sonderkamp, Freie Universität Berlin and, slightly later, Bonn Universität; and Simone Van Riet, Université catholique de Louvain.

Activity has been greatly facilitated thanks to the collaboration of Marie Louise Cauwelaert in Louvain-la-Neuve (Belgium) in 1986–1988; Emanuela Appetiti in Barcelona and Madrid (Spain) in 1993–1999, and Washington, DC (USA) in 2002–2014; and Patricia Kellogg and Külly Pitsal in Washington, DC (USA) in 2007–2009 and 2009–2011 respectively.

From 1986 until recently, the curators of manuscripts in the many libraries preserving medical manuscripts have provided invaluable information and responded to my many queries, particularly during the years 2007–2014, as did also several colleagues. I am pleased to acknowledge here the assistance I have received from all of them (alphabetical order of last names): Maria Luisa Agati, Università degli Studi di Roma Tor Vergata, Rome; Anna Agostini, Biblioteca Capitolare Fabroniana, Pistoia; Monica Maria Angeli, Biblioteca Marucelliana, Florence; Aspasia Angelikopoulou, Εθνική Βιβλιοθήκη της Ελλάδος, Athens; Alexandra Antonova, Българска Академия на Науките, Sofia; Toby Appel, Harvey Cushing/John Hay Whitney Medical Library, Yale University, New Haven, CT; Antonia Arahova, Εθνική Βιβλιοθήκη της Ελλάδος, Athens; Franca Arduini, Biblioteca Universitaria di Bologna; Patricia Aske, Pembroke College, Cambridge; Robert Babcock, Beinecke Rare Book and Manuscript Library, Yale University, New Haven, CT; Pedro Bádenas de la Peña, Consejo Superior de Investigaciones Científicas, Madrid; Sylvie Ballester-Radet, Médiathèque Jean-Christophe Ruffin, Sens; Bruce C. Barker-Benfield, Bodleian Library, Oxford; Guglielmo Bartoletti, Biblioteca Riccardiana, Florence; Athina Bazou, Ακαδημία Αθηνών; Marianthi Bella, Εθνική Βιβλιοθήκη της Ελλάδος, Athens; Friederike Berger, Bayerische Staatsbibliothek, Munich; Giulia Bologna, Biblioteca Trivulziana, Milan; Mirna Bonazza, Biblioteca Comunale Ariostea, Ferrara; Daniel Bornemann, Bibliothèque nationale et universitaire, Strasbourg; Ivan Boserup, Det Kongelige Bibliotek, Copenhagen; André Th. Bouwman, Universiteitsbibliotheek, Leiden; Clare Brown, Lambeth Palace Library, London; Anna-Elisabeth Bruckhaus, Universitätsbibliothek Tübingen; Dylan Sean Burns, The Rare Book and Manuscript Library, University of Illinois at Urbana-Champaign, IL; Pierrette Casseyre, Bibliothèque interuniversitaire de médecine, Paris; Annaclara Cataldi Palau, King's College, London; Soňa Černoká, Lobkowiczká Knihovna, Nelahozeves; Gioconda Chiademi, Biblioteca centrale della Regione siciliana "Alberto Bombace", Palermo; Guy Cobolet, Bibliothèque Interuniversitaire Santé, Paris; Pierre Cockshaw, Bibliothèque royale de Belgique, Brussels; Grazia Maria De Rubeis, Biblioteca Palatina, Parma; Rita De Tata, Biblioteca Comunale dell'Archiginnasio, Bologna; Dietmar Debes, Karl-Marx Universität, Leipzig; Jean-François Delmas, Bibliothèque Municipale Inguimbertine, Carpentras; Denes Dienes, Sárospataki

---

[1] All personal names are in Latin alphabet, whereas institution names are in the original alphabet. As for the city names, they are not mentioned if they are included in the institution name. When they are provided, they are Anglicized.

Református Teológiai Akadémia; Ueli Dill, Öffentliche Bibliothek der Universität Basel; Mark Dimunation, Library of Congress, Washington, DC; Rita Di Natale, Biblioteca centrale della Regione siciliana "Alberto Bombace", Palermo; Gabriela Dumitrescu, Academia Română, Bucharest; Valentina D'Urso, Biblioteca Vallicelliana, Rome; Jack Eckert, Francis Countway Library, Harvard University, Boston, MA; Natacha Elagina, Российская национальная библиотека, Saint Petersburg; Thomas Elsmann, Staats- und Universitätsbibliothek Bremen; Ángel Escobar Chico, Universidad de Zaragoza; Phillip K. Escreet, Glasgow University Library; Sabine Fahrenback, Karl-Marx Universität, Leipzig; Raffaele Farina, Biblioteca Apostolica Vaticana; Christian Förstel, Bibliothèque nationale de France, Paris; Maria Bianca Foti, Università degli studi, Messina; Vasiliki Frangou, Εθνική Βιβλιοθήκη της Ελλάδος, Athens; Pálma Füsti-Molnár, Sárospataki Református Kollégium; Jill Gage, Newberry Library, Chicago, IL; Enrico Galbiati, Biblioteca Ambrosiana, Milan; Ernst Gamillscheg, Österreichische Nationalbibliothek, Vienna; Dagmar Geithner, Universität Leipzig; Chrysoula Georgaki, Εθνική Βιβλιοθήκη της Ελλάδος, Athens; Martin Germann, Bibliothèque de la Bourgeoisie, Berne; Stefanos Geroulanos, Athens; Dorotei Getov, Българска Академия на Науките, Sofia; Gary Gillum, Brigham Young University, Provo, UT; Estelle Gittins, Trinity College Dublin; Claudia Giuliani, Istituzione Biblioteca Classense, Ravenna; Claude Gleyze, Bibliothèque municipale, Lyon; Håkan Hallber, Uppsala Universitetsbibliothek; Jonathan Harrison, St. John's College, Cambridge; Christian Heitzmann, Herzog August Bibliothek, Wolfenbüttel; Kurt Heydek, Staatsbibliothek zu Berlin-Preussischer Kulturbesitz, Berlin; Christopher Hilton, Wellcome Library for the History and Understanding of Medicine, London; Eva Horvath, Staats- und Universitätsbibliothek Hamburg Carl von Ossietzky; Basilio Intrieri, Biblioteca Statale del Monumento Nazionale di Grottaferrata; Sinziana Ionescu, Universitatea din Bucureşti; Donald Jackson, University of Iowa, Iowa City, IA; Jaroslava Kašparová, Národní Knihovna České Republiky, Praha; Nadezhda Kavrus-Hoffmann, Glenmont, NY; Ann Kelders, Bibliothèque royale de Belgique, Brussels; Sigrid Kohlmann, Universitätsbibliothek Erlangen-Nürnberg; Eleni Kondyli, Εθνικό και Καποδιστριακό Πανεπιστήμιο Αθηνών; Yannis Konstantellis, Μήθυμνα Λέσβου; Maria Kouli, Βιβλιοθήκη της Βουλής των Ελλήνων, Athens; Anna Koulikourdi, Γενικά Αρχεία του Κράτους, Athens; Anna Kozlowska, Biblioteca Jagiellońska, Uniwersytet Jagiellońska w Krakowie; Rallou Kralli-Konstantelli, Μήθυμνα Λέσβου; Ekaterina Krushelnitskaya, Российская национальная библиотека, Saint Petersburg; Stefan Kubów, Biblioteka Uniwersytecka we Wrocławiu; Erich Lamberz, Ludwig-Maximilians-Universität München; Zoe Lamproulou, Εθνική Βιβλιοθήκη της Ελλάδος, Athens; Patrick Latour, Bibliothèque Mazarine, Paris; Anastasia Lazaridou, Βυζαντινό και Χριστιανικό Μουσείο, Athens; Elisabeth Leedham-Green, Cambridge University; Julien Leroy, Biblioteca Apostolica Vaticana; Óscar Lilao, Biblioteca universitaria, Salamanca; Francesco Lo Monaco, Università degli Studi di Bergamo; Perk Loesch, Sächsische Landesbibliothek, Dresden; Vivien Longi, Bibliothèque Interuniversitaire Santé, Paris; Santo Lucà, Università degli Studi di Roma "La Sapienza"; Caroline Macé, Katholieke Universiteit Leuven; Christoph Mackert, Universitätsbibliothek "Bibliotheca Albertina", Leipzig; Scott Mandelbrote, Peterhouse, Cambridge; Marilena Maniaci, Università delgi Studi di Cassino e del Lazio Meridionale; Susy Marcon, Biblioteca Nazionale Marciana, Venice; Carlo Maria Mazzucchi, Università cattolica del Sacro Cuore, Milan; Muriel McCarthy, Marsh's Library, Dublin; David McKitterick, Trinity College, Cambridge; Janet McMullin, Christ Church, Oxford; Ulrike Mehringer, Universitätsbibliothek Tübingen; Jean Marc Meylan, Bibliothèque publique et universitaire, Geneva; Heidrun Mieter, Universitätsbibliothek Tübingen; Ernesto Milano, Biblioteca estense universitaria, Modena; Claudia Minners-Knaup, Herzog August Bibliothek, Wolfenbüttel; Marietta Minotos, Γενικά Αρχεία του Κράτους, Athens; Valerio Montanari, Biblioteca Comunale dell'Archiginnasio, Bologna; Janet Morris, Cambridge Antiquarian Society; David Morrison, Worcester Cathedral; Maria Moussoura, Εθνική Βιβλιοθήκη της Ελλάδος, Athens; Haralampos

Moutsopoulos, Εθνική Βιβλιοθήκη της Ελλάδος, Athens; Manfred Mühlner, Sächsische Landesbibliothek, Dresden; Claudia Musto, Civica Biblioteca-Archivi Storici "Angelo Mai", Bergamo; András Németh, Országos Széchényi Könyvtár, Budapest; Manuel Nin, Pontificio Collegio Greco Sant' Anastasio, Rome; Laura Nuvoloni, The British Library, London; Eva Nyström, Uppsala Universitet; Jean-Marie Olivier, Olivet; Luciano Osbat, Biblioteca capitolare, Centro diocesano di documentazione per la storia e la cultura religiosa, Viterbo; Joachim Ott, Thüringer Universitäts- und Landesbibliothek, Jena; Ralph Päsler, Philipps-Universität Marburg; Claudio Paolocci, Biblioteca Franzoniana, Genoa; Niki Papavramidou, Αριστοτέλειο Πανεπιστήμιο Θεσσαλονίκης; Cesare Pasini, Biblioteca Apostolica Vaticana; Domenico Pellegrino, Università degli studi, Messina; Erik Petersen, Det Kongelige Bibliotek, Copenhagen; Anna Plattner, Österreichische Nationalbibliothek, Vienna; Marzia Pontone, Archivio Storico Civico e Biblioteca Trivulziana, Milan; Barbara Prout, Bibliothèque de Genève; Claudia Rapp, Universität Wien; Diether Roderich Reinsch, Freie Universität Berlin; Alexa Renggli, Zentralbibliothek Zürich; Anne Richard, Bibliothèque royale de Belgique, Brussels; Ludwig Ries, Universitätsbibliothek, Heidelberg; Jayne Ringrose, University Library, Cambridge; Maria Teresa Rodriquez, Biblioteca Regionale Universitaria Giacomo Longo di Messina; Dieter Rohlfing, Niedersächsische Staats- und Universitätsbibliothek Göttingen; Maria Rosaria Romano Vicenzo, Biblioteca Nazionale Vittorio Emanuele III, Naples; Barbara Roth, Bibliothèque de Genève; Lawrence Schoenberg, Longboat Key, FL; Helmut Schröer, Badische Landesbibliothek, Karlsruhe; Friedrich Simader, Österreichische Nationalbibliothek, Vienna; Georgia Skalochoritou, Πρωτότυπο Πειραματικό Γενικό Λύκειο Μυτιλήνης του Πανεπιστημίου Αιγαίου, Mytilini, Lesvos; Petr Slouka, Lobkowiczká knihovna, Nelahozeves; Claudia Sode, Köln Universität; Apostolos Spanos, Universitetet i Agder; Mark Statham, Gonville and Caius College, Cambridge; Walther Stein, Sächsische Landesbibliothek, Dresden; Frank-Joachim Stewing, Stiftsbibliothek und Stiftsarchiv Zeitz; Hans-Walter Storck, Staats- und Universitätsbibliothek Hamburg Carl von Ossietzky; Wojciech Swieboda, Biblioteca Jagiellońska, Uniwersytet Jagiellońska w Krakowie; Valéria Szeli, Országos Széchényi Könyvtár, Budapest; Slawomir Szyller, Biblioteka Narodowa, Warszaw; Andrei Tarlescu, Academia Română, Bucharest; Russ Taylor, Brigham Young University, Provo, UT; Barbara Tellini Santoni, Biblioteca Vallicelliana, Rome; Alan Thomas, Bookseller, London; Tony Trowles, Westminster Abbey, London; Agamemnon Tselikas, Μορφωτικό Ίδρυμα Εθνικής Τραπέζης, Athens; Costas Tsiamis, Εθνικό και Καποδιστριακό Πανεπιστήμιο Αθηνών; Filippos Tsimpoglou, Εθνική Βιβλιοθήκη της Ελλάδος, Athens; Georgia Tsouri, Γενικά Αρχεία του Κράτους, Athens; Elizabeth Tunis, History of Medicine Division, National Library of Medicine, Bethesda, MD; Ubaldo Valentini, Biblioteca del Capitolo Metropolitano, Milan; Christiane Van den Bergen-Pantens, Bibliothèque royale de Belgique, Brussels; Steven Van Impe, Erfgoedbibliotheek Hendrik Conscience, Antwerpen; Naomi van Loo, New College, Oxford; Silvana Verdini, Biblioteca Angelica, Rome; Francesco Vergara, Biblioteca centrale della Regione siciliana "Alberto Bombace", Palermo; Michiel Verweij, Bibliothèque royale de Belgique, Brussels; Maryse Viviand, Bibliothèque Sainte-Geneviève, Paris; William M. Voelkle, The Morgan Library and Museum, New York, NY; Christoph von Steiger, Bibliothèque de la Bourgeoisie, Berne; Colin Wakefield, Bodleian Library, Oxford; Pierre-E. Wagner, Médiathèque du Pontiffroy, Metz; Marie-Claire Waille, Bibliothèque municipale de Besançon; Julia Walworth, Merton College, Oxford; Birgit Wendel, Badische Landesbibliothek Karlsruhe; David Weston, Glasgow University Library; Jan Just Witkam, Universiteitsbibliotheek Leiden; Martin Wittek, Bibliothèque royale de Belgique, Brussels; Lawrence Witten, Rare Books, Southport; Roland Wittwe, Corpus Medicorum Graecorum, Berlin; Christopher Wright, Lambeth Palace Library, London; Helen C. Wüstefeld, Bibliotheca Philosophica Hermetica, Amsterdam; Maria Zervou, Πρότυπο Πειραματικό Γενικό Λύκειο

Μυτιλήνης του Πανεπιστημίου Αιγαίου, Mytilini, Lesvos; Marian Zwiercan, Biblioteca Jagiellońska, Uniwersytet Jagiellońska w Krakowie.

In past and recent times, Roland Folter, then at HP Kraus, New York, NY; Jeffrey Eger, Auction catalogues, Morristown, NJ; Christopher de Hamel, then at Sotheby's, London; Camille Previte and Joshua Lipton at Sotheby's, New York, NY; and Paul Grinke, Bernard Quaritch Ltd, London, provided invaluable help to ascertain the provenance and new location of several manuscripts.

Professors John Duffy, Harvard University; Ann-Ellis Hanson, Yale University; Jutta Kollesch, Berlin Academy of Sciences; Vivian Nutton, University College London; and Nancy Siraisi, Hunter College and the Graduate Center of the City University of New York, NY, gave advice on some aspects of this research program. Mgr. Paul Canart, Scriptor emeritus, Biblioteca Apostolica Vaticana, read the whole mansucript, spotted many typos and other errors, and helped identify a couple of misidentified codices that had resisted my efforts.

Finally, special thanks go to the editors of my manuscript, Marisa Gomez, Patricia Kellogg, Jim Kelly and Jenny Rogers.

CENSUS OF BYZANTINE AND RENAISSANCE MANUSCRIPTS

Ἅγιον Ὄρος (Μοναστική Πολιτεία Ἁγίου Ὄρους) (Holy Mountain, Monastic State of the Holy Mountain) (GR)

Ἱερά Βατοπεδινή Σκήτη Ἁγίου Δημητρίου (Skiti Agiou Dimitriou)

55/VI	Gregorius Nyssenus, *De hominis opificio* (frg.). Lamberz and Litsas 1978: 95-97.

Ἱερά Μονή Ἁγίου Παντελεήμονος (Agiou Panteleimonos Monastery)

72 (5578)	See [0090].
535 (6042)	(pp. 126 et seq.) Nicephorus Blemmydes, *De corpore*. Lampros 1895-1900: 2.391.
649 (6156)	(ff. 105r et seq.) Johannes Damascenus, *Quid est homo?* Lampros 1895-1900: 2.410.

Ἱερά Μονή Βατοπεδίου (Vatopedi Monastery)

12/I	(ff. 16v-18r) Epiphanius, *De duodecim gemmis*. Lamberz 2006: 72-87 (especially 73).
12/IV	(ff. 220r-221v) *Lexica botanica et medica*. Lamberz 2006: 72-87 (especially 85).
13	(ff. 170v-174r) Epiphanius, *Physiologus*. Lamberz 2006: 87-94.
29	See [0027]. Lamberz 2006: 128-130.
42	(ff. 141v-144v, 148r-153r) *Formulae medicinarum*; (ff. 153r-155v) Hippocrates et Galenus; (ff. 161r-163r) *De aegrotantibus*; (ff. 163r-171r) *Formulae medicinarum*. Lamberz 2006: 191-203.
54	(ff. 83r-146r) Gregorius Nyssenus, *De hominis opificio*. Lamberz 2006: 238-239.
61	(f. 1r-v) Gregorius Nyssenus, *De hominis opificio* (frg.). Lamberz 2006: 285-287.
120	Gregorius Nazianzenus, *De humana natura*. Eustratiades and Arcadios 1924: 30-31 (does not specifically identify the text); Domiter 1999: 22.
128	(ff. 76r et seq.) Gregorius Nyssenus, *De hominis opificio*. Eustratiades and Arcadios 1924: 32.
131	(ff. 28r-88v) Gregorius Nyssenus, *De hominis opificio*. Eustratiades and Arcadios 1924: 33.

594   (ff. 228r et seq.) Gregorius Nyssenus, *De hominis opificio*.

Eustratiades and Arcadios 1924: 116-117.

621   Paulus Aegineta, *Epitome medica*.

Eustratiades and Arcadios 1924: 122.

985   (ff. 10r et seq.) *Praecepta medica et medicinarum formulae*.

Eustratiades and Arcadios 1924: 179.

Ιερά Μονή Διονυσίου (Dionysiou Monastery)

Shelfmarks are according to Papazoglou 1990: 495-501 (table of concordance of shelfmarks according to Lampros 1895-1900: 1. 319-436, and current shelfmarks)

59   See [0028].

168   See [0034].

195   (no. 6) *Plantae medicinales*.

Lampros 1895-1900: 1.417 with shelfmark 355 (3889).

263   See [0029].

297   See [0033].

402   See [0035].

414   (no. 1) *De plantarum nominibus*; (no. 2) *Formulae medicinarum*; (no. 3) *Antidota*.

Lampros 1895-1900: 1.414 with shelfmark 346 (3880).

465   See [0030].

471   (no. 3) *De hominis septem aetatibus*.

Lampros 1895-1900: 1.373-374 with shelfmark 226 (3760).

521   (no. 5) *De stomachi dolore*.

Lampros 1895-1900: 1.435 with shelfmark 584 (4118).

Ιερά Μονή Εσφιγμένου (Esfigmenou Monastery)

131 (2144)   (no. 33) Epiphanius, *De duodecim gemmis*.

Lampros 1895-1900: 1.186-187.

317 (2330)   See [0040].

Ιερά Μονή Ιβήρων (Iviron Monastery)

28 (735)   (ff. 255v-258v) Epiphanius, *De mensuris et ponderibus*.

Sotiroudis 1998: 49-53.

38 (536)   Nemesius Emesenus, *De natura hominis* (frg.).

Sotiroudis 1998: 71-73; Morani 1981: 29.

78 (401)	(f. 67v) *De hominis septem aetatibus*.
	Sotiroudis 1998: 149-155.
80 (499)	(ff. 76r-102r) Symeon Seth, *De alimentorum facultatibus*.
	Sotiroudis 1998: 159-160.
83 (455)	(f. 55r-v) *De corporis partium nominibus*.
	Björck 1938: 144; Sotiroudis 1998: 162-166.
92 (792)	See [0042].
	Sotiroudis 1998: 182-192.
151 (4271)	See [0041] and [0043].
152 (4272)	See [0044].
164 (4284)	See [0045].
165 (4285)	(ff. 146r et seq.) Achmet, *Oneirocriticon*.
	Lampros 1895-1900: 2. 43-44.
181 (4301)	See [0048].
182 (4302)	See [0050] and [0049].
184 (4304)	See [0051].
187 (4307)	(no. 1) Gregorius Nazianzenus, *De humana natura*.
	Lampros 1895-1900: 2.51-52; Domiter 1999: 21.
189 (4309)	See [0052].
190 (4310)	See [0053].
206 (4326)	(ff. 1r et seq.) Symeon Seth, *De alimentorum facultatibus*.
	Lampros 1895-1900: 2.59.
207 (4327)	*Iatrosofion* (16th century).
	Lampros 1895-1900: 2.59.
210 (4330)	(ff. 44v et seq.) Hippocrates, *Epistula ad Ptolemaeum*; (ff. 95v et seq.) *Medicamenta*.
	Lampros 1895-1900: 2.60-61.
	See [0055].
214 (4334)	(no. 1) Symeon Seth, *De alimentorum facultatibus*; (nos. 2-4) *Iatrosofia tria*; (no. 5) Galenus, *Protrepticum* (?).
	Lampros 1895-1900: 2.61-62.
216 (4336)	See [0056].
217 (4337)	See [0057].
218 (4338)	See [0058].
222 (4342)	*Iatrosofion* (16th century).
	Lampros 1895-1900: 2.63.

329 (4449)	(no. 5) Symeon Seth, *De alimentorum facultatibus*. Lampros 1895-1900: 2.84-87.
348 (4468)	See [0064].
377 (4497)	See [0065].
381 (4501)	See [0066].
382 (4502)	(ff. 445r et seq.) *De hominis genitura*. Lampros 1895-1900: 2.109-118.
388 (4508)	See [0067].
475 (4595)	Nemesius Emesenus, *De natura hominis* (frg.). Lampros 1895-1900: 2.150; Morani 1981: 62.
494 (4614)	(f. 12v) *De hominis quinque sensibus*. Lampros 1895-1900: 2.155-156.
520 (4640)	(no. 10) *De hominis vita*. Lampros 1895-1900: 2.162-163.
692 (4812)	(no. 11) *Formula medicinae*. Lampros 1895-1900: 2.205-206.
695 (4815)	See [0074].
698 (4818)	(no. 2) *Distinctio infirmitatum*. Lampros 1895-1900: 2.208.
765 (4885)	(ff. 5r et seq.) *Definitiones physicae*. Lampros 1895-1900: 2.223.
1332 (5452)	(no. 3) Maximus Planudes, *De urinis*. Lampros 1895-1900: 2.271.
1359 (5479)	(no. 7) *Nomina plantarum*. Lampros 1895-1900: 2.277.

Ιερά Μονή Κουτλουμουσίου (Koutloumousiou Monastery)

4 (3073)	(no. 2) Gregorius Nyssenus, *De hominis opificio*. Lampros 1895-1900: 1.270-271.
9 (3078)	(pp. 347-358) Nemesius Emesenus, *De natura hominis*. Lampros 1895-1900: 1.271; Morani 1981: 29.
187 (3260)	See [0079].
263 (3336)	(ff. 10v et seq.) *De hominis septem aetatibus*. Lampros 1895-1900: 1.307.
269 (3342)	(no. 5) *Praescriptiones medicae*; (no. 12) Nemesius Nyssenus (vel Emesenus [?]), *De natura hominis*. Lampros 1895-1900: 1.307-308; Morani 1981: 29.

Ιερά Μονή Μεγίστης Λαύρας (Great Lavra Monastery)

B 77   (ff. 66v et seq.) Gregorius Nyssenus, *De hominis opificio.*

Spyridon and Eustratiades 1925: 22.

B 105   (ff. 78r et seq.) Gregorius Nyssenus, *De hominis opificio.*

Spyridon and Eustratiades 1925: 27.

Γ 88   (ff. 1r et seq.) Basilius Caesariensis, *De hominis opificio.*

Spyridon and Eustratiades 1925: 45.

Γ 90   Paulus Aegineta, *Epitome medica.*

Spyridon and Eustratiades 1925: 45.

E 168   Aetius Amidenus, *Libri medicinales.*

Spyridon and Eustratiades 1925: 95 (where the content is identified as a *iatrosofion*); Mavroudis and Sakellaridou-Sotiroudi 1987 for the identification of the content.

E 192   Nicolaus Myrepsus, *Antidotarium.*

Spyridon and Eustratiades 1925: 103.

H 49   *Capitula de pathologia.*

Spyridon and Eustratiades 1925: 110-111.

Θ 4   (ff. 12r et seq.) Gregorius Nyssenus, *De hominis opificio* (frg.).

Spyridon and Eustratiades 1925: 132.

Θ 29   *Iatrosofion ex Hippocrate, Galeno et Meletio* (16th century).

Spyridon and Eustratiades 1925: 137.

M 38   (ff. 1r et seqq.) *Formulae medicinarum*; (ff. 42v et seq.) Paulus Aegineta, *Epitome medica,* 7.25 (*De succedaneis*).

Spyridon and Eustratiades 1925: 309.

M 68   (pp. 143 et seq.) Gregorius Nyssenus, *De hominis opificio.*

Spyridon and Eustratiades 1925: 314-315.

Ω 6^β (pp. 193v et seq.) Epiphanius, *Physiologus.*

Spyridon and Eustratiades 1925: 325.

Ω 23   (ff. 429v et seq.) Nicephorus Gregoras, *Scholia in Synesii de insomniis.*

Spyridon and Eustratiades 1925: 328.

Ω 56   (f. 81) Aetius Amidenus, *De astrorum signis.*

Spyridon and Eustratiades 1925: 337-338.

Ω 63   Aetius Amidenus, *Libri medicinales.*

Spyridon and Eustratiades 1925: 340.

Ω 64   Aetius Amidenus, *Libri medicinales.*

Spyridon and Eustratiades 1925: 340.

Ω 65   Aetius Amidenus, *Libri medicinales.*

            Spyridon and Eustratiades 1925: 340.

Ω 66   (ff. 1r et seq.) Paulus Aegineta, *Epitome medica*, 5 et 6; (ff. 120r
            et seq.) Aetius Amidenus, *Libri medicinales*, 16.

            Spyridon and Eustratiades 1925: 340.

Ω 69   See [0087].

Ω 70   See [0088].

Ω 71   Galenus, *De medendi methodo.*

            Spyridon and Eustratiades 1925: 342.

Ω 72   See [0089].

Ω 73   Paulus Aegineta, *Epitome medica.*

            Spyridon and Eustratiades 1925: 342.

Ω 74   (ff. 97r et seq.) Paulus Aegineta, *Epitome medica*, 7.

            Spyridon and Eustratiades 1925: 343.

Ω 75   See [0082].

            Spyridon and Eustratiades 1925: 343.

Ω 76^{α} *Physiologus.*

            Spyridon and Eustratiades 1925: 343-344.

Ιερά Μονή Παντοκράτορος (Pantokrator Monastery)

46 (1080)   (no. 2) Gregorius Nyssenus, *De hominis opificio.*

            Lampros 1895-1900: 1.97.

234 (1268) See [0100].

247   (ff. 319r et seq.) Gregorius Nyssenus, *De hominis opificio.*

            Politis and Manousakas 1973: 146.

Ιερά Μονή Σταυρονικήτα (Stavronikita Monastery)

160 (1025) (no. 2) *De hominis membris.*

            Lampros 1895-1900: 1.89-90.

Ιερά Μονή Ξηροποτάμου (Xiropotamou Monastery)

554/ς   Gregorius Nyssenus, *De hominis opificio.*

            Xiropotaminos and Sotiroudis 2012: 230.

Αλεξάνδρεια (الإسكندرية, Alexandria) (EG)

Πατριαρχείο, Πατριαρχική Βιβλιοθήκη Αλεξανδρείας (Patriarchate, Patriarchal Library of Alexandria)

–

71	(ff. 152r-158r) Symeon Seth, *De alimentorum*; (ff. 158r-162r) Nicephorus Constantinopolitanus Patriarcha, *Oneirocriticon*.
	Moschonas 1945: 77-79 (1965: 57-59).
87	(ff. 273v-279v) Aristoteles, *De insomniis*.
	Moschonas 1945: 88-89 (1965: 65-66); *Aristoteles graecus* 1976: 1-2.
124	(ff. 282v-284r) Hippocrates, *Epistula ad Ptolemaeum regem*.
	Moschonas 1945: 112 (1965: 82).
172	Gregorius Nazianzenus, *De humana natura*.
	Moschonas 1945: 162-163 (1965: 117-118) (does not mention the work specifically); Domiter 1999: 20.
175	(ff. 1r-66v) Aristoteles, *Problemata*; (ff. 75r-299v) Galenus, *Capitula medica*.
	Moschonas 1945: 165 (1965: 119); *Aristoteles graecus* 1976: 3-4.
196	(ff. 127r-148v) *De generatione*.
	Moschonas 1945: 184-186 (1965: 133-134).
325	(f. 66r-v) *De pulsu*.
	Moschonas 1945: 281 (1965: 199).

[Amsterdam] (NL)

[Universitäts-Bibliothek] (Universiteitsbibliotheek [University Library])

[Amstelodam.] (*Amstellodamensis*)

[?]   I.109.

This manuscript of Galen, *Linguarum seu dictionum exoletarum Hippocratis explicatio*, without shelfmark in Diels' catalogue is not in Amsterdam, but in Oxford, Bodleian Library, where it is MS. D'Orville 3 (= [0865]).

In Perilli 1999: 431 and n8, 434, 437, it is identified as Leiden, D'Orville 3 (correction in Perilli 2000: 28n1, and Perilli 2011: 177-179).

Ἄνδρος (Andros) (GR)

    Ιερά Μονή Ζωοδόχου Πηγής ή της Αγίας (Monastery of the Zoodochou Pigis or Agias)

        58   (ff. 90v et seq.) Epiphanius, *Physiologus.*

                    Lampros 1898: 57-58.

        72   (ff. 98r et seq.) Epiphanius, *Physiologus.*

                    Lampros 1898: 65-67.

Ankara (TR)

    Türk Tarih Kurumu (Turkish Historical Society)

        3   (ff. 245v-246r) Athanasius Alexandrinus, *De hominis quinque sensibus.*

                    Moraux 1964: 7-15.

Ἄντισσα (Antissa, Lesvos) (GR)

    Μονή Αγίου Ιωάννου Ὑψηλού (Ypsilou Monastery of St. John)

        6   (ff. 92r-104v, 121r-128r) Gregorius Nyssenus, *De hominis opificio* (frg.).

                    Papadopoulos-Kerameus 1884-1888: 147 (1970 reprint: 134-136).

Antwerpen (Antwerp) (BE)

    Stadtbibliothek (Stadsbibliotheek [City Library]), now Erfgoedbibliotheek Hendrik Conscience (Hendrik Conscience Heritage Library)

        Antverp. (*Antverpensis*)

[0002]   **426**   I.12.

                    Omont 1885: 41-42.

                    Current shelfmark: B. 426 (Dermul 1939: 41).

                    According to Magdelaine 1994: 200-201 and 338, this is a copy of Rabelais' printed edition of Hippocrates, *Aphorismi* (Lyon, 1532, with several reeditions).

                    The manuscript is copied by Lambert Hortensius (1501-1574) (Dermul 1939: 41).

Athen (Ἀθῆναι, Athens) (GR)

    Bibl. tês Boulês (Βιβλιοθήκη τῆς Βουλῆς [Parliament Library]), now Βιβλιοθήκη της Βουλής των Ελλήνων (Greek Parliament Library)

        –

        32   (f. 2r) *De hominis septem aetatibus.*

                    Lampros 1905: 226-230; Karas 1994: 378.

[0003]	**39**	N.26 (7).
		Lampros 1905: 359.
		18th-century *iatrosofion*.
[0004]	**43**	N.58.
		Lampros 1905: 364.
[0005]	**68**	N.25, 28 (2), 46, 49, 62, 63.
		Lampros 1906: 471-473; Karas 1994: 382, 386, 410-411.
		18th-century *iatrosofion*.
	84	*Varia medica* (Aetius Amidenus; Dioscorides; Galenus, *in Hippocratis Aphorismos*; Hippocrates; Symeon Seth; Theophanes [Chrysobalantes] et alia).
		Lampros 1907: 229-236.

Nationalbibl. (Nationalbibliothek, Ἐθνικὴ Βιβλιοθήκη [National Library]), now Εθνική Βιβλιοθήκη της Ελλάδος ΕΒΕ (National Library of Greece – ΕΒΕ)

	–	
	329	(γ ́) Nemesius Emesenus, *De natura hominis*.
		Sakkelion and Sakkelion 1892: 55 (does not list the text); Morani 1981: 29.
[0006]	**375**	II.66.
		Sakkelion and Sakkelion 1892: 64.
	415	(ff. 80r, col. 1, l. 13-94v, col. 2, l, 9) Basilius Caesariensis, *De hominis opificio*.
		Sakkelion and Sakkelion 1892: 73-74.
[0007]	**433 (132)**	II.39.
		Sakkelion and Sakkelion 1892: 79-80.
[0008]	**447 (146)**	II.66.
		Sakkelion and Sakkelion 1892: 85.
	1070	(ff. 201r-204r) Diocles, *Ad Antigonum regem epistula de tuenda valetudine*.
		Sakkelion and Sakkelion 1892: 190 (does not mention the text); *CCAG* X (Delatte) 1924: 8-9; *CMAG* V (Zuretti and Severyns) 1928: 149.
[0009]	**1180**	II.44.
		Sakkelion and Sakkelion 1892: 214.
		18th-century *iatrosofion*.
[0010]	**1236**	II.27.
		Sakkelion and Sakkelion 1892: 224.
		18th-century *iatrosofion*.

[0011]   **1444**   II.27.

Codex *Atheniensis* 1444 does not contain Diocles, *Ad Antigonum regem epistula de tuenda valetudine*, but rather a *nomokanon* (see Sakkelion and Sakkelion 1892: 258). This is probably a mistake for *Atheniensis* 1494 (= [0021]), which contains the *Epistula*.

[0012]   **1477**   I.3, 11.

Sakkelion and Sakkelion 1892: 265; Karas 1994: 380.

[0013]   **1478**   N.60.

Sakkelion and Sakkelion 1892: 265; Karas 1994: 397.

17th-century *iatrosofion*.

[0014]   **1479**   I.123; II.34, 79.

Sakkelion and Sakkelion 1892: 265; Karas 1994: 193.

19th-century *iatrosofion*.

[0015]   **1480**   II.29.

Sakkelion and Sakkelion 1892: 265.

19th-century *iatrosofion* (1861).

[0016]   **1481**   II.55, 68.

Sakkelion and Sakkelion 1892: 265; Karas 1994: 148, 388, 402.

1482   (ff. 56v-76v) Meletius, *Iatrosofion*.

Sakkelion and Sakkelion 1892: 265; Alexopoulou 1998: 4-6.

1484   *Iatrosofion*

Sakkelion and Sakkelion 1892: 266; Karas 1994: 219.

15th-16th century manuscript.

[0017]   **1486**   I.12.

Sakkelion and Sakkelion 1892: 265; Alexopoulou 1998: 4-6.

Iatrosofion dated 1793.

[0018]   **1488**   I.10.

Sakkelion and Sakkelion 1892: 266.

19th-century *iatrosofion*.

1489   (ff. 1r-3r) *Tabula capitulorum* (acephala); (ff. 9r-131r) *Iatrosofion*, including: (ff. 108v-111v) Alexander, *De septem herbarum facultate*.

On ff. 7v and 8v, drawing of a horse; ff. 132r-140v, additional notes.

Sakkelion and Sakkelion 1892: 266; *CCAG* X (Delatte) 1924: 30.

[0019]   **1491**   I.78 (2), 79 (2).

Sakkelion and Sakkelion 1892: 266-267; Karas 1994: 351.

18th-century *iatrosofion*.

[0020]	**1493**	I.99, 121.
		Sakkelion and Sakkelion 1892: 267.
[0021]	**1494**	I.91; II.102.
		Sakkelion and Sakkelion 1892: 267.
		Also [0011].
[0022]	**1498**	I.12.
		Sakkelion and Sakkelion 1892: 268; Karas 1994: 94-95.
		18th-century *iatrosofion*.

| | 1499 | (ff. 1r-29v, l. 3) *Collectio remediorum*; (ff. 30r, l. 11-52r) *Collectio alia remediorum in tribus columnis ordinata* (et non *Lexicon plantarum nominum* ut Sakkelion et Sakkelion); (ff. 53r-111r, l. 14) Symeon Seth, *De alimentorum facultatibus*; (ff. 111r, l. 15-113v, l. 15) *Lexicon plantarum*; (ff. 113v, l. 16-115r, l. 10) *De succedaneis*; (ff. 115r, l. 11-118v) *Collectio remediorum*; (ff. 119r-124v, l. 13) *Tabula capitulorum*; (ff. 124v, l. 14-127v, l. 6) *De dentibus*; (ff. 127v, l. 8-186v, l. 8) Theophanes [Chrysobalantes], *Epitome de curatione morborum, Synopsis de remediis, De alimentis*; (ff. 186v, l. 8-172 [= 193]r) *Remedia hospitalis*; (ff. 173 [= 194]v-187 [= 208]r, l. 9) *De diaeta*; (ff. 187[= 208]r, l. 9 - 194 [= 215]r, l. 3) *Prognostica*; (f. 194 [215r, ll. 4-15] *De vino et aqua potabili*; (ff. 194 [= 215]v-224 [= 245]v) *Notulae medicae variae*. |
| | | Sakkelion and Sakkelion 1892: 268; Sonderkamp 1987: 73-75; Karas 1994: 166, 247, 409. |

[0023]	**1500**	I.12.
		Sakkelion and Sakkelion 1892: 268; Karas 1994: 131.
		19th-century *iatrosofion*.
[0024]	**1502**	I.100.
		Sakkelion and Sakkelion 1892: 269; Karas 1994: 191-192, 352.
		18th-century *iatrosofion*.
[0025]	**1504**	I.44.
		Sakkelion and Sakkelion 1892: 269; Karas 1994: 147-148.
		19th-century *iatrosofion*.
[0026]	**1506**	II.64.
		Sakkelion and Sakkelion 1892: 269; Karas 1994: 32-33.
		19th-century *iatrosofion*.
	2045	(f. 80v) *Iatrosophica* (14th/15th century).
		Politis and Politi 1991: 93-94.

2086	(ff. 376r-377r) *Iatrosofion*; (ff. 382r-387) [Râzî], *De pestilentia* (frg.).
	Politis and Politi 1991: 120-121.
	Formerly Θεσσαλονίκη, Ἑλληνικὸν Γυμνάσιον (Thessalonica, Greek Gymnasium), 17 (Serruys) (= [1613]).
2146/I	(ff. 1r-71v) Theophanes [Chrysobalantes], *Epitome de curatione morborum.*
	Politis and Politi 1991: 174-176 (especially 174).
	Formerly Θεσσαλονίκη, Ἑλληνικὸν Γυμνάσιον (Thessalonica, Greek Gymnasium), 79 (Serruys).
2187	(f. 71r-v) *De graviditate*; (f. 79v) *De quattuor elementis ex quibus homo constituitur.*
	Politis and Politi 1991: 213-220.
2429	(ff. 1-3v) Nemesius Emesenus, *De natura hominis* (frg.).
	Politis and Politi 1991: 427-433.
2479	(ff. 203r-205r) Symeon Seth, *De alimentorum facultatibus* (frg.).
	Politis and Politi 1991: 481-482.
2490	Tegumentum anterior: *Formulae medicinarum.*
	Politis and Politi 1991: 491-492.
2492	(ff. 124r, l. 11-125r, l. 7) Epiphanius, *De duodecim gemmis* (frg.).
	Politis and Politi 1991: 493-496.
2583	(ff. 344v-345) Gregorius Nyssenus, *De hominis opificio* (frg.).
	Politis n. d./1: 14-18.
2786	(ff. 1r-28r) Galenus, *De crisibus* (acephalus); (ff. 30r-33r, l. 15) Galenus, *Commentarius ad Hippocratis de humoribus* (frg.); (ff. 33r, l. 16-34v, l. 13) Hippocrates, *De natura hominis* (frg.); (ff. 34v, l. 14-35r, l. 22) *Tabula capitulorum*; (ff. 35v, l. 21-130v) Meletius, *De hominis natura* (mutilus).
	Kougeas n. d.
2922	(ff. 8r-59v) *Liber medicinalis ex lingua persica translatus*; (ff. 60r-62v) *Lexicon plantarum*; (ff. 63r-88v) *Remedia variorum morborum ex Promoti libro*; (ff. 89r-98v) *Lexicon plantarum*; (ff. 98v-99v) *De mensuris et ponderibus*; (ff. 100r-104r, l. 18) Philagrius, *De pulsibus*; (ff. 104r, l. 19-110v, l. 18) Magnus Emesenus, *De urinis*; (ff. 110v, l. 19-112r, l. 17) *Liber alius de urinis*; (f. 112r, l. 17-112v) Hippocrates, *Prognosticon* (frg.); (ff. 184r-185r, l. 12); *De bile*; (ff. 185r, l. 13-202v) *Collectio remediorum.*
	Politis n. d./2.
3113	(f. 128r-v) *Iatrosofion ex Galeno, Hippocrate et aliis* (frg.); (ff. 131r-261v) *Iatrosofion.*
	Kournoutou n. d.: 149-150.

Αθήνα (Athens) (GR)

Βιβλιοθήκη της Βουλής των Ελλήνων (Greek Parliament Library)

See **Athen**, **Bibl. tês Boulês** (see above, p. 10).

Εθνική Βιβλιοθήκη της Ελλάδος ΕΒΕ (National Library of Greece – ΕΒΕ)

See **Athen, Nationalbibl.** (see above, p. 11).

Μετόχιον Παναγίου Τάφου-ΜΠΤ (Metochion of the Holy Sepulchre, MPT)

179	See [0410].
199	See [0412].
273	See [0413].

274   Nemesius Emesenus, *De natura hominis* (*Florilegium Hierosolymitanum*).

Papadopoulos-Kerameus 1891-1915: 4.252-253 (does not list Nemesius); Morani 1981: 32.

303   (ff. 366r et seq.) Manuel Philes, *De animalium proprietate* (frg.)

Papadopoulos-Kerameus 1891-1915: 4.271-283.

357	See [0415].
363	See [0416].

462   (ff. 3r-133r) *Physiologus*.

Papadopoulos-Kerameus 1891-1915: 5.32-33.

565   (ff. 1r-85v) Meletius, *De hominis natura*.

Papadopoulos-Kerameus 1899: 5.120; Karas 1994: 390.

Μουσείο Μπενάκη (Benaki Museum)

Μπ (Mp)

7   (ff. 292v-293r) Lucas, *Sales*.

Tselikas 1977: 25; Lappa-Zizica and Rizou-Kouroupou 1991: 19-20.

49   (pp. 1-229) *Iatrosofion*; (pp. 229-237) *Medicinalia varia*; (pp. 262-281) *Physiologus*; (pp. 331-343, 355, 358, and ff. I, VIr-VIIIv) *Iatrosofion*.

Lappa-Zizica and Rizou-Kouroupou 1991: 44-49; Karas 1994: 223-226.

ΤΑ (TA)

44   (ff. 60v-65r) Nicephorus Blemmydes, *De urinis*.

Tsakona n.d.: 6.

176   (ff. 1r-36v) Symeon Seth, *De alimentorum facultatibus*; (ff. 37r-42v) *Iatrosofion*; (ff. 43r-82v) Galenus, *De simplicium medicamentorum temperamentis et facultatibus* (frg.).

Lappa-Zizica and Rizou-Kouroupou 1991: 146-147; Karas 1994: 346, 408-409.

239   (ff. 10v and 13r) *De hominis septem aetatibus.*

Tselikas 1977: 30-32; Lappa-Zizica and Rizou-Kouroupou 1991: 169-172.

Εθνικό και Καποδιστριακό Πανεπιστήμιο Αθηνών (National and Kapodistrian University of Athens)

Τμήμα Φιλολογίας, Σπουδαστήριο Βυζαντινής και Νεοελληνικής Φιλολογίας (Department of Philology, Seminary of Byzantine and Neo-Hellenic Philology)

7   (ff. 51v-60r) Epiphanius, *Physiologus*; (ff. 65r-80v) Manuel Philes, *De animalium proprietate.*

Zoras and Bouboulidis 1964: 21-23.

Athos (Ἄθως, Mount Athos) (GR)

Apart from Vatopedi ([0027]) and Lavra ([0081]-[0089]), and also two exceptions ([0038] and [0041]), identifiers in Diels are the sequential numbers in Lampros 1895-1900, followed by the actual shelfmarks of the manuscripts.

Bibl. Mon. Batopediou (Βιβλιοθήκη Μονῆς Βατοπεδίου [Library of Vatopedi Monastery]), now Ιερά Μονή Βατοπεδίου (Vatopedi Monastery)

–

[0027]   **A 29**   II.5; N.43.

Eustratiades and Arcadios 1924: 11.

Current shelfmark: 29.

Bib. Mon. Dionysiou (Βιβλιοθήκη Μονῆς Διονυσίου [Library of Dionysiou Monastery]), now Ιερά Μονή Διονυσίου (Dionysiou Monastery)

The manuscripts of this monastery have received new shelfmarks. For a table of concordance between shelfmarks according to Lampros 1895-1900: 1.319-436, and current shelfmarks, see Papazoglou 1990: 495-501.

–

[0028]   **3701. 167**   I.40, 124.

Lampros 1895-1900: 1.352-353 with shelfmark 167 (3701).

Current shelfmark: 59.

[0029]   **3748. 214**   II.39, 40.

Lampros 1895-1900: 1.363-364 with shelfmark 214 (3748).

Current shelfmark: 263.

[0030]   **3758. 224**   I.47.

Lampros 1895-1900: 1.368-373 with shelfmark 224 (3758).

Current shelfmark: 465.

[0031]   **3766. 232**   II.35.

Lampros 1895-1900: 1.379-380 with shelfmark 232 (3766).

17th-century manuscript.

[0032]   **3778. 244**   II.35.

Lampros 1895-1900: 1.382 with shelfmark 244 (3778).

17th-century manuscript.

[0033]   **3799. 265**   II.66.

Lampros 1895-1900: 1.390 with shelfmark 265 (3799).

Current shelfmark: 297.

[0034]   **3808. 274**   II.39.

Lampros 1895-1900: 1.392-396 with shelfmark 274 (3808).

Current shelfmark: 168.

[0035]   **3881. 347**   II.58.

Lampros 1895-1900: 1.414-416 with shelfmark 347 (3881).

Current shelfmark: 402.

[0036]   **3897. 363**   II.35.

Lampros 1895-1900: 1.418-419 with shelfmark 363 (3897).

18th-century excerpts.

Bibl. Mon. Docheiariou (Βιβλιοθήκη Μονῆς Δοχειαρίου [Library of Dochiariou Monastery]), now Ιερά Μονή Δοχειαρίου (Dochiariou Monastery)

–

[0037]   **2917. 243**   I.47.

Lampros 1895-1900: 1.260 with shelfmark 243 (2917); Karas 1994: 376, 379.

17th-century manuscript.

Bibl. Mon. Esfigmenou (Βιβλιοθήκη Μονῆς Ἐσφιγμένου [Library of Esfigmenou Monastery]), now Ιερά Μονή Εσφιγμένου (Esfigmenou Monastery)

–

[0038]   **41**   I.12, 41, 104; II.5.

This manuscript is listed among the copies of the following texts (listed according to the sequential number of pages in Diels' catalogue):

- Hippocrates, *Aphorismi* (I.12);
- Hippocrates, *Sententiae de vita et morte* (I.41);
- Galenus, *In Hippocratis Aphorismos commentarius* (I.104);
- Aetius Amidenus, *Libri medicinales* (II.5).

According to Lampros 1895-1900: 1.175, Esfigmenou 41 (2054) does not contain medical texts but Gregorius Nazianzenus.

Diels' catalogue probably reproduces information taken from the following publications by Costomiris (explicitly cited at II.5):

- 1889: 352-353, on Hippocrates, *Aphorismi*;
- 1889: 358, about two *Commentarii in Hippocratis Aphorismos* (one anonymous and the other by Galen);
- 1890: 177, on Aetius Amidenus, *Libri medicinales*.

Costomiris' information, in turn, comes from a catalogue of the manuscripts in the Esfigmenou collection by Minoïde Mynas (1790-1860) contained in the codex Paris, *Supplementum graecum* 675 (on which see Omont 1886-1888: 3.294-295). According to Costomiris 1889, this catalogue contains the following information about the manuscript Esfigmenou 41:

- f. 83r: Hippocrates, *Aphorismi* (see Costomiris 1889: 353) and *Commentarii in Hippocratis Aphorismos* (*ibid.*: 358);
- f. 83v: Aetius Amidenus, *Libri medicinales* (see Costomiris 1890: 177).

In the 1890 article, however, Costomiris mentioned that he could not find this manuscript (that is, the manuscript mentioned by Minas) in Lampros' catalogue then in preparation (see Costomiris 1890: 177n2: "Dans le catalogue manuscrit du Mont-Athos dressé par M. Lambros, qui a eu la bonté de le prêter, je n'ai pu trouver ce manuscrit").

Esfigmenou 41 is not listed in Olivieri 1935: V-X (Aetius Amidenus), but is mentioned in Magdelaine 1994: 227 and n5 (Hippocrates, *Aphorismi*), who seems to consider that its absence in Lampros' catalogue results from an omission by Lampros.

There seem to have been two manuscripts identified by the same number (41), unless Mynas' information is incorrect. Whatever the case, current manuscript Esfigmenou 41 is not the one referred to here, and the one identified by Mynas as no. 41 cannot be identified.

[0039]   **2323. 310**   I.12.

Lampros 1895-1900: 1.199 with shelfmark 310 (2323).

18th-century item.

[0040]   **2330. 317**   I.21.

Lampros 1895-1900: 1.199.

Current shelfmark: 317 (2330).

Bibl. Mon. Ibêrôn (Βιβλιοθήκη Μονῆς ᾽Ιβήρων [Library of Iviron Monastery]), now Ιερά Μονή Ιβήρων (Iviron Monastery)

–

[0041]   **151**   II.109.

See [0043].

[0042]   **4212. 92**   I.40.

Lampros 1895-1900: 2.14-18.

Current shelfmark: 92 (792)

[0043]   **4271. 151**   I.40, 48, 93, 99-100, 117, 121, 132; II.14, 41, 58, 69, 70, 78.

Lampros 1895-1900: 2.34-35 with shelfmark 151 (4271).

See [0041].

[0044]   **4272. 152**   II.35.

Lampros 1895-1900: 2.35-36.

Current shelfmark: 152 (4272).

[0045]   **4284. 164**   I.61, 91.

Lampros 1895-1900: 2.43.

Current shelfmark: 164 (4284).

[0046]   **4294. 174**   I.42, 123.

Lampros 1895-1900: 2.46-47 with shelfmark 174 (4294); Karas 1994: 174.

17th-century *iatrosofion*.

[0047]   **4300. 180**   I.100.

Lampros 1895-1900: 2.48 with shelfmark 180 (4300); Karas 1994: 49-50.

17th-century manuscript.

[0048]   **4301. 181**   II.3.

Lampros 1895-1900: 2.48-49.

Current shelfmark: 181 (4301).

[0049]   **4302. 181**   II.27, 39, 73.

Mistake for 4302.182 (= [0050]).

[0050]   **4302. 182**   I.17, 47; II.91.

Lampros 1895-1900: 2.49.

Current shelfmark: 182 (4302).

Also [0049].

[0051]   **4304. 184**   I.102.

Lampros 1895-1900: 2.49-50.

Current shelfmark: 184 (4304).

[0052]   **4309. 189**   I.89, 90, 94, 102.

Lampros 1895-1900: 2.52.

Current shelfmark: 189 (4309).

| [0053] | **4310. 190** | I.56, 148; II.35. |

Lampros 1895-1900: 2.53-54.

Current shelfmark: 190 (4310).

| [0054] | **4325. 205** | II.35. |

Lampros 1895-1900: 2.58 with shelfmark 205 (4325).

17th-century manuscript.

| [0055] | **4330. 310** | I.41. |

This manuscript is referenced as a copy of Hippocrates, *Ad Ptolemaeum regem epistula.*

Codex Iviron 310 (= 4430 and not 4330) does not contain such text, but rather a νόμιμον (Lampros 1895-1900: 2.81). This is a mistake for 4330.210, which contains the letter on ff. 44v et seq.

See Άγιο Όρος, Ιερά Μονή Ιβήρων, 210 (4330) (see p. 5).

| [0056] | **4336. 216** | II.29, 39. |

Lampros 1895-1900: 2.62.

Current shelfmark: 216 (4336).

| [0057] | **4336. 217** | II.32, 34. |

This manuscript is referenced as having the copies of the following two texts:

- (f. 10) Dioscorides, *Euporista* (II.32);
- (f. 51B) Dioscorides, *Excerpta* (II.34).

Codex Iviron 217 (whose sequential number in Lampros 1895-1900: 2.62, is not 4336, but 4337) does not contain these texts, but the following that seem to have been incorrectly identified:

- (ff. 10r et seq.) βίβλος διοσκορίδους καὶ θεραπείας ἁπλῶν καὶ συνθέτων φαρμάκων;
- (ff. 51v et seq.) ἑρμηνεία τοῦ διοσκορίδους περὶ τοῦ καριοφάλου καὶ ἄλλων ἑτέρων.

Lampros 1895-1900: 2.62; Wellmann 1914: 6; Karas 1994: 159.

| [0058] | **4338. 218** | I.39. |

Lampros 1895-1900: 2.62.

Current shelfmark: 218 (4338).

| [0059] | **4339. 219** | I.99, 132. |

Lampros 1895-1900: 2.63 with shelfmark 219 (4339); Karas 1994: 114.

18th-century *iatrosofion.*

[0060]   **4340. 220**   I, 44; II.7.

Lampros 1895-1900: 2.63 with shelfmark 220 (4340); Karas 1994: 159, 240.

17th-century *iatrosofion*.

[0061]   **4436. 316**   II.71, 72, 77.

Lampros 1895-1900: 2.82 with shelfmark 316 (4436); Karas 1994: 254, 402.

17th-century *iatrosofion*.

[0062]   **4450. 330**   II.35.

Lampros 1895-1900: 2.87-88 with shelfmark 330 (4450); Karas 1994: 324.

18th-century codex.

[0063]   **4463. 343**   I.42, 44.

Lampros 1895-1900: 2.91 with shelfmark 343 (4463).

19th-century manuscript.

[0064]   **4468. 348**   II.35.

Lampros 1895-1900: 2.92-93.

Current shelfmark: 348 (4468).

[0065]   **4497. 377**   II.35.

Lampros 1895-1900: 2.102.

Current shelfmark: 377 (4497).

[0066]   **4501. 381**   I.40.

Lampros 1895-1900: 2.103-109.

Current shelfmark: 381 (4501).

[0067]   **4508. 388**   I.132.

Lampros 1895-1900: 2.122-138.

Current shelfmark: 388 (4508).

[0068]   **4655. 535**   I.42, 123; II.64.

Lampros 1895-1900: 2.166 with shelfmark 535 (4655); Karas 1994: 163-164.

16th-century *iatrosofion*.

[0069]   **4671. 551**   I.12.

Lampros 1895-1900: 2.169 with shelfmark 551 (4671). Also Magdelaine 1994: 202.

17th-century copy.

[0070]   **4720. 600**   II.35.

Lampros 1895-1900: 2.181-182 with shelfmark 600 (4720).

17th-century copy.

[0071]   **4788. 668**   II.35.

Lampros 1895-1900: 2.195-196 with shelfmark 668 (4788).

18th-century item.

[0072]   **4789. 669**   I.136.

Lampros 1895-1900: 2.196 with shelfmark 669 (4789); Karas 1994: 350.

18th-century manuscript.

[0073]   **4799. 679**   II.35.

Lampros 1895-1900: 2.199 with shelfmark 679 (4799).

18th-century manuscript.

[0074]   **4815. 695**   II.35.

Lampros 1895-1900: 2.207.

Current shelfmark: 695 (4815).

[0075]   **4871. 751**   II.36.

Lampros 1895-1900: 2.218-220 with shelfmark 751 (4871).

17th-century codex.

[0076]   **4925. 805**   II.35.

Lampros 1895-1900: 2.226-227 with shelfmark 805 (4925).

17th-century item.

[0077]   **5034. 914**   I.40, 124.

Lampros 1895-1900: 2.236-237 with shelfmark 914 (5034); Karas 1994: 246, 349, 375.

17th-century manuscript.

[0078]   **5437. 1317**   I.136.

Lampros 1895-1900: 2.263-265, with shelfmark 1317 (5437); Karas 1994: 281-282.

18th-century codex.

Bibl. Mon. Koutloumousiou (Βιβλιοθήκη Μονῆς Κουτλουμουσίου [Library of Koutloumousiou Monastery]), now Ιερά Μονή Κουτλουμουσίου (Koutloumousiou Monastery)

–

[0079]   **3260. 2**   II.35.

This item is listed as a copy of Epiphanius, *Physiologus*.

Manuscript Koutloumousiou 2 is not numbered 3260 in Lampros 1895-1900: 1.270, but 3071, and it does not contain Epiphanius, *Physiologus*.

As for the manuscript with sequential number 3260 in Lampros 1895-1900: 1.294, it is Koutloumousiou 187. This manuscript contains Epiphanius, *Physiologus*, under no. 2. It is probably this number 2 attributed to the text in the description of its content in Lampros, *ibid.*, that provoked the incorrect number attributed to the manuscript in Diels' catalogue.

Current shelfmark: 187 (3260).

[0080]   **3321. 248**   I.111; II.34, 73.

Lampros 1895-1900: 1.305 with shelfmark 248 (3321); Karas 1994: 106, 349.

17th-century copy.

Bibl. Mon. Lauras (Βιβλιοθήκη Μονῆς Μεγίστης Λαύρας [Library of the Great Lavra Monastery]), now Ἱερά Μονή Μεγίστης Λαύρας (Great Lavra Monastery)

–

[0081]   –   II.107.

Diels' catalogue adds the following information about this manuscript of Timotheus Gazaeus, *De animalibus quadrupedibus physicisque eorum facultatibus* listed without shelfmark:

Vgl. Parisin. Suppl. 799. f. 18. Costomiris, Rev. des ét. gr. IV [1892] p. 99.

In Costomiris' article (in *Revue des études grecques* 4 [1891] and not 4 [1892] as referenced in Diels' catalogue), the following can be read:

Son ouvrage [of Timotheus of Gaza] ... se trouve incomplet dans un ms. de la bibliothèque de saint Athanase de Laura au Mont-Athos. Voir *Suppl. grec* de Paris 799, fol. 18.

The manuscript of Paris, *Supplementum graecum* 799 contains (ff. 18r-27v) a catalogue of some manuscripts of the monastic libraries at Mount Athos (title f. 18r, ll. 1-2: Βίβλων τινῶν ἐκ τῶν πολλῶν καὶ διαφόρων τῶν ἐν τοῖς μοναστηρίοις τοῦ Ἄθω κατάλογος). The catalogue of the Lavra (ff. 18r, l. 3-20v, l. 11) lists a copy of Timotheus, *De animalibus* (f. 18r, ll. 10-11) identified as follows:

Τιμοθέου γραμματικοῦ πρὸς τὸν αὐτοκράτορα Ἀναστάσιον περὶ ζώων · ἀτελές.

The catalogue by Spyridon and Eustratiades 1925 does not make it possible to identify this manuscript.

[0082]   –   II.29, 31, 32, 33, 38, 39 (2).

This item is a 12th-century copy of the following texts (listed according to the sequential number of pages in Diels' catalogue):

• Dioscorides, *De materia medica* (II.29);

• Pseudo-Dioscorides, *Thêriaka* (II.31);

• Pseudo-Dioscorides, *Alexipharmaka* (II.32);

• Pseudo-Dioscorides, *De mensuris et ponderibus* (II.33);

• Eutecnius, *Paraphrasis in Dionysii Ixeutica* (II.38);

• Eutecnius, *Paraphrasis in Nicandri Theriaca* (II.39);

• Eutecnius, *Paraphrasis in Nicandri Alexipharmaca* (II.39).

The list of content corresponds to that of Athous, Lavrae Ω 75, on which see above, p. 8, Ἅγιο Ὄρος, Ἱερά Μονή Μεγίστης Λαύρας.

12th century (instead of 11th) corresponds to the period proposed for the manuscript at Diels' time and does not invalidate the identification.

[0083]   –   II.5.

[0084]

[0085]   Four manuscripts of Aetius Amidenus, *Libri medicinales*, without shelfmark

[0086]   identified as follows:

Ausser Ω 70 und 72 noch 4 weitere Hdss. bei Costomiris Rev. des ét. gr. III p. 166 und 127.

The reference to Costomiris is to Costomiris 1890:

- at 166, the author briefly refers to 6 Aetius Amidenus manuscripts at Lavra;

- at 177-178 (and not 127 as in Diels) he mentions that there are six manuscripts of Aetius Amidenus (none identified by means of a shelfmark) in the Lavra library. He has not personally inspected these manuscripts, but mentions them on the basis of the Paris manuscript *Supplementum graecum* 675, ff. 192r, 194r, 199r, 216r, 217r and 217v (which is actually a catalogue of manuscripts of the Lavra monastery by Minoïde Mynas on which, see Omont 1886-1888: 3.294-295).

On each of these six manuscripts Costomiris' 1890: 177-178 provides the following information to which I add, between parentheses, the reference to manuscript Paris *Supplementum graecum* 675. It must be noted that Costomiris' transcription of the data in Paris, *Supplementum graecum* 675 does not exactly reproduce the content of the manuscript and is erroneous on more than one point.

In Costomiris article, the manuscripts are identified by a number in either Arabic or Greek numerals.

Those identified by Arabic numerals appear in a catalogue contained ff. 168r-171v and 173r-200r and entitled (f. 168r, ll. 1-2): "Catalogue de la bibliotheque de Laura". Data are as follows (translation is mine):

- ms. 12°, 14th century, paper, in-folio, incomplete (books 8-13), Αετίου [*sic*] ὀφφικίου (Paris, *Supplementum graecum* 675, f. 192r, ll. 3-4);

- ms. 22, 14th century, paper, in-4°, book 12, Αετίου [*sic*] Ἀμιδηνοῦ κομητος [*sic*] τοῦ ὀψικίου λόγος ιβ^{ος} (Paris, *Supplementum graecum* 675, ff. 193v-194r; for the identification of Aetius' text, see f. 194r, ll. 27-29);

- ms. 46: 13th century, paper, in-folio, incomplete, books 1-8 (ἐκ τῶν τοῦ Αετίου [*sic*]). Book 1 ends at ὤκιμον; this codex ends at f. 64 (Paris, *Supplementum graecum* 675, f. 199r, ll. 28-33).

Those identified by Greek numerals appear in a brief catalogue (ff. 209r-217r) entitled (f. 209r, ll. 1-3) "Catalogue de la Grande bibliotheque [*sic*] de Laura. Ici ouvrages seulement classiques":

- ms. Δ: dated 1395, paper, books 1-16, Ἀετίου Ἀμιδηνοῦ σύνοψις τῶν τρίων βιβλίων Ὀριβασίου ... (Paris, *Supplementum graecum* 675, f. 216r, l. 13-216v);

- ms. E: paper, small in-folio, books 2-16 (book 16 incomplete) (Paris, *Supplementum graecum* 675, f. 217v, ll. 1-3);

- ms. ΣΤ: 13th century, paper, in-8°, book 16 (Paris, *Supplementum graecum* 675, f. 217r, ll. 4-16).

On the basis of Costomiris' descriptions, the manuscripts in these two groups do not seem to correspond to, nor to duplicate each other.

None of the manuscripts (whatever the group) seems to correspond to any of the Aetius Amidenus codices in Spyridon and Eustratiades 1925: 340, other than Ω 70 and Ω 72 mentioned regarding these four manuscripts and listed in Diels (= [0088] and [0089] respectively):

- Ω 63 (1873);
- Ω 64 (1874);
- Ω 65 (1875);
- Ω 66 (1876).

Olivieri 1935: V, lists only the manuscripts Ω 63 and Ω 64.

On these manuscripts, see Ἅγιον Ὄρος, Μεγίστη Λαύρα (see pp. 7-8).

[0087]	**Ω 69**	II.110.
		Spyridon and Eustratiades 1925: 341.
[0088]	**Ω 70**	II.5; N.43.
		Spyridon and Eustratiades 1925: 342.
[0089]	**Ω 72**	II.5; N.43.
		Spyridon and Eustratiades 1925: 342.

Bibl. Mon. Panteleêmonos (Βιβλιοθήκη Μονῆς Παντελεήμονος [Library of Panteleimonos Monastery]), now Ἱερά Μονή Ἁγίου Παντελεήμονος (Agiou Panteleimonos Monastery)

–

[0090]	**5578. 72**	I.148.
		Lampros 1895-1900: 2.288-289.
		Current shelfmark: 72 (5578).
[0091]	**5752. 245**	II.35.
		Lampros 1895-1900: 2.341 with shelfmark 345 (5752).
		17th-century copy.
[0092]	**5768. 261**	II.64.
		Lampros 1895-1900: 2.342 with shelfmark 261 (5768).
		18th-century manuscript.
[0093]	**5769. 262**	I.42, 123; II.64, 79.
		Lampros 1895-1900: 2.342-343 with shelfmark 262 (5769); Karas 1994: 71-72.
		18th-century *iatrosofion*.
[0094]	**5796. 289**	I.12.
		Lampros 1895-1900: 2.354 with shelfmark 289 (5796).
		18th-century codex.

[0095]   **6342. 835**   I.12.

Lampros 1895-1900: 2.442 with shelfmark 835 (6342); Karas 1994: 381-382, 385.

17th-century manuscript.

[0096]   **6351. 844**   II.91.

Lampros 1895-1900: 2.443 with shelfmark 844 (6351); Karas 1994: 206.

18th-century copy.

[0097]   **6372. 865**   II.64.

Lampros 1895-1900: 2.447-448 with shelfmark 865 (6372).

19th-century copy.

Bibl. Mon. Xêropotamou (Βιβλιοθήκη Μονῆς Ξηροποτάμου [Library of Xiropotamou Monastery]), now Ιερά Μονή Ξηροποτάμου (Xiropotamou Monastery)

–

[0098]   **2342.99**   I.125.

Mistake for 2432.99 (= [0099]).

[0099]   **2432. 99**   I.39, 46, 124; II.34.

Lampros 1895-1900: 1.206 with shelfmark 99 (2432); Karas 1994: 169-170.

17th-century codex.

Also [0098].

Pantokratoros (Παντοκράτορος [Pantokrator Monastery]), now Ιερά Μονή Παντοκράτορος (Pantokrator Monastery)

–

[0100]   **1268. 234**   I.148.

Lampros 1895-1900: 1.112-113.

Current shelfmark: 234 (1268).

Stauronikêta (Σταυρονικήτα [Stavronikita Monastery]), now Ιερά Μονή Σταυρονικήτα (Stavronikita Monastery)

–

[0101]   **951. 86**   II.35.

Lampros 1895-1900: 1.84 with shelfmark 86 (951).

17th-century manuscript.

Xenophôntos (Ξενοφώντος [Xenophontos Monastery])

–

[0102]   **739. 37**   II.39.

Lampros 1895-1900: 1.65 with shelfmark 37 (739); Karas 1994: 353.

18th-century manuscript.

Basel (CH)

Bibl. univ. (*Bibliotheca universitatis* [University Library]), now Öffentliche Bibliothek der Universität Basel (Public Library of Basel University)

–

[0103]   **F VI 46**   II.77.

Omont 1886: 416.

Now Mscr F VI 46.

Öffentliche Bibliothek der Universität Basel (Public Library of Basel University)
Mscr F VI 46. See [0103].

Bergamo (IT)

Biblioteca Civica (City Library)

Cassaforte

1.8   Palimpsest.

Scriptio superior: Boethius, *Commentarius in Porphyrii Isagogem.*

Scriptio inferior: *In Hippocratis Aphorismos commentarius.*

Harlfinger, Brunschön and Vasiloudi 2006: 145, 163; Lo Monaco 2007 and 2008.

Berlin (DE)

–

–

[0104]   **Pap. 6934**   I.37.

A papyrus, not a manuscript (= Mertens/Pack 542).

Marganne 1981: 3.

[0105]   **Pap. 7094**   I.37.

A papyrus, not a manuscript (= Mertens/Pack 541).

Marganne 1981: 1-2.

Königl. Bibl. (Königliche Bibliothek [Royal Library]), now Staatsbibliothek zu Berlin-Preussischer Kulturbesitz SBB-PKB (Berlin State Library-Prussian Cultural Heritage)

In most items of the folio (= [0109]-[0115]), quarto (= [0106]-[0108] and [0152]-[0153]) and Hamilton (= [0116]) collections, Diels' catalogue includes a three-digit number in Arabic numerals between parentheses. This number is the sequential number in the catalogue by de Boor 1897; it is not part of the shelfmark of the manuscripts.

4°. (quarto)

[0106]   **2 (301)**   II.61.

de Boor 1897: 165-166.

17th-century copies of printed works.

[0107]	**5 (304)**	II.36, 63.
		de Boor 1897: 167-168.
		Now Kraków (PL), Biblioteka Jagiellońska (see p. 103).
		Also [0152].
[0108]	**21 (319)**	I.96.
		de Boor 1897: 179-180.
		This manuscript was destroyed during World War II.

fol. (folio)

[0109]	**7 (247)**	II.109.
		de Boor 1897: 125.
		Now Kraków (PL), Biblioteka Jagiellońska (see p. 103).
[0110]	**35 (271)**	II.70.
		de Boor 1897: 140.
		Now Ms. graec. fol. 35.
[0111]	**37**	N.43.
		de Boor 1897: 140-142.
		Now Kraków (PL), Biblioteka Jagiellońska (see p. 103).
		Also [0112].
[0112]	**37 (273)**	II.5, 8.
		Same as [0111].
[0113]	**38**	N.43.
		de Boor 1897: 142.
		18th-century scholars' notes.
		Also [0114].
[0114]	**38 (274)**	II.5.
		Same as [0113].
[0115]	**39 (275)**	II.7, 10, 13, 15, 16, 17 (2), 18 (2), 20, 22, 34, 37, 73, 79-80, 91, 109.
		de Boor 1897: 142-144.
		This manuscript in fact contains notes by Carl Weigel (1769-1845) on Greek medical texts (see Cutolo 2012: 27, who identifies the manuscript as Berlin 275).

Hamilton. (*Hamiltonienses*)

[0116]	**270 (401)**	I.74.
		de Boor 1897: 231-232; Merolla 2010: 108-109.
		Now Ms. Ham. 270.
		Formerly [1652].

Phillips. [*sic*] (Phillipps, *Phillippici*)

All the manuscripts in this collection are now identified as "Ms. Phill." followed by the four-digit number from the Phillipps collection as in the catalogue by Studemund and Cohn 1890. Their sequential number in this catalogue is not a shelfmark.

References to the Meerman collection as in Diels ([0120]-[0123], [0125], [0127]-[0128], [0130]-[0134], [0141]-[0143], [0146]-[0148] and [0151]) are not part of the shelfmarks. They come from the catalogue of the Meerman collection published in 1824 (*Bibliotheca Meermanniana* 1824, vol. 4).

[0117]	**1432**	II.39.
		Studemund and Cohn 1890: 9.
		Now Ms. Phill. 1432.
[0118]	**1462**	I.40, 124.
		Studemund and Cohn 1890: 18-19.
		Now Ms. Phill. 1462.
	Ms. Phill. 1478	(ff. 27r-34v) Meletius, *De natura hominis* (frg.).
		Studemund and Cohn 1890: 27-28.
[0119]	**1487**	I.47.
		Studemund and Cohn 1890: 33.
		Now Ms. Phill. 1487.
	Ms. Phill. 1507	(ff. 209r-212v) Aristoteles, *De insomniis*.
		Studemund and Cohn 1890: 44; *Aristoteles graecus* 1976: 40-42.
	Ms. Phill. 1508	(ff. 1r et seq.) Aristoteles, *Problemata*.
		Studemund and Cohn 1890: 44; *Aristoteles graecus* 1976: 42-43.
	Ms. Phill. 1523	(ff. 1r-234v) Cassianus Bassus, *Geoponica*.
		Studemund and Cohn 1890: 48.
[0120]	**1524 (ol. Meerm. 214)**	I.86; II.102, 104.
		Studemund and Cohn 1890: 48-49.
		Now Ms. Phill. 1524.
[0121]	**1525 (ol. Meerm. 215)**	I.109; II.76; N.61.
		Studemund and Cohn 1890: 49.
		Now Ms. Phill. 1525.
[0122]	**1526 (ol. Meerm. 216)**	I.100, 111.
		Studemund and Cohn 1890: 49-50.
		Now Ms. Phill. 1526.
[0123]	**1527 (ol. Meerm. 217)**	I.47, 68; II.40, 85, 101.
		Studemund and Cohn 1890: 50.
		Now Ms. Phill. 1527.

[0124]	**1528**	II.109.
		Studemund and Cohn 1890: 50-51.
		Now Ms. Phill. 1528.
[0125]	**1529 (ol. Meerm. 220)**	I.32, 98; II.98.
		Studemund and Cohn 1890: 51.
		Now Ms. Phill. 1529.
[0126]	**1530**	II.29, 31, 32.
		Studemund and Cohn 1890: 51.
		Now Ms. Phill. 1530.
[0127]	**1531 (Meerm. 223)**	II.17 (2), 18 (2), 64, 102, 109.
		Studemund and Cohn 1890: 51-52.
		Now Ms. Phill. 1531.
		Same as [1644] and possibly also [1647].
[0128]	**1532 (ol. Meerman. 225)**	I.12; II.17 (2), 18 (2), 70, 83, 92, 97, 102.
		Studemund and Cohn 1890: 52-53.
		Now Ms. Phill. 1532.
[0129]	**1533**	II.15, 70, 92.
		Studemund and Cohn 1890: 53.
		Now Ms. Phill. 1533.
[0130]	**1534 (Meerm. 229)**	II.5.
		Studemund and Cohn 1890: 53.
		Now Ms. Phill. 1534.
[0131]	**1535 (ol. Meerm. 229)**	II.11.
		Studemund and Cohn 1890: 53-54.
		Now Ms. Phill. 1535.
[0132]	**1536 (ol. Meerm. 231)**	II.88, 89 (2), 90.
		Studemund and Cohn 1890: 54.
		Now Ms. Phill. 1536.
		Also [0716].
[0133]	**1537 (ol. Meerman. 233)**	I.12.
		Studemund and Cohn 1890: 54.
		Now Ms. Phill. 1537.
		Formerly [0212].
[0134]	**1538 (ol. Meerm. 233)**	I.56; II.24.
		Studemund and Cohn 1890: 55.
		Now Ms. Phill. 1538.
[0135]	**1539**	II.29.
		Studemund and Cohn 1890: 56-57.
		Now Ms. Phill. 1539.

[0136]	**1540**	II.24, 95, 98, 100, 111, 112 (2).
		Studemund and Cohn 1890: 57-59.
		Now Ms. Phill. 1540.
[0137]	**1547**	II.93.
		Studemund and Cohn 1890: 60-61.
		Now Ms. Phill. 1547.
	Ms. Phill. 1552	(ff. 1r-2v) Aristoteles, *Problemata* (frg.).
		Studemund and Cohn 1890: 63-64; *Aristoteles graecus* 1976: 43-45.
[0138]	**1557**	II.66.
		Studemund and Cohn 1890: 66.
		Now Ms. Phill. 1557.
[0139]	**1558**	II.9.
		Studemund and Cohn 1890: 66-67.
		Now Ms. Phill. 1558.
[0140]	**1562**	N.47.
		Studemund and Cohn 1890: 67-68.
		Now Ms. Phill. 1562.
	Ms. Phill. 1563	(ff. 1r-35r) Manuel Philes, *De animalium proprietate*.
		Studemund and Cohn 1890: 68.
	Ms. Phill. 1564	*Geoponica*.
		Studemund and Cohn 1890: 68.
	Ms. Phill. 1565	(ff. 1r et seq.) *Geoponica*.
		Studemund and Cohn 1890: 68-69.
[0141]	**1566 (ol. Meerm. 269)**	I.41, 75, 97, 113, 124; II.102.
		Studemund and Cohn 1890: 69-70.
		Now Ms. Phill. 1566.
[0142]	**1567 (ol. Meerm. 270)**	I.67.
		Studemund and Cohn 1890: 70-71.
		Now Ms. Phill. 1567.
[0143]	**1568 (ol. Meerm. 271)**	II.49, 72.
		Studemund and Cohn 1890: 71.
		Now Ms. Phill. 1568.
	Ms. Phill. 1569	Râzî, *De pestilentia*.
		Studemund and Cohn 1890: 71.
[0144]	**1570**	I.117; II.68, 78.
		Studemund and Cohn 1890: 71-72.
		Now Ms. Phill. 1570.

[0145]	**1571**	I.112; II.20, 79, 100.
		Studemund and Cohn 1890: 72.
		Now Ms. Phill. 1571.
	Ms. Phill. 1572	(ff. 1r-2v) *Remedia varia*; (ff. 3r-v) *De lapidum facultate* (frg.); (ff. 4r-5r) *Remedia varia*; (ff. 5r-6r) *De lapidibus*; (f. 7r-v) *Collectio medica*; (ff. 13r and 9r-10r) *Medicamina*; (f. 11r) Nicephorus Constantinopolitanus Patriarcha, *Oneirocriticon* (frg.); (f. 11v) *Oneirocriticon* (frg.).
		Studemund and Cohn 1890: 72-73.
	Ms. Phill. 1574	(f. 132v) Nicephorus Constantinopolitanus Patriarcha, *Oneirocriticon*; (f. 189r) *Geoponica* (frg.).
		Studemund and Cohn 1890: 73-75.
	Ms. Phill. 1575	Achmet, *Oneirocriticon*.
		Studemund and Cohn 1890: 75.
[0146]	**1576 (Meerm. 286)**	N.58.
		Studemund and Cohn 1890: 75.
		Now Ms. Phill. 1576.
[0147]	**1577 (Meerm. 287)**	N.36, 51, 52.
		Studemund and Cohn 1890: 75-77.
		Now Ms. Phill. 1577.
	Ms. Phill. 1580	Manuel Philes, *De animalium proprietate*.
		Studemund and Cohn 1890: 77.
[0148]	**1581 (ol. Meerm. 297)**	II.71.
		Studemund and Cohn 1890: 77-78.
		Now Ms. Phill. 1581.
[0149]	**1582**	II.108, 109 (2).
		Studemund and Cohn 1890: 78.
		Now Ms. Phill. 1582.
[0150]	**1583**	I.40; II.7, 69, 78; N.46, 56, 67.
		Studemund and Cohn 1890: 78-79.
		Now Ms. Phill. 1583.
	Ms. Phill. 1591	(ff. 119v-120r) Splenus philosophus, *De generatione hominis* (*sub nomine* Damna sophistes).
		Studemund and Cohn 1890: 80-81.
	Ms. Phill. 1617	(ff. 197r-198v) Nemesius Emesenus, *De natura hominis* (frg.).
		Studemund and Cohn 1890: 92-94.

[0151]	**1991**	I.78 (2), 79 (2).
	(ol. Meerm. 218)	Studemund and Cohn 1890: 103.
		Now Ms. Phill. 1991.
	qu. (quarto)	
[0152]	**5 (304)**	I.39, 124.
		Same as [0107].
[0153]	**46 (348)**	II.64.
		de Boor 1897: 194-201.
		Now Kraków (PL), Biblioteka Jagiellońska (see p. 103).

Staatsbibliothek zu Berlin-Preussischer Kulturbesitz SBB-PKB (Berlin State Library-Prussian Cultural Heritage).

See **Königl. Bibl.** (see above, pp. 27-33).

Ms. graec. fol., see **fol.** (see above, p. 28).

Ms. graec. qu., see **4°** and **qu.** (see above, pp. 27-28 and 33).

Ms. Ham., see **Hamilton.** (see above, p. 28).

Ms. Phill., see **Phillips.** [*sic*] (see above, pp. 29-33).

Bern (CH)

Burgerbibliothek Bern/Bibliothèque de la Bourgeoisie de Berne (Burgerbibliothek Bern)

See **Stadtbibliothek.**

Stadtbibliothek (City Library), now Burgerbibliothek Bern/Bibliothèque de la Bourgeoisie de Berne (Burgerbibliothek Bern)

	–	
	135	(pp. 43-48) Aristoteles, *De insomniis*.
		Andrist 2007: 140-145; *Aristoteles graecus* 1976: 52-53, 464.
[0154]	459	II.89 (2).
		Andrist 2007: 206-215.
[0155]	579	I.26, 37.
		Andrist 2007: 232-254; *CMAG* IV (Goldschmidt) 1932: 321.
[0156]	691	I.72.
		Andrist 2007: 295-299.

Berne (CH)

Bibliothèque de la Bourgeoisie de Berne/Burgerbibliothek Bern (Burgerbibliothek Bern)

See **Bern, Stadtbibliothek.**

Besançon (FR)

Bibliothèque municipale (Municipal Library)

408	(ff. 156r-164v) Theophylactus Simocatta, *Quaestiones physicae*.
	Omont 1886-1888: 3.363, no. 13; Gollob 1908/2: 12-14.

Bethesda, MD (US)

U.S. National Institutes of Health, National Library of Medicine, History of Medicine Division

MS. 81 Census	Stephanus Atheniensis, *In Hippocratis prognosticum*.
	Tunis 1989: 6.
MS. 82 Census	Tunis 1989: 6.
	Formerly [0221].

Bologna (IT)

Bibl. Comunale (Biblioteca Comunale [Municipal Library]), now Biblioteca Comunale dell'Archiginnasio (Archiginnasio Municipal Library)

–

[0157]	**Bonon. A I 13**	II.66-67.
		The abbreviated term "Bonon." (= *Bononiensis*, "from Bologna") is not part of the shelfmark.
		Olivieri and Festa 1895: 475-476.
		Current shelfmark: A 13.

Biblioteca Comunale dell'Archiginnasio (Archiginnasio Municipal Library)

–

	A 13	See [0157].

Bibl. Universitaria (Biblioteca Universitaria [University Library])

Bonon. (*Bononienses*)

[0158]	**457 vol. XXIV no. 1**	II.24.
		Puntoni 1896/2: 367-368; *CMAG* II (Zuretti et al.) 1927: 130-143.
[0159]	**1808**	I.115, 116, 117, 120, 122, 126, 131, 132; II.5, 20, 34, 38, 41, 58, 73, 76, 83, 91, 106.
		Olivieri and Festa 1895: 389-396; *CMAG* II (Zuretti et al.) 1927: 143-144.
[0160]	**2294**	II.9.
		Olivieri and Festa 1895: 401-402.
[0161]	**2678**	I.96.
		Puntoni 1896/2: 375.
[0162]	**2911**	II.21.
		Olivieri and Festa 1895: 419-429.

[0163]   **3232**   I.12.

This copy of Hippocrates, *Aphorismi* is not manuscript 3232, which does not contain Greek texts (it is not listed in Olivieri and Festa 1895).

The item referred to here is 3632 (= [0165]) (see also Magdelaine 1994: 88 n1).

[0164]   **3563**   I.37.

Olivieri and Festa 1895: 432-433.

[0165]   **3632**   I.4, 5, 17, 18, 20, 28, 31, 39, 40, 80, 111, 113, 114, 115, 117, 130, 132; II.5, 7, 13, 15, 16, 20, 25, 29, 34, 41, 45 (2), 56, 59, 60, 73, 75, 80, 86, 87, 91, 100, 102, 106 (2), 110.

Olivieri and Festa 1895: 442-456; *CMAG* II (Zuretti et al.) 1927: 144, 298-321.

Also [0163].

[0166]   **3633**   I.40; II.28.

Olivieri and Festa 1895: 456.

               3634   *Curationes variae.*

Olivieri and Festa 1895: 456-457 (where the manuscript is mistakenly numbered 8634).

[0167]   **3635**   II.9, 22.

Olivieri and Festa 1895: 457-458.

[0168]   **3636**   I.12, 61, 64, 94, 127, 129, 136; II.27, 77, 80, 92, 102.

Olivieri and Festa 1895: 458-460.

[0169]   **3637**   I.70.

Olivieri and Festa 1895: 461-463.

Biblioteca Universitaria (University Library)

See above **Bibl. Universitaria.**

Boston, Mass. (US)

Harvard University, Medical School, Francis A. Countway Library of Medicine

Rare Books and Special Collections

          736 Ballard   Dioscorides, *De materia medica.*

Faye and Bond 1962: 206, no. 39; Kavrus-Hoffmann 2012: 77-84.

Bremen (DE)

Staats- und Universitätsbibliothek Bremen (State and University Library Bremen)

   -

          msb 0023   (ff. 244v-248v) Symeon Seth, *Conspectus rerum naturalium.*
Stahl 2004: 123-126.

          msb 0106   (ff. 1r-36r) Manuel Philes, *De animalium proprietate.*
Stahl 2004: 155-158.

Breslau (now Wrocław) (PL)

–

–

[0170]   **?**   N.50.

This manuscript mentioned without library name, collection or shelfmark contains Epiphanius, *De mensuris et ponderibus*.

It was Rehd. 240 of the former *Bibliotheca urbana Vratislaviensis* (Vratislava City Library, now Biblioteka Uniwersytecka we Wrocławiu [University Library Wrocław]). The manuscript contained Epiphanius' text on ff. 249r-254r.

Catalogus Vratislaviensis 1889: 63-65.

This item was destroyed during World War II (Alland 1956: 37).

bibl. urb. (*Bibliotheca urbana [Vratislaviensis]* [Vratislava City Library]), now Biblioteka Uniwersytecka we Wrocławiu (Wrocław University Library)

–

[0171]   **34**   II.67.

This copy of Nemesius, *De natura hominis* is contained in current codex Rehd. 34.

This manuscript is made of 4 different codices of which the first (ff.1-55) is referred to here (see ff. 1r-54r for Nemesius' text).

The third codex in the same manuscript (ff. 88-149) contains (ff. 124r-135r) Synesius Cyrenensis, *De insomniis*, and also (ff. 120v-123v, 125v, 132r et in marginibus ff. 124r-135r) Nicephorus Gregoras, *Explicatio in librum Synesii De insomniis*.

Catalogus Vratislaviensis 1889: 42-45 for the whole manuscript, 43 for the first codex (see also Morani 1981: 11) and 44-45 for the third codex.

Brüssel (Bruxelles) (BE)

Königl. Bibl. (Königliche Bibliothek [Royal Library]), now Bibliothèque royale de Belgique (Royal Library of Belgium)

Bruxell. (*Bruxellenses*)

[0172]   **1871-77**   I.37.

Omont 1885: 19; Calcoen 1965-1975: 1.45.

[0173]   **5362-64**   II.63.

Omont 1885: 32; Calcoen 1965-1975: 2.16-17.

[0174]   **11337-41**   II.108, 109-110.

Omont 1885: 18; Calcoen 1965-1975: 3.54-55.

[0175]   **11345-48**   I.109; II.37.

Omont 1885: 18; Calcoen 1965-1975: 3. 55-58.

[0176]   **11351-52**   II.67.

Omont 1885: 14; Calcoen 1965-1975: 3. 58-59.

Humanist copy of Nemesius Emesenus, *De natura hominis*, used by Nicaise van Ellebode (d. 1577) for his *editio princeps* (Antverpiae, Ex officina Christophori Plantini, 1565), together with a Latin translation (Morani 1981: 53).

[0177]   **11354**   II.39.

Omont 1885: 12.

18170-73   Nicander, *Theriaca* et *Alexipharmaca*.

Omont 1885: 26; Calcoen 1980: 54.

II.4837   Nemesius Emesenus, *De natura hominis* (frg.).

Morani 1981: 58-59.

IV.459   Palimpsest.

Scriptio superior: Hagiographico-homiletica.

Scriptio inferior: Paulus Aegineta, *Epitome medica*.

Quinze années 1969: 30-32; Wittek 1975: 247; Noret 1979; Foti 1987; Harlfinger, Brunschön and Vasiloudi 2006: 145, 158-159; Rodriquez 2008: 207.

Formerly Phillipps 22406 (*Phillipps manuscripts* 1837-1871: 417).

See also Messina, Biblioteca Regionale Universitaria, S. Salvatore, 2 (see below, p. 137).

IV.488   Symeon Seth, *De alimentorum facultatibus*.

Quinze années 1969: 151-152; Wittek 1975: 251.

Formerly Phillipps 2355 (*Phillipps manuscripts* 1837-1871: 28)

Bruxelles (BE)

Bibliothèque royale de Belgique (Royal Library of Belgium)

See **Brüssel, Königl. Bibl.**

București (Bucharest) (RO)

Biblioteca Academiei Române (Romanian Academy Library)

–

165   (ff. 95r-104r) Gregorius Nyssenus, *De hominis opificio*.

(Litzica 559)   Litzica 1909: 237-239.

452   (pp. 203 et seq.) Nemesius Emesenus, *De natura hominis*.

(Litzica 602)   Litzica 1909: 289-294.

Budapest (HU)

Mus. nat. Hungar. (*Museum nationale Hungaricum* [National Museum of Hungary]), now Országos Széchényi Könyvtár (National Széchényi Library)

–

[0178]   **9 fol.**   II.70, 71, 72, 73.

Now National Széchényi Library, Manuscript collection, Fol. Graec. 9.

[Bibl. Regia] (*Bibliotheca Regia* [Royal Library])

–

[0179]   **[Cod. Matthiae Corvini]**   I.102.

This copy of Galenus, *In Hippocratis librum de alimento commentarii IV* in the collection of the king of Hungary Matthias Corvinus (1443-1490) seems to be lost. It does not appear in Csapodi and Csapodi-Gárdony 1982, Bono et al. 2002, or in the list provided by Tanner 2008: 216-224.

Országos Széchényi Könyvtár (National Széchényi Library)

Kéziratar (Manuscript collection)

Fol. Graec. 4   (ff. 23v et seq.) Iohannes Zacharias Actuarius, *De dieta*.

Kubinyi 1956: 16-17.

Fol. Graec. 9   See [0178].

Kubinyi 1956: 23-24.

Quart. Graec. 6   (ff. 2r et seq.) Ioannes Prisdyanus, *De intestinis*; (ff. 6r et seq.) Theophilus, *De urinis*; (ff. 27r et seq.), Aetius Amidenus, *De excrementis*; (ff. 29r et seq.) Ioannes Prisdyanus, *De excrementis*; (ff. 54r et seq.) Hippocrates, *Prognosticon* (frg.); (ff. 75v et seq.) *Capitula medica varia*; (ff. 88r et seq.) *Collectio alphabetica medicinarum*.

Kubinyi 1956: 36-38.

Quart. Graec. 14   (ff. 70r-79v) Hippocrates, *Epistula ad Ptolemaeum regem*.

Kubinyi 1956: 47-48.

Cairo (EG)

Ad. Cattaui

[0180]   –   N.52.

This is a papyrus, believed to be in Alexandria University, P. Cairo Crawford 1 (= 2377 Pack²).

Marganne 1981: 140-143.

Patriarch. Alexandrin. (*Patriarchatus Alexandrinus* [Patriarchate of Alexandria]), now Πατριαρχική Βιβλιοθήκη Αλεξανδρείας (Patriarchal Library of Alexandria).

The Greek Orthodox Patriarchate of Alexandria was in Cairo until 1928, when it was moved back to Alexandria.

For other manuscripts, see Αλεξάνδρεια (الإسكندرية, Alexandria), Πατριαρχείο, Πατριαρχική Βιβλιοθήκη Αλεξανδρείας (Patriarchate, Patriarchal Library of Alexandria) (see p. 9).

[0181]   **46**   N.41, 68.

This item appears among the copies of Galen, *Excerpta varia* (N.41) and Theophilus, *De excrementis* (N.68).

Manuscript 46 of the Patriarchate in Alexandria does not seem to contain either Galen or Theophilus, or any other medical text, but rather a bilingual Greek-Arabic euchologion (Moschonas 1945: 61-62 [1965: 45-46]).

According to Moschonas 1945: XXX, no manuscript of Alexandria collection contains any works by Theophilus. The data in Diels might refer to codex 36 (ff. 1r-3r) Galenus, *Regimen ex quattuor elementis et de preservatione sanitatis* (Moschonas 1945: 54-55 [1965:41]). This is a 17th-century manuscript (Moschonas, *ibid.*; Karas 1994: 348).

Cambridge (GB)

The four-digit numbers used in Diels' catalogue to identify manuscripts in the several libraries of Cambridge are not shelfmarks, but sequential numbers in *C.M.A.* 1697.

[Ashmol.] (Ashmolean)

[0182]   **[7751]**   I.5.

This is not a Greek copy of Hippocrates, *Prognosticon*, but rather a Latin one at Oxford, Bodleian Library, MS. Ashmole 1285 (Alexanderson 1963 does not mention it. See also, about the *Aphorismi* contained in the same codex, Kibre 1985: 44, and Magdelaine 1994 who does not mention it among the Greek codices).

The same information appears in Ackermann 1825: XLVII (without brackets).

Number 7751 comes from *C.M.A.* 1697: tome 1, part 1 (devoted to the libraries at Oxford and not Cambridge contrary to Ackermann and Diels), p. 341, in a catalogue of manuscripts collected by Elias Ashmole (1617-1692) and preserved in the *Bibliotheca Ashmoliana* (for the catalogue, see *C.M.A.* 1697: 1.1.315-357). These manuscripts were transferred from the Ashmolean Museum to the Bodleian Library in 1860 (Morgan 1973: 159). The manuscript referred to here is listed among the

"Medici Lat(ini)" (see *C.M.A.* 1697: 1.1.341) and described as follows (*ibid.*):

7751. Theophili Liber Urinarum, & pulsuum.

Liber Prognosticorum, &c. Hippocratis, 1285, 6. 8. 9.

Madan, Craster and Denholm-Young 1937: 1143.

Caius Coll. (Caius College), now Gonville and Caius College

In [0189]-[0195], numbers come from *C.M.A.* 1697, tome 1, part 3, pp. 114-115, in the catalogue of manuscripts of *Collegii Caio-Gonvillensis in Cantabrigia* (*ibid.*: 1.3.107-130).

Numbers [0189]-[0191] are included in a list of medical manuscripts (*C.M.A.* 1697: 1.3.114-115) donated to the College by John Kays, best known as Caius (1510-1573).

Numbers [0192]-[0194] are in a section (*C.M.A.* 1697: 1.3.115-116) entitled "Libri Latine Conscripti" (*ibid.*: 1.3.115).

A table of concordance between the numbers in *C.M.A.* 1697 and the current shelfmarks is in James 1907: xviii-xx.

The numbers from *C.M.A.* 1697 are used in Ackermann 1821 and 1825.

[0183]	**47**	I.68, 74, 91, 122.
		Now Gonville and Caius College Library, 47/24.
		Also [0189].
[0184]	**50**	I.4, 11, 12, 17, 18, 19, 20, 21, 22, 23 (2), 24 (2), 25, 26 (2), 27, 28, 29 (2), 33, 34 (2), 35 (2), 48 (2); II.93.
		Now Gonville and Caius College Library, 50/27.
[0185]	**76**	I.11, 29, 80; II.109.
		Now Gonville and Caius College Library, 76/43.
		Also [0191].
[0186]	**77**	II.11.
		Now Gonville and Caius College Library, 77/44.
[0187]	**355**	I.5, 12, 73, 79 (2), 111.
		Now Gonville and Caius College Library, 355/582.
		Also [0190].
[0188]	**360**	I.63, 65, 91.
		Now Gonville and Caius College Library, 360/587.
[0189]	**[946]**	I.68, 120.

This item is supposed to contain Galenus, *De usu partium corporis humani libri XVII* (I.68) and *De abortivo foetu* (I.120).

Information in Diels' catalogue reproduces data in Ackermann 1821 (where there are no brackets):

- XCV, no. 29 ctd., *De usu partium*;
- CLXXXVIII, *sub titulo*, and CCVI, *De abortivo foetu* (in both passages the text is attributed to Galen).

The information comes from *C.M.A.* 1697: 1.3.114, where the manuscript is described as follows:

946.2. Galeni de methodo sanandi lib. 14. Juxta titulum in hoc tamen volumine reperiuntur tantummodo quinque libri & pars Sexti Caeteri habentur in prox. Vol.

2. Idem de usu partium, opus imperfect. sumens initium à capite. 3.

3. De Hippocratis & Platonis dogmatibus lib. 4. imperf.

4. De Abortivo foetu tractatus imperf. L. 48.

This manuscript is Gonville and Caius College Library, 47/24 (= [0183]). It is made of four parts, each with its own page or folio numbering.

De usu partium (frg.) is contained in the second part (starting after p. 160; the first folio is numbered 0). Codex Gonville and Caius 47/24 appears in Diels' catalogue I.68 (with shelfmark 47) among the manuscripts containing *De usu partium* (= [0183]).

The text identified in *C. M. A.* 1697 as *De abortivo foetu* (without author's name and title) and attributed to Galen in subsequent literature (from Ackermann 1821 on; see also rencently Fichtner 2012: 84) can be read in the fourth part of Gonville and Caius 47/24, which is made of two folios at the end of the manuscript numbered 10 and 11 (following the third part, made of nine folios). This text in the present manuscript is recorded a second time in Diels' catalogue (I.122), but under the shelfmark "Caius College 47" (= [0183]) and another title:

De XII portis. Frgm. Inc. In porta XVII καὶ βλάβης εἶδον. Expl. in porta XIX ἰατροὶ τοῦ κόπτειν τὴν αἴεραν.

This text, which also appears in [0196] and [0486], is not a Galenic work, but a fragment of the *Efodia* made of three chapters (6.17, 18, and 19 [*partim*] in the version of *Vaticanus graecus* 300). In *C.M.A.* 1697 (followed by all the subsequent literature) it has been misidentified on the basis of the title of the first chapter (6.17: *On abortifacient and anticonceptional substances*), whereas the other two deal with placenta's elimination (6.18) and sciatica (6.19). In Diels, its identification as a fragment of the text known as *De XII portis* (and also as *De spermate* and *Zagonia* [Fichtner 2012: 115 no. 330]) is incorrect as is also the transcription of its *explicit* (... ἄκραν instead of αἴεραν in Diels).

The other two texts contained in the manuscript according to *C. M. A.* 1697 are listed in Diels' catalogue under "Gonville and Caius 47" (= [0183]) as follows:

- *De placitis Hippocrates et Platonis* (= part 3 of the manuscript). See Diels I.74;
- *Methodi medendi libri XIV* (= part 1 of the manuscript). See Diels I.91.

Same as [0183].

[0190]   **[948]**   I.111.

This copy of Galenus, *Definitiones medicae*, is Gonville and Caius College Library, 355/582 (= [0187].

This manuscript is listed by *C.M.A.* 1697: 1.3.114-115 (where the text referred to here is entitled *De terminis medicis*), followed by Ackermann 1821: CCVI (where there are no brackets).

[0191]   **[949]**   I.80.

This manuscript of Galenus, *De differentiis febrium libri II*, is Gonville and Caius College Library, 76/43.

It is listed in *C.M.A.* 1697: 1.3.115 (with the title *de differentia febricitantium lib 2*), and this entry is reproduced in Ackermann 1821: CCVI (where there are no brackets).

Same as [0185].

[0192]   **[954]**   I.5.

This is not a Greek, but rather a Latin copy of Hippocrates, *Prognosticon* (see Kibre 1985: 208; Alexanderson 1963 does not mention it).

James 1907: 51-52.

It is listed in *C.M.A.* 1697: 1.3.115, among the "Libri Latine Conscripti" of the Collegium Gaio-Gonvillense, and, further on, in Ackermann 1825: XLVII (without brackets).

Now Gonville and Caius College Library, 59/153.

[0193]   **[959]**   I.21.

This is a copy of Hippocrates, *De natura humana*. It is not in Greek, but in Latin (see Kibre 1985: 195).

James 1907: 94-96.

The manuscript appears in *C.M.A.* 1697: 1.3.115, among the "Libri Latine Conscripti" of the Collegium Gaio-Gonvillense, and again in Ackermann 1825: CXLVII (without brackets, however).

Now Gonville and Caius College Library, 95/47.

[0194]   **[962]**   I.12.

This manuscript listed as a copy of Hippocrates, *Aphorismi*, is not in Greek but in Latin (see Kibre 1985: 46; Magdelaine 1994 does not list it). It is Gonville and Caius College Library, 345/620.

James 1907: 388-390.

It appears in *C.M.A.* 1697: 1.3.115, among the "Libri Latine Conscripti" of the Collegium Caio-Gonvillense, and, further on, in Ackermann 1825: LXVI (who includes it [without brackets] among the Latin copies of the *Aphorismi*).

[0195]   **[1134]**   I.5.

This codex is referenced as a copy of Hippocrates, *Prognosticon*, at Gonville and Caius College in Cambridge.

Number 1134 appears in *C.M.A.* 1697: 1.3.124, in a list (1.3.120-129) included in the catalogue of Gonville and Caius College and entitled as follows (1.3.120):

Catalogus librorum MSS. ex Donatione Magistri More quondam Socii hujus Collegii.

This item contains 17 texts, none of which is medical.

The manuscript numbered 1134 probably referred to here appears in *C.M.A.* 1697, tome 1, part 2 (about Oxford, and not Cambridge), in a catalogue (1.2.31-38) entitled as follows (2.1.31):

Librorum Manuscriptorum Collegii Novi in Oxonia catalogus.

In the section *Libri Medicinae* (1.2.34-35), number 1134 reads as follows (1.2.35):

1134.170 Isagogoe Joannitti.

Philaretus de pulsuum negotio.

Tegni Galeni cum Commentario Haly.

Theophilus de Urinis.

Aphorismi Hippocratis, cum Commentario Galeni, Lat.

Prognostica Hippocratis, cum Commentario Galeni, Lat.

Regimen Acutorum Hippocratis, cum Commentario Galeni, Lat.

Aegidii versus de Urinis, cum Commentario Gilberti.

This item is codex 170 in the collection of New College at Oxford (= [0882]), and is a Latin manuscript (see Kibre 1985: 14 [*Acutorum regimen*], 56 [*Aphorismi*], 210 [*Prognostica*]; neither Alexanderson 1963 [*Prognosticon*], nor Magdelaine 1994 [*Aphorismi*] list it).

The same information (without brackets) appears in Ackermann 1825: XLVII, where the text contained in the manuscript is identified as follows:

Cum aphor. et Galeni comm. Latin.

Same as [0882].

[0196]   **[6605]**   I.120.

This is supposed to be a copy of Galenus, *De abortivo foetu* (on which see [0189]).

No number 6605 appears in the catalogue of Gonville and Caius College at Cambridge in *C.M.A.* 1697: 1.3.107-130. It appears, instead, in two other catalogues in *C.M.A.* 1697:

- a short catalogue in *C.M.A.* 1697: 1.1.301, with 20 manuscripts in the collections of the Bodleian Library. This catalogue is entitled as follows:

  Accedunt Annotationes viri summi Henrici Savilli in scriptores Mathematicos.

  Number 6605 contains Cl. Ptolemaei Geographia Gr. cum Notis.

- the second catalogue (*C.M.A.* 1697: 2.1.198-203) is entitled as follows (2.1.198):

  Librorum Manuscriptorum Caroli Theyeri Generosi in Comitatu Glocestriensi catalogus.

Number 6605 is described as follows (2.1.202):

Pantegni Constantini.

Anatomia Galeni, & de interioribus.

Megategni Galeni. Alkind. de gradibus.

Alfarabius de tempore.

Aristoteles de animalibus; de anima, &c.

Tract. de substantia orbis.

De terra & Elementis.

No mention of a treatise *De abortivo foetu* by Galenus is made.

These being the only two occurrences of number 6605 in *C.M.A.* 1697, this information cannot be explained. It appears in Ackermann 1821: CLXXXVIII, *sub titulo* (without brackets).

Information about the manuscripts numbered 6605 in *C.M.A.* 1697 has been incorrectly recorded in the scholarly literature. The codex 6605 listed in *C.M.A.* 1697: 2.1.202, appears in Ackermann 1821: CXXVI, no. 56, with an explicit and correct reference to "Cat. MSS. Angl.", but a mistaken mention of Galenus, *Methodi medendi*.

Cambridge University Library

–

Ee. 5. 7	Imagines plantarum ex Dioscorides, *De materia medica*.	
	Browne 1900: 307.	
Ff. 3. 30	See [0199].	
	Catalogue ULCambridge 1856-1867: 2.426-429.	
Gg. 1. 2	See [0200].	
	Catalogue ULCambridge 1856-1867: 3.8-14.	
Kk. 5. 7	See [0197].	
Ll. 4. 12	See [0201].	
	Catalogue ULCambridge 1856-1867: 4.61-66.	
Ll. 5. 4	See [0202].	
	Catalogue ULCambridge 1856-1867: 4.88-92.	
Mm. 1. 17	Index in Dioscoridis, *De materia medica*.	
	Catalogue ULCambridge 1856-1867: 4.109-110.	

Cantabr. (*Cantabrigenses* [Cambridge])

–

[0197]   **2049 (Kk V 7)** II.37.

This is a copy of Erotianus, *Vocum Hippocraticarum conlectio*.

Number 2049 is not a shelfmark but a sequential number in the *Catalogue ULCambridge* 1856-1867: 3.677.

Catalogue ULCambridge 1856-1867: 3.677.

Current shelfmark: Kk. 5. 7 (see p. 44).

[0198] **[2329]** I.5.

This is not a Greek, but rather a Latin copy of Hippocrates, *Prognosticon* (see Kibre 1985: 208, where this item is identified as 1738 [Ii.II.5]; Alexanderson 1963 does not mention it).

Number 2329 is not a shelfmark but a sequential number in *C.M.A.* 1697: 1.3.169, in a catalogue (*ibid.*: 1.3.164-171) entitled as follows (see 1.3.164):

Librorum manuscriptorum in Bibliotheca Publica celeberrimae Academiae Cantabrigiensis catalogus.

The contents of item 2329 is the following (*ibid.*: 1.3.169):

Prognosticon Hippocratis, cum Commentario Galeni

2. Thesaurus pauperum, editus a Petro Hispano.

3. Tacuyn, id est, regimen sanitatis, liber editus per Albuchasin. Hoc exemplar est imperfectum.

A manuscript of the *Prognosticon* with the same number, but without brackets, is quoted in Ackermann 1825: XLVII.

It is now Cambridge, University Library, Ii. 2. 5.

Cantabrig. Bibl. Univ. (*Cantabrigensis Bibliotheca Universitatis* [Cambridge University Library])

On all these manuscripts see p. 44.

–

[0199] **F. F. 3. 30** I.96, 118; II.9, 27.

Current shelfmark: Cambridge, University Library, Ff. 3. 30.

[0200] **Gg I 2** II.36.

Current shelfmark: Cambridge, University Library, Gg. 1. 2.

[0201] **L l IV 12** I.21, 25, 26, 37; II.39.

Current shelfmark: Cambridge, University Library, Ll. 4.12.

[0202] **L. L. 5, 4** I.11.

Current shelfmark: Cambridge, University Library, Ll. 5. 4 .

[Cath. Metens.] (*Cathedralis Metensis*)

–

[0203] **[226]** I.5.

This copy of Hippocrates, *Prognosticon*, referenced as a Greek manuscript in a collection at Cambridge, is actually a Latin manuscript once in the library of Metz Cathedral in France.

The same information as in Diels' catalogue (together with a reference to "Montf. II. p. 1380" [= Montfaucon 1739]) appears in Ackermann 1825: XLVII (without brackets):

in bibl. cathed. Metensi cum antiqua translatione et commento no. 226 secundum Montf. II. p. 1380.

The appellation *Cath. Metens.* (= *Cathedralis Metensis*) does not designate any cathedral at Cambridge. Instead, it designates the cathedral church in Metz (France), which had a collection of manuscripts until 1791. A catalogue of this collection is provided in Montfaucon 1739: 2.1376-1384.

Number 226 (which is not a shelfmark but a sequential number in Montfaucon) referred to here contains the following texts (*ibid.*: 2.1380) :

Hippocratis liber prognosticorum cum antiqua translatione & commento. Ejusdem Regimentum acutorum, cum commento Galieni, in pergameno 500. circiter ann.

On the basis of this information, it appears that this manuscript is also referred to in Ackermann 1821: CLXXXIV, no. 15 ctd., as follows:

... cum commento Galieni est in biblioth. cathedr. Metens. n. 226. Montf. II. p. 1380.

This is a Latin manuscript (see Kibre 1985: 56, where the shelfmark is accompanied by a * meaning "not examined"; Alexanderson 1963 [*Prognosticon*] does not mention this manuscript).

Further to the confiscation of the belongings of religious communities in the wake of French Revolution, the collection of Metz Cathedral library was transferred to the city library in Metz (now Bibliothèque-Médiathèque Pontiffroy). There, the present item was no. 174 (see *Catalogue général des manuscrits* 1879: 78, where its provenance is identified as "De la cathédrale de Metz").

This manuscript is listed in Diels I.6, among the copies of the Latin translation of Hippocrates, *Prognosticon*, with the specification "Comm. sup. Progn.", and also at I.15, among the copies of the Latin translation of Hippocrates, *Aphorismi*, with the specification "c. comm. Gal."

This manuscript was destroyed in 1944 during World War II (*Catalogue général des manuscrits* 1962: 7 for the fire of the collection, and 12 for this item).

Coll. St. Johann. (*Collegium Sancti Johannis* [St. John's College]), now St. John's College

–

[0204]   **A6**   II.70.

James 1913: 7-8.

Now St. John's College Library, MS A. 6.

Gonville and Caius College Library

47/24	See [0183] and [0189].	
	James 1907: 39-40.	
50/27	See [0184].	
	James 1907: 41-43.	
76/43	See [0185] and [0191].	
	James 1907: 73-75.	
77/44	See [0186].	
	James 1907: 75-76.	
355/582	See [0187] and [0190].	
	James 1908: 402-404.	
360/587	See [0188].	
	James 1908: 407-408.	

[**Pembroch.**] ([*Collegium*] *Pembrochianum* [Pembroke College]), now Pembroke College

–

[0205]

[2055]   I.5, 12.

This is not a Greek, but rather a Latin copy of Hippocrates, *Prognosticon* (I.5) and *Aphorismi* (I.12).

Number 2055 is not a shelfmark but a sequential number in *C.M.A.* 1697: 3.1.159, in the catalogue of manuscripts "in Aula Pembrochiana apud Cantabrigiam" (3.1.156-161), where the content of the manuscript is described as follows (1.3.159):

2055. 127. Comment. super Tegni secundum Galenum

2. Regimen acutorum, cum Comment.

3. Liber Aphorismorum, cum Comment.

4. Liber Prognosticorum, cum Comment.

This Latin manuscript is listed by Ackermann 1825: LXVI, among the Latin copies of the *Aphorismi*. See also Kibre 1985: 51 (*Aphorismi*), 203 and 208 (*Prognosticon*). Neither Alexanderson 1963 (*Prognosticon*) nor Magdelaine 1994 (*Aphorismi*) mention it. Similarly, Ackermann 1825: XCIX, lists it among the Latin manuscripts of *Regimen acutorum*, as does also Kibre 1985: 12. Nevertheless, Ackermann 1825: XLVII, mentions it among the Greek copies of *Prognosticon*. In no case, however, does Ackermann 1825 use brackets.

James 1905: XXXIII (table of concordance of *C.M.A.* 1697 and current shelfmark of this item) and 206-207 (description of the manuscript).

Now Pembroke College Library MS 228.

St. John's College Library

–

A. 6	See [0204].

[St. Petri] ([*Collegium*] *Sancti Petri* [St. Peter's College]), now Peterhouse

–

[0206]   **[1866]**   I.5, 12.

This manuscript of Hippocrates, *Prognosticon* (I.5) and *Aphorismi* (I.12), is in Latin.

Number 1866 is not a shelfmark, but rather a sequential number in the catalogue of manuscripts *Domus S. Petri apud Cantabrigiam* published in *C.M.A.* 1697: 1.3.147-155, where the present item is described as follows (*ibid.*: 1.3.153):

1866. 204. Aphorismi Hippocratis, cum commentario Galeni, interprete Constantino Aphricano Montis Cassinensis Monacho, medicinae perito.

2. Prognostica ejusdem, cum comment.

3. Liber de regimine acutorum, cum comment.

4. Tegni Galeni, cum comment. Haly.

This is not a Greek manuscript, but rather a Latin one. Ackermann 1825: XLVII (*Prognosticon*) and LXVI (*Aphorismi*), in both cases without brackets, lists it among the Latin copies of the works, and neither Alexanderson 1963 nor Magdelaine 1994 mention it (for the *Prognosticon* and the *Aphorismi*, respectively). See also Kibre 1985: 55 (*Aphorismi*), 208 (*Prognosticon*), and also 12 (*Regimen acutorum*).

James 1899: xii (table of concordance *C.M.A.* 1697 and James' catalogue) and 37-38 (for the present item).

Now Peterhouse Library Ms. 14.

Trinity Coll. (Trinity College)

–

[0207]   **1386**   II.109.

This is a copy of Ioannes Zacharias Actuarius, *De urinis*.

Number 1386 is not a shelfmark but a sequential number in James 1902: 398.

For a description of the manuscript, see James 1902: 398.

This manuscript is now Trinity College Library, O.8.11.

Trinity College Library

–

B.9.1   (ff. 20r et seq.) Gregorius Nyssenus, *De hominis opificio*.
James 1900: 257-259.

O.2.12   (no. III) Andromachus, *Carmen de antidotis*.
James 1902: 96-97.

O.8.11   See [0207].

Cambridge, Mass. (US)

Harvard University, Houghton Library

Ms. gr.

17/6   (ff. 144r-154r) Aristoteles, *Physiognomica*.
Kavrus-Hoffmann 2010: 211-222; *Aristoteles graecus* 1976: 110-117 (especially 113-114).

| 17/7 | (ff. 155r-173r) [Galenus], *De historia philosophica.* |
| | Kavrus-Hoffmann 2010: 211-222; *Aristoteles graecus* 1976: 110-117 (especially 114). |

Typ.

46	(ff. 1r-7r, 17r-40v, 45r-51v) Nemesius Emesenus, *De natura hominis.*
	Morani 1981: 60-61; Kavrus-Hoffmann 2011: 17-29.
222	Manuel Philes, *De animalium proprietate.*
	Kavrus-Hoffmann 2011: 46-52.

Carpentras (FR)

Bibl. Inguimbertine (Bibliothèque Inguimbertine [Inguimbertine Library]), now Bibliothèque municipale Inguimbertine (Municipal Inguimbertine Library)

–

[0208]   **nr. 1774**   I.115; II.73.

Catalogue général des manuscrits 1899: 205-214.

Current shelfmark: Ms 1774.

Also [0209].

17th-century collection of extracts on metrology from manuscripts of the *Bibliotheca Regia* (*Parisina*) and the *Bibliotheca Vaticana* (see [0209]).

[0209]   **nr. 1774**   II.3, 24, 36, 38, 61.

(P., V)   The letters **P.** and **V** that follow the shelfmark in Diels' catalogue as in the *Catalogue général des manuscrits* 1901: 205, do not pertain to the shelfmark of the manuscript but indicate its provenance and an old shelfmark: **P.** refers to Peiresc (that is, Nicolas-Claude Fabri de Peiresc [1580-1637]) and **V** is not the letter V but the Roman numeral digit 5. This manuscript comes from the collection of Peiresc (partially preserved at Carpendras library; see Lambert 1862: 2.XVII-XV, and *Catalogue général des manuscrits* 1901: XXVI-XXXIII). In the catalogue of Carpentras collection compiled by Charles-Godefroy-Alphonse Lambert (b. 1795) (3 volumes, 1862), the manuscript now with shelfmark 1774 is identified as number 5 in the Peiresc collection in Carpentras (Lambert 1862: 2.23-31; see *Catalogue général des manuscrits* 1901: LVIII, for a table of concordance between Lambert's identifier and the current shelfmark).

Same as [0208].

Castellorizo (Μεγίστη) (Καστελλόριζο) (GR)

–

[0210]   **nr. -**   I.123.

This item listed without library name and shelfmark is a copy of Galenus, *Iatrosofia.*

The only collection known to have been in the Greek island of Καστελλόριζο is that of the local teacher Achilleas L. Dimantaras (1852-1930).

His library and archives were given to the Γενικά Αρχεία του Κράτους (General State Archives of Greece) in Athens by his family (see Gkinis 1963: 113, and also Olivier 1995: no. 1646).

In the current state of research, this item cannot be located in the collections of the General State Archives of Greece in Athens. At any rate, from its description in Diels' catalogue, it seems to be a recent *iatrosofion* rather than a copy of an authentic Galenic treatise.

Chalke (Χάλκη) (former Ottoman Empire, now Heybeli Ada [TR])

Bibl. Mon. Theotokou (Βιβλιοθήκη Μονῆς Θεοτόκου [Library of the Theotokou Monastery], actually Μονή Παναγίας Καμαριωτίσσης [Monastery of the Panagia Kamariotissa])

The manuscripts of this library were transferred in 1936 to the Greek Orthodox Patriarchate in Istanbul

–

[0211]   **82**   I.41.

This manuscript is now in Istanbul, Οικουμενικό Πατριαρχείο Κωνσταντινουπόλεως, Πατριαρχική Βιβλιοθήκη, Μονή Παναγίας Καμαριωτίσσης, 82 (Ecumenical Patriarchate of Constantinople, Patriarchal Library, Monastery of the Panagia Kamariotissa) (see below, p. 90).

Cheltenham (GB)

Mediom. (*Mediomontani* [Middlehill])

–

[0212]   **1537**   II.20.

Phillipps Manuscripts 1837-1871: 18.

See [0133].

Phillipps. (Phillipps collection)

–

[0213]   **3084**   II.30.

Phillipps Manuscripts 1837-1871: 35.

Now New Haven, CT (USA), Yale University, Harvey Cushing/ John Hay Whitney Medical Library, Manuscript 31 vault (see p. 165).

[0214]   **3892**   II.63.

Phillipps Manuscripts 1837-1871: 53.

Now New Haven, CT (USA), Yale University, Harvey Cushing/John Hay Whitney Medical Library, Manuscript 33 vault (see p. 165).

[0215]   **4614**   I.64, 65, 71 (2), 76, 83, 84, 93.

Phillipps Manuscripts 1837-1871: 75.

Now New Haven, CT (USA), Yale University, Beinecke Rare Book and Manuscript Library, MS 1121 (see p. 165).

[0216]   **6665=6765**   I.96.

Phillipps Manuscripts 1837-1871: 99, no. 6665, described as follows among the "MSS. de ignoto":

6665 Simeon Sethus de Ciborum proprietate. ⁋ Galeni Synopsis. Graecé. 12*mo. V. S.* xiii.

See also *ibid.*: 101, no. 6765, described as follows in the section entitled "Supplement ad Bibl. Meerman. Codices MSS. Graeci.":

6765 298 Simeonis Sethi, Antiocheni, de Ciborum proprietatibus. ⁋ Anonymus in Galenum de Simplicibus. 18*mo. V.S.* xii. 172 *leaves.*

In spite of their differences, these two entries are about the same item (on the current location of which, see below), as the presence of the two numbers on f. Ir in the manuscript indicates.

Contrary to Petit 2010: 146, this manuscript is no longer at Cheltenham (see Touwaide 2009: 534).

It is now in Munich, Bayerische Staatsbibliothek, *Monacensis graecus* 633 (see p. 157).

Also [0218].

[0217]   **6763**   II.70 (2), 96.

Phillipps Manuscripts 1837-1871: 101.

Now New Haven, CT (USA), Yale University, Harvey Cushing/John Hay Whitney Medical Library, Manuscript 34 vault (see p. 165).

[0218]   **6774**   I.96.
          (ol. Meerm. 298)

According to Diels' catalogue, this manuscript contains Galenus, *De simplicium medicamentorum temperamentis et facultatibus.*

There is a mistake in Diels' catalogue and, probably on this basis, also in Petit 2010: 146. According to *Phillipps Manuscripts* 1837-1871: 101, the manuscript Phillipps 6774 contains *Bedae Martyrologium.* On the other hand, the manuscript Meerman 298 (*Bibliotheca Meermanniana* 1824: 4.47, *sub numero*) contains the following works:

Simeonis Sethi Protovestiarii, Antiocheni, de ciborum proprietatibus et virtute syntagma. – Anonymi synopsis in quaedam Galeni capita de simplicibus.

Manuscript Meerman 298 became Phillipps 6765, described as follows in *Phillipps Manuscripts* 1837-1871: 101, *sub numero*:

Simeonis Sethi, Antiocheni, de Ciborum proprietatibus. ⁋ Anonymus in Galenum de Simplicibus." (see above, [0216]).

Thus there is confusion between Phillipps 6774 and 6765, the latter of which is referred to here.

Same as [0216].

[0219]   **21975**   II.30, 31, 32, 34, 39 (2).

Phillipps Manuscripts 1837-1871: 408.

Now New York, NY (US), Morgan Library, MS M. 652 (see p. 166).

[0220]   **23007**   II.44.

Phillipps Manuscripts 1837-1871: 425, where this item is described as follows:

Hierocles in Carmen Pythagorae.

❡ Galeni Historia de Philosophis.

❡ Hermetis *vel* Mercuri Trismegisti opus Medico-Mathematicum *Graecè*. 8*vo. brn. cf. ch.* s. xv. *Ex Bibl.* Guilford.

In 1978 and 1979, the manuscript was offered for sale by Kraus in New York, NY (US) Since it was a composite volume, it was divided into three different codices:

• Kraus 1978: no. 16: text 2 above corresponding to item 2 below;

• Kraus 1979: 76, no. 63: text 1 above corresponding to item 1 below;

• Kraus 1979: 94, no. 81: text 3 above corresponding to item 3 below.

Its three parts are now:

• Pythagoras, *Carmen aureum*: until 2011, it was Amsterdam, Bibliotheca Philosophica Hermetica, BPH 107; it is now Paris, Chicago, and New York, Les Enluminures, TM 540;

• Galen, *De historia philosophica*: Provo, UT (US), Brigham Young University, Lee Library, L. Tom Perry Special Collections, Vault 091 G13 1475 (see below, p. 266);

• *Iatromathematica*: private collection in Paris (see below, p. 262).

[0221]   **24, 386**   I.89.

This manuscript is a copy of Galenus, *Synopsis librorum suorum sedecim de pulsibus*.

The catalogue of the Phillipps collection ends with number 23,837 (*Phillipps Manuscripts* 1837-1871: 436). The manuscript is not listed in Munby 1960.

Now Bethesda, MD (USA), National Library of Medicine, MS. 82 Census (see above, p. 34).

Chicago, IL (US)

> Newberry Library
>
> > Case
> >
> > > 103   Hippocrates, *Epistulae*.
> > >
> > > de Ricci and Wilson 1935: 543 (where the manuscript is identified as Ry. 9).
> > >
> > > The manuscript will be re-catalogued with a Greek MS shelfmark.

Città del Vaticano (Vatican City) (VA)

> Biblioteca Apostolica Vaticana (Vatican Apostolic Library)
>
> > Archivio di San Pietro (San Pietro Archive)
> >
> > > H 45   See [1443].
> >
> > *Barberiniani graeci*
> >
> > > 5   Capocci 1958: 6-7.
> > >
> > > See [1422].
> > >
> > > 11   Capocci 1958: 11-12.
> > >
> > > See [1423] and [1437].
> > >
> > > 17   Capocci 1958: 18-19.
> > >
> > > See [1424].
> > >
> > > 39   (ff. 85v-87r) *Lexicon botanicum*.
> > >
> > > Capocci 1958: 39-42.
> > >
> > > 49   Capocci 1958: 52-53.
> > >
> > > See [1425]. Also [1426].
> > >
> > > 80   Capocci 1958: 99-100.
> > >
> > > See [1428].
> > >
> > > 81   (ff. 114v-129r) Synesius Cyrenensis, *De insomniis*.
> > >
> > > Capocci 1958: 100-102.
> > >
> > > 91   Capocci 1958: 124-125.
> > >
> > > See [1429] and also [1439].
> > >
> > > 118   Capocci 1958: 163-164.
> > >
> > > See [1430].
> > >
> > > 127   See [1431] and [1438].
> > >
> > > 147   (ff. 1r-32r) Cassius iatrosophista, *Problemata*; (ff. 48r-161r) Galenus, *De remediis parabilibus*; (ff. 162r-188v) Galenus, *De motu musculorum*.
> > >
> > > Capocci 1958: 253-256.

152/III	See [1432].
212	(ff. 2v-3v) *De mensuris et ponderibus*; (ff. 3v-3ar) Diodorus, *De ponderibus et mensuris*.
	Mogenet 1989: 52.
213	(ff. 265v-275v) Nicephorus Blemmydes, *De corpore*.
	Mogenet 1989: 52-55.
220	(f. I) Hippocrates, *Aphorismi* (frg.).
	Mogenet 1989: 161 (for the text) and 161-165 (for the manuscript).
221	(ff. 1r-42v) Galenus, De *diebus decretoriis*; (ff. 47r-55r) Galenus, *Fragmenta varia*.
	Mogenet 1989: 65-67.
222	(ff. 7r-21v and 24r-25r) Dioscorides, *De materia medica*, recensio alphabetica (frg.).
	Mogenet 1989: 67-68.
237/IV	See [1433].
272	(ff. 6r-142v) Galenus, *In Hippocratis Aphorismos commentarii et Galeni in eos commentarii VII*; (ff. 142ar-144r) Hippocrates, *Prorrheticum*, I.
	Mogenet 1989: 116-117, 166.
278	(ff. 3v-4v) Rufus Ephesius, *De membrorum hominis appellationibus*.
	Mogenet 1989: 122-125.
289	(ff. 188v-192v) Aristoteles, *Physiognomonica*.
	de Ricci 1907: 102-103.
344	de Ricci 1907: 107; Alexopoulou 1998: 8-9.
	See [1434].
438	Epiphanius, *Physiologus*.
	de Ricci 1907: 114 (under the title "De natura animalium").
522	de Ricci 1907: 119-120.
	See [1435].
566	de Ricci 1907: 123.
	See [1436].

Chigiani graeci

For the shelfmarks of the Chigi manuscripts, see Canart and Peri 1970: 172, and, more recently D'Aiuto and Vian 2011: 1.408.

R.IV.11	Palimpsest (Canart 2004: 47, where the manuscript is identified as no. 11).
	Scriptio inferior: unidentified text.

Scriptio superior: (ff. 90v-104v) Epiphanius, *Physiologus.*

Franchi de' Cavalieri 1927: 12-15, no. 11.

R.IV.13   (ff. 1r-121v) Nemesius Emesenus, *De natura hominis.*

Franchi de' Cavalieri 1927: 21-22, no. 13.

R.IV.16   (ff. 57r et seq.) Gregorius Nazianzenus, *De humana natura.*

Franchi de' Cavalieri 1927: 23-25, no. 16; Domiter 1999: 22.

F.VII.159   *Ex Dioscuridis libro de materia medica, herbarum animaliumque figurae coloribus pictae.*

Franchi de' Cavalieri 1927: 104-106, no. 53.

Ottoboniani graeci, see **Rom, Bibl. Vaticana, Ottobon.** (see below, pp. 276-278).

Palatini graeci, see **Rom, Bibl. Vaticana, Palat.** (see below, pp. 278-281).

Palatinus latinus

24   (ff. 41-42) Palimpsest.

Scriptio superior: *Vetus testamentum.*

Scriptio inferior: *Formulae medicinarum.*

Fohlen 1979; Fohlen et al. 1982: 19n1; Harlfinger, Brunschön and Vasiloudi 2006: 146, 159-161.

On the manuscript, see Vattasso and Franchi de' Cavalieri 1902: 20-22; more recently, Fohlen et al. 1982: 19-26.

Reginenses graeci, see **Rom, Bibl. Vaticana, Reg. Suec.** (see below, p. 282).

Rossiani, see **Wien, Bibl. Colleg. S. J. Rossia** (= [1742]).

After their transfer to the Vatican Library in 1921, the *Rossiani* manuscripts have received new shelfmarks (table of concordance in Canart and Peri 1970: 322-323).

736   (ff. 153v-154r) Nemesius Emesenus, *De natura hominis* (frg.).

Van de Vorst 1906: 496-498, no. 10 (X. 116); Gollob 1910:17-29, no. 10 (Sign. X. 116).

927   (ff. 25 et seq.) *Geoponica.*

Van de Vorst 1906: 544, no. 36 (XI. 77).

982   Galenus, *De usu partium.*

Van de Vorst 1906: 548, no. 41 (XI. 132); Gollob 1908: 12-13, no. II. (Sign. XI. 132).

It was [1442].

See also *Rossianus* 1018 (below) and [1742].

986   (f. 381r et seq.) Astrampsychus, *Epistula ad Ptolomaeum regem.*

Van de Vorst 1906: 501-508, no. 16 (XI.136) .

1018

(ff. 3r-7v) Maximus Planudes, *De urinis*; (f. 7v) *Phlebotomia*; (ff. 7v-9v) Hippocrates, *De quattuor elementis et humoribus ex quibus homo fit*; (ff. 9v-11v) Hippocrates, *De quattuor elementis mundi*; (ff. 11v-13r) *De affectibus*; (ff. 12v-135v) Paul Nicaeus, *De cognitione et curatione variorum morborum*; (ff. 136r-156v) *Preparationes medicamentorum*.

Van de Vorst 1906: 547-548, no. 40 (XI. 167); Gollob 1908: 1-12, no. I. (Sign. XI. 167).

It was [1742] and has been confused with current manuscript *Rossianus* 982 (above) in Diels' catalogue.

Urbinates graeci, see **Rom, Bibl. Vaticana, Urbin.** (see below, pp. 282-284).

Vaticani graeci, see **Rom, Bibl. Vaticana, Vatic.** (see below, pp. 284-307).

Vaticani latini, see **Rom, Bibl. Vaticana, Vatic. lat.** (see below, p. 307)

[Corbie] (FR)

[Bibl. S. Petri Corbeiens.] (*Bibliotheca Sancti Petri Corbeiensis* [Library of St. Peter at Corbie])

–

[0222]

[Montf. p. 1407]   I.148.

This is supposed to be a copy of Galenus, *Excerpta varia* in the collection of a "Bibl. S. Petri Corbeiens[is]" not better identified in Diels' catalogue.

Reference is to Montfaucon 1739: 2.1407, in the catalogue of manuscripts "in Bibliotheca Monasterii Sancti Petri Corbeiensis" (*ibid.*: 2.1406-1408), that is the library of the Benedictine monastery of St. Peter at Corbie. The manuscript appears among *Philosophi & Medici* and is described as follows (2.1407):

Collectiones ex Galeno Fratris Joan. Ordinis Minorum, cod. memb. saec. 15.

The information in Diels' catalogue comes from Ackermann 1821: CLXXXVIII, where the following can be read (without brackets):

Collectiones ex Galeno fratr. Joann. ordin. minor. exstant in bibl. S. Petri Corbeiensis. Montfautc. p. 1407.

With the French Revolution, the library of Corbie Monastery was closed and its manuscripts were transferred to Amiens sometimes during the year 1791 (Delisle 1861: 320-322). They are now among the holdings of the Bibliothèque of Amiens (now identified as "Bibliothèques d'Amiens Métropole").

The item referred to in Diels' catalogue seems to be the current manuscript Amiens, 303 C coming from Corbie (see f. 1r for the note of provenance "Monasterii Sti Petri Corbeiensis"). Its content has been incorrectly identified by Montfaucon and in the subsequent literature. It is not by Galen, but by *Iohannes Galenus* as an addition on f. 1r indicates:

Incipit communeloquium (add man. rec.: compilatum a fratre Johanne Galeno ordinis fratrum minorum)

It is not a copy of any ancient Greek or Byzantine medical work, but the *Communiloquium Margarita doctorum sive Summa collationum ad omne genus hominum sive Summa de regimine vitae humanae* by John of Wales (Iohannes Guallensis [ca. 1220; fl. 1257-1285; d. 1285]). The work is known through several manuscripts and was published in an incunabulum edition as early as 1472 (on John of Wales, see Waddingus 1650: 209-211, and, more recently, Glorieux 1933-1934: 2, no. 332a, and Sharpe 1997: 338).

On manuscript Amiens 303 C, see Garnier 1843: 236-237; *Catalogue général des manuscrits* 1893: 142-145.

Darmstadt (DE)

Hessische Landes- und Hochschulbibliothek (State and University Library of Hesse)

Misc. gr.

2773   (f. 216r) Pseudo-Dioscorides, *Praecepta salubria*.

Denig 1899: 21-22; Voltz and Crönert 1897: 553; *Aristoteles graecus* 1976: 122-124.

Δημητσάνα (Dimitsana) (GR)

Δημόσια Ιστορική Βιβλιοθήκη και Μουσείο της Ελληνικής Σχολής Δημητσάνας (Public Historical Library and Museum of the Hellenic School of Dimitsana)

-

12   ff. 153r et seq.) Hippocrates, *Aphorismi*.

Gritsopoulos 1952: 193-196; Karas 1994: 38.

16th/18th-century copy.

Dresden (DE)

Königl. Bibl. (Königliche Bibliothek [Royal Library]), now Sächsische Landesbibliothek–Staats- und Universitätsbibliothek Dresden (Saxe State Library–Dresden State and University Library)

This collection has been heavily damaged during World War II. For the current state of its holdings, see the 1979 reprint of Schnorr von Carolsfeld 1882, with handwritten notes about the state of preservation of each item (see [0225] and [0227]). Furthermore, the volumes that were brought from Moscow to Dresden by Christian Friedrich Matthaei (1744-1811) were returned to Moscow in 1947 (see [0223] and [0224]).

-

[0223]   **Da 1**   I.61, 100.

Schnorr von Carolsfeld 1882 (1979): 282.

This item is a part (41 ff.) of manuscript Москва (Moskva), Государственный Исторический Музей (ГИМ), Синодальная Библиотека Московского Патриархата (Gosudarstvennyi Istoricheskii Muzei (GIM), Sinodal'naia

Biblioteka Moskovskoi Patriarkhii [State Historical Museum [GIM], Synodal Library of Moscow Patriarchate]), Sinod. 51 (464 Vlad.) (= [0731]; see also [0722] and [0723], and possibly [0720]), which was brought to Dresden by Christian Friedrich Matthaei (von Gebhardt 1898: 537) and sold by him to Dresden Library (Ebert 1822: 241).

In 1947 this manuscript was returned to Russia and is now Москва (Moskva), Российский Государственный Архив Древних Актов (РГАДА) (Rossiiskii Gosudarsdarstvennyi Arkhiv Drevnikh Aktov [RGADA], Russian State Archive of Ancient Documents [RGADA]), Фонд (Fond.) 1607, Dresden Da 01 (see below, p. 150).

According to Boudon 2002: 198n110, the location of this manuscript is unknown, whereas Petit 2009: LXXXIII, identifies it as a *Dresdensis*, but remains imprecise about its location.

[0224]   **D a 5**   II.64, 73, 78, 108, 109, 110, 111; N.69.

Schnorr von Carolsfeld 1882 (1979): 283-284.

This item might be a part of the current Москва (Moskva), Государственный Исторический Музей (ГИМ), Синодальная Библиотека Московского Патриархата (Gosudarstvennyi Istoricheskii Muzei (GIM), Sinodal'naia Biblioteka Moskovskoi Patriarkhii [State Historical Museum [GIM], Synodal Library of Moscow Patriarchate]), Sinod. 187 (= [0737]). It had probably been brought from Moscow (Synodal Library) to Dresden by Christian Friedrich Matthaei (von Gebhardt 1898: 537-538) and sold by him to Dresden Library (Ebert 1822: 242).

In 1947 it was returned to Russia and it is now Москва (Moskva), Российский Государственный Архив Древних Актов (РГАДА) (Rossiiskii Gosudarsdarstvennyi Arkhiv Drevnikh Aktov [RGADA], Russian State Archive of Ancient Documents [RGADA]), Фонд (Fond.) 1607, Dresden Da 05 (see below, p. 150).

[0225]   **Da 57**   II.67.

Schnorr von Carolsfeld 1882 (1979): 297-298.

Current shelfmark: Da. 57.

According to the 1979 reprint of Schnorr von Carolsfeld, *ibid.*, this volume is seriously damaged and its text cannot be read.

[0226]   **Da 58**   II.67.

Schnorr von Carolsfeld 1882 (1979): 298.

According to von Gebhardt 1898: 554, this item of only 5 folios might be a quire from the current manuscript Москва (Moskva), Государственный Исторический Музей (ГИМ), Синодальная Библиотека Московского Патриархата (Gosudarstvennyi Istoricheskii Muzei (GIM), Sinodal'naia Biblioteka Moskovskoi Patriarkhii [State Historical Museum [GIM], Synodal Library of Moscow Patriarchate]), Sinod. 316 (= 459 in Vladimir 1894: 695-697) (see below, p. 149).

Current shelfmark: Da 58.

[0227]   **Da 67**   II.108.

Schnorr von Carolsfeld 1882 (1979): 299.

Printed edition of Iohannes Zacharias Actuarius, *De spiritu animali libri II*, by Johann Friedrich Fischer (1626-1799) (Leipzig: J. F. Langenhemii, 1774), with a collation of the manuscript Da. 5 (= [0224]) by Christian Friedrich Matthaei (1744-1811).

According to the 1979 reprint of Schnorr von Carolsfeld, *ibid.*, this item is no longer present among the holdings of Dresden Library as a consequence of World War II.

[0228]   **Ed. Aldine**   II.114.

This item listed in the *Addenda* is a copy of the 1525 Aldine edition of Galenus, *Opera omnia*.

The *Addenda* specify that this copy is "... conspicuum, quod et in textu ipso nonnulla atramento sunt correcta et in margine librorum plurimorum adnotantur argumenta brevia, versiones latinae, variae denique lectiones haud paucae".

Ilberg 1889.

[Dublin] (IE)

[Bibl. Narcissi] (*Bibliotheca Narcissi* [Narcissus Library]), now Marsh Library

Numbers are not shelfmarks, but sequential numbers in *C.M.A.* 1697. Items [0229] and [0230] were in the collection of Narcissus Marsh (1638-1713).

–

[0229]   **[1218]**   I.148.

This manuscript is referenced as a Greek copy of Galenus, *Excerpta*.

Number 1218 appears in the catalogue of manuscripts of Narcissus March (*C.M.A.* 1697: 2.2.52-56) among the "Libri MSS Arabi" (2.2.53) and is described as follows (2.2.55):

1218.22. Fragmenta medica ex Galeno & Hippocrate, 4t°.

It is an Arabic ms., now Oxford, Bodleian Library, MS. Marsh 158.

Savage-Smith 2011: 186-188 (entry 48B).

[0230]   **[1709]**   I.42.

This is supposedly a copy of Hippocrates, *De methodo medendi libri VI* in Greek.

The same information appears in Ackermann 1825: CLXXVII, *sub titulo Methodus curandi Hippocratica* (without brackets).

Number 1709 appears in the same catalogue as [0229] where it is described as follows (2.2.61):

1709.34. Methodus curandi Hippocratis; item Commentarii Hunein Ibn Ishak in Anatomem Galeni. Arab.

It is an Arabic ms., now Oxford, Bodleian Library, MS. Marsh 379.

Savage-Smith 2011: 331-334 (entry 75), 371-373 (entry 85), 401-405 (entry 99).

[0231]   **[cod. Brit. 502]**   I.10, 19.

This manuscript is a copy of Hippocrates, *De morbis popularibus I et III* (I.10) and *De morbis popularibus II, IV-VII* (I.19).

Same as [0232].

[Coll. Trinit.] (*Collegium* [*Sanctae*] *Trinitatis* [Trinity College])

–

[0232]   **[502]**   I.5, 12.

This manuscript is listed among the copies of Hippocrates, *Prognosticon* (I.5) and *Aphorismi* (I.12).

The same information appears in Ackermann 1825: XLVII (among the "CODICES MSS." without precision of the language), and LXV (in the section "*Latini* exstant"), respectively (without brackets, however).

Number 502 appears in the catalogue of manuscripts "Collegi Sanctae Trinitatis apud Dublinum" in *C.M.A.* 1697: 2.2.16-48. It is a Latin manuscript containing 17 works including the following medical ones (*ibid.*: 2.2.34):

502.362. Hippocratis, Aphorismi, f. 1.

2. Prognostica Hippocratis, 12.

3. Liber Hippocratis de regimine acutorum, 19.

4. Liber Epidemiorum Hippocratis, 29.

5. Ejusdem Astronomia de infirmitatibus, 37.

6. Isagoge Jo. ad Tegni Galeni, 43.

7. Secreta Hippocratis, 53.

This manuscript is listed among the Latin copies of the *Aphorismi* in Ackermann 1825: LXV (without brackets). Neither Alexanderson 1963 nor Magdelaine 1994 mention it. See Kibre 1985: 13 (*Regimine acutorum*), based on Diels.

Abbott 1900: 62-63.

Now Trinity College Library Dublin, TCD MS 403.

Also [0231].

Edinburgh (GB)

University Library

–

230   Cassianus Bassus, *Geoponica*.

Borland 1916: 323.

Edschmiadzin (AM)

–

–

[0233]   nr. ?   II.30.

This manuscript listed without any element of identification (library, collection and shelfmark) under the name of Armenia's Etchmiadzin Cathedral (Էջմիածնի Մայր Տաճար [Ējmiatsni Mayr Tačar]) in Vagharshapat (in the Armavir Province of Armenia) is a copy of Dioscorides, *De materia medica*.

It is now Երևան (Yerevan) (AM), Մատենադարան. Մ. Մաշտոցի անվան հին ձեռագրերի գիտահետազոտական ինստիտուտ (Matenadaran. M. Maštoc'i anvan hin jeřagreri gitahetazotakan institut [Matenadaran. Mesrop Mashtots Institute of Ancient Manuscripts]), M 141 (see p. 372).

Ελασσόνα (Elassona) (GR)

Ιερά Μονή Παναγίας Ολυμπιώτισσας (Monastery of Panagia Olympiotissa)

–

189   (f. 33r) *De hominis aetatibus*; (ff. 115v et seq.) *De foetus formatione*; (ff. 133v et seq.) *De elementis et sanitatis conservatione*; (ff. 139r et seq.) *De phlebotomia*.

Skouvaras 1967: 369-371.

Erlangen (DE)

Universitätsbibliothek (University Library), now Universitätsbibliothek Erlangen-Nürnberg (University Library of Erlangen-Nuremberg)

–

[0234]   **Bibl. Univ. 89** II.44, 45; N.53 (4).

Current shelfmark: Ms. A 4.

[0235]   **90**   I.12; II.7, 104.

Current shelfmark: Ms. A 3.

Universitätsbibliothek Erlangen-Nürnberg (University Library of Erlangen-Nuremberg)

Handschriften Abteilung (Department of Manuscripts)

Ms. A 3   Thurn 1980: 22-24.

See [0235].

Ms. A 4   Thurn 1980: 24-28.

See [0234].

Escurial (San Lorenzo de El Escorial) (ES)

Scorial. (*Scorialenses*)

[0236]   **Puschm. I p. 90**   II.12.

This is a manuscript of Alexander Trallianus, *Therapeutica*.

The reference is to Puschmann 1878-1879: 1.90, where a manuscript of the Escorial is mentioned with no element of identification other than a reference to "Miller (Catal. des MSS. grecs de l'Escurial, pag. 140)" (= Miller 1848).

On this basis this manuscript can be identified as Φ. I. 2.

Same as [0263].

[0237]   **III 14**   II.20.

This manuscript is mentioned in reference to codex Oxford Baroccian. 88 (= [0817]) containing Athenaeus, *Synopsis de urinis*. It is Escorial T. II. 14.

Supplementary information in Diels' catalogue provides a list of manuscripts (including the Escorial item) and a reference to "Daremberg Not. et Extr. I 17."

In Daremberg 1853: 17, we find the same list of manuscripts as in Diels' catalogue for this specific entry. The Escorial manuscript mentioned in Daremberg is "T, III, 14 [*sic*], f. 197" (instead of III 14 in Diels' catalogue), with a reference to "Catal. des mss. de l'Escurial, par M. Miller, p. 130" (= Miller 1848).

In Miller 1848: 130, an anonymous *Synopsis de urinis* is listed as being on f. 197r of a manuscript that is not T. III. 14 as in Daremberg, but T. II. 14.

There is a series of mistakes: III 14 in Diels' catalogue is a mistake for T. III. 14 in Daremberg 1853, and T. III. 14 in Daremberg, in turn, is a mistake for T. II. 14, as the reference to Miller 1848: 130 reveals.

The text contained at ff. 192r-198r is not Athenaeus, *Synopsis de urinis* as stated in Diels' catalogue, but the *Synopsis* edited by Ideler 1841-1842: 2.305-306 (see Revilla 1936: 487-495).

Same as [0251].

[0238]   **III. R. 3**   I.73, 132; II.13, 30, 32.

          See R.III.3 (below).

[0239]   **C. II.11**   I.96.

          Mistake (typo [?]) for Σ.II.11 (= [0247]).

[0240]   **C.III.17**   I.96.

          Mistake (typo [?]) for Σ.III.17 (= [0248]).

[0241]   **R.I.12**   II.5, 77, 78, 79.

          Revilla 1936: 17-21.

          R.III.3   See [0238].

          Revilla 1936: 150-159.

	R.III.22	(ff. 21r-165r) Nicephorus Gregoras, *Scholia in Synesii de insomniis.*
		Revilla 1936: 197-199.
[0242]	**Σ.I.12**	I.81; II.50, 89.
		Revilla 1936: 252-256.
[0243]	**Σ.I.17**	II.30, 31, 32, 38, 39 (3).
		Revilla 1936: 268-271.
[0244]	**Σ.II.3**	I.69.
		Revilla 1936: 284-293.
[0245]	**Σ.II.5**	I.17, 79 (2), 102.
		Revilla 1936: 294-299.
[0246]	**Σ.II.10**	I.97.
		Revilla 1936: 312-316.
[0247]	**Σ.II.11**	I.100, 103.
		Revilla 1936: 316-318.
		Also [0239].
	Σ.III.1	(ff. 202r-203r) Nemesius Emesenus, *De natura hominis* (frg.).
		Revilla 1936: 337-342; Morani 1981: 62.
	Σ.III.3	(ff. 1r-18r) Nicander, *Theriaca*; (ff. 18r-29r) Nicander, *Alexipharmaca.*
		Revilla 1936: 343-346.
[0248]	**Σ.III.17**	I.100, 111, 117, 127; II.5, 7, 67, 105.
		Revilla 1936: 376-383.
		Also [0240].
[0249]	**T.II.12**	I.44; II.30.
		Revilla 1936: 483.
	T.II.13	(ff. 85v-89v) Aristoteles, *De insomniis.*
		Revilla 1936: 484-487; *Aristoteles graecus* 1976: 161-162.
[0250]	**T.II 14**	II.47.
		Same as [0251].
[0251]	**T.II.14**	I.26; II.5, 53, 75, 97-98, 109.
		Revilla 1936: 487-495.
		Also [0237] and [0250].
[0252]	**T.III.7**	I.67 (3), 69, 108.
		Revilla 1936: 518-519.

[0253]	**Υ.I.9**	II.9.
		de Andrés 1965: 89-92.
	Υ.III.5	(ff. 13r-275r) *Efodia*; (f. 275r) *De urinis*; (ff. 275v-284v) Johannes Damascenus, *De purgantibus*.
		de Andrés 1965: 150-151.
[0254]	**Υ.III.10**	I.47.
		de Andrés 1965: 155-157.
[0255]	**Υ.III.14**	I.114, 127; II.28, 42, 53, 59, 77, 78, 102 (2), 110.
		de Andrés 1965: 161-164; *CMAG* V (Zuretti and Severyns) 1928:3-4.
[0256]	**Υ III 17**	I.5.
		Same as [0257].
[0257]	**Υ.III.17**	I.104, 107; II.24.
		de Andrés 1965: 167-169.
		Also [0256] and [0277].
[0258]	**y.I.8**	I.12, 17, 18; II.17 (2), 18 (2), 76, 104.
		de Andrés 1965: 185-186.
		In Baffioni 1963, this manuscript is incorrectly identified as Y.I.8.
[0259]	**y.I.9**	II.37, 71.
		de Andrés 1965: 186-187.
[0260]	**y.I.15**	II.62, 63.
		de Andrés 1965: 192-193.
	y.III.9	(ff. 214r-216v) *Lexicon botanicum*.
		de Andrés 1965: 227-229; Touwaide 1999: 217, 228.
[0261]	**y.III.16**	I.32.
		de Andrés 1965: 237-239.
[0262]	**y.III.18**	II.95.
		de Andrés 1965: 240-241; *CMAG* V (Zuretti and Severyns) 1928: 39-42, 96-99.
[0263]	**Φ.I.2**	II.4, 8, 11, 12, 71, 77, 89 (2).
		de Andrés 1965: 2-4.
		Also [0236].
[0264]	**Φ.I.6**	II.5.
		de Andrés 1965: 9.
[0265]	**Φ.I.10**	I.151; II.27, 34, 62.
		de Andrés 1965: 15-17.

[0266]	**Φ.I.11**	II.24, 95.
		de Andrés 1965: 18; *CMAG* V (Zuretti and Severyns) 1928: 4-39; 96-99.
	Φ.II.14	(f. 1r) Astrampsychus, *Epistula ad Ptolomaeum regem.*
		de Andrés 1965: 41-42.
[0267]	**Φ.II.15**	II.5.
		de Andrés 1965: 42-43.
[0268]	**Φ.III.7**	I.5, 12, 104, 107; II.33, 57.
		de Andrés 1965: 56-57; *CMAG* V (Zuretti and Severyns) 1928: 42-44.
[0269]	**Φ III 11**	I.73.
		Same as [0270].
[0270]	**Φ.III.11**	I.43, 78 (2), 79 (2), 82, 93, 96, 100, 113; II.40, 102.
		de Andrés 1965: 60-64.
		Also [0269].
[0271]	**Φ.III.12**	I.5, 12, 22, 44, 127; II.77, 78, 108, 109, 110 (2), 111.
		de Andrés 1965: 64-66.
	Φ.III.15	(ff. 293r-306v) Iohannes Argyropoulos, *Responsa ad quaestiones.*
		de Andrés 1965: 68-71.
[0272]	**X.I.11**	II.9, 67.
		de Andrés 1965: 250-251.
[0273]	**X.II.2**	II.36.
		de Andrés 1965: 263-265.
	X.II.4	*Efodia.*
		de Andrés 1965: 266-268.
[0274]	**X.II.9**	II.67.
		de Andrés 1965: 274.
	X.III.10	(in tegumento anteriori) Thessalus, *De morbis* (frg.).
		de Andrés 1965: 311-313.
	X.IV.6	Palimpsest (Pérez Martin 2008).
		Scriptio inferior:

- (ff. 84-99, passim) unidentified text;
- (ff. 84-91, passim; 107-121, passim) Homiliarium;
- (ff. 99b-106) unidentified text;
- (ff. 107-121, passim; 127-134) Hymni liturgici;
- (ff. 122-136) Musica.

Scriptio superior:

- (ff. 76r-101v et 101v-113r) *Duae collectiones medicae*;
- (ff. 113r-132v, 134r-v, 133r-v) *Excerpta ex Dioscuride et aliis medicis iuxta alphabetum.*

de Andrés 1965: 329-331.

[0275]	**Ψ.I.13**	II.24, 95.

de Andrés 1967: 18-19; *CMAG* V (Zuretti and Severyns) 1928: 44-60.

Ψ.II.12 (ff. 74r-126v) Gregorius Nyssenus, *De hominis opificio*.

de Andrés 1967: 36-39.

Ψ.II.17 (ff. 40v-43r) Aetius Amidenus, *De astrorum signis*.

de Andrés 1967: 43-44 (on the manuscript, but without mention of the text here); *CCAG* XI.2 (Zuretti) 1934: 27-35.

Ψ.II.18 (ff. 72v-118v) Gregorius Nyssenus, *De hominis opificio*.

de Andrés 1967: 45.

Ψ.III.5 (ff. 126v-215r) Gregorius Nyssenus, *De hominis opificio*.

de Andrés 1967: 59-60.

[0276] **Ψ.III.7** II.39.

de Andrés 1967: 62-64.

[0277] **Ψ.III.17** I.12.

Mistake (typo [?]) for Y III 17 (= [0257]).

[0278] **Ψ.IV.14** II.5.

de Andrés 1967: 99-100.

Ψ.IV.27 (ff. 24r-82ᵃv) Symeon Seth, *De alimentorum facultatibus*.

de Andrés 1967: 115-116.

[0279] **Ω.I.8** II.3, 5, 13, 20, 34, 77.

de Andrés 1967: 126-128.

Ω.III.3 (ff. 76v-146v) Gregorius Nyssenus, *De hominis opificio*.

de Andrés 1967: 176-178.

Ω.IV.7 (ff. 1r-98r) Gregorius Nyssenus, *De hominis opificio*.

de Andrés 1967: 212-213.

Ferrara (IT)

Biblioteca comunale Ariostea (Ariostea Municipal Library)

Classe II

117 (ff. 4v-79v) Meletius, *De hominis natura*; (ff. 145r-155r) Theophanes [Chrysobalantes], *De victus ratione*.

Mioni 1965: 1.99-100.

Firenze (Florence) (IT)

    See **Florenz** (below).

    Biblioteca Medicea Laurenziana (Medicea Laurenziana Library)

        See **Bibl. Mediceo Laurentiana** (below).

        Antinori

           101   See [0372].

                        Rostagno and Festa 1893: 213-218; *CCAG* I (Olivieri) 1898: 74.

        Ashburnhamiani

           1639   Synesius Cyrenensis, *De insomniis*.

                        Rostagno and Festa 1893: 209.

        Conventi soppressi

           See **Conv. soppr.** (below).

        plutei

           See **Laurent.** (see below, pp. 68-80).

    Biblioteca Nazionale

    Magliabechiani

        1   See [0374] and [0375].

        44   See [0376].

    Biblioteca Riccardiana

        See **Bibl. Riccardiana.** (see below, pp. 80-81).

Florenz (Firenze) (IT)

    Bibl. Marucell. (Biblioteca Marucelliana [Marucelliana Library])

        –

[0280]   **A 109**   I.18.

                        Copy of Hippocrates, *Lex*, by Anton Maria Salvini (1653-1729).

                        Vitelli 1894: 561.

    Bibl. Mediceo Laurentiana (*Bibliotheca Mediceo Laurentiana*) now Biblioteca Medicea Laurenziana [Medicea Laurenziana Library])

        Conv. soppr. (Conventi soppressi [Suppressed Convents])

[0281]   **59**   II.30.

                        Rostagno and Festa 1893: 145-146.

        85   (ff. 78r et seq.) Basilius Caesariensis, *De hominis opificio*.

                        Rostagno and Festa 1893: 149.

[0282]   **153**   I.37.

                        Rostagno and Festa 1893: 161.

[0283]   **163**   I.120.

Rostagno and Festa 1893: 164.

[0284]   **627 (Abb. 2728)**   II.94.

The abbreviation **Abb.** is a mistake for AF in the old shelfmark AF 2728 (Rostagno and Festa 1893: 172).

Rostagno and Festa 1893: 172-76.

Laurent. (*Laurentiani*)

[0285]   –   II.73.

This is a reference to one or more Oribasius manuscripts containing *Praecepta salubria* (frg.).

Although this text does not seem to appear in any Florentine manuscript under Oribasius' name, it can be found in the following three codices:

- plut. 57.50 (= [0301]) (f. 577v) under the title ὑγιεινὰ παραγγέλματα σύντομα (Bandini 1764-1770: 2.432);
- plut. 59.17 (= [0305]) (f. 74r) under the title περὶ διαίτης (Bandini 1764-1770: 2.533);
- plut. 87.16 (= [0371]) (f. 14r) under the title ὑγιεινὰ παραγγέλματα σύντομα (Bandini 1764-1770: 3.397).

These three manuscripts are listed in Diels' catalogue (II.20) under Asclepiades, *Praecepta salubria* (= [0301], [0305], and [0371], respectively). The present item duplicates one or more of these numbers.

[0286]   **[ap. Bandini III 122]**   I.117.

This is a copy of a Pseudo-Galenic treatise entitled, *De sero lactis*.

Reference is to Bandini 1764-1770: 3.121-122 (and not 122 only as listed in Diels) about plut. 74.19 (= [0332]). The text is listed at § XI, where it is attributed to Johannes Damascenus and entitled *De sero lactis et eius facultate*.

The same information (including the incorrect page number) appears in Ackermann 1821: CLXXXVI, chapter XIV, *sub titulo* (without brackets).

[0287]   **plut. 4, 10**   II.94.

Bandini 1764-1770: 1.530-532.

plut. 4.18   (ff. 111v et seq.) Basilius Caesariensis, *De hominis opificio*; (ff. 137r et seq.) Gregorius Nyssenus, *De hominis opificio*.

Bandini 1764-1770: 1.541-542.

plut. 4.27   (ff. 186v et seq.) Gregorius Nyssenus, *De hominis opificio*.

Bandini 1764-1770: 1.550-551.

plut. 5.18   Palimpsest.

Scriptio superior: Psalterium.

Scriptio inferior: Hippocrates, *Prognosticum*.

Harlfinger, Brunschön and Vasiloudi 2006: 145, 164.

On the manuscript, see Bandini 1764-1770: 1.41.

[0288]   **plut. 7, 2**   II.67.

Bandini 1764-1770: 1.198-202.

plut. 7.4   (ff. 1 et seq.) Gregorius Nyssenus, *De hominis opificio*.

Bandini 1764-1770: 1.203-205.

plut. 7.10   (ff. 85v et seq.) Gregorius Nazianzenus, *De humana natura*.

Bandini 1764-1770: 1.216-240; Mossay and Coulie 1998: 120-121; Domiter 1999: 21.

plut. 7.15   *Variae sententiarum collectiones ex medicis antiquis inter quos* (f. 91v) Galenus; (f. 209v) Metrodora; (ff. 131v, 139v, 150r, 151r, 169v, 178r, 182r, 196v, 210v, 240r, 242v) Moschion.

Bandini 1764-1770: 1.252-254.

plut. 7.18   (ff. 210r et seq.) Gregorius Nazianzenus, *De humana natura*.

Bandini 1764-1770: 1.257-261; Domiter 1999: 21.

plut. 7.19   (ff. 75r-115r) Symeon Seth, *De alimentorum facultatibus*; (ff. 137v-201v) *De morbis et eorum cura* (forse eodem Setho); (ff. 202r-221v) *Medicamina composta a variis medicis secundum rationem xenonis*; (ff. 222r-224r) Diocles, *Ad Antigonum regem epistula de tuenda valetudine*; (ff. 224v-225v) Galenus, *De ponderibus et mensuris*; (f. 226r) *Remedia*; (f. 226v) *Prognosticum de aegroto*; (f. 226v) *De infirmo non negligendo*; (ff. 226v-227r) *Unguentum Zoes reginae*; (ff. 230r-231v) *De moderamine gravidae et embyronis*; (f. 239r) *Compendium de urinis*; (ff. 239r-242r) *Formulae medicinarum*; (ff. 242r-266v) *Hiera Galeni*; (ff. 267r-268v) Galenus, *De succedaneis*.

Bandini 1764-1770: 1.262-266.

Also [0300].

[0289]   **plut. 7, 35**   II.67.

Bandini 1764-1770: 1.295-298.

plut. 10.12   (ff. 121r et seq.) Gregorius Nyssenus, *De hominis opificio*.

Bandini 1764-1770: 1.482.

plut. 10.21   (ff. 150r et seq.) Nicephorus Gregoras, *Scholia in Synesii de insomniis*.

Bandini 1764-1770: 1.488-489.

[0290]   **[plut. 25, ?]**   I.20.

[0291]   **[plut. 25 (?)]**   I.33.

These two items are referred to as copies of Hippocrates, *Prorrêtikos A'-Praesagiorum liber I* (I.20) and *B'-liber II* (I.33).

The Florentine manuscripts of the *pluteus* 25 are in Latin (Bandini 1774: 741/742-755/756).

Equally imprecise information (without brackets or question mark) appears in Ackermann 1825: LVIII, about "*Praedictionum liber II.* (et I.)" ([*sic*] p. LV for this title):

... in bibl. Medic. plut. 25, p. 45. 142 ...

In spite of its imprecision, this reference makes it possible to identify the two manuscrits referred to here as 74.1 (= [0313]) and 75.4 (= [0347]), in which the Hippocratic *Praenotiones* can be found according to Bandini 1764-1770: 3.45 and 142.

Same as [0313] and [0347].

[0292]	**plut. 28, 13**	N.36, 53.
		Bandini 1764-1770: 2.25-27.
[0293]	**plut. 28, 14**	I.112; II.82; N.36, 52.
		Bandini 1764-1770: 2.27-31.
	plut. 28.16	(f. 236r) *Medicomathematica Mercurii Trismegisti ad Ammonem Aegyptium*; (f. 240v) Galenus, *De decubitu infirmorum prognostica ex mathematica disciplina.*
		Bandini 1764-1770: 2.31-34; *CCAG* I (Olivieri) 1898: 38-39, and also 19 (cod. 7, ff. 221 and 225).
	plut. 28.23	*Geoponica.*
		Bandini 1764-1770: 2.42-43.
[0294]	**plut. 28, 33**	N.53.
		Bandini 1764-1770: 2.58.
[0295]	**plut. 28, 34**	I.112, 135; II.82; N.36, 53, 62, 69.
		Bandini 1764-1770: 2.59-62.
[0296]	**plut. 28, 44**	II.3.
		Bandini 1764-1770: 2.66-67.
	plut. 32.16	(ff. 299 et seq.) Nicander, *Theriaca*; (ff. 307r et seq.) Nicander, *Alexipharmaca*; (ff. 352 et seq.) Gregorius Nazianzenus, *De humana natura.*
		Bandini 1764-1770: 2.140-146; Domiter 1999: 21.
	plut. 32.19	(ff. 45r et seq.) Manuel Philes, *De animalium proprietate.*
		Bandini 1764-1770: 2.147-173.
	plut. 55.6	(ff. 35v et seq.) Synesius Cyrenensis, *De insomniis.*
		Bandini 1764-1770: 2.240-244.
	plut. 55.7	(f. 211r) Marcellus Sidetes, *De piscibus.*
		Bandini 1764-1770: 2.244-268.
	plut. 55.8	(ff. 170v et seq.) Synesius Cyrenensis, *De insomniis.*
		Bandini 1764-1770: 2.269-270.
[0297]	**plut. 56, 1**	II.3.
		Bandini 1764-1770: 2.289-294.

[0298]	**plut. 56, 15**	I.72, 134.

[0298]   **plut. 56, 15**   I.72, 134.

Bandini 1764-1770: 2.314-315.

[0299]   **plut. 56, 21**   II.67.

Bandini 1764-1770: 2.320.

plut. 57.12   (ff. 52v et seq.), Hippocrates, *Epistulae*.

Bandini 1764-1770: 2.350-354.

[0300]   **plut. 57 (?), 19**   I.115.

This item with uncertain identification contains Galenus, *De ponderibus et mensuris* on f. 224 verso.

The manuscript *Florentinus* plut. 57, 19 does not contain medical texts, but rather Libanius, *Epistolae* (see Bandini 1764-1770: 2.359). It is not listed in Schilbach 1970 among the sources for metrological texts.

This is a mistake. Although Mercati 1917: 17-18, suggested that it is Oxford, Bodleian Library, Laud 58 (= [0848]), it is more probably *Florentinus Laurentianus* plut. 7.19 (see p. 69), which contains (ff. 224v-225v) Galenus, *De ponderibus et mensuris* (Bandini 1764-1770: 1.262-266 for the manuscript, and 265, no. XXVIII for the text).

plut. 57.22   (ff. 104 et seq.) Demetrius Pepagomenus, *De podagra*.

Bandini 1764-1770: 2.364-365.

plut. 57.33   (ff. 80r-92v) Aristoteles, *Physiognomonica*.

Bandini 1764-1770: 2.385-387; *Aristoteles graecus* 1976: 203-205.

plut. 57.45   (ff. 256v et seq.) Hippocrates, *Epistulae*.

Bandini 1764-1770: 2.423-425.

[0301]   **plut. 57, 50**   II.20.

Bandini 1764-1770: 2.431-433.

Also [0285].

[0302]   **plut. 58, 2**   I.110.

Bandini 1764-1770: 2.438-440.

[0303]   **plut. 58, 24**   II.94.

Bandini 1764-1770: 2.464-466.

plut. 59.5   (ff. 4v et seq.) Hippocrates, *Epistulae*.

Bandini 1764-1770: 2.491-493.

[0304]   **plut. 59, 14**   I.12, 29, 70, 82, 89, 101 (2); II.51, 83, 96; N.34, 36, 37, 63.

Bandini 1764-1770: 2.524-526.

[0305]   **plut. 59, 17**   II.20.

Bandini 1764-1770: 2.529-535.

Also [0285].

plut. 59.27   (ff. 169v et seq.) Hippocrates, *Epistulae.*

Bandini 1764-1770: 2.546-547.

plut. 60.4   (ff. 72v et seq.) Hippocrates, *Epistulae.*

Bandini 1764-1770: 2.588-589.

plut. 60.6   (ff. 387r et seq.) Synesius Cyrenensis, *De insomniis.*

Bandini 1764-1770: 2.590-592.

plut. 60.16   (ff. 90 et seq.) *De mensuris et ponderibus.*

Bandini 1764-1770: 2.605-607.

[0306]   **plut. 71, 1**   I.33.

The treatise *De alimento* by Hippocrates does not appear on f. 61 in *Florentinus* pluteus 71, 1 (which contains Simplicius, *In decem praedicamenta Aristotelis*; see Bandini 1764-1770: 3. 1). It appears in pluteus 74.1 (= [0313]).

Bandini 1764-1770: 3.41-46; see 43 for *De alimento.*

[0307]   **[plut. 73, 1]**   I.48.

This manuscript is referenced as a copy of *Remedia* by Hippocrates.

The codex *Florentinus* 73.1 is a Latin manuscript (it is not mentioned in Fryde 1996) that does not contain Hippocratic works in Latin translation (it is not listed in Kibre 1985), but it does contain Celsus, *De medicina* (see Marx 1915: XXV-XXVI; Serbat 1995: LXVIII; Mazzini 1999: 45) as well as a list of authors of formulae for medicines, including *Ypocrates* (Bandini 1776: 11-22).

Other manuscripts may have been referred to. Three mentions of Florentine manuscripts of the pluteus 73 containing texts with a similar content appear in Ackermann 1825 (without brackets) with a reference to "Montfauc. I" (= Montfaucon 1739, vol. 1):

- CLXXVI: *Hippocratis de regimine medicorum* ("Montfauc. I. p. 383"), where an annotation "quis sit nescio" appears.

  In Montfaucon 1739: 1.383, this is plut. 73.30, which corresponds to the current plut. 73.33 as Bandini 1776: 64 established (for the manuscript, see *ibid.*: 60-64). In the manuscript plut. 73.30, see ff. 85 et seq., for the text *Hippocras de regimine Medicorum* (Bandini 1776: 63);

- CLXXVI-CLXXVII: *Hippocratis de diversis herbarum generibus* ("Montfauc. I. p. 381").

  In Montfaucon 1739: 1.381, this is plut. 73.1, which corresponds to the current plut. 73.16 (see Bandini 1776: 41, and 35-41 for the description of the manuscript). The manuscript contains Pseudo-Apuleius, which may have been mistakenly identified as a Hippocratic treatise as in Montfaucon;

- CLXXVII: *Hippocr[atis] antidotarium* ("Montfauc. p. 382").

  In Montfaucon 1739: 1.382, this is plut. 73.11, which corresponds to the current plut. 73.23 (Bandini 1776: 49, and 48-49 for the whole manuscript). It contains an *antidotarium* (ff. 68 et seq. [Bandini 1776: 48]), which is not by Hippocrates as in Montfaucon 1739 and Ackermann 1825, but by Râzî (Bandini 1776: 48).

[0308]   **[plut. 73, 7]**   I.12.

This manuscript of Hippocrates, *Aphorismi* is not in Greek, but in Latin. It is not mentioned by either Magdelaine 1994 or Fryde 1996.

A manuscript "Laur. Med. plut. 73. no. VII" is mentioned by Ackermann 1825: LXV (without brackets) among the Latin manuscripts of the *Aphorismi* with a reference to "Montf. I. p. 382" (= Montfaucon 1739: 1.382) in which the content of the manuscript is identified as follows:

VIII. [falso pro VII] Membr. liber Isagogarum Joannitii ad * Tegni Galeni.

Liber Aphorismorum Hippocratis particul. VII.

Philareti de Pulsibus.

Aphorismi Joannis Damasceni.

Liber Tegni Galieni.

Acutorum Hippocratis.

This item in Montfaucon 1739 corresponds to the current plut. 73.21 as Bandini 1776: 46 established (stressing the typo VIII pro VII in Montfaucon). The description of the content provided by Montfaucon 1739 for plut. 73.7 corresponds to that of plut. 73.21 in Bandini 1776 (on plut. 73.21, see Bandini 1776: 45-46). *Florentinus* 73.21 is listed in Kibre 1985: 62.

[0309]   **[plut. 73, 8]**   I.12.

This copy of Hippocrates, *Aphorismi* is not a Greek, but a Latin manuscript. It is not mentioned by either Magdelaine 1994 or Fryde 1996.

A manuscript "Laur. Med. plut. 73. no. VIII" is mentioned by Ackermann 1825: LXV (without brackets) among the Latin manuscripts of the *Aphorismi*, with a reference to "Montf. I. p. 382 (= Montfaucon 1739: 1.382) in which the content of the manuscript is identified as follows:

VIII. Membr. Hippocratis Aphorismata particul. VII.

Manuscript plut. 73.8 according to Montfaucon 1739 corresponds to the current plut. 73.13 as Bandini 1776: 32 established. This manuscript contains "Hippocratis Aphorismi particulae VII. Anonymo interprete" (Bandini 1776: 32). Codex plut. 73.13 is listed in Kibre 1985: 48. On it, see also Fryde 1996: 827.

[0310]   **plut. 73, 9**   I.111.

Whereas this manuscript is listed among the Greek copies of Galenus, *Definitiones medicae* in Diels' catalogue, it is a Latin codex (see Bandini 1776: 26-28; the codex is not mentioned in Fryde 1996).

This is a translation by Euphrosyno Bonino *philosopho Florentino* (Frosino Bonino [*fl.* 1497-1525]) (Durling 1967: 466, no. 48, and Rice 1980: 157).

[0311]   **[plut. 73, 22]** I.12.

This is not a Greek copy of Hippocrates, *Aphorismi* (it is not mentioned by Fryde 1996), but a Latin one, which is plut. 73.28.

A manuscript "Laur. Med. plut. 73. no. XXII" is mentioned by Ackermann 1825: LXV (without brackets) among the Latin manuscripts of the *Aphorismi* with a reference to "Montf. I. p. 382" (= Montfaucon 1739: 1.382, for plut. 73 XXII; however, see p. 383 instead of 382).

Manuscript pluteus "73 XXII" in Montfaucon 1739 does not contain the *Aphorismi*, but instead contains the following text:

XXII. Membr. antiq. Rosea spina Chirurgiae, quae est colligens dicta sapientum composita a Magistro Bongiannae de Orto Cive Aretino particularis III.

There seems to be a mistake in Ackermann 1825 (followed by Diels), possibly for plut. 73 XXIV in Montfaucon 1739: 383, which contains the following works:

XXIV. Membr Isagoge in medicinam magistri Joannicii, sine titulo.

Hippocratis Aphorismata, sine titutlo.

Ejusdem prognosticorum libri sive parculae [*sic*] III.

Libri Philareti de pulsibus sine titulo.

Liber de differentia urinarum The .... [*sic*] sine titulo.

Ars Galeni lib. tribus, sine titulo.

Hippocrates de morbis acutis.

Liber Medicus, sine titulo: omina cum schol. & gloss. interlin.

Codex plut. 73 XXIV in Montfaucon 1739 corresponds to the current plut. 73.28, which contains the Latin works listed by Montfaucon for 73 XXIV (Bandini 1776: 52-53).

[0312]   **[plut. 74, (?)]** I.81.

This item of uncertain identification is listed among the copies of Galenus, *De morborum temporibus*.

The same information (without brackets) appears in Ackermann 1821: CII, no. 33 ("in Medicea plut. 74").

No *Florentinus* codex seems to contain the Galenic treatise referred to here (see Bandini 1764-1770: 3.507-509, *sub nomine* Galenus).

This may be a confusion with the Galenic treatise *De totius morbi temporibus* contained in codex pluteus 74.5 (= [0317] on which see Bandini 1764-1770: 3.51-53, especially 51, § IX).

[0313]   **plut. 74, 1**   I.4, 5, 8, 10, 11 (3), 12 (2), 17, 18, 19 (2), 20 (3), 21, 22, 23 (2), 24 (3), 25 (2), 26 (2), 27 (3), 28 (2), 29 (3), 30 (2), 31 (2), 33, 34 (3), 35 (2), 38, 109; II.37, 93.

Bandini 1764-1770: 3.41-46.

Also [0290] and [0306].

[0314]   **plut. 74, 2**   I.121; II.26, 50, 75, 77; N.47, 61.

Bandini 1764-1770: 3. 46-48.

[0315]   **plut. 74, 3**   I.17, 59 (2), 60 (2), 68, 69, 70, 71, 72, 73, 74 (2), 83, 95, 106 (2), 109-110, 110 (3), 111, 121; N.36.

Bandini 1764-1770: 3.48-50.

[0316]   **plut. 74, 4**   I.68.

Bandini 1764-1770: 3.50-51.

[0317] **plut. 74, 5**   I.60, 63, 64, 65, 70, 72, 73, 81, 83 (2), 86, 99 (2), 100.

Bandini 1764-1770: 3.51-53. On I.86 (Galenus, *De pulsibus ad tirones*), see Garofalo 2010: 89-91, who indicates that the 74.5 is a mistake for 75.5 (= [0348]).

Also [0312].

[0318] **plut. 74, 6**   I.91.

Bandini 1764-1770: 3.53.

[0319] **plut. 74, 7**   I.10, 11 (3), 67, 91, 106, 107, 126; II.15 (2), 16, 20, 42, 71, 73, 76, 77, 89, 90, 91, 92 (2); N.61, 65.

Bandini 1764-1770: 3.53-93.

[0320] **plut. 74, 8**   I.104, 107.

Bandini 1764-1770: 3.93-94.

[0321] **plut. 74, 9**   I.68.

Bandini 1764-1770: 3.94.

[0322] **plut. 74, 10**   I.39, 66, 124-125, 130, 132; II.11, 32, 102; N.30, 49.

Bandini 1764-1770: 3.95-98, 136-138.

According to Petit 2010: 146, who lists the manuscripts of Galenus, *De simplicium medicamentorum temperamentis ac facultatibus*, this manuscript is lost or cannot be found (*ibid.*: 146n5).

This may result from some confusion: the text described in Bandini 1764-1770: 3.95, is not Galenus, *De simplicium medicamentorum temperamentis ac facultatibus* as Bandini's description may suggest, but Dioscorides, *De remediis parabilibus*, as the appendix in Bandini 1764-1770: 136-138 explicitly specifies (see also Fryde 1996: 799). This text is followed by a collection of formulae for medicines identified as a post-Galenic anthology (Scarborough 1981: 24n119).

In the inventory of the Medici collection compiled by Fabio Vigili (d. 1553) between 1508 and 1510 (codex *Vaticanus Barberinianus latinus* 3185), number 365 (in *Vat. Barb. lat.* f. 320v; see Fryde 1996: 654, and 819, no. 365) is identified as follows:

Galeni περὶ ἁπλῶν φαρμάκων, sive περὶ τῆς τῶν ἁπλῶν φαρμάκων δυνάμεως, id est de simplicibus libri undecim.

Such description may have prevented the identification of Vigili's item 365 as current plut. 74, 10 and has given the impression that the Vigili manuscript is lost (Fryde 1996: 654) or unidentifiable (*ibid.*: 817).

Jackson 1998: 204, *sub* Vig. 365, identifies Vigili's number 365 as Paris, *graecus* 2159.

[0323] **plut. 74, 11**   I.5, 12, 82; II.75, 76, 91, 102, 104; N.61.

Bandini 1764-1770: 3.98-100.

[0324] **plut. 74, 12**   I.63, 68, 74, 79, 82, 90, 91, 101; N.34.

Bandini 1764-1770: 3.100-101.

See also [0325].

[0325]   **[plut. 74, 12]** I.56.

This manuscript is supposed to contain *Excerpta Hippocratica varia*.

Although this designation is not precise enough to identify any specific text, plut. 74, 12 contains, according to Bandini 1764-1770: 3.100-101, fragments of Galenic commentaries on Hippocratic treatises identified as follows in Bandini, *ibid.*:

- (ff. 1r et seq.) Excerpta quaedam ..., *e Galeni Libris IX. de Placitis Hippocratis et Platonis* (see Diels I.74 where plut. 74, 12 is mentioned, as well as De Lacy 2005: 26-28);

- (f. 28v) *Galeni ex Commentariis in Hippocratem de natura hominis* (see Diels I.101, where 74, 12 is mentioned, as well as Mewaldt 1914: XIII);

- (f. 30) Alia Galeni *ex primo Libro de elementis iuxta Hippocratis sententiam* ... (see Diels I.63 where plut. 74, 12 is listed, as well as De Lacy 1996: 33).

If so, this item is the same as [0324].

[0326]   **plut. 74, 13**   I.12, 17; II.50, 93, 109.

Bandini 1764-1770: 3.102-115.

[0327]   **plut. 74, 14**   I.100, 111.

Bandini 1764-1770: 3.115-116.

[0328]   **plut. 74, 15**   II.71.

Bandini 1764-1770: 3.116-117.

[0329]   **plut. 74, 16**   I.78 (2), 79 (2), 85.

Bandini 1764-1770: 3.117-118.

[0330]   **plut. 74, 17**   I.96; II.30, 71 (2), 77.

Bandini 1764-1770: 3.118-120.

[0331]   **plut. 74, 18**   I.68, 87 (2), 88 (2).

Bandini 1764-1770: 3.120-121.

[0332]   **plut. 74, 19**   I.61.

Bandini 1764-1770: 3.121-122.

See also [0286].

[0333]   **plut. 74, 20**   II.32; N.49.

Bandini 1764-1770: 3.122.

[0334]   **plut. 74, 21**   I.24; II.77.

Bandini 1764-1770: 3.122-124.

[0335]   **plut. 74, 22**   I.74, 94-95, 95, 112.

Bandini 1764-1770: 3.124-125.

[0336]   **plut. 74, 23**   II.8, 30, 32 (2), 77, 78, 79; N.49 (2).

Bandini 1764-1770: 3.125-127.

[0337]   **plut. 74, 24**   II.77.

Bandini 1764-1770: 3.128.

[0338]   **plut. 74, 25**   I.77, 98, 104; N.32.
                                     Bandini 1764-1770: 3.128-129.

[0339]   **plut. 74, 26**   II.77.
                                     Bandini 1764-1770: 3.129-130.

[0340]   **plut. 74, 27**   II.77.
                                     Bandini 1764-1770: 3.130.

[0341]   **plut. 74, 28**   I.87 (2), 88 (2).
                                     Bandini 1764-1770: 3.130-131.

[0342]   **plut. 74, 29**   II.77.
                                     Bandini 1764-1770: 3.131.

[0343]   **plut. 74, 30**   I.85.
                                     Bandini 1764-1770: 3.131.

[0344]   **plut. 74, 31**   I.35, 82, 87, 107, 127; II.77, 101, 102.
                                     Bandini 1764-1770: 3.132-134.

[0345]   **plut. 75, 2**   II.5.
                                     Bandini 1764-1770: 3.139-140.

[0346]   **plut. 75, 3**   I.5; II.61, 65.
                                     Bandini 1764-1770: 3.141-142.

[0347]   **plut. 75, 4**   II.78.
                                     Bandini 1764-1770: 3.142-145.
                                     Also [0291].

[0348]   **plut. 75, 5**   I.102, 107; II.5-6; N.35, 43.
                                     Bandini 1764-1770: 3.145-147.
                                     See also [0317].

[0349]   **plut. 75, 6**   II.29.
                                     Bandini 1764-1770: 3.147-151.

[0350]   **plut. 75, 7**   I.95, 119; II.6, 15, 90 (2), 92; N.43.
                                     Bandini 1764-1770: 3.151-152.

[0351]   **plut. 75, 8**   I.97; II.7, 27, 33, 34, 110.
                                     Bandini 1764-1770: 3.153-155.

[0352]   **plut. 75, 9**   I.93; II.78-79, 108, 109.
                                     Bandini 1764-1770: 3.155-156.

[0353]   **plut. 75, 10**   I.44, 114, 117; II.6, 52; N.43 (2).
                                     Bandini 1764-1770: 3.156-158.
                                     Also [0354].

[0354]   **[plut. 75, 10]** I.5.

This item is listed among the copies of the Hippocratic *Prognosticon*.

The codex pluteus 75, 10 contains only a fragment of the treatise on ff. 9v-11v (see Alexanderson 1963: 73).

It is mentioned without any information on the extent of its content in Ackermann 1825: XLVII (without brackets), where it is listed "teste Montfauc. ... I. p. 388" (= Montfaucon 1739: 1.388: "Hippocratis praenotiones, & alia excerpta medica de Phlebotomia, & herbis quibusdam capit. XXIX").

Same as [0353].

[0355]   **plut. 75, 11**   II.79, 108, 109, 110.

Bandini 1764-1770: 3.158-159.

[0356]   **plut. 75, 12**   II.6.

Bandini 1764-1770: 3.159-160.

[0357]   **plut. 75, 13**   II.6, 9.

Bandini 1764-1770: 3.160-161.

[0358]   **plut. 75, 14**   I.63, 80; II.10.

Bandini 1764-1770: 3.161-162.

[0359]   **plut. 75, 15**   II.17 (2), 18 (2).

Bandini 1764-1770: 3.162-163.

[0360]   **plut. 75, 16**   I.93; II 22, 79, 108, 109, 110.

Bandini 1764-1770: 3.164-165.

[0361]   **plut. 75, 17**   I.97, 132.

Bandini 1764-1770: 3.165-166.

[0362]   **plut. 75, 18**   II.6; N.43.

Bandini 1764-1770: 3.166.

[0363]   **plut. 75, 19**   I.56, 121, 127; II.24, 63, 101.

Bandini 1764-1770: 3.166-1168; *CMAG* II (Zuretti et al.) 1927: 321-324.

[0364]   **plut. 75, 20**   II.6; N.43.

Bandini 1764-1770: 3.168.

[0365]   **plut. 75.21**   II.6, 76; N.61.

Bandini 1764-1770: 3.169-170.

[0366]   **plut. 75.22**   II.76; N.61.

Bandini 1764-1770: 3.170.

                plut. 80.19   (ff. 22v et seq.) Synesius Cyrenensis, *De insomniis*.

Bandini 1764-1770: 3.208.

                plut. 81.1   (ff. 125r-126v) Aristoteles, *De insomniis*.

Bandini 1764-1770: 3.219-221; *Aristoteles graecus* 1976: 257-260.

	plut. 85.4	Theodorus Metochita, *In Aristotelis de insomniis commentarius.* Bandini 1764-1770: 3.249.
	plut. 86.1	(ff. 157v et seq.) Meletius, *De natura hominis.* Bandini 1764-1770: 3.283-285.
[0367]	**plut. 86.6**	II.67. Bandini 1764-1770: 3.293-296.
	plut. 86.9	(f. 190r-v) [Dioscorides], *De antifarmacis*; (ff. 190v-194r) *Carmen de viribus herbarum*; (ff. 220r et seq.) Hippocrates, *Aphorismi cum Theophili commentario.* Bandini 1764-1770: 3.327-332; Magdelaine 1994: 274 and n3, 279.
	plut. 86.12	(ff. 1v et seq.) Gregorius Nyssenus, *De natura hominis.* Bandini 1764-1770: 333-334.
	plut. 86.13	(ff. 3r et seq.) Gregorius Nyssenus, *De natura hominis.* Bandini 1764-1770: 3.335-338.
[0368]	**plut. 86.14**	II.82 (2). Bandini 1764-1770: 3.338-345.
[0369]	**plut. 86.16**	II.100, 115. Bandini 1764-1770: 3.347-360; *CMAG* II (Zuretti et al.) 1927: 35-39.
[0370]	**plut. 86.20**	II.98, 105; N.66. Bandini 1764-1770: 3.364-365.
	plut. 86.23	Nicephorus Gregoras, *Expositio in librum de insomniis Synesii.* Bandini 1764-1770: 3.366-367.
	plut. 87.4	(ff. 145r-190r) Aristoteles, *Problemata.* Bandini 1764-1770: 3.384-385; *Aristoteles graecus* 1976: 291-293.
	plut. 87.11	(ff. 303v-308) Aristoteles, *De insomniis.* Bandini 1764-1770: 3.292; *Aristoteles graecus* 1976: 301-302.
	plut. 87.15	Aristoteles, *Problemata.* Bandini 1764-1770: 3.396; *Aristoteles graecus* 1976: 310-311.
[0371]	**plut. 87.16**	II.20. Bandini 1764-1770: 3.396-403. Also [0285].
	plut. 87.20	(ff. 134r-136v) Aristoteles, *De insomniis*; (ff. 225r-241r) Aristoteles, *Problemata.* Bandini 1764-1770: 3.404-406; *Aristoteles graecus* 1976: 319-323.

plut. 87.21   (ff. 34v-40v) Aristoteles, *De insomniis.*

Bandini 1764-1770: 3.407-408; *Aristoteles graecus* 1976: 323-324.

plut. 91.10   (ff. 145-162) Nicander, *Theriaca*; (ff. 162-171v) Nicander, *Alexipharmaca.*

Bandini 1764-1770: 3.427-432.

Laurent. App. *(Laurentiana Appendix)*

[0372]   2   I.22, 42 (2), 43 (2), 122, 123, 125, 127; II.3, 12, 13, 14, 22, 27, 33, 35, 38, 42, 47, 64, 79, 80, 98, 100.

Rostagno and Festa 1893: 213-218.

Current shelfmark: Antinori 101 (see p. 67).

bibl. naz.[1] (Biblioteca nazionale [National Library])

In Diels' catalogue, these manuscripts are identified in two different ways:

- in [0373] and [0374], old shelfmarks made of three elements (two Roman numerals followed by an Arabic numeral);
- in [0375] and [0376], the new shelfmarks, which correspond to the sequential numbers in Vitelli 1894 and Olivieri 1897.

–

[0373]   **II.III.304**   II.39.

Olivieri 1897: 403.

18th-century scholarly copy.

Current shelfmark: *Magliabechianus* 30.

[0374]   **II.III.428**   I.44, 56.

Current shelfmark: *Magliabechianus* 1.

Same as [0375].

Magliabech. *(Magliabechiani)*

[0375]   1   I.44, 127.

Vitelli 1894: 543-544.

Also [0374].

[0376]   44   II.79.

Olivieri 1897: 409-410.

Bibl. Riccardiana (Biblioteca Riccardiana [Riccardiana Library])

Riccard. *(Riccardiani)*

Diels' catalogue adds the old shelfmarks between parentheses to the current ones (in Arabic numerals).

---

[1]   = Magliabecchiana [*sic*] in I.XV.

Old shelfmarks are made of three elements:

- the capital letter "K";
- a number in Roman numerals;
- a number in Arabic numerals.

They appear in Lami 1756 alphabetical catalogue of the Riccardiana Library. They are no longer used and have been replaced by the sequential numbers of Vitelli 1894.

[0377]   **10 (K I 12)**   II.11.

Vitelli 1894: 479-481; *CCAG* I (Olivieri) 1898: 74-75.

Current shelfmark: Riccard. 10.

12   (f. 1r) *Formulae medicinarum*; (ff. 1v et seq.) *De lapidum et planetarum virtutibus.*

Vitelli 1894: 481-485, *CCAG* I (Olivieri) 1898: 75; Elsheikh 1990: 3.

14   (ff. 163v-168r) Aristoteles, *De insomniis.*

Vitelli 1894: 485; *Aristoteles graecus* 1976: 354-356.

[0378]   **17 (K I 24)**   I.107.

Vitelli 1894: 486; Elsheikh 1990: 3.

Current shelfmark: Riccard. 17.

[0379]   **31 (K II 4)**   II.108.

Vitelli 1894: 490-493; Elsheikh 1990: 3-4.

Current shelfmark: Riccard. 31.

[0380]   **41 (K II 2)**   I.12, 44; N.37.

Vitelli 1894: 498-500; Elsheikh 1990: 4.

Current shelfmark: Riccard. 41.

[0381]   **44 (K II 5)**   I.5, 12, 77, 104, 107, 112.

Vitelli 1894: 501-502; Elsheikh 1990: 4.

Current shelfmark: Riccard. 44.

56   (ff. 1r et seq.) Nicander, *Theriaca*; (ff. 29r et seq.) Nicander, *Alexipharmaca.*

Vitelli 1894: 507; Elsheikh 1990: 4-5.

64   Gregorius Nazianzenus, *De humana natura.*

Vitelli 1894: 516-517; Domiter 1999: 22.

[0382]   **71 (K II 16)**   II.79.

Vitelli 1894: 520-522; Elsheikh 1990: 5.

Current shelfmark: Riccard. 71.

81   (ff. 94r-105v) Aristoteles, *De insomniis.*

Vitelli 1894: 527; *Aristoteles graecus* 1976: 362-363.

[0383]   **91 (K II 7)**   II.32; N.49.

Vitelli 1894: 531; Elsheikh 1990: 5.

Current shelfmark: Riccard. 91.

Gallipoli (Καλλίπολη, former Ottoman Empire, now Gelibolu [TR])

Ekkl. Ag. Nikolaou (Ἐκκλησία Ἁγίου Νικολάου [St. Nicolas Church])

–

[0384]   **38**   I.5, 41, 127, 131; II.7, 59-60, 96, 102.

This manuscript is listed for the following texts (listed here in the order of the folios according to Diels' catalogue, except the first one, which has no folio numbering in Diels' catalogue; references to Diels' catalogue follow the titles):

Stephanus Alexandrinus, *In Hippocratis praenotiones* (II.96);

f. 39: Hippocrates, *Epistula ad Ptolemaeum (2)* (I.41);

ff. 39 and 41v: Galenus, *De pulsibus* (I.131);

ff. 52 and 57v: Galenus, *De urinis* (I.127);

f. 58: Magnus Emesenus, *De urinis* (II.59-60);

f. 64v: Theophilus, *De urinis* (II.102);

f. 81: Aetius Amidenus, *Excerpta* (II.7);

f. 81v: Hippocrates, *Prognosticon* (I.5).

This manuscript and its content are mentioned in Diels' catalogue on the basis of Papadopoulos-Kerameus 1887: 8-9 (Papadopoulos-Kerameus' work is listed among the sources consulted to compile Diels' catalogue in Diels I.XXIII).

Number 38 comes from Papadopoulos-Kerameus 1887: 6-12, specifically 8-9. It does not reproduce a shelfmark of the library, but was attributed by Papadopoulos-Kerameus as he states in the article (*ibid.*: 7).

Whereas Diels' catalogue lists this item as in the library of St. Nicolas Church, the article by Papadopoulos-Kerameus 1887 listing the manuscripts in Gallipoli mentions this item (p. 8-9) among the holdings of the Βιβλιοθήκη Κοινότητος (*Community Library*), and not of St. Nicolas Church (see p. 6 for a first mention of the *Community Library* and pp. 7-12 for a list and a short description of some of its manuscripts including the present one).

This identification in Diels' catalogue results from confusion among the three collections in Gallipoli mentioned in Papadopoulos-Kerameus 1887: 6-12, including a collection at a St. Nicolas Church, which contained at least one manuscript (below).

In spite of the 1915-1916 Gallipoli campaign, manuscripts from St. Nicolas Church and the collection of the Βιβλιοθήκη Κοινότητος have been preserved. The codex of St. Nicolas Church mentioned by Papadopoulos-Kerameus 1887: 6-7, is now in Ἀθήνα, Μουσείο Μπενάκη (Athens, Benaki Museum), TA 316 (see Lappa-Zizica and Rizou-Kouroupou 1991: 220-221); another manuscript from Gallipoli is Athens, Benaki Museum, TA 150 (see Lappa-Zizica and Rizou-Kouroupou 1991: 133-135).

Although the library of the Institut Français d'Etudes Byzantines (IFEB) in Paris contains one medical manuscript from Gallipoli, Βιβλιοθήκη Κοινότητος (IFEB manuscript 34 [corresponding to number 35 in Papadopoulos-Kerameus 1887: 8], which contains at ff. 129r-150r a copy of the *Physiologus* dated 1599), this manuscript (on which see Bingeli et al. 2014: 58-60, and below, p. 262) is not the item mentioned in Diel's catalogue.

In the current state of research, the location of the manuscript referred to here is unknown (in this sense, see Alexanderson 1963: 73-74 about Hippocrates, *Prognosticon*, and Duffy 1983: 18-19 about Stephanus' commentary on the same treatise). It might be in a private collection (see Olivier 1995: 306, *sub nomine* Gelibolu).

Genf (Geneva) (CH)

Genev. Bibl. Urb. (*Genevensis Bibliotheca Urbis* [Geneva City Library]), now Bibliothèque de Genève (Geneva Library)

-

[0385]   42   I.96.

Omont 1886: 438.

Now Ms. grec 42.

Genève (Geneva) (CH)

Bibliothèque de Genève (Geneva Library)

CL

241   Plantarum imagines ex Dioscoride, *De materia medica*.

Sotheby's 1990: 124-128.

Ms grec

42   See [0385].

Genova (Genoa) (IT)

Biblioteca Franzoniana (Franzoniana Library)

Urbani

17   See [0386].

Cataldi Palau 1990: 98-104.

Biblioteca universitaria (University Library)

–

F.VI.9   (ff. 3r-5r) Aristoteles (= Ps.-Alexander Aphrodisiensis), *Problemata* (frg.).

Martini 1896: 324-326; *Aristoteles graecus* 1976: 364-365.

Genua (Genova) (IT)

Bibl. della Missione urbana (Biblioteca della Missione urbana [Urban Mission Library]), now Biblioteca Franzoniana (Franzoniana Library)

–

[0386]   **17**   II.39.

Ehrhard 1893: 275-276.

Current shelfmark: Urbani 17.

Glasgow (GB)

Glasgow University Library, Special Collections Department

Hunter

271 (U.5.11)   See [0387] and also [1548].

447 (V.5.17)   (ff. 1r-3r) Gregorius Nyssenus, *De hominis opificio* (frg.).

Young 1908: 370-372.

Hunterian. ([*Bibliotheca*] *Hunteriana* [Hunterian Library])

–

[0387]   **V. 5. 11**   II.108.

Young 1908: 218-219.

Now Glasgow, Glasgow University Library, Special Collections Department, Ms Hunter 271 (U.5.11).

Göttingen (DE)

Niedersachsische Staats-und Universitätsbibliothek (Lower Saxony State and University Library)

8° Cod. Ms. phil.

73   (pp. 410 et seq.) Hermes Trismegistus, *Ratio iudicandi de morbis et infirmorum decubitu.*

Meyer 1893: 1.18.

Univ. -Bibl. (Universitäts-Bibliothek [University Library]), now Niedersachsische Staats-und Universitätsbibliothek (Lower Saxony State and University Library)

Hist. nat. (*Historia naturalis*)

[0388]   **3**   I.3.

Meyer 1893: 2.287-288, with the following description:

Hippocratis opera omnia, Venet. 1526, das Handexemplar des Janus Cornarius aus Zwickau ... Am Rande stehen Conjecturen, theils des Cornarius selbst theils anderer, und viele Variante ...

Current shelfmark: 4° Cod. Ms. hist. nat. 3.

Venetian edition of Hippocrates annotated by Janus Cornarius (ca. 1500-1558).

[0389]   **4**   I.3.

Meyer 1893: 2.288, with the following description:

Hippocrates ... libri omnes, Basil. 1538. Handexemplar des Joh. Oporinus, an dessen Rand Bemerkungen, Conjecturen und Lesarten eingetragen sind ...

Basel edition of Hippocrates with handwritten notes by Johannes Herbster, better known as Oporinus (1507-1568).

Current shelfmark: 4° Cod. Ms. hist. nat. 4.

[0390]   **5**   II.104.

Meyer 1893: 2.288.

17th-century copy.

Current shelfmark: 4° Cod. Ms. hist. nat. 5.

[0391]   **6**   II.34.

Meyer 1893: 2.288, where the following description can be read:

Simplicium facultates medicae ex antiquis (Dioscoride), opera et studio G. H. V. 1670.

Manuscript of Georg Hieronymus Welsch (1624-1677).

Now 8° Cod. Ms. hist. nat. 6.

[0392]   **90**   II.30.

Meyer 1893: 2.311, with the following description:

Dioscoridis opera 1598, darin, wie es scheint, von der Hand Joh. Gramm's (1685-1749), der sich auch auf dem Titelblatt eingetragen hat, "variae lectiones ... excerptae ... ex codice vetusto bibliothecae S. Johannis Neapoli", einer Bilderheft des 5. Jahrh., seit 1717 in Wien (vgl. Lambecius supplem. I Sp. 343 ff.).

Collation of variant readings from codex now Napoli, Biblioteca Nazionale, ex *Vindobonensis graecus* 1 (see p. 158 and [1832]) by Johannes Gramm (1685-1749).

Current shelfmark: 2° Cod. Ms. hist. nat. 90.

Philol. (*Philologici*)

[0393]   **2**   I.49.

Meyer 1893: 1.2, with the following description:

Excerpte aus Leidener Handschriften, 18. Jahrh.

Now 8° Cod. Ms. philol. 2.

[0394]   **21**   I.49.

Meyer 1893: 1.7, with the following description:

Hauptsächlich Abschriften aus Leidener Handschriften ... Von verschiedenen geschrieben im 17. und 18. Jahrh.

Collations of manuscripts from the collection of Leiden library.

Now 8° Cod. Ms. philol. 21.

29   (ff. 139r-182v) Nicander, *Theriaca* et *Alexipharmaca*.

Meyer 1893: 1.9-10.

Current shelfmark: 8° Cod. Ms. philol. 29.

Grottaferrata (IT)

Biblioteca del Monumento nazionale di Grottaferrata (Library of Grottaferrata National Monument)

–

Z.γ.VI (GR. 81)   See [0395].

Klosterbibliothek (Biblioteca del Monastero [Convent Library]), now Biblioteca del Monumento nazionale di Grottaferrata (Library of Grottaferrata National Monument)

Diels' identification of the manuscript includes the old shelfmark of the codex (with a mistake), followed by a reference to the catalogue by Rocchi 1883, that is, the following elements in Rocchi's catalogue:

• chapter ("Series nona: Codices philosophici");

• sequential number of the manuscript in this chapter ("Codex quadragesimus sextus").

Such reference to Rocchi's catalogue is not part of the shelfmark of the manuscript. On the shelfmark system at Grottaferrata Library, see Rocchi 1893: 285-289.

The Grottaferrata manuscripts are now identified by means of a shelfmark made of three elements separated by a period sign:

• a Greek majuscule letter;

• a Greek minuscule letter;

• a Roman numeral.

The three elements are followed by the abbreviation "GR." and an Arabic numeral between parentheses.

The Greek Grottaferrata manuscripts have received a new numeration (continuous through the collection, in Arabic numerals), which has not been published yet, although it has already been used in some works (for example Lucà 2003).

–

[0395]   **2 γ VI (series IX cod. 46)**   I.67 (3), 109.

Rocchi 1883: 492-493.

Current shelfmark: Z.γ.VI (GR. 81).

Hamburg (DE)

–

–

[0396]   **v. Fabricius, IX. 454-474**   II.108.

This item, listed without a library name and a shelfmark, is a copy of Xenocrates, *De alimento ex aquatilibus*.

The reference is to Fabricius, *Bibliotheca graeca*, vol. 9 (1719), pp. 454-474, where the text of Xenocrates, *De alimento ex aquatilibus* can be found (Greek text and Latin translation by Giovanni Battista Rasario [1517-1578]). See also *ibid.* p. 453, where Xenocrates is listed in the "Index Scriptorum ex quibus Oribasius libros ex ἑβδομηκονταβίβλῳ superstites composuit" (see pp. 452-453 for the index, and 452 for this title). There is no mention of any Greek manuscript.

The only *codex Hamburgensis* that contains Xenocrates' text is now at the Staats- und Universitätsbibliothek Hamburg "Carl von Ossietzky", philol. 313 (see below, p. 88).

Same as [0397].

Stadtbibliothek (City Library), now Staats- und Universitätsbibliothek Hamburg "Carl von Ossietzky" (Hamburg "Carl von Ossietzky" State and University Library)

Hamburgens. (*Hamburgensis*)

[0397]   **200**   N.68.

A reference is made to the "Philologica Hamburgensia, Hambg. 1905". As Diels' catalogue mentions this is the codex *Hamburgensis philol. 313*.

Number 200 is the sequential number in Münzel 1905: 37-38 (that is, the *Philologica Hamburgensia* mentioned in Diels' catalogue), where the correspondence with the current philol. 313 is provided.

Same as [0396].

Uffenbach. (*Uffenbachianus*)

This is a reference to the collection owned by Zacharias Konrad von Uffenbach (1683-1734). For its catalogue, see Uffenbach 1720.

[0398]   **105**   I.71.

This codex of Galenus, *De optima corporis nostri constitutione*, also appears at I.65 among the Latin translations of Galenus, *De temperamentis*.

This is a Latin manuscript described as follows in Uffenbach 1720: 4.114, under number CV:

Vol. CV. Duod.

Chartaceum recentissimum, sistens:

1. Galeni libros Tres de Temperamentis diligentius recognitos Thoma Linacro interprete.

2. Eiusdem Galeni de optima nostri corporis constitutione librum unum Ferdinando Balamio interprete ad graecorum exemplarium fidem castigatum.

On these translations by Thomas Linacre (1460-1524) and Ferdinando Balami (d. after 1552 [?]), see Durling 1961: 291 no. 114b, and 288 no. 75d, respectively.

Franke 1967: 193, identifies this manuscript as *medicus* 914. According to the same, *ibid.*, and Kristeller 1983: 562 (for whom it is a 16th/17th-century codex), this manuscript is in Berlin (on the Hamburg manuscripts in Berlin after World War II, see Carter 1966).

During the winter of 1989-1990, the Hamburg manuscripts then-preserved in Berlin were returned to Hamburg (see Molin Pradel 2001: 15).

The present item is now at the Staats- und Universitätsbibliothek Hamburg "Carl von Ossietzky", with the shelfmark *medicus* 914.

No recent printed catalogue is available.

Staats- und Universitätsbibliothek Hamburg "Carl von Ossietzky" (Hamburg "Carl von Ossietzky" State and University Library)

in scrin.

50a	(f. 1v) *Remedia contra tussim.*
	Molin Pradel 2002: 32-37.

philol.

313	Molin Pradel 2002: 213-220.

This is a humanistic manuscript by several hands. The folios containing Xenocrates (ff. 21r-27r) are by Heinrich Lindenbruch (1570-1642) (Molin Pradel 2002: 219 for the identification of the hand; on his collection of manuscripts, *ibid.*, 7-10).

Same as [0396] and [0397].

Heidelberg (DE)

Bibl. Univ. (*Bibliotheca Universitatis* [University Library]), now Universitätsbibliothek (University Library)

Abteilung Handschriften und Alte Drucke (Department of Manuscripts and Early Printed Books)

All of the manuscripts are identified as Cod. Pal. graec. with the sequential numbers they have in Stevenson 1885.

	129	(ff. 69r et seq.) Gregorius Nyssenus, *De hominis opificio.*
		Stevenson 1885: 61-62.
		Now Cod. Pal. graec. 129.
[0399]	**132**	I.38.
		Stevenson 1885: 63-64.
		Now Cod. Pal. graec. 132.
[0400]	**155**	I.41.
		Stevenson 1885: 83-84.
		Now Cod. Pal. graec. 155.
	356	(ff. 168v et eq.) Epiphanius, *De duodecim gemmis* (frg.).
		Stevenson 1885: 203-207.
		Now Cod. Pal. graec. 356.

[0401]	**375**	II.71.
		Stevenson 1885: 242.
		Now Cod. Pal. graec. 375.
[0402]	**398**	I.38.
		Stevenson 1885: 254-257.
		Now Cod. Pal. graec. 398.

Universitätsbibliothek, Abteilung Handschriften und Alte Drucke (University Library, Department of Manuscripts and Early Printed Books)

Cod. Pal. graec.

See **Bibl. Univ.**

Holkham (GB)

Bibl. des Gr. Leicester (Bibliothek des Greifes Leicester [Library of the Earl of Leicester])

The collection of 108 Greek manuscripts owned by the Earl of Leicester, originally held at Holkham Hall, was acquired in 1960 by the Bodleian Library in Oxford (Barbour 1960) where today it is identified as the Holkham Gr. collection.

On these manuscripts, see below, pp. 181-182, Oxford, Bodleian Library, Holkham Gr. MSS.

—

[0403]	**nr. 282**	I.4, 5, 8, 10 (2), 11 (3), 12-13, 19, 21, 22, 23, 27 (2), 28 (2), 29 (2), 30, 31 (2), 32 (3), 33, 34, 35, 46; N.25 (3), 26 (3) (on both pages of the Supplement [= N], the manuscript is listed under Padua, S. Joann. in Viridario).
		Foerster 1884: 163.
		Now Oxford, Bodleian Library, MS. Holkham Gr. 92.
		Formerly [0886] and [0903].
[0404]	**nr. 283**	II.6; N.43 (under Padua, S. Joann. in Viridario).
		Foerster 1884: 163.
		Now Oxford, Bodleian Library, MS. Holkham Gr. 108.
		Formerly [0901].
[0405]	**nr. 289**	II.36.
		This manuscript is listed among the copies of Epiphanius, *De mensuris et ponderibus*.
		The presence of this text in current manuscript Oxford, Bodleian Library, MS. Holkham Gr. 112 (corresponding to former item 289 of Holkham collection) cannot be confirmed in the current state of cataloguing of the Holkham collection (Barbour 1960: 612-613).
		At any rate current Holkham Gr. 112 contains (ff. 163v et seq.) a medical lexicon (probably a lexicon of medicinal plants) (Barbour 1960: 612).

Foester 1884: 164 (does not mention either Epiphanius or the medical lexicon).

[0406]   **nr. 293**   I.13; II.99.

Foerster 1884: 164-165 (does not list the texts referred to here, Hippocrates, *Aphorismi* [frg.], or Synesius, *De insomniis*).

Now Oxford, Bodleian Library, MS. Holkham Gr. 106.

Ιερουσαλήμ (Jerusalem) (IL)

Πατριαρχείο, Πατριαρχική Βιβλιοθήκη (Patriarchate, Patriarchal Library). For all the collections, see below **Jerusalem** (see below, pp. 92-95).

Ιερά Μονή Αγίου Σάββα (Agios Savva)

See **Bibl. Mar-Saba.** (see below, p. 93)

Πανάγιος Τάφος (Holy Sepulchre)

See **Bibl. patriarch.** (see below, pp. 94-95).

Πατριαρχείο (Patriarchate)

See **Bibl. patriarch.** (see below, pp. 94-95).

Ιερά Μονή Τιμίου Σταυρού (Holy Cross)

See **Bibl. d. hl. Kreuz.** (see below, p. 93)

Istanbul (TR)

Οικουμενικό Πατριαρχείο Κωνσταντινουπόλεως, Πατριαρχική Βιβλιοθήκη (Ecumenical Patriarchate of Constantinople, Patriarchal Library)

The Patriarchal Library preserves several collections, identified by the name of their earlier location.

Ιερά Μονή Αγίας Τριάδος (Holy Trinity [Agia Trias] Monastery)

107   (no. 3) Gregorius Nyssenus, *De hominis opificio.*

Tsakopoulos 1956: 118-119, no. 99.

Ιερά Μονή Παναγίας Καμαριωτίσσης (Monastery of the Panagia Kamariotissa)

82   See [0211].

Kouroupou and Géhin 2008: 245-247.

139   tegumentum anterior Nemesius Emesenus, *De natura hominis* (frg.).

Kouroupou and Géhin 2008: 353-355.

153   (ff. 3v-67v) *Physiologus.*

Kouroupou and Géhin 2008: 372-373.

157   (ff. 304r-305v) Epiphanius, *De duodecim gemmis.*

Kouroupou and Géhin 2008: 376-388 (especially 383, no. 24).

160   (ff. 80r-86v) Hermes Trismegistus, *Liber ad Ammonem* (frg.).

Kouroupou and Géhin 2008: 393-394.

Topkapı Sarayı Kütüphanesi (Topkapi Sarayi Library)

Gayri İslâmî Eserler (G. İ.) (Non-Islamic Works)

9	*Geoponica.*
	Deissmann 1933: 56-57.
10	(ff. 124 et seq.) Hippocrates, *Testamentum.*
	Deissmann 1933: 57.
11	See [0444].
	Its current location is unknown.
12	*De lapidibus et animalibus.*
	Deissmann 1933: 58.
19	(ff. 247v-250v) *Hygiena et anatomia*; (ff. 251r-273r) Adamantios, *Physiognomica* (*De oculis*).
	Deissmann 1933: 61-63; *Aristoteles graecus* 1976: 373-375.
64	Adamantios, *Physiognomica* (*De oculis*).
	Deissmann 1933: 96.

Jena (DE)

Thüringer Universitäts- und Landesbibliothek (Thuringia University and State Library)

Ms. Bos.

f. 1	See [0407].
	Stockhausen 2001: 685-689.

Ms. G.B.

f. 31	See [0719].

Universitätsbibliothek (University Library), now Thüringer Universitäts- und Landesbibliothek (Thuringia University and State Library)

–

[0407]   –   N.50.

This copy of Epiphanius, *De mensuris et ponderibus* mentioned here without collection name and shelfmark is now Ms. Bos. f. 1 (above).

[0408]   **Aldina c. nott. Cornarii**   I.58.

This is the 1525 Aldine edition of Galen with handwritten notes by Janus Cornarius (1500-1588). It is mentioned in Ackermann 1821: CCV, ll. 28-37.

See Perilli 2011: 180.

Jerusalem (IL)

With the exception of the library identified as **Bibl. d. hl. Grabes**, the several libraries listed in Diels' catalogue are not independent libraries, but rather collections within the Patriarchal Library (Πατριαρχική Βιβλιοθήκη).

Bibl. d. hl. Grabes (Bibliothek des heiligen Grabes, Βιβλιοθήκη τοῦ Παναγίου Τάφου [Library of the Holy Sepulchre], actually Μετόχιον Παναγίου Τάφου [Collection of the Metochion of the Holy Sepulchre]).

When Diels' catalogue was compiled, these manuscripts were not in Jerusalem, but at the Patriarchate in Constantinople as Papadopoulos-Kerameus 1891-1915: 4.[a] and 4.1 already mentioned. Most of them are currently in Αθήνα, Εθνική Βιβλιοθήκη της Ελλάδος EBE (Athens, National Library of Greece – EBE). See above, p. 15.

–

[0409]	38	II.88.
		Rufus, *De vesicae renumque affectibus*.
		It is actually no. 83 of the same collection (see Sideras 1977: 14n2).
		Papadopoulos-Kerameus 1891-1915: 4.93-94.
		This is a 17th-century manuscript (Karas 1994: 403).
[0410]	179	I.126.
		Papadopoulos-Kerameus 1891-1915: 4.150.
[0411]	189	I.32.
		Papadopoulos-Kerameus 1891-1915: 4.161.
		18th-century manuscript (Karas 1994: 379).
[0412]	199	I.125.
		Papadopoulos-Kerameus 1891-1915: 4.174-175.
[0413]	273	II.67.
		Papadopoulos-Kerameus 1891-1915: 4.251-252; Morani 1981: 62.
[0414]	304	II.63.
		Papadopoulos-Kerameus 1891-1915: 4.283-284.
		17th-century manuscript (1615) (Karas 1994: 390-391).
[0415]	357	II.63.
		Papadopoulos-Kerameus 1891-1915: 4.332.
[0416]	363	I.125.
		Papadopoulos-Kerameus 1891-1915: 4.335-337.
[0417]	405	II.67.
		Papadopoulos-Kerameus 1891-1915: 4.362-363; Morani 1981: 62.
		18th-century manuscript (1717) copied on the basis of no. [0413] according to Papadopoulos-Kerameus (*ibid.*) followed by Morani.

Bibl. d. hl. Kreuzes (Bibliothek des heiligen Kreuzes, Βιβλιοθήκη τοῦ Τιμίου Σταυροῦ [Library of the Holy Cross]), actually Ιερά Μονή Τιμίου Σταυρού (Holy Cross Collection)

–

[0418]   68   I.125.

This manuscript (Galenus, *De hominis natura testamentum*) is not in the collection of the Ιερά Μονή Τιμίου Σταυρού, but at the Πατριαρχείο. The codex is listed in Papadopoulos-Kerameus 1891-1915: 1.154-156 as in the collection of the Patriarchate, with a supplement in Id., *ibidem*: 3. 324-334, where the text referred to here appears (3.325). This supplement follows the catalogue of the manuscripts in the collection of the Ιερά Μονή Τιμίου Σταυρού (Papadopoulos-Kerameus 1891-1915: 3.1-175), something that may have caused the mistake in Diels' catalogue. See below, p. 94.

[0419]   85   I.148.

Papadopoulos-Kerameus 1891-1915: 3.138-143.

Bibl. Mar-Saba (Bibliothek Mar-Saba, Βιβλιοθήκη Μαρ-Σάββα [Mar-Sabba Library]), actually Ιερά Μονή Αγίου Σάββα (Agios Savva Collection)

–

121   (no. 6, ff. 211r-213v) Maximus Planudes, *De urinis*; (no. 7, ff. 214r et seq.) Hippocrates, *De quattuor elementis et humoribus*.

Papadopoulos-Kerameus 1891-1915: 2.201-203.

332   (ff. 151 et seq.) Basilius Caesariensis, *De hominis origine*.

Papadopoulos-Kerameus 1891-1915: 2.457-459; Smets and Van Esbroeck 1970: 129.

[0420]   366   II.39.

Papadopoulos-Kerameus 1891-1915: 2.482-492.

416   (ff. 1r-178r) Aristoteles, *Problemata*.

Papadopoulos-Kerameus 1891-1915: 2.533; *Aristoteles graecus* 1976: 387-388.

419   Gregorius Nazianzenus, *De humana natura*.

Papadopoulos-Kerameus 1891-1915: 2.539-540 (does not identify the work); Domiter 1999: 21.

[0421]   432   I.42, 123; II.64.

Papadopoulos-Kerameus 1891-1915: 2.546-547.

17th-century (1662) *iatrosofion*.

[0422]   481   I.13, 105.

Papadopoulos-Kerameus 1891-1915: 2.562-563.

18th-century copy (1713 [?]).

[0423]   498   I.5, 13, 20, 33.

Papadopoulos-Kerameus 1891-1915: 2.567.

18th-century manuscript.

Bibl. patriarch. (Bibliothek des Patriarchates, Βιβλιοθήκη τοῦ Πατριαρχείου [Patriarchal Library]), actually Πατριαρχείο (Patriarchal Collection) or Πανάγιος Τάφος (Collection of the Holy Sepulchre)

—

[0424]	**15**	II.67.
		Papadopoulos-Kerameus 1891-1915: 1.65-68; Morani 1981: 32.
	68	Galenus, *De hominis natura testamentum*.
		Papadopoulos-Kerameus 1891-1915: 1.154-156 and 3.325.
		See [0418].
[0425]	**102**	I.3, 13, 104-105.
		Papadopoulos-Kerameus 1891-1915: 1.175.
		18th-century copy (Karas 1994: 93).
[0426]	**108**	II.9.
		Papadopoulos-Kerameus 1891-1915: 1.186-192.
[0427]	**148**	I.42, 115, 136; II.41, 97.
		Papadopoulos-Kerameus 1891-1915: 1.250.
[0428]	**203**	II.63.
		Papadopoulos-Kerameus 1891-1915: 1.283.
	208	(ff. 1r-68r) *Physiologus*.
		Papadopoulos-Kerameus 1891-1915: 1.287.
	254	Gregorius Nazianzenus, *De humana natura*.
		Papadopoulos-Kerameus 1891-1915: 1.323 (does not explicitly identify the text); Domiter 1999: 21.
	261	(ff. 1 et seq.) *De dieta*; (ff. 35 et seq.) Leo Imperator, *Physiognomonia*.
		Papadopoulos-Kerameus 1891-1915: 1.325-326.
	271	(ff. 1r et seq.) *Physiologus*.
		Papadopoulos-Kerameus 1891-1915: 1.328-329.
[0429]	**273**	II.7, 77, 91.
		Papadopoulos-Kerameus 1891-1915: 1.329-330.
		18th-century manuscript (Karas 1994: 273).
	281	(no. 4) Splenius philosophus, *De generatione hominis*.
		Papadopoulos-Kerameus 1891-1915: 1.354-356.
[0430]	**339**	II.79.
		Papadopoulos-Kerameus 1891-1915: 1.378.
[0431]	**463**	I.56.
		Papadopoulos-Kerameus 1891-1915: 1.432-433.
		18th-century manuscript.

[0432]	**470**	II.63.
		Papadopoulos-Kerameus 1891-1915: 1.435-436;
		18th-century copy (Karas 1994: 392).
[0433]	**511**	II.63.
		Papadopoulos-Kerameus 1891-1915: 1.461-462.
		18th/19th century (Karas 1994: 95, 392).

Καλλονή Λέσβου (Kalloni, Lesvos) (GR)

    Ιερά Μονή Λειμώνος (Limonos Monastery)

        See **Lesbos** ([0472] and [0473])

Καρδίτσα (Karditsa) (GR)

    Ιερά Μονή Κορώνης (Koronis Monastery)

        4   Dioscorides, *De materia medica*.

              Politis 1976: 59; Karas 1994: 354-355.

Karlsruhe (DE)

    Badische Landesbibliothek Karlsruhe (Baden State Library Karlsruhe)

        See **Großherzogl. Hof. u. Landesbibliothek.**

    Großherzogl. Hof. u. Landesbibliothek (Großherzogliche Hof- und Landesbibliothek [Library of Grand Duchy Court and State]), now Badische Landesbibliothek Karlsruhe (Baden State Library Karlsruhe)

        –

[0434]	**449**	I.8, 13, 28, 29.
		Badische Landesbibliothek 1896/1970: 82, 301.
		Current shelfmark: K 449.
[0435]	**451**	II.67.
		Badische Landesbibliothek 1896/1970: 82-83, 302; Morani 1981: 10.
		Current shelfmark: K 451.

Königsberg Pr. (now Kaliningrad [RU])

    –

    Regimont. (*Regimontani*)

[0436]	**S. 35**	I.151.
		This item is listed in the *Addenda* in volume I, with a reference to I.113 (*De urinis ex Hippocrate, Galeno aliisque quibusdam*, identified as Kühn 19.609-628).

According to the description on I.151, this text appears on f. 273v and is fragmentary (*explicit* = Kühn 19.611, 7).

Although no institution is provided at I.151, the information in N.37 (= [0437]) seems to be about the same item and specifies that this manuscript was in the collections of the **bibl. urb.** (*Bibliotheca urbis* = Stadtbibliothek [City Library]).

A catalogue of this collection was compiled by Seraphim 1909. Manuscript S 35 is actually S 35. 8° (on which see Seraphim 1909: 302 and 346) and is a 14th/15th-century codex of 274 ff., containing mainly Sextus Empiricus (p. 302).

Some supplementary information is provided by Seraphim 1909: 346 (that is, in the *Nachträge*):

Hinter den Dialexeis auf Bl. 273/274 und den hinteren Innendeckel Aufzeichnungen und Notizen medicinischen Inhalts.

This information is referred to at N.37 (= [0437]).

On this manuscript, see Mutschmann 1909, particularly 246 (short description); Canart 1977-1979: 309 (short description and history of the manuscript) and 313-314 (who hypothesizes that this manuscript might have been copied by Demetrius Damilas and originally belonged to the Vatican Library); Diller 1983: 387, *sub* Kaliningrad (*in ima pagina*), who confirms Canart's hypothesis, that is, that this manuscript strayed from the Vatican Library.

Whatever the copyist and the previous location of this manuscript, the text referred to in Diels' catalogue is a late addition, probably not by the merchant, mayor of Gdansk (1664-1675) and book collector Nicolas von Bodeck (1611-1676) who marked it with his ex-libris in 1652 or 1657. It might rather be a Galenic extract by a practicing physician who owned the codex between 1527 (when it may have left the Biblioteca Vaticana during the sack of Rome) and 1652/7 (when von Bodeck wrote his ex-libris).

The current location of this item is unknown (Canart 1977-1979: 313n2). It is believed to have been destroyed during World War II.

bibl. urb. (*Bibliotheca urbis* [Stadtbibliothek, City Library])

This library was heavily damaged during World War II.

–

[0437]   **16 *b* 12**   N.37.

From the information provided here, the text on f. 273v (*De urinis ex Hippocrate, Galeno aliisque quibusdam*) is by a recent hand.

This is the same item as [0436].

A copy of this text was made by M. Odau for the *Corpus Medicorum Graecorum*.

Kgl. u. Univ. Bibl. (Königlich- und Universitätsbibliothek [Royal and University Library])

This library was heavily damaged during World War II. Holdings can be found in the collections of libraries in (alphabetical order of country names): Germany, Lithuania, Netherlands, Poland, and Russia (Päsler 2007).

Dietz-Nachlaß (Dietz's Legacy)

These were volumes owned by Friedrich Reinhold Dietz (1804-1836), which have been bequeathed by his widow to Königsberg University Library.

On the two items below, see Touwaide 2009: 494-495 (particularly n332).

According to Rivier 1962: 285n3, reporting information provided at that time by Karl Deichgräber (1903-1984), these items are considered lost "since the events of 1945" (translation is mine).

[0438]   **I 1-3**   I.3.

This is a copy of Kühn's edition of Hippocrates, *Opera omnia* (3 vols., Leipzig, 1825-1827) with collations of manuscripts by Dietz.

On the manuscripts collated by Dietz, see Touwaide 2009: 492n310.

[0439]   **I 4**   I.3.

According to Diels' catalogue, this is a copy of the edition of Hippocrates, *De morbo sacro* by Dietz (Leipzig, 1827; on this edition, see Touwaide 2009: 492n310), with Dietz's handwritten notes and collations of manuscripts.

Konstantinopel (former Byzantine empire. Currently Istanbul [TR])

The items [0440]-[0443] mentioned without library name or collection in Constantinople are listed in two of the eight catalogues of Constantinopolitan libraries contained in the manuscript *historicus graecus* 98 of the Österreichische Nationalbibliothek in Vienna (on which see Hunger 1961: 107).

Items [1752], [1753] and [1754] (listed in Diels' catalogue under Wien, Hofbibliothek) need to be added to these four numbers. [1752] and [1753] appear in the same catalogue as [0440] and [0441]. [1753] is a duplicate of [0440]. [1754] is listed in the same catalogue as [0442] and [0443].

These catalogues were first published anonymously in 1578 by the German scholar Iohannes Hartung (1505-1579) in a booklet entitled *Bibliotheca Sive Antiquitates Urbis Constantinopolitanae* (= Hartung 1578). They have been reproduced ("plagiarized" according to Lauxtermann 2013: 272n9) by several humanists among whom the French Antoine du Verdier (1544-1600), cited in Diels' catalogue ([0440] and [0441]) (du Verdier, *Supplementum Epitomes Bibliothecae Gesnerianae*, 1585, pp. 56-64). du Verdier's edition has been corrected by Adam František Kollar (1718-1783) in his edition of Peter Lambeck's catalogue of the manuscripts in the imperial library in Vienna (Kollar 1766-1782; see vol. 1 [1766]: 268-276) referred to in numbers [1752] and [1753]. A new edition of these catalogues was published in 1877 by Richard Foerster (1843-1922) in his work *De antiquitatibus et libris manuscriptis Constantinopolitanis commentatio*, 1877, referred to in [0442]. More recently Georgios K. Papazoglou has republished these lists with a study (Papazoglou 1983; for the edition of the lists, see 371-412). On these catalogues, see recently Lauxtermann 2013.

For items [0440] and [0441] Diels' catalogue refers to du Verdier's edition of one of the library catalogues of manuscripts that is entitled as follows (du Verdier 1585: 57, col. 2, ll. 9-11):

Ex catalogo librorum hinc inde extantium à Grammatico exhibito, continenti libros 174.

Corrections to du Verdier's edition can be found in Kollar (ed. Lambeck) 1776: 269-273. They are referred to in [1752] and [1753].

The first edition of this catalogue is by Hartung 1578: [Bi]v-Ciiv. For more recent editions, see Foerster 1877: 19-23; Przychocki 1938: 34-42; Papazoglou 1983: 379-389.

As early as 1897, Karl Krumbacher deemed this catalogue (as well as all the others in the manuscript *Vindobonensis historicus graecus* 98) as a forgery (Krumbacher 1897: 411-412). All subsequent studies have confirmed that the catalogue of the collection owned by the *Grammaticus* is a forgery (Przychocki 1938; Maas 1938; Lauxtermann 2013: 278-279).

Item [0442] includes references to Foerster 1877 and Costomiris 1889.

Foerster 1877: 27-29, provides an edition of all the catalogues contained in the manuscript *Vindobonensis historicus graecus* 98, including the following (Foerster 1877: 27, col. 1, ll. 1-2):

ταῦτά εἰσι τὰ βιβλία τοῦ ἐνδοξοτάτου ἄρχοντος κυροῦ μιχαὴλ τοῦ καντακουζηνοῦ

This is the catalogue of the library owned by Michael Cantacuzenus nicknamed Şeytanoğlu (d. 1578). For a more recent edition, see Papazoglou 1983: 397-403. On him, see Papazoglou 1983: 327-329, and Papazoglou 1988.

In Diels' catalogue item [0443] does not include a reference to any previous literature. However, this item probably reproduces the information of Ackermann 1821: CLX, no. 104 (without brackets or question mark), where the manuscript is identified as having been in the collection of Michael Cantacuzenus. Furthermore, a reference to du Verdier (i.e. du Verdier 1585) appears in Ackermann ("Verdier p. 62"). Indeed, du Verdier 1585: 62, provides the edition of the catalogue of the library of Michael Cantacuzenus (p. 62 for the catalogue, and 62, col. 1, ll. 3-5 for its title). This catalogue was first published by Hartung 1578: Eir-Eiiir. Corrections to du Verdier's edition are found in Kollar (ed. Lambeck) 1776: 275-276. Besides Foerster 1877: 27-29, the catalogue has been reedited by Papazoglou 1983: 397-403. This collection was auctioned after the owner's death.

Item [1754] is explicitly identified in Diels' catalogue as possibly coming from Michael Cantacuzenus' collection.

–

[0440]   **[apud Verdier]**   I.124.

This is a copy of Galenus, *Hippocratis liber resolutionis, quem Galenus explicat.*

Some slightly more complete information appears in Ackermann 1821: CLXXXVII, ll. 22-24:

Hippocratis liber resolutionis, quem Galenus explicat, et Galenum Mich. Psellus. Verdier.

The reference to "[apud Verdier]" in Diels' catalogue and to "Verdier" in Ackermann is to du Verdier 1585: 59, col. 1, ll. 48-49:

Hippocratis in libros Resolutionis quattuor quos Galenus explicat, & in Galeni explicationem Michael Psellus.

Kollar 1766-1782: 1.273, ll. 12-17, provides the Greek version of this title:

Ibidem: (i.e., "In Catalogo librorum 174, a Grammatico quodam exhibito [Id.: 1.269, ll. 1-2]) *Hippocratis in libros resolutionis quattuor, quos Galenus explicat.* In Codice Caesareo (i.e. in *Vindobonensis historicus graecus* 98) legitur: Τοῦ Ἱπποκράτους εἰς τὰ ἀναλυτικὰ βιβλία δεκατέσσερα. Καὶ ἐξεγεῖται αὐτὰ ὁ Γαληνός.

This notice of Kollar is reproduced in Ackermann 1821: CLXXXIX, § 3, including the reference to Kollar.

In the first edition of the catalogue by Hartung 1578: Ciir, no. 154, this item is identified as follows:

154. Hippocratis in libros Resolutionis quattuor, quos Galenus explicat, et in Galeni Explicationem Michaël Psellus.

In Foerster 1877: 23, col. 1, no. ρνγ´ this item is described as follows:

τοῦ Ἱπποκράτους εἰς τὰ ἀναλυτικὰ βιβλία δεκατέσσαρα, καὶ ἐξηγεῖται αὐτὰ ὁ γαληνός, καὶ πάλε εἰς τοῦ γαληνοῦ τὴν ἐξήγησιν ἔχει ἑρμηνεία ὁ σοφώτατος μιχαὴλ ὁ ψελλός

Recent edition by Przychocki 1938: 41, and Papazoglou 1983: 388.

See also Costomiris 1889: 382, which repeats the information of Kollar 1766-1782, and Foerster 1877.

The correction to du Verdier 1585 by Kollar 1766-1782 (above) is referred to in Diels' catalogue (= [1753]) as if it were about another copy of the same text in Vienna, when it actually duplicates the present item.

Since this catalogue is considered to be a forgery, this item probably does not correspond to any preserved manuscript. See also Papazoglou 1983: 193, no. 153.

[0441]   **[ap. Verdier II 57]**   I.148.

According to Diels' catalogue, this item contains Galenus, *Excerpta*.

The reference to "Verdier II 57" is to du Verdier 1585: 57, that is, the list of the manuscripts owned by an unidentified Constantinopolitan *Grammaticus*, where, however, no manuscript identified as in Diels' catalogue can be found.

No such item appears in the other editions of the same catalogue: Hartung 1578: [Bi]v-Ciiv; Foerster 1877: 19-23; Przychocki 1938: 34-42; Papazoglou 1983: 379-389.

[0442]   **[Cod. Mich. Cantacuzeni]**   I.116, 123, 132.

These three mentions of a manuscript owned by Michael Cantacuzenus in Diels' catalogue include references to Foerster 1877 and Costomiris 1889. The texts they are related to are identified as follows in Diels' catalogue (including the bibliographical information):

- Galenus, *De ventis, igne, aquis, terra* (I.116) ("bei Foerster de antiquit. et libr. mss. Constantinopol. p. 27 und Costomiris Rev. des ét. gr. II p. 382/383 no. ΛΔ' ");

- Galenus, *De medicis* (I.123) ("bei Foerster de antiquit. et libr. mss. Constantinopol. p. 27 und Costomiris Rev. des ét. gr. II p. 382/3 no. ΛΓ' Γαλ. Π. ἰατρῶν διδασκάλων καὶ μαθητῶν");

- Galenus, *De materia medica* (I.132) ("bei Foerster de antiquit. et libr. mss. Constantinopol. p. 27 und Costomiris Rev. des ét. gr. II p. 382/383 no. Λ' ").

The references to Foerster are to Foerster 1877: 27-29, that is, the edition of the list of books owned by Michael Cantacuzenus, with the following items (together with references to Costomiris 1889 as provided in Diels' catalogue):

- λδ΄ τοῦ αὐτοῦ γαληνοῦ περὶ ἀνέμων, περὶ πυρός, περὶ ὕδατος ὀμβρίου καὶ ὕδατος ποταμοῦ καὶ ὕδατος θαλασσίου καὶ ὕδατος λίμνης καὶ ὕδατος φρέατος, ἔτι καὶ γῆς λευκῆς καὶ κοκκίνης · καὶ τὸ χαρτὶ ἔνε βεβράϊνο (reproduced in Costomiris 1889: 382, no. λδ΄);

- λγ΄ τοῦ αὐτοῦ γαληνοῦ περὶ ἰατρῶν διδασκάλων καὶ μαθητῶν · καὶ τὸ χάρτι ἔνε βεβράϊνο (reproduced in Costomiris 1889: 382, no. λγ΄);

- λ΄ τοῦ αὐτοῦ γαληνοῦ περὶ ὕλης ἰατρικῆς · καὶ τὸ χάρτι ἔνε βεβράϊνο (reproduced in Costomiris 1889: 382, no. λ΄).

For a more recent edition, see Papazoglou 1983: 400.

The current location of this manuscript (or these manuscripts) is unknown. See also Papazoglou 1983: 344-345, no. 34 (about item λδ΄), and 344, no. 30 (about item λ΄), and below [1754].

[0443]   **[Cod. Mich Cantacuzeni ?]**   I.116.

This is supposed to be a copy of Galenus, *De anatomia vivorum*.

A treatise *De anatomia vivorum* by Galen is mentioned in Ackermann 1821: CLX, no. 104 (without brackets or question mark), with the following reference to a manuscript (*ibid.*, ll. 5-4 *ab imo*):

Codex erat in bibl. Mich. Cantacuzeni. Verdier p. 62.

The reference is to du Verdier 1585: 62, col. 1, l. 2 *ab imo*, where the following item is listed among the books "illustriss. Domini Michaelis Cantacuzeni" (62, col. 1, ll. 3-5):

Galenus de Anatome animalium vivorum.

The same description is provided by Hartung 1578: Eiir, l. 9.

Foerster 1877: 27, col. 2, ll. 35-36 provides the Greek title of this item:

κε΄ ἰατροσόφιον γαληνοῦ περὶ ἀνατομῆς τῶν ζώντων · καὶ τὸ χάρτι ἔνε βιββάκινο.

Recent edition in Papazoglou 1983: 400.

The current location of this item is unknown. See also Papazoglou 1983: 344, no. 25, and also below [1754].

Bibl. d. Serail (Bibliothek der Serail [Serail Library]), actually Topkapı Sarayı Kütüphanesi (Topkapi Serail Library)

–

[0444]   **11**   I.3, 58.

Deissmann 1933: 57.

The current location of this item is unknown.

København (Copenhagen) (DK)

  See **Kopenhagen** (see below, p. 102).

  Det Kongelige Bibliotek (The Royal Library)

    Add. (= Additional)

      277, 4°   Schartau 1994: 463-464.

                See [0449].

    e don. var. (= e donatione varirorum)

      14, 2°   Schartau 1994: 453-454.

                See [0450].

      29, 2°   Schartau 1994: 455-456.

                See [0451]. Also [0899] and possibly [0894].

      42, 4°   Schartau 1994: 457.

                See [0448]. Also [0890].

    Fabr. (= *Fabricii* or Fabricius' Samling [Collection of Johann Albert Fabricius [1668-1736])

      60, 4°   (ff. 33r-49v) Aristoteles, *Physiognomica*.

                Aristoteles graecus 1976: 390-391 and 488; Schartau 1994: 389-390.

      61, 4°   (pp. 98-101) Democritus, *Physica et mystica*.

                Schartau 1994: 391-394.

      93, 4°   Xenocrates, *De alimentis ex fluviatilibus*.

                Schartau 1994: 414.

  Gamle kongelige Samling (GkS) (General royal Collection)

      224, 2°   Schartau 1994: 84-87.

                See [0445].

      225, 2°   Schartau 1994: 88-90; Karas 1994 (where the manuscript is mistakenly identified as "245").

                See [0446].

      1628, 4°   Aristoteles, *Problemata* (frg.).

                Aristoteles graecus 1976: 389; Schartau 1994: 135-137.

      1648, 4°   Schartau 1994: 138-139.

                See [0447].

      2140, 4°   (pp. 105-128) Hero Alexandrinus, *De mensuris*.

                Schartau 1994: 218-219.

  NkS (Ny kongelig Samling [New royal Collection])

      5, 8°   (ff. 3r-6v) Epiphanius, *De duodecim gemmis*.

                Schartau 1994: 345-346.

Thott (Thottske Samling [collection of Otto Thott [1703-1785])

190   *Picturae plantarum desuntae ex Dioscoridis, De materia medica.*

Jørgensen 1926: 441-442; Touwaide 2006.

207, 2°   (ff. 66v-73r) Democritus, *Physica et mystica.*

Schartau 1994: 243-252.

Kopenhagen (Copenhagen) (DK)

See København (see above, p. 101).

Königl. Bibliothek (Königliche Bibliothek [Royal Library]), now Det Kongelige Bibliotek (The Royal Library)

Hauniens. ant. fund. reg. (*Hauniense antiquum fundum regis* [Haunia Ancient Collection of the King]), now Gamle kongelige Samling (GKS) (General royal Collection)

[0445]   **224**   I.4, 5, 8, 10, 11 (3), 12, 13, 17, 18, 19 (2), 20 (3), 21, 22 (2), 23 (2), 24 (3), 25 (2), 26 (2), 27 (3), 28 (2), 29 (3), 30 (2), 31 (2), 33 (2), 34 (3), 35 (2), 38, 39, 110; II.93.

Current shelfmark: GkS 224, 2°.

[0446]   **225**   I.66, 98, 99 (2), 148.

Current shelfmark: GkS 225, 2°.

[0447]   **1648**   I.111.

Current shelfmark: GkS 1648, 4°.

Bibl. Univ. (*Bibliotheca Universitatis* [University Library]), now at Det Kongelige Bibliotek (The Royal Library)

e donatione variorum 4°

[0448]   **42**   I.61.

Current shelfmark: e don. var. 42, 4°.

Also [0890].

[0449]   **277**   II.32.

Contrary to Diels' catalogue, this is not a manuscript of the e donatione variorum collection, but rather of the Additional collection.

Schartau 1994: 463-464.

Current shelfmark: Add. 277, 4°.

e donatione variorum Fol.

[0450]   **14**   I.89.

Current shelfmark: e don. var. 14, 2°.

[0451]   **29**   II.97.

Current shelfmark: e don. var. 29, 2°.

Same as [0899] and, possibly also, [0894].

Krakau (Kraków) (PL)

Bibl. Univ. Jagellon. (*Bibliotheca Universitatis Jagiellonensis* [Jagiellonian University Library]), now Biblioteca Jagiellońska, Uniwersytet Jagiellońska w Krakowie (Jagiellonian Library, Jagiellonian University, Kraków)

–

[0452]   **2526 FF VI 5** II.55, 63, 82, 102.

Gollob 1903: 23-25.

Current shelfmark: BJ 2526.

Kraków (PL)

Biblioteca Jagiellońska, Uniwersytet Jagiellońska w Krakowie (Jagiellonian Library, Jagiellonian University, Kraków)

BJ

2526   See [0452].

Ms. Graec. (aus der ehemaligen Preussischen Staatsbibliothek zu Berlin, zur Zeit in der Biblioteca Jagiellońska, Uniwersytet Jagiellońska w Krakowie [formerly at the Preussische Staatsbibliothek in Berlin, currently at the Jagiellonian Library, at the Jagiellonian University, Kraków])

folio

7   See [0109].

37   See [0111] and [0112].

quarto

5   See [0107] and [0152].

46   See [0153].

Leiden (NL)

Universiteitsbibliotheek (University Library)

Bibliothecae Publicae Graecae (BPG)

BPG 2A   See [0475].

BPG 6   See [0476].

BPG 16   See [0477].

BPG 62 A   See [0478].

BPG 67 B   (ff. 113v-135v) Synesius Cyrenensis, *De insomniis*.

de Meyïer and Hulshoff Pol 1965: 106-109.

BPG 67 O   See [0479].

BPG 100   Epiphanius, *De mensuris et ponderibus*.

de Meyïer and Hulshoff Pol 1965: 188.

Gronoviani (GRO)

> GRO 12   See [0480].

Perizoniani (PER)

> PER F. 6/I   (ff. 1r-2r) Demetrius Pepagomenus, *De podagra*.
> de Meyïer 1946: 5-6.

> PER F.6/II   (ff. 17v-18r) Aristoteles, *Physiognomonica*.
> de Meyïer 1946: 6-7.

> PER F. 7 A.   (ff. 143r-159r, 159r-169v, 175r-214r, 214r-239v) Nicander,
> *Theriaca* et *Alexipharmaca* (cum scholiis).
> de Meyïer 1946: 10-12.

Scaligeriani (SCA)

> SCA 18   See [0482] and [0483].

> SCA 71   See [0484].

Vossiani graeci folio (VGF)

> VGF 10   See [0506].

> VGF 10 III   Hippocrates: (ff. 1r-13v) *Aphorismi*; (ff. 13v-22r) *Prognostica*;
> (ff. 22r-26v) *De flatibus*; (ff. 26v-35r) *Vectiarius*; (ff. 35r-40r)
> *De natura ossium*; (ff. 40v-58r) *De fracturis*; (ff. 58r-61r) *De
> officina medici*; (ff. 61r-62r) *De exsectione foetus*; (ff. 62r-128r)
> *De mulierum affectibus*; (ff. 128r-138r) *De sterilibus*; (ff.
> 138r-143v) *De superfoetatione*; (ff. 143v-146r) *De septimestri
> partu*; (ff. Ff. 146r-147r) *De octimestri partu*; (ff. 147v-148r) *De
> virginum morbis*; (ff. 148r-166v) *De natura muliebri*; (f. 167r-
> v) *De exsectione pueri*; (ff. 167v-184v) *Praesagiorum libri II*; (ff.
> 184v-187r) *De fistulis*; (ff. 187r-188v) *De haemorrhoidibus*;
> (ff. 188v-195v) *Coa praesagia*; (ff. 196r-242v) *De morbis
> popularibus libri I-VI*.
> de Meyïer 1955: 13-14.
> See [0506] and possibly [0496].

> VGF 11   See [0487] and [0507].

> VGF 22   See [0508].

> VGF 25   See [0509].

> VGF 27   See [0510].

> VGF 29   See [0492].

> VGF 31   See [0511] and possibly [0493].

> VGF 32   See [0512].

> VGF 53   See [0513] and possibly [0488].

> VGF 58   See [0494] and [0514].

> VGF 59   See [0495] and [0515].

> VGF 65   See [0516].

Vossiani graeci octavo (VGO)

VGO 1	(f. 76r-76v, l. 3) Nemesius Emesenus, *De natura hominis* (frg.). de Meyïer 1955: 198-200; Morani 1981: 62.
VGO 7	See [0503].
VGO 10	Gregorius Nazianzenus, *De humana natura*. de Meyïer 1955: 210-211; Domiter 1999: 21.
VGO 18	See [0504].
VGO 19	See [0485].
VGO 20	See [0505].

Vossiani graeci quarto (VGQ)

VGQ 9	See [0497]. Also [0474].
VGQ 17	See [0491] and [0498].
VGQ 18/VIII	(ff. 94r-101v) Demetrius Pepagomenus, *De podagra*. de Meyïer 1955: 112-117 (especially 116).
VGQ 20/II	(f. 239v) Aetius Amidenus, *Libri medicinales*, 3.114. de Meyïer 1955: 118-124 (especially 120-121).
VGQ 28	(ff. 1r-13r) Adamantius, *Physiognomonica*; (f. 23r-v) *Fragmentum de colore sanguinis*. de Meyïer 1955: 131-132.
VGQ 38	See [0499].
VGQ 45	See [0500].
VGQ 49	(ff. 1r-130v) Achmet, *Oneirocriticon*. de Meyïer 1955: 157-158.
VGQ 50	See [0501] and also [0489].
VGQ 51	(ff. 39r-53v) Aristoteles, *Physiognomonica*; (frg.); (ff. 143v-144v) *Epistula Artaxerxis* (Hippocrates, 1-5). de Meyïer 1955: 159-161; *Aristoteles graecus* 1976: 403-404.
VGQ 54	See [0502].
VGQ 59	(ff. 135r-162r) Nicander, *Theriaca;* (ff. 162r-178r) Nicander, *Alexipharmaca*. de Meyïer 1955: 175-178.
VGQ 76	(f. 101v) *Nomina medicorum et philosophorum graecorum*. de Meyïer 1955: 192-196.

Vossiani miscellanei (VMI)

VMI 1	See [0517].
VMI 11	See [0518].
VMI 16/I	(ff. 18r-25v) Aristoteles, *Problemata* (frg.). de Meyïer 1955: 254-256.

VMI 18/V	(ff. 47r-49v) Maximus Planudes, *De urinis.*
	de Meyïer 1955: 257-260 (especially 259).
VMI 22	See [0519].

Vulcaniani (VUL)

VUL 43	See [0520].
VUL 53 B	*Excerpta brevissima ex Auctoribus medicis Graecis et Latinis.*
	Molhuysen 1910: 23.
VUL 56	See [0521].
VUL 57	See [0522].
VUL 90 B	"Videtur esse ex *Tractatu de Medicina* capitulum "Rusticis cura secundum Graecos", scil. quae prosunt contra pestem."
	Molhuysen 1910: 33.

Leipzig (DE)

Institut f. Geschichte der Medizin (Institute for the History of Medicine)

–

[0453]   –   N.29.

This item without a shelfmark is Galenus, *Opera varia.* It is actually a copy of the five-volume 1538 printed edition (Basel) with variant readings and collations by Leo Allatius (ca. 1586-1669).

This manuscript is now at the Universitätsbibliothek (University Library), shelfmark Sudhoff III 815 a-e.

Universitätsbibliothek (University Library), now Universitätsbibliothek "Bibliotheca Albertina" (University Library "Albertina Library")

Manuscripts are now identified as Cod. graec. with the number they have below.

–

[0454]   **50**   I.75, 85.

Gardthausen 1898: 71.

Current shelfmark: Cod. graec. 50.

[0455]   **51**   I.79, 96.

Gardthausen 1898: 71-72.

Current shelfmark: Cod. graec. 51.

[0456]   **52**   I.66, 100, 111.

Gardthausen 1898: 72-73.

Current shelfmark: Cod. graec. 52.

[0457]   **53**   I.93.

Gardthausen 1898: 73-74; von Gebhardt 1898: 464-465.

This manuscript is no longer available. It seems to have been destroyed during World War II.

[0458]   **54**   I.109.

Gardthausen 1898: 74.

19th-century manuscript (Karas 1994: 353).

[0459]   **55**   I.61.

Gardthausen 1898: 74; Karas 1994: 346.

Current shelfmark: Cod. graec. 55.

[0460]   **56**   I.103.

Gardthausen 1898: 74.

19th-century codex (Karas 1994: 353).

[0461]   57   I.58, 148.

Gardthausen 1898: 74-75.

18th/19th-century manuscript.

[0462]   **58**   I.58.

Gardthausen 1898: 75.

Recent scholarly manuscript.

[0463]   **59**   II.15, 71.

Gardthausen 1898: 75:

"Moderne Abschrift von Oribasius de laqueis et machinamentis und Apollonius Citiensis, Commentar zum Hippocrates, angefertigt von Fr. del Furia [Francisco del Furia (1777-1856)] in Florenz und K. G. Kühn [Karl Gottlob Kühn (1754-1840)]."

See Kollesch, Kudlien and Nickel 1965: 7.

[0464]   **60**   II.110.

Gardthausen 1898: 75.

18th-century copy (1786 and 1787) (Karas 1994: 385).

[0465]   **61**   I.3.

Gardthausen 1898: 75-76.

19th-century copy (Karas 1994: 383).

[0466]   **62**   II.77.

Gardthausen 1898: 76.

19th -century copy.

[0467]   **63 (ol. 1109 ?)** II.17, 17-18, 18 (2).

Gardthausen 1898: 76-77.

Number 1109 is an old shelfmark (it is written on the spine of the codex). It is not part of the current shelfmark of the manuscript.

Current shelfmark: Cod. graec. 63.

[0468]   **64**   II.15.

Gardthausen 1898: 77.

18th-century copy (Karas 1994: 340).

[0469]   **65**   II.6.

Gardthausen 1898: 77-78.

19th-century copy (Karas 1994: 340).

[0470]   **66**   II.24, 95.

Gardthausen 1898: 78-81; *CMAG* IV (Goldschmidt) 1932: 222-246.

17th-century copy.

            70   (f. 29r-v) Epiphanius, *De duodecim gemmis* (frg.).

Gardthausen 1898: 85-86.

Current shelfmark: Cod. graec. 70.

      Rep. I 92   *Iatrosofion* (15th century).

Naumann 1838: 126 no. CCCXCII.

Bibl. senat. (*Bibliotheca senatus* [Senate Library])

–

[0471]   **391**   II.6; N.43.

This manuscript is now at the Universitätsbibliothek (University Library), with the shelfmark Rep. I 36aa.

Naumann 1838: 126, no. CCCXCI.

18th-century copy.

Lesbos (Lesvos) (GR)

Bibl. tês tou Leimônos monês (Βιβλιοθήκη τῆς τοῦ Λειμῶνος Μονῆς [Library of the Limonos Monastery]), actually Καλλονή Λέσβου, Ιερά Μονή Λειμώνος (Kalloni, Lesvos, Limonos Monastery)

–

[0472]   **175**   I.56, 148; II.36, 40, 64.

Papadopoulos-Kerameus 1888: 101.

17th-century *iatrosofion*.

[0473]   **268**   II.20.

Papadopoulos-Kerameus 1888: 124-128; Karas 1994: 321, 341; Karas 1994: 341.

This is a 1552 codex containing a collection of theological texts, some of which include discussions on the human nature in the way of *iatrosofia*.

Leyden (Leiden) (NL)

   Universitäts-Bibliothek (Universiteitsbibliotheek [University Library])

     –

[0474]   **(Catal. p. 395)** II.88, 90.

> This item without collection name or shelfmark is listed among the copies of Rufus, *De vesicae renumque affectibus* (II.89) and *De corporis humani appellationibus* (II.90).

> The imprecise reference in Diels is to the catalogue by Senguerdii et al. 1716: 395, col. 2, ll. 35-37, where this item is described as follows:

> Rufi Ephesi Monobiblon [*sic*], de purgando. Ejusdem de affectionibus ἐν κύστει καὶ νεφροῖς. Manu recente. In charta. 9

> A reference as in Diels' catalogue is found in Daremberg 1879: X.

> This manuscript is *Vossianus graecus* Q 9 (= [0497]) (in this sense [about *De vesicae renumque affectibus*], see Sideras 1977: 14n2).

   B.P. (*Bibliotheca Publica* [Public Library]), now Bibliotheca Publica Graeca (BPG)

[0475]   **2 A**   I.93; II.97.

> de Meyïer and Hulshoff Pol 1965: 4.

> Current shelfmark: BPG 2 A.

[0476]   **6**   II.6.

> de Meyïer and Hulshoff Pol 1965: 9-10.

> Current shelfmark: BPG 6.

[0477]   **16**   I.96.

> de Meyïer and Hulshoff Pol 1965: 15-16.

> Current shelfmark: BPG 16.

[0478]   **62 A**   II.66.

> de Meyïer and Hulshoff Pol 1965: 95-96.

> Current shelfmark: BPG 62 A.

[0479]   **670**   I.3.

> Mistake (typo?): this is not 670, but rather 67 O.

> de Meyïer and Hulshoff Pol 1965: 121.

> Current shelfmark: BPG 67 O.

   Gron. (= *Gronoviani*, Abraham Gronow, also known as Gronovius [1695-1775])

[0480]   **12**   II.39.

> Geel 1852: 3-4.

> Current shelfmark: GRO 12.

Ruhnken (David Ruhnken [1723-1798])

[0481]   **11**   II.63.

Bibliotheca Academiae Lugduno-Batavae 1932: 78, no. 11.

18th-century collation of manuscripts of Erotianus by David Ruhnken (Geel 1852: 35, no. 120).

Current shelfmark: RUH 11.

Scal. (*Scaligerani*, Joseph Justus Scaliger [1540-1609])

[0482]   **18**   I.63, 64, 65, 78, 79 (2).

Molhuysen 1910: 4-5.

Copy by Joseph Justus Scaliger.

Current shelfmark: SCA 18.

Also [0483].

[0483]   **18 (?)**   I.78.

This copy of Galenus, *De differentiis morborum*, is the current codex *Scaligeranus* 18, ff. 60-65 (Molhuysen 1910: 4).

Same as [0482].

[0484]   **71**   I.5, 13, 56.

Molhuysen 1910: 27.

Current shelfmark: SCA 71.

Voss. (*Vossian,* Isaak Voss, also known as Vossius [1618-1689])

[0485]   –   II.44.

This manuscript without shelfmark is a copy of Hermes Trismegistus, *De succis plantarum.*

This is *Vossianus graecus* Octavo 19 (current shelfmark: VGO 19).

CCAG IX.2 (Weinstock) 1953: 96.

[0486]   [-]   I.120.

This item without shelfmark is a copy of Galenus, *De abortivo foetu* (on which text see [0189]). The same information (without brackets) appears in Ackermann 1821: CLXXXVIII, *sub titulo.*

No manuscript containing a text identified as *De abortivo foetu* can be found in the catalogue of Vossius' collection either in *C.M.A.* 1697: 2.1.57-72, or in the Leiden catalogue of Vossius' manuscripts, which predates Diels' catalogue (Senguerdii et al. 1716: 391-403).

[0487]   [?]   I.79.

This copy of Galenus, *De symptomatum differentiis* without shelfmark probably corresponds to the current *Vossianus graecus* F 11 (now VGF 11 = [0507]).

[0488]   [?]   I.92.

This manuscript without shelfmark is a copy of Galenus, *De methodo medendi* ("in. et fin. mut."). It probably corresponds to the current *Vossianus graecus* F 53 (current shelfmark: VGF 53) (= [0513]).

[0489]   **[Cat. bibl. Lugd. Bat. p. 398 n. 50]**   I.123.

This copy of Galenus, *Hippiatrosofion* is described as follows in the "Cat. bibl. Lugd. Bat." (= Senguerdii et al. 1716: 398, col. 1, ll. 4-11):

Hippiatrica cum figuris, & multum discrepantia ab editis ... 50

It corresponds to the current *Vossianus graecus* Q 50 (current shelfmark: VGQ 50) (= [0501]).

de Meyïer 1955: 158-159.

[0490]   **9**   II.71.

This codex is listed as a copy of Oribasius, *Medicae collectiones ad Iulianum*.

No *Leidensis Vossianus* contains Oribasius, either in Greek or in Latin (see the *Index auctorum* in de Meyïer 1955: 286-298 [Greek] and 299-301 [Latin]). This is probably *Vossianus Latinus* Q 9, which contains medical texts, though no mention of Oribasius (see de Meyïer 1975: 20-25).

[0491]   **[16]**   I.61.

This item is supposed to be a copy of Galenus, *Ars medica*.

No *Vossianus graecus* 16 (either folio or quarto) contains this work (see de Meyïer 1955: 19 [F 16] and 110-111 [Q 16]).

The only *Vossianus graecus* containing the treatise is the current *Vossianus graecus* Q 17 (current shelfmark: VGQ 17), ff. 1r-79v (= [0498]) (see de Meyïer 1955: 111-112).

See also Boudon 2002: 197n109 ctd. about this item, and 200 about VGQ 17.

[0492]   **29**   II.4.

This codex is a copy of Aelius Promotus, *Physica et Antipathetica*.

The only *Vossianus* manuscript containing such a text is the current *Vossianus graecus* F 29 (VGF 29), ff. 3-5 (de Meyïer 1955: 31; on the manuscript: *ibid.*: 31-32).

[0493]   **[31]**   I.127.

This copy of Galenus, *De urinis* is probably *Vossianus graecus* F 31 (current shelfmark: VGF 31 = [0511]), which contains at ff. 8v-10v a treatise *De urinis*, attributed, however, to Theophilus instead of Galen as in Diels' catalogue.

de Meyïer 1955: 33-34.

[0494]   **[58]**   I.99.

This manuscript is referenced among the copies of Galenus, *De theriaca ad Pisonem liber*.

The only *Vossianus* manuscript containing this text (actually a fragment) is the current *Vossianus graecus* F 58 (current shelfmark: VGF 58 = [0514]), ff. 232v-233.

de Meyïer 1955: 290; for the manuscript: *ibid.*: 66-68.

[0495]   **[2168]**   I.87.

This manuscript with an identifier that does not correspond to the shelfmark system of Leiden library, is a codex of Galenus, *De pulsuum differentiis libri IV*.

Number 2168 is not a shelfmark, but a sequential number in the catalogue of the manuscript collection of "doctissimi Isaaci Vossii canonici windesoriensis" published in *C.M.A.* 1697: 2.1.57-72 (the table of contents of *C.M.A.*1697, f. ****2r, col. 2, ultimae duo lineae adds "... qui [sc. codices] nunc servantur Lugduni Batavorum"). At 2.1.59, the content of codex 2168 is described as follows:

2168.57. Dioscorides de Plantis, ordine alphabetico digestus, & multum ab editis discrepans.

Idem de Venenatis & Alexipharmacis.

De divisione partium & stationum anni, & quaenam medicinae singulis conveniant temporibus secundum Aegyptios. Auctore ut videtur, Michaële Psello.

De Discrepantia pulsuum, quorum cognitio clarior facta post Galenum. Horum singulae formae & figurae in singulis describuntur morbis.

Ad varios morbos remedia utilissima.

This description allows for the identification of this item as *Vossianus graecus* F 59 (VGF 59) (= [0515]) in spite of the difference in the title *(De discrepantia pulsuum ...* for *De pulsuum differentiis).*

[0496]   **[2324]**   I.121.

This manuscript with an identifier that does not correspond to the shelfmark system in Leiden library, is a copy of Galenus, *De septimestri partu.*

Number 2324 is not a shelfmark, but a sequential number in the same catalogue as [0495] published in *C.M.A.* 1697: 2.1.57-72. At 2.1.62, the content of manuscript 2324 is identified as follows:

2324.213. Galenus de partu Septimestri.

The identification of this item is problematic. It seems that no *Vossianus graecus* contains such a treatise (de Meyïer 1955: 290 *sub nomine* Galenus). However, item 2124 (and not 2324) in *C.M.A.* 1697: 2.1.58, corresponding to the current *Vossianus graecus* F 10 (VGF 10) (= [0506]), was a set of four volumes described as follows in *C.M.A., ibid.*:

2124.13. Hippocratis opera omnia, cum expositionibus Galeni, Tomis IV.

Codex *Vossianus graecus* F 10 is currently made of 3 volumes (VGF 10^{I}, VGF 10^{II} and VGF 10^{III}), which contain most of the Hippocratic treatises (with some duplications). It may be the case that the fourth volume containing "Galeni expositiones" (as per *C.M.A., ibid.*) is now lost or that the identification of the author of the text referred to here is incorrect: instead of Galenus, it should be Hippocrates, since *De septimestri partu* is contained in VGF 10^{III}, ff. 143v-146r.

Information in Diels' catalogue comes from Ackermann 1821: CXLI, no. 70 (without brackets).

Possibly same as [0506].

Voss. 4° (*Vossiani* in quarto)

[0497]   **9**   II.88, 90.

de Meyïer 1955: 104.

Current shelfmark: VGQ 9.

Also [0474].

[0498]	**17**	I.61.
		de Meyïer 1955: 111-112.
		Current shelfmark: VGQ 17.
		See [0491].
[0499]	**38**	I.38.
		de Meyïer 1955: 145-147.
		Current shelfmark: VGQ 38.
[0500]	**45**	I.77, 78, 89, 95, 109, 112 (2).
		de Meyïer 1955: 154.
		Current shelfmark: VGQ 45.
[0501]	**50**	I.43.
		de Meyïer 1955: 158-159.
		Current shelfmark: VGQ 50.
		Also [0489].
[0502]	**54**	II.50.
		de Meyïer 1955: 163-172.
		Current shelfmark: VGQ 54.

Voss. 8° (*Vossiani* in octavo)

[0503]	**7**	I.49.
		de Meyïer 1955: 204-208.
		Current shelfmark: VGO 7.
[0504]	**18**	II.7, 92, 93.
		de Meyïer 1955: 220-221.
		Current shelfmark: VGO 18.
[0505]	**20**	II.108.
		de Meyïer 1955: 221-222.
		Current shelfmark: VGO 20.

Voss. fol. (*Vossiani* in folio)

[0506]	**10**	I.4, 5, 8, 10, 11 (2), 12, 17, 18, 19 (2), 20 (2), 21, 22 (2), 23, 24 (3), 25 (2), 26, 27, 29 (2), 30, 31 (2), 33, 34 (3), 35, 44, 46, 48 (2), 49; II.93.
		de Meyïer 1955: 11-14.
		Current shelfmark: VGF 10.
		Possibly [0496].
[0507]	**11**	I.79.
		de Meyïer 1955: 14-15.
		Current shelfmark: VGF 11.
		Also [0487].

[0508]   **22**   II.77.

de Meyïer 1955: 25-26.

Current shelfmark: VGF 22.

[0509]   **25**   II.26, 42.

de Meyïer 1955: 28.

Current shelfmark: VGF 25.

[0510]   **27**   I.66.

de Meyïer 1955: 29-30.

Current shelfmark: VGF 27.

[0511]   **31**   II.101.

de Meyïer 1955: 33-34.

Current shelfmark: VGF 31.

Possibly [0493].

[0512]   **32**   II.108, 109, 110.

de Meyïer 1955: 34-37.

Current shelfmark: VGF 32.

[0513]   **53**   I.85, 93.

de Meyïer 1955: 61.

Current shelfmark: VGF 53.

Possibly [0488].

[0514]   **58**   II.6, 30.

de Meyïer 1955: 66-68.

Current shelfmark: VGF 58.

Contrary to Petit 2010: 146 (according to whom this manuscript is lost or cannot be found), this item still is on the shelves of Leiden Universiteitsbibliotheek.

Also [0494].

[0515]   **59**   II.33 (2), 34, 101.

de Meyïer 1955: 68-72.

Current shelfmark: VGF 59.

Also [0495].

[0516]   **65**   N.66.

de Meyïer 1955: 76-77.

Current shelfmark: VGF 65.

Voss. Miscell. (*Vossiani miscellanei*)

[0517]   **1 pars 13**   I.110.

This is a copy of Galenus, *Linguarum s. dictionum exoletarum Hippocratis explicatio.*

The mention "pars 13" is not an element of the shelfmark, but refers to the fact that, in the manuscript *Vossianus miscellaneus* 1, the text under consideration is the 13th.

de Meyïer 1955: 222-226 (especially 224-225).

Current shelfmark VMI 1.

[0518]   **11**   I.91-92, 93.

de Meyïer 1955: 245-246.

Current shelfmark: VMI 11.

[0519]   **22**   II.108.

de Meyïer 1955: 267-269.

Current shelfmark: VMI 22.

Vulc. (*Vulcaniani*, Bonaventura de Smet, also known as Vulcanius [1538-1614])

[0520]   **43**   I.87 (2), 88 (2).

Molhuysen 1910: 16-17.

Current shelfmark: VUL 43.

[0521]   **56**   I.40.

Molhuysen 1910: 23-25.

Current shelfmark: VUL 56.

[0522]   **57**   I.66.

Molhuysen 1910: 25.

Current shelfmark: VUL 57.

[0523]   **108 pars 15**   I.49.

The mention "pars 15" does not belong to the shelfmark, but indicates that the text referred to here is the 15th in the volume.

Molhuysen 1910: 49-51.

Fragments copied by Bonaventura Vulcanius.

Current shelfmark: VUL 108.

[Warnerian.] (*Warneriani*, Levinus Warner [ca. 1618-1665])

[0524]   **[53]**   I.127.

This is supposed to be a Greek manuscript of Galen, *De urinis*.

The information (without brackets) comes from Ackermann 1821: CLXVI, no. 119 ctd., ll. 6-9:

Collectanea ex Galeno de variis urinae quoad colorem generibus exstant inter libros legati Warneriani in bibl. Ac. Lugd. B. p. 407. no. 53.

This is an Arabic manuscript, with shelfmark Warner 53 (Or. 4791).

This item appears in the list of "Manuscripti Hebraici, Quos Bibliothecae legavit Nobilissimus Levinus Warnerus" (Senguerdii et al. 1716: 405; for the list, see 405-408), that is, the donation by Levinus Warner.

Number 53 (Senguerdii et al. 1716: 407, col. 2, ll. 24-22 *ab imo*, no. 53, as Ackermann correctly mentions) reads as follows:

Joannis Mesuae Medici Arabis Medicina. Ejusdem Antidota. Collectanea ex Galeno de variis Urinae quoad colorem generibus. 53.

Van Der Heide 1977: 37.

Livorno (IT)

Biblioteca Labronica (Labronica Library)

–

853 (12 d 18) (ff. 213r-223r) Serapion, *Simplicium medicinarum nomina graeca et latina.*
Mioni 1965: 1.123.

London (GB)

[Bibl. eccl. Westmonast.] (*Bibliotheca ecclesiae Westmonasteriensis* [Library of Westminster Church]), now Westminster Abbey Library

–

[0525]   **[1100]**   I.89.

This is supposed to be a manuscript of Galenus, *De crisibus.*

The same information (without brackets) appears in Ackermann 1821: CVIII, no. 43, where the manuscript is listed among the Greek codices of the treatise.

Number 1100 is not a shelfmark, but a sequential number in *C.M.A* 1697: 2.1.27 in the catalogue of manuscripts "ecclesiae Westmonasteriensis" (2.1.27-29). The manuscript is described as follows:

1100.10. Galenus περὶ κρίσεων

This item was lost in the fire that destroyed part of the Westminster Abbey collections in 1694. No mention of it appears in Alexanderson 1967.

Robinson and James 1909: 52, no. 1100 for the manuscript, and 21, 26 for the fire.

British Library

See **British Museum**, with the following collections:

Additional: see **Addit.** and **Addit. (Brit. Mus.)** (see below, pp. 117-118)

Arundel: see **Arundel.** (see below, p. 118).

Burney: see **Burneian.** (see below, p. 118).

Egerton

3154   *Geoponica.*
McKendrick 1999: 281.

Harley: see **Harleian.** (see below, pp. 118-119).

Royal: see **Regius.** (see below, p. 120).

Sloane: see **Sloan.** (see below, p. 120).

Stowe: see **Stowe.** (see below, p. 120).

British Museum (library collections are now at the British Library)

    Addit. (Additional)

      See also below **Addit. (Brit. Mus.).**

[0526]	**5108**	II.29.
		Richard 1952: 3.
	5119	(ff. 1r et seq.) *Tractatus de hominis anatomia*; (ff. 12r et seq.) *Glossarii medici et pharmaceutici fragmenta*; (ff. 15v, 22v) *Prescripta varia*; (ff. 32v et seq.) *Medicamenta e diversis medicis composta secundum expositionem Zenonis* [*sic*].
		Richard 1952: 4.
[0527]	**6898**	I.13, 92.
		Richard 1952: 6; Merolla 2010: 93.
		Formerly [1651].
[0528]	**8231**	II.34.
		Richard 1952: 8.
	8240	Nicephorus Constantinopolitanus Patriarcha, *Oneirocriticon*.
		Richard 1952: 9.
[0529]	**10,058**	I.114, 124, 125, 132-133; II.7, 14, 41, 58, 79, 80, 93.
		Richard 1952: 12-13.
[0530]	**11,888**	I.68, 111.
		Richard 1952: 20-21.
	14620	See [0534].
	17148	See [0535].
[0531]	**17,900**	I.127-128, 134; II. 10, 33, 54, 102 (2).
		Richard 1952: 29.
	23.927	Aristoteles, *Problemata*.
		Richard 1952: 43; *Aristoteles graecus* 1976: 456-458.
[0532]	**28,830**	I.42, 123.
		Richard 1952: 52.
[0533]	**34,060**	I.41.
		Richard 1952: 57-60.

    Addit. (Brit. Mus.) (Additional, British Museum)

[0534]	**14620**	N.50.
		Catalogue of Additions 1850: 83.

[0535]   **17148**   N.50.

Catalogue of Additions 1864: 372.

Arundel. (*Arundeliani*, Thomas Howard, 2nd Earl of Arundel [1585-1646])

[0536]   –   I.93.

The text referred to in this manuscript listed without shelfmark is Galenus, *Ad Glauconem de medendi methodo*, with the following information: "incipit f. 114".

This is Arundel 537, and the text can be found at ff. 114r-156r.

McKendrick 1999: 19.

Same as [0537].

516   (f. 356v) *De hominis natura.*

McKendrick 1999: 1-3.

[0537]   **537**   II.108, 109, 110.

McKendrick 1999: 19.

Also [0536].

[0538]   **538**   I.13, 17, 18, 20-21, 28, 29.

McKendrick 1999: 19-20.

Burneian. (*Burneiani*, Charles Burney [1757-1817])

52   (ff. 88v-130r) Gregorius Nyssenus, *De hominis opificio.*

McKendrick 1999: 38.

[0539]   **75**   II.61.

McKendrick 1999: 47-48.

[0540]   **94**   I.119; II.59, 71, 89 (2).

McKendrick 1999: 57-58.

97   (ff. 2r-45v) Manuel Philes, *De animalium proprietate.*

McKendrick 1999: 61-62.

[0541]   **523**   I.58.

McKendrick 1999: 83.

Harleian. (*Harleiani*, Robert Harley [1661-1724])

1686   *Geoponica.*

McKendrick 1999: 88.

1868   *Geoponica.*

McKendrick 1999: 92.

5564   (ff. 2r-20r) Epiphanius, *De duodecim gemmis*; (ff. 20v-21v) *De myrrhae praeparatione.*

McKendrick 1999: 111.

5576   (ff. 53r-72r) Gregorius Nyssenus, *De hominis opificio.*

McKendrick 1999: 116-117.

	5596	(ff. 50v-51r) *Plantae astrologicae.*
		McKendrick 1999: 123-124.
	5597/II	(ff. 9r-19v, 22r-42v) Artemidorus, *Oneirocritica.*
		McKendrick 1999: 124.
	5604	(ff. 1r-20v) Heron, *Geoponica*; (ff. 20v-164r) *Geoponica.*
		McKendrick 1999: 127.
[0542]	**5611**	I.105.
		McKendrick 1999: 129-130.
[0543]	**5625**	I.87 (2), 88 (2).
		McKendrick 1999: 138.
[0544]	**5626**	I.13, 41, 42, 75, 118, 123; II.3, 6, 15, 16-17, 56, 58, 91.
		McKendrick 1999: 139.
[0545]	**5635**	I. 38.
		McKendrick 1999: 143-145.
[0546]	**5651**	I.85.
		McKendrick 1999: 156.
[0547]	**5652**	I.68.
		McKendrick 1999: 156.
[0548]	**5679**	II.30, 32.
		McKendrick 1999: 169.
[0549]	**5685**	II.67.
		McKendrick 1999: 170.
	5726	*Geoponica.*
		McKendrick 1999: 178-179.
[0550]	**6295**	I.5, 13, 41, 46; II.9, 40, 65.
		McKendrick 1999: 197-198.
	6299	(ff. 46r-58r) Adamantius, *Physiognomonica.*
		McKendrick 1999: 200.
[0551]	**6301**	I.38.
		McKendrick 1999: 201.
[0552]	**6305**	I.89, 90, 117; II.7, 33, 79 (2), 106.
		McKendrick 1999: 202-203.
	6322	(ff. 252v-266v) Synesius Cyrenensis, *De insomniis.*
		McKendrick 1999: 208.
[0553]	**6326**	II.17, 18 (3).
		McKendrick 1999: 209-210.
		See possibly [0887] and [0904].

Regii (now Royal)

[0554]   **12 F III**   I.111.

This is not a Greek, but a Latin translation of [Galen], *Definitiones medicae*.

Warner and Gilson 1921: 2.62.

16.C.ii   *Praescriptiones medicae.*

McKendrick 1999: 228.

[0555]   **16 C XI**   I.90.

McKendrick 1999: 232.

Current shelfmark: Royal. 16.C.xi.

[0556]   **16. C. XVI**   I.5; II.19.

McKendrick 1999: 235.

Current shelfmark: Royal. 16.C.xvi.

16.D.i   (ff. 117v-143r) Gregorius Nyssenus, *De hominis opificio*.

McKendrick 1999: 240-242.

[0557]   **[1734, 4]**   I.5.

This seems to be a mistake, apparently referring to Harley 1734, ff. 105-105v (previously pp. 205-206), which contains an English version of Hippocrates, *Prognostic*. The number 4 following the shelfmark might refer to the fact that the *Prognostic* is the fourth text in the codex.

This manuscript does not appear in Alexanderson 1963.

Sloan. (Sir Hans Sloane [1660-1753])

[0558]   **804**   II.32.

Richard 1952: 1.

[0559]   **2434**   II.6.

Richard 1952: 2.

Stowe (collection of Richard Temple-Nugent-Brydges-Chandos-Grenville, 1st Duke of Buckingham and Chandos [1776-1839]), at Stowe House, near Buckingham)

[0560]   **1073**   I.5, 13, 17, 18, 77.

Richard 1952: 89.

Lambeth Palace, Archiepiscopal Library

1204   (ff. 1r-58v) Aristoteles, *Problemata*.

Aristoteles graecus 1976: 459-462.

Medical Society

This collection was purchased in 1984 by the Wellcome Library. The manuscripts are identified with a shelfmark MSL = Medical Society, London.

[0561]   –   I.150.

This manuscript listed without shelfmark in Diels' catalogue, which contains *Indices in Galenum*, is now London, Wellcome Library, MS. MSL 83. It is listed in Diels' catalogue with a reference to "Costomiris Revue des études grecques II [1889] p. 381."

According to Costomiris 1889: 381, this is "a very detailed table of author names cited by Galen with references to the Basel edition ... in a recent script." (translation is mine).

Costomiris (381n3) referencing Daremberg 1853: 164, states that the hand is "recent".

[0562]   **AA a 1 = Xa 32**   I.40, 41, 47.

Current shelfmark: London, Wellcome Library, MS. MSL 14.

[0563]   **A Ac 2 = Wf 15**   II.77.

Current shelfmark: London, Wellcome Library, MS. MSL 114.

[0564]   **HHi 17 = We 30**   I.5, 13, 48, 100, 115, 125, 128, 131, 132-133; II.7, 79, 80, 98, 101, 102, 109.

Current shelfmark: London, Wellcome Library, MS. MSL 60.

[0565]   **HH i 21. 22 = We 28. 29**   I.41, 131; II.7, 102, 108-109, 109, 110.

Current shelfmark: London, Wellcome Library, MS. MSL52 A&B.

See also [0568].

[0566]   **H Hi 23 = We 32a**   II.17, 18 (3), 89 (2).

Current shelfmark: London, Wellcome Library, MS. MSL 62.

[0567]   **NNa 11 = Wf 8**   II.110.

Current shelfmark: London, Wellcome Library, MS. MSL 112.

[0568]   **We 29**   II.48.

Same as [0565], vol. B.

[0569]   **Wf 6**   II.71.

Current shelfmark: London, Wellcome Library, MS. MSL 126.

[0570]   **Wf 7**   II.6.

Current shelfmark: London, Wellcome Library, MS. MSL 109.

[0571]   **Wf 16**   II.109.

Current shelfmark: London, Wellcome Library, MS. MSL 124.

Natural History Museum

Banks MSS (Sir Joseph Banks [1734-1820])

63   Dioscorides, *De materia medica*, imagines plantarum.

No printed catalogue is currently available.

Wellcome Library

MS. 289   *Definitiones medicae (graecae)*

Moorat 1962: 184; Bouras-Vallianatos 2015: 316-317.

MS. 354   (ff. 1r-18v) Damascius, *Commentarius in Hippocratis Aphorismos* (frg.); (ff. 18v-21v) Hippocrates, *Prognosticon*; (ff. 22r-107v) Stephanus Alexandrinus, *Commentarius in Hippocratis Prognosticon*.

Moorat 1962: 225-226; Bouras-Vallianatos 2015: 317-318.

MS. MSL 14   See [0562].

Dawson 1932: 24; Bouras-Vallianatos 2015: 283-286.

MS. MSL 52   See [0565]; also [0568].

A&B   Dawson 1932: 59-60; Bouras-Vallianatos 2015: 286-292.

MS. MSL 60   See [0564].

Dawson 1932: 68-72; Bouras-Vallianatos 2015: 292-302.

MS. MSL 62   See [0566].

Dawson 1932: 74; Bouras-Vallianatos 2015: 302-305.

MS. MSL 83   See [0561].

Dawson 1932: 91.

MS. MSL 109   See [0570].

Dawson 1932: 112; Bouras-Vallianatos 2015: 305-307.

MS. MSL 112   See [0567].

Dawson 1932: 114; Bouras-Vallianatos 2015: 307-308.

MS. MSL 114   See [0563].

Dawson 1932: 115-116; Bouras-Vallianatos 2015: 308-311.

MS. MSL 124   See [0571].

Dawson 1932: 120-121; Bouras-Vallianatos 2015: 311-313.

MS. MSL 126   See [0569].

Dawson 1932: 122-123; Bouras-Vallianatos 2015: 316.

MS. MSL 135 — Theophanes Nonnus (Chrysobalantes): (ff. 4-96) *Epitome*; (ff. 96-110) *Synopsis de remediis*; (ff. 110v-154) Psellus, *De victu ratione*.

Dawson 1932: 130-131; Bouras-Vallianatos 2015: 314-316.

Los Angeles, CA (US)

The J. Paul Getty Museum

Ms. Ludwig

XV 2 — (ff. 3r-41v) Angelus Gregorius, *Physiologia* (with a table of content on f. 1r-v).

von Euw and Plotzek 1985: 155-171 (+ ills. 51-66).

Former Phillipps 7715 (Sotheby 1971: 78-81, lot 515 [+ plates 18-20]).

University of California, Louise M. Darling Biomedical Library

History and Special Collections, Benjamin MSS

MS 14 — (ff. 1r-20v) *Lexicon plantarum*; (ff. 21r-29v) *Iatrosofion*; (ff. 29v-34r) Diocles, *Epistula de sanitate tuenda*; (ff. 36r-42r) *De pulsibus*; (f. 42r-v) *De urinis*; (ff. 42v-56r) *Aphorismata medica*; (ff. 56r-60v) *De excrementis*; (ff. 60v-64r) *Formulae antidotorum*; (ff.64r-70v) *Iatrosofion*; (ff.71r-79v) Symeon Seth, *De alimentorum facultatibus* (frg.); (ff. 80r-91v) *Iatrosofion*; (ff. 92r-131r) *Iatrosofion*; (ff. 132r-142v) *Phlebotomia*.

Faye and Bond 1962: 408-409, where the manuscript is listed under Rochester, NY, "The Library of Dr. J. A. Benjamin, Strong Memorial Hospital, The University of Rochester". It was donated in 1963 to the University of California, Los Angeles (Ferrari 1991: 26). Also O'Malley and Gnudi 1968: 4.

Lyon (FR)

Bibliothèque de la ville (City Library), now Bibliothèque municipale (Municipal Library)

–

[0572]   **52**   II.67.

Omont 1886/2: 38-39 (no. 47 [52]) followed by Omont 1886-1888: 3. 371, no. 52 [52], and *Catalogue général des manuscrits* 1900: 18-19 (where the manuscript has an incorrect sequential number: 51 instead of 52 [Olivier 1995: 511n1]).

This is now manuscript 122 in the collection of the Bibliothèque municipale.

16th/17th century scholarly manuscript.

Madrid (ES)

–

–

[0573]   **Matrit. 166**   II.53.

This manuscript listed without library name or collection in Diels' catalogue, is mentioned regarding codex Escurial, I II 14, which contains Johannes Damascenus, *Excerpta*. The manuscript is listed as a copy of these excerpts.

The identification "Matrit. 166" is a deformation of N 166, which is an earlier shelfmark of the current manuscript Vitr. 26-1 in the collection of the Biblioteca Nacional (National Library; see p. 127) (see de Andrés 1987: 530-532).

This is not a manuscript of Ioannes Damascenus, *Excerpta*, as Diels' catalogue suggests, but a copy of the *Efodia*, whose text contains a fragment of Ioannes Damascenus' work on f. 212r, as Diels' catalogue rightly indicates.

Same as Madrid, Biblioteca Nacional, Vitr. 26-1 (see p. 127), and also [0586] and [0587].

Bibl. Univ. (*Biblioteca universitaria* [University Library]), now Biblioteca de la Universidad Complutense (Library of Complutense University)

–

[0574]   **30**   II.36.

Villa-Amil y Castro 1878: 8.

Now Biblioteca de la Universidad Complutense, 116-zo-22.

Biblioteca Nacional (National Library)

See **Nationalbibliothek** (below).

Biblioteca de la Universidad Complutense (Library of Complutense University)

–

116-z°-22   See [0574].

de Andrés 1974: 239-244.

Nationalbibliothek (Biblioteca Nacional [National Library])

Except for [0581], [0585] and [0586], the shelfmark of the items of the Biblioteca Nacional in Diels' catalogue include a previous shelfmark between parentheses (identified as "olim" or "ol." except in [0575] and [0579]). These old shelfmarks are made of a capital Latin letter ("N" and "O") followed by a number in Arabic numerals. [0587] is identified by means of a shelfmark according to this system without the recent one. In [0575], [0577], and [0580] this old shelfmark is incorrect.

These old shelfmarks can be found in Iriarte 1769 (for shelfmarks N 1-N 125), Miller 1886 (for shelfmarks N 126-N 141 and O 1-O 103), and Vieillefond 1934 (for shelfmarks N 142-N 175 and O 100-O 132). A table of concordance between these and the current shelfmarks can be found in de Andrés 1987: 619-621.

–

4552   (ff. 29r-33r) *Physiologus* (frg.).

de Andrés 1987: 11-15.

[0575]	**4557 (N 119)**	I.38.
		The old shelfmark was N 19 and not N 119 (Iriarte 1769: 71-81 for N 19).
		de Andrés 1987: 26-27.
	4563	(ff. 103r-105v) Aristoteles, *De insomniis*.
		Wartelle 1963: 61, no. 862 (the manuscript is identified as N 26); de Andrés 1987: 38-40.
[0576]	**4581 (olim N 45)**	II.77.
		de Andrés 1987: 65-66.
	4610	(ff. 25v-60v) Gregorius Nyssenus, *De hominis opificio*.
		de Andrés 1987: 115-116.
[0577]	**4616 (olim N 48)**	II.82.
		Mistake for 4616 (olim N 84) (= [0578]).
[0578]	**4616 (olim N 84)**	II.9, 22, 34, 77, 80, 87.
		de Andrés 1987: 126-130; *CMAG* V (Zuretti and Severyns) 1928: 93.
		Also [0577].
	4622	(ff. 219r-220v) Adamantius, *Physiognomonica*.
		de Andrés 1987: 142-143.
	4624	(ff. 62v-78v) Synesius Cyrenensis, *De insomniis*.
		de Andrés 1987: 145-146.
[0579]	**4631 (N 110)**	I.126; II.7, 34, 36, 41 (2), 43, 77, 79, 80, 87.
		de Andrés 1987: 158-160; *CMAG* V (Zuretti and Severyns) 1928: 75-92, 100-110.
[0580]	**4634 (olim N 112)**	I.5, 13.
		The old shelfmark was N 113 and not N 112 (Iriarte 1769: 447 for N 113).
		de Andrés 1987: 164-165.
[0581]	**4636**	II.50.
		de Andrés 1987: 169-174.
		Also [0582].
[0582]	**4636 (ol. N 115)**	II.89.
		Same as [0581].
	4681	(ff. 18r-64v) Michael Psellus, *Syntagma diaeteticum*.
		de Andrés 1987: 232-234.
	4684	(ff. 254-256) Aristoteles, *Problemata* (frg.).
		Wartelle 1963: 61, no. 867 (the manuscript is identified as N 54); de Andrés 1987: 238-240.

	4758	(ff. 75r-86v) Nemesius Emesenus, *De natura hominis* (frg.)
		de Andrés 1987: 352-354.
[0583]	**4759**	II.28, 67.
	(olim N 138)	de Andrés 1987: 354-356.
[0584]	**4783**	I.112.
	(olim O 67)	de Andrés 1987: 383-385.
	4806	(ff. 155r-242v) Gregorius Nyssenus, *De hominis opificio.*
		de Andrés 1987: 420-423.
	4818	(ff. 1v-6v) Antonius Calosynas, *De alimentis.*
		de Andrés 1987: 435-436.
	4848	(ff. 111r-124v) Basilius Caesariensis, *De hominis opificio.*
		de Andrés 1987: 463-464.

4850   (ff. 1r-31v) Symeon Seth, *De alimentorum facultatibus*; (ff. 35r-113v) *Remedia et antidota morborum*; (ff. 113v-120r) Michael Psellus, *De diaeta*; (ff. 146r-147v) *Quid est homo?*; (ff. 148r-163v) Hippocrates, *Prognosticon*; (ff. 164r-169v) Theophilus, *De excrementis*; (ff. 170r-173r) Palladius, *De febribus*; (ff. 175r-184v) *Cataplasmata*; (ff. 185r-194r) Hippocrates, *Aphorismi*; (ff. 196r-197v) *Synopsis de urinis*; (ff. 197v-207v) Galenus, *De signis et causis morborum et de methodo medendi* (frg.); (ff. 208r-235v) Michael Psellus, *De alimentorum facultatibus*; (ff. 245r-256v, 264r-284v, 257r-v) *Remedia*; (ff. 257v-261r) *Synopsis de urinis.*

de Andrés 1987: 465-468.

[0585]	**4861**	II.39.
		de Andrés 1987: 480-482.
[0586]	**9715**	II.110.

The number 9175 is not a shelfmark in the collections of the Biblioteca Nacional (National Library) in Madrid, but an incorrect reproduction of the shelfmark 97.15 that the manuscript had when it was preserved in the collection of the Biblioteca del Cabildo de Toledo (Chapter's Library, Toledo Cathedral) (see Graux, ed. Martin 1892: 275-278, and also Vieillefond 1935: 210). Shelfmark 97.15 is correctly mentioned in [0587].

This is the current Vitr. 26-1, on which see [0573] and [0587], and also below.

[0587]   **N 116 (ol. Tolet. 97.15)**   II.85.

These are shelfmarks from two different collections in which the manuscript was preserved:

- N 116 refers to the collection of the former *Regia Biblioteca Matritensis* (Royal Library in Madrid). However, it is mistaken, as the codex formerly identified as N 116 (corresponding to the current 4637 of the Biblioteca Nacional; see de Andrés 1987: 174-177) contains a *Collectio epistularum* (Iriarte 1769: 466-475). Exact shelfmark is N 166 (on which see Vieillefond 1935: 210).

  Number 166 is mentioned in [0573] in a partially incorrect way (the initial capital letter "N" is missing) and without location.

- The shelfmark "olim Toletanus 97.25" refers to the collection of the Biblioteca del Cabildo de Toledo (Chapter's Library, Toledo Cathedral) (see Graux, ed. Martin 1892: 275-278, and Vieillefond 1935: 210).

This is the current Vitr. 26-1.

Same as [0573], [0586], and Vitr. 26-1 (below).

Vitr. 26-1   See [0573], [0586] and [0587].

de Andrés 1987: 530-532.

Privatbibliothek des Königs (Real Biblioteca [Royal Library], actually Biblioteca del Palacio [Palace Library])

These manuscripts once belonged to the Colegios Mayores at Salamanca, which were suppressed in 1798. Their books were confiscated under King Carlos IV (king 1789-1809) and sent to the royal palace in Madrid. They were returned to Salamanca University in 1954, and are now at the Biblioteca universitaria (University Library) (see Fink-Errera 1959), on which see below, pp. 309-310.

Their shelfmarks in Diels' catalogue are not those of the codices in the royal library (which can be found on the ex-libris dating back to King Ferdinand VII [king 1808 and 1813-1833] on the back of the anterior cover; on these shelfmarks, see Beaujouan 1962: 48-51), but, rather, are those attributed to the manuscripts by Charles Graux (1852-1882) in the printed version of his catalogue of this collection (Graux, ed. Martin 1892).

The shelfmarks between parentheses with the mention "ol." (= olim) that follows the shelfmark as above in Diels' catalogue, are not old shelfmarks as the term *olim* indicates. Instead, they are those attributed to the manuscripts by Graux in the first version of his catalogue (on which see Graux 1879: 121-122).

Both these first and second shelfmarks have been written in the manuscripts: the first on the ex-libris dating back to King Ferdinand VII and the second on the guard leaves.

[0588]   **14 (ol. 13)**   II.39-40.

This copy of Gregorius Nyssenus, *De hominis opificio* is now Salamanca, Biblioteca universitaria, 2710 (see p. 310).

Graux, ed. Martin 1892: 76-77, no. 14;

[0589]   **44 (ol. 23)**   I.122; II.30, 32 (2).

This copy of Galenus, *De theriaca*, and Dioscorides, *De materia medica* (followed by the two treatises *De venenis* and *De animalibus venenosis* ascribed to Dioscorides) is now Salamanca, Biblioteca universitaria, 2659 (see p. 310).

Graux, ed. Martin 1892: 114-115, no. 44.

Mailand (Milano [Milan]) (IT)

Arch. del Capitolo Metropolitano (Archivio del Capitolo Metropolitano [Archives of the Metropolitan Chapter])

–

[0590]   **2**   I.117; II.30, 32 (2), 33, 34, 68, 79, 100.

Martini 1893: 42-45.

Current shelfmark: II, E 2, 17.

Bibl. Ambrosiana (Biblioteca Ambrosiana [Ambrosiana Library])

–

[0591]   –   N.36.

Refers to I.111, where *Ambrosianus* Q 3 sup. (= [0647]), f. 202, is listed about Galenus, *Quod qualitates incorporeae sint*, and corrects the folio number into 202v.

[0592]   **v. Berthelot Ruelle, p. 56**   II.100.

This manuscript of Synesius Cyrenensis, *Ad Dioscorum, scholia in librum Democriti*, listed without shelfmark is identified by means of a reference to Berthelot and Ruelle, *Alchimistes grecs, Texte grec* (1888), p. 56, who identify it as "le cod. *Ambrosianus* de Milan", without any other element of identification.

Based on Martini and Bassi 1906, this item could correspond to three *Ambrosiani*:

- E 37 sup., ff. 301r et seq. (Martini and Bassi 1906: 313-315) (= [0625]);
- A 57 inf., ff. 65v et seq. (Martini and Bassi 1906: 887-891) (= [0663]);
- A 193 inf. olim N 299, ff. 64r et seq. (Martini and Bassi 1906: 910-912) (= [0665]).

[0593]   **[ap. Montf. p. 497]**   I.58.

This is a codex of Galenus, *Opera varia*.

The reference is to Montfaucon, 1739: 1.491-505:

Index Bibliothecae Manuscriptorum Ambrosianae Mediolanensis MSS Graeci ...

At 1.497 the present item is identified as follows without shelfmark or other element of identification:

Galeni opera varia volumina XVIII.

The description is not precise enough to allow for identification.

[0594]   **Vgl. Montfaucon I p. 504**   II.89.

This manuscript listed without precise identification in Diels' catalogue is referred to among the copies of Rufus, *De corporis humani appellationibus*.

The reference is to the same catalogue of the Ambrosiana library in Montfaucon as above ([0593]), where the item is described as follows (1.504) without shelfmark or other element of identification:

Rufi Ephesi nomenclatura partium humani corporis, bomb. bis.

Based on Martini and Bassi 1906, this item could correspond to two *Ambrosiani*:

- H 22 sup., ff. 11r et seq. (= [0634]).

Martini and Bassi 1906: 505-515;

- & 141 sup. (= [0660]).

Martini and Bassi 1906: 872-873.

[0595]	**A 45 Sup.**	N.27 (2), 31, 38, 64.
		Martini and Bassi 1906: 1-5.
[0596]	**A 80 Sup.**	N.41.
		Martini and Bassi 1906: 15-17.
[0597]	**A 92 Sup.**	N.46.
		Martini and Bassi 1906: 22-23.
[0598]	**A 95 Sup.**	I.40, 41, 126; II.30, 32, 33, 102, 104; N.41, 46.
		Martini and Bassi 1906: 23-28; *CMAG* II (Zuretti et al.) 1927: 100-101.
[0599]	**A 110 Sup.**	I.41.
		Martini and Bassi 1906: 37-38.
[0600]	**A 156 Sup.**	I.5, 13, 20, 77, 105, 107, 112.
		Martini and Bassi 1906: 64.
[0601]	**A 157 Sup.**	II.7; N.43.
		Martini and Bassi 1906: 65.
[0602]	**A 162 Sup.**	N.44.
		Martini and Bassi 1906: 73-74; *CMAG* II (Zuretti et al.) 1927: 102.
	A 174 sup.	(ff. 199v et seq.) Aristoteles, *De insomniis*; (ff. 226r et seq.) Aristoteles, *Physiognomonica*.
		Martini and Bassi 1906: 80; Wartelle 1963: 64, no. 905.
[0603]	**A 175 Sup.**	N.43.
		Martini and Bassi 1906: 80-82.
[0604]	**B 39 Sup.**	II.67.
		Martini and Bassi 1906: 103-105.
[0605]	**B 63 Sup.**	N.51.
		Martini and Bassi 1906: 110.
[0606]	**B 72 Sup.**	I.41; N.27, 67.
		Martini and Bassi 1906: 115.
[0607]	**B 82 Sup.**	N.51.
		Martini and Bassi 1906: 122.

[0608]   **B 90 Sup.**   I.111.

Martini and Bassi 1906: 126.

B 98 sup.   (ff. 168v et seq.) Orpheus, *Lithica*.

Martini and Bassi 1906: 129-130.

[0609]   **B 108 Sup.**   I.25, 27, 33, 76, 94 (2), 95, 99; N.31.

Martini and Bassi 1906: 144-145.

[0610]   **B 113 Sup.**   I.5, 18 (2), 22, 38, 43, 49; II.76, 104; N.62.

Martini and Bassi 1906: 147-151.

[0611]   **B 126 Sup.**   I.23, 100; II.77.

Martini and Bassi 1906: 160-162.

[0612]   **B 157 Sup.**   I.132; II.17, 18 (2), 18-19.

Martini and Bassi 1906: 172.

Possibly [0887] and [0904].

[0613]   **C 4 Sup.**   I.49, 68, 96; N.39.

Martini and Bassi 1906: 178.

C 32 sup.   (ff. 70r-109v) Nicander, *Theriaca*; (ff. 111r-124r) Nicander, *Alexipharmaca*.

Martini and Bassi 1906: 186.

[0614]   **C 69 Sup.**   N.47.

Martini and Bassi 1906: 194-200.

[0615]   **C 85 Sup.**   I.11, 12, 19, 22, 23, 24 (2), 25, 26 (2), 27(2), 28, 29 (2), 30 (2), 31(2), 33, 34, 35.

Martini and Bassi 1906: 202-203.

[0616]   **C 88 Sup.**   N.51.

Martini and Bassi 1906: 204-205.

[0617]   **C 89 Sup.**   II.109.

Martini and Bassi 1906: 205.

[0618]   **C 102 Sup.**   II.30; N.30, 34.

N.30, 34 correct the erroneous identification of this manuscript as C 102 inf. (= [0667]) at I.61 (at N.30 reference is made to I.63 instead of I.61), about Galenus, *Ars medica*, and I.100, about Galenus, *De remediis parabilibus libri III*.

Boudon 2002: 196n109, noticed the mistake at I.61, but not the correction at N.30.

On C 102 sup. see Martini and Bassi 1906: 217-218.

[0619]   **C 118 Sup.**   I.103.

This manuscript is listed among the copies of Galenus, *In Hippocratis de humoribus librum commentarii III*.

Mediolanus C 118 sup. does not contain this text, but rather Procopius, *Historia arcana* (Martini and Bassi 1906: 223-224).

This is a mistake for C 119 sup. (= [0620]). A correction is made at N.35 (see [0620]).

[0620]   **C 119 Sup.**   II.30; N.35.

N.35 mentions that the reference to *Mediolanensis* C 118 Sup. (= [0619]) is incorrect and should be C 119 sup. instead.

Martini and Bassi 1906: 224.

[0621]   **C 120 Sup.**   I.89.

Martini and Bassi 1906: 224-225.

[0622]   **D 13 Sup.**   II.55, 71, 73-74.

Martini and Bassi 1906: 234-235.

    D 15 sup.   (f. 134v) *De plantis nonnullis.*

Martini and Bassi 1906: 235-237.

[0623]   **D 33 Sup.**   N.59.

Martini and Bassi 1906: 253-254.

[0624]   **E 6 Sup.**   N.41.

Martini and Bassi 1906: 297.

    E 16 sup.   (ff. IIIr, 1 et seq.) *Physiologus*; (f. 47r) *Pronosticum de infirmis.*

Martini and Bassi 1906: 303-304.

[0625]   **E 37 Sup.**   N.37, 44, 66, 67, 69.

Martini and Bassi 1906: 313-315; *CMAG* II (Zuretti et al.) 1927: 339-340.

Possibly [0592].

[0626]   **E 105 Sup.**   I.96.

Martini and Bassi 1906: 358.

    E 112 sup.   (ff. 1r-22r) Nicander, *Theriaca*; (ff. 22r-30v) Nicander, *Alexipharmaca.*

Martini and Bassi 1906: 361.

[0627]   **F 23 Sup.**   N.27, 29.

Martini and Bassi 1906: 379-382.

[0628]   **F 88 Sup.**   II.67.

Martini and Bassi 1906: 401-404.

[0629]   **F 107 Sup.**   N.51.

Martini and Bassi 1906: 425-426.

[0630]   **F 112 Sup.**   N.32 (2).

Martini and Bassi 1906: 428.

[0631]   **G 69 Sup.**   N.61.

Martini and Bassi 1906: 488-493.

[0632]   **G 97 Sup.**   I.61, 78 (2), 79 (2), 92.

Martini and Bassi 1906: 499.

[0633]   **H 11 Sup.**   N.51.

Martini and Bassi 1906: 500-502.

[0634]   **H 22 Sup.**   N.65.

Martini and Bassi 1906: 505-515.

Possibly [0594].

[0635]   **H 43 Sup.**   N.44.

Martini and Bassi 1906: 520-521.

H 45 sup.   (ff. 13v et seq.) Gregorius Nazianzenus, *De humana natura*.

Martini and Bassi 1906: 522-524.

[0636]   **H 49 Sup.**   II.28.

Martini and Bassi 1906: 524-525.

H 50 sup.   (ff. 89v et seq.) Aristoteles, *De insomniis*.

Martini and Bassi 1906: 525-526; Wartelle 1963: 68, no. 946.

[0637]   **L 30 Sup.**   II.96, 104.

Martini and Bassi 1906: 566.

[0638]   **L 44 Sup.**   N.67.

Martini and Bassi 1906: 576-579.

[0639]   **L 110 Sup.**   I.4, 11, 18, 20, 21 (2), 22, 23 (2), 24 (2), 26, 28, 29 (2), 33, 34, 35; II.97, 101, 102, 104; N.65.

Martini and Bassi 1906: 596-598.

[0640]   **L 119 Sup.**   II.32 (2); N.48.

Martini and Bassi 1906: 605.

[0641]   **M 41 Sup.**   N.44.

Martini and Bassi 1906: 613-616.

M 50 sup.   (ff. 143r et seq.) Basilius Caesariensis, *De hominis opificio*.

Martini and Bassi 1906: 619-620.

N 150 sup.   (ff. 1r-54r) Nicander, *Theriaca*; (ff. 57r-91v) Nicander, *Alexipharmaca*.

Martini and Bassi 1906: 661.

N 248 sup.   (ff. 30r et seq.) *Communis lapidum doctrina*; (f. 31v) Demosthenes, *De lapidibus* (frg.) et Dioscorides, *De materia medica* (frg.).

Martini and Bassi 1906: 671-672.

[0642]	**O 50 Sup.**	I.87; N.33.
		Martini and Bassi 1906: 679-680.
	O 94 sup.	(ff. 39r et seq.) Nicephorus Constantinopolitanus Patriarcha, *Oneirocriticon*; varia ex Indis et Persis ut, exempli gratia: (f. 52v) *De emeto*; (f. 53r) *De catharticis*; (f. 53v) *Aliud de catharticis*.
		Martini and Bassi 1906: 682-685.
[0643]	**O 117 Sup.**	I.125; N.50.
		Martini and Bassi 1906: 687-688.
[0644]	**O 123 Sup.**	N.69.
		Martini and Bassi 1906: 689-694.
[0645]	**P. 32 Sup.**	N.39.
		Martini and Bassi 1906: 703.
	P 34 sup.	(ff. 181r et seq.) Aristoteles, *Physiognomonica*.
		Martini and Bassi 1906: 704-705; Wartelle 1963: 70, no. 970.
[0646]	**P 90 Sup.**	N.25, 38, 58.
		Martini and Bassi 1906: 716-717.
	Q 1 sup.	(ff. 146r et seq.) Nicephorus Gregoras, *Scholia in Synesii de insomniis*.
		Martini and Bassi 1906: 737.
[0647]	**Q 3 Sup.**	I.72, 73, 74, 79, 79-80, 82 (2), 85, 95, 100 (2), 103, 109 (2), 111, 119.
		Martini and Bassi 1906: 738-740.
		See [0591].
[0648]	**Q 13 Sup.**	I.5; N.49.
		Martini and Bassi 1906: 747-751.
[0649]	**Q 14 Sup.**	N.51.
		Martini and Bassi 1906: 751-754.
[0650]	**Q 52 Sup.**	I.85.
		Martini and Bassi 1906: 766.
	Q 74 sup.	(ff. 9v-16v) Nemesius Emesenus, *De natura hominis*.
		Martini and Bassi 1906: 767-780; Morani 1981: 29-30.
[0651]	**Q 87 Sup.**	I.67, 109; II.80; N.30, 41, 49.
		Martini and Bassi 1906: 791-794.
[0652]	**Q 94 Sup.**	I.90-91, 100; II.23, 40, 98; N.34, 39, 46 (2), 65.
		Martini and Bassi 1906: 798-800.
[0653]	**R 20 Sup.**	II.65, 79, 109 (2), 110 (2); N.69 (2).
		Martini and Bassi 1906: 818-819.
[0654]	**R 111 b**	II.68.
		Mistake for R 111 Sup. (= [0655]).

[0655]   **R 111 Sup.**   N.45, 48, 60.

Martini and Bassi 1906: 833-834.

See also [0654].

R 119 sup.   (ff. 359v et seq.) Aristoteles, *De insomniis*.

Martini and Bassi 1906: 839-841; Wartelle 1963: 71, no. 984.

[0656]   **S 3 Sup.**   I.67; II.4 (3), 12, 26, 42, 68; N.30, 42 (3).

Martini and Bassi 1906: 842-844.

[0657]   **S 19 Sup.**   II.97, 104.

Martini and Bassi 1906: 846-847.

[0658]   **T 19 Sup.**   I.13, 111; N.25, 36.

Martini and Bassi 1906: 854.

[0659]   **T 141 (v. Daremberg, Rufus. XXIII)**   II.89.

Mistake dating back to Daremberg 1879: XXIII, for & 141 sup. (= [0660]), correctly referenced at N.65.

Y 132 sup.   (ff. 1r et seq.) *Propositiones et praescriptiones excerptae ex opere quodam de re medica*.

Martini and Bassi 1906: 859.

[0660]   **& 141 Sup.**   N.65.

Martini and Bassi 1906: 872-873.

See [0659]. Possibly also [0594].

& 143 sup.   Epiphanius, *Physiologus* (frg.).

Martini and Bassi 1906: 873.

[0661]   **& 147 Sup.**   II.110.

Martini and Bassi 1906: 875.

[0662]   **A 27 Inf.**   II.96.

Martini and Bassi 1906: 881-882.

[0663]   **A 57 Inf.**   N.47, 52, 66, 67, 69 (2).

Martini and Bassi 1906: 887-891.

Possibly [0592].

A 61 inf.   (ff. 63r-64v) *Medica quaedam per schemata graeco-latina*.

Martini and Bassi 1906: 892.

[0664]   **A 81 Inf.**   I.96.

Martini and Bassi 1906: 896-897.

[0665]   **A 193 Inf.**   N.47, 52, 66, 67, 69 (2).

Martini and Bassi 1906: 910-912; *CMAG* II (Zuretti et al.) 1927: 71-91.

Possibly [0592].

A 270 inf.   (ff. 51r et seq.) Gregorius Nyssenus, *De hominis opificio*.

Martini and Bassi 1906: 928-929.

[0666]   **C 80 Inf.**   I.66.

Martini and Bassi 1906: 950-951.

[0667]   **C 102 Inf.**   I.61, 100; N.30, 34.

This manuscript is referred to among the copies of Galenus, *Ars medica* (I.61) and *De remedis parabilibus libri II* (I.100).

This shelfmark does not exist (see Martini and Bassi 1906: 951).

At N.30 (about *Ars medica*), there is a reference to I.63 (whereas the manuscripts of Galen's *Ars medica* are listed at I.61).

At N.34 (about *De remedis parabilibus*), this item is correctly identified as C 102 Sup. (= [0618]).

Indeed, *Ars medica* appears in C 102 Sup., ff. 128r-152v (see also Boudon 2002: 198 and 196n109). *De remediis parabilibus* is not contained in C 102 sup. This might be an incorrect identification of one of the botanical texts in the manuscript (Martini and Bassi 1906: 217-218).

See [0618].

[0668]   **C 222 Inf.**   II.85.

Martini and Bassi 1906: 984-990.

C 255 inf.   (ff. 152r et seq.) Epiphanius, *Physiologus*.

Martini and Bassi 1906: 997-998.

C 296 inf.   *Cyranides*.

Martini and Bassi 1906: 1025; *CMAG* II (Zuretti et al.) 1927: 278-294.

D 134 inf.   *Cyranides*.

Martini and Bassi 1906: 1037; *CMAG* II (Zuretti et al.) 1927: 278-294.

[0669]   **D 293 Inf.**   I.89.

Martini and Bassi 1906: 1049.

[0670]   **D 338 Inf.**   II.67.

Martini and Bassi 1906: 1053-1054.

D 474^4 [olim 125] inf.   *Efodia*.

Martini and Bassi 1906: 1063.

[0671]   **D 477 Inf.**   II.34.

As Diels' catalogue mentions, this is a copy of Dioscorides, *Excerpta*, "In partem D. notae M. Ant. Maranthae".

These are notes on Dioscorides, *De materia medica*, by Bartholomaeus Marantha (d. after 1570) and not by "M. Ant. Marantha" (= [?] Marcus Antonius) as described in Diels' catalogue.

Kristeller 1963: 288; Riddle 1980: 105-106; Kristeller 1991: 34.

[0672]   **D 518 Inf.**   I.89.

Martini and Bassi 1906: 1069.

D 529 inf.   (ff. 81r-93r) Nicander, *Theriaca*; (ff. 93v-102v) Nicander, *Alexipharmaca*.

Martini and Bassi 1906: 1071-1072.

[0673]   **E 10 Inf.**   N.51.

Martini and Bassi 1906: 1081-1082.

[0674]   **H 2 Inf.**   N.27, 28, 43, 44, 63, 64.

Martini and Bassi 1906: 1096-1101; *CMAG* II (Zuretti et al.) 1927: 97-100.

[0675]   **I 166 Inf.**   N.43.

Martini and Bassi 1906: 1137.

[0676]   **S.Q.E. VIII 13** I.3.

This is not a manuscript, but is instead a copy of the printed edition of Hippocrates, *Opera omnia* (in Greek), Venice, 1526.

Its exact shelfmark is S.Q.E.VIII.13.

[0677]   **S.Q.E. VIII 14** I.3, 49.

This is not a manuscript, but is instead a copy of the same 1526 printed edition of Hippocrates as [0676].

Its exact shelfmark was S.Q.E.VIII.14.

It is no longer among the holdings of the Biblioteca Ambrosiana.

[0678]   **S.Q.J. VII 9**   I.3.

This is not a manuscript, but is instead a copy of the same 1526 printed edition of Hippocrates as [0676].

Its exact shelfmark was S.Q.I.VII.9.

It is no longer among the holdings of the Biblioteca Ambrosiana.

[0679]   **S.Q.T. VIII 9**   I.4.

This is not a manuscript, but is instead a copy of the printed edition of Hippocrates, *Opera* (in Greek), Basel, 1538.

Its exact shelfmark is S.Q.T.VIII.9.

Trotti

373   (ff. 118r-119v and 117r) Stephanus Alexandrinus, *In Hippocratis Prognosticum commentaria*, chapter 1, section IV.

Pasini 1997: 73-80.

Bibl. Trivulziana (Biblioteca Trivulziana [Trivulziana Library]), now Archivio Storico Civico e Biblioteca Trivulziana (City Historical Archives and Trivulziana Library)

–

[0680]   **685**   I.64, 65, 71 (2), 83, 93, 102, 103, 118, 120.

Martini 1896: 377-381; Santoro 1965: 153.

Messina (IT)

Biblioteca Regionale Universitaria Giacomo Longo di Messina (Giacomo Longo Regional University Library of Messina)

Fondo Vecchio (Old Collection)

F. V. 2	(ff. 2r-49v) Gregorius Nyssenus, *De hominis opificio*.
	Mioni 1965: 1.137.
F. V. 11	(f. 7v, ll. 9-33) Epiphanius, *De duodecim gemmis* (frg.).
	Mioni 1965: 1.130-140.
F. V. 12	(ff. 173r-176r) Michael Psellus, *De lapidum virtutibus*; *De duodecim gemmis*.
	Mioni 1965: 1.140-142.

S. Salvatore (San Salvatore [Collection of St. Salvatore Monastery])

2	Palimpsest.
	Scriptio superior: Hagiographico-homiletica.
	Scriptio inferior: Paulus Aegineta, *Epitome medica*.
	Noret 1979; Foti, 1987; Harlfinger, Brunschön and Vasiloudi 2006: 145, 158-159; Rodriquez 2008: 207.
	On the manuscript: Mancini 1907: 2-6.
	See also Bruxelles, Bibliothèque royale, IV.459 (see p. 37).
50	(ff. 64r-66v.) Gregorius Nyssenus, *De hominis opificio*.
	Mancini 1907: 98-99.
84	See [0681] and [0682].
114	(ff. 1r-5r, l. 14) *Infirmitates et medicinae*.
	Mancini 1907: 177-180.
162	(f. 198v) *Formula ad emplastrum conficiendum*.
	Mancini 1907: 219-229.
F 4/4B	See [0683].

Bibl. S. Salvatoris (*Biblioteca Sanctissimi Salvatoris* [S. Salvatore Library]), now at the Biblioteca Regionale Universitaria Giacomo Longo di Messina (Giacomo Longo Regional University Library of Messina)

–

[0681]	**84**	II.6.
		Now Messina, Biblioteca Regionale Universitaria, S. Salvatore, 84.
		Same as [0682].

Universität (Università [University]). These manuscripts are now at the Biblioteca Regionale Universitaria Giacomo Longo di Messina (Giacomo Longo Regional University Library of Messina)

–

[0682]	**84**	I.148; II.74.

Fraccaroli 1897: 491; Mancini 1907: 144-145.

Same as [0681].

[0683]	**111**	I.92.

This item is referred to among the copies of Galenus, *Medendi methodus.*

The manuscript of Messina S. Salvatore 111 contains the Gospels (Mancini 1907: 174-175). In addition, it contained a folio from an 11th-century manuscript containing Galen, *Medendi methodus.* This folio has been extracted from the manuscript and is now identified with the shelfmark F 4/4B (see p. 137).

Μετέωρα (Meteora) (GR)

Ιερά Μονή Αγίου Στεφάνου (St. Stephen's Monastery)

–

85   (ff. 12r et seq.) Hippocrates et Galenus, *Capitula medica.*
Sofianos 1986: 259-269.

135   (ff. 1r et seq.) *Iatrosofion*; (ff. 43r et seq.) *Iatrosofion.*
Both 16th century.
Sofianos 1986: 396-397.

Ιερά Μονή Βαρλαάμ (Varlaam Monastery)

–

178   (ff. 155r et seq.) Galenus, *De somniis.*
Bees 1984: 245-247.

194   (ff. 172r et seq.) Epiphanius, *De duodecim gemmis.*
Bees 1984: 269-271.

204   (ff. 103r-162r) *Physiologus.*
Bees 1984: 321-325.

Ιερά Μονή Μεταμορφώσεως του Σωτήρος (or: Ιερά Μονή Μεγάλου Μετεώρου) (Monastery of the Transfiguration of the Savior, or: Great Meteora Monastery)

–

67   (ff. 48v et seq.) *De phlebotomia.*
Bees 1967: 86-91.

68   (ff. 32v et seq.) Epiphanius, *De duodecim gemmis.*
Bees 1967: 91-94.

91	(f. 14r) Hippocrates, *De anno*; (ff. 15r et seq.) *De creatione mundi et hominis*; (ff. 15v et seq.) Nicephorus Constantinopolitanus Patriarcha, *Oneirocriticon*.
	Bees 1967: 122-124.
151	(ff. 106r et seq.) Synesius Cyrenensis, *De insomniis*.
	Bees 1967: 174-183.
349	(ff. 72r et seq.) Βότανον τῶν Σωχάδων.
	Bees 1967: 361-363.
399	(ff. 91r et seq.) Epiphanius, *Physiologus* (frg.).
	Bees 1967: 413-416.
403	(ff. 5r et seq.) *Collectio medica*; (ff. 40r et seq.) Symeon Seth, *De alimentorum facultatibus*; (ff. 119r et seq.) *Iatrosofion*; (ff. 327v et seq.) *Prognostica medica*.
	Bees 1967: 419-422.
409	(ff. 19r et seq.) *De creatione mundi et hominis*; (ff. 20v et seq.) Hippocrates, *Ad Galenum ipsius discipulum*.
	Bees 1967: 428-432.
589	(ff. 307v et seq.) *Medicina*.
	Bees 1967: 619-620.
593	(ff. 280v et seq.) Epiphanius, *De duodecim gemmis*; (ff. 340v et seq.) *Iatrosofion*; (ff. 345r et seq.) *Iatrosofion*.
	Bees 1967: 684-688.
620	(f. 10r-v) *Materia medica*.
	Bees 1967: 691-692.

Milano (Milan) (IT)

See **Mailand** (see above, pp. 128-136).

Archivio Storico Civico e Biblioteca Trivulziana (Historical Archives and Trivulziana Library)

See **Bibl. Trivulziana** (see above, p. 136).

Biblioteca Ambrosiana (Ambrosiana Library)

See **Bibl. Ambrosiana** (see above, pp. 128-136).

Biblioteca e Archivio del Capitolo Metropolitano (Library and Archives of the Metropolitan Chapter)

See **Arch. del Capitolo Metropolitano** (see above, p. 128).

Mileae (Μηλεαί [now Μηλιές, Milies]) (GR)

Bibl. Mileens. (*Bibliotheca Mileensis* [Βιβλιοθήκη Μηλεῶν, Mêleai Library], now Δημόσια Βιβλιοθήκη Μηλεών [Public Library of Milies])

–

[0684]   78   II.30.

Papadopoulos-Kerameus 1901: 50.

Manuscript dated 1774 (Karas 1994: 360).

Mitylene (Μυτιλήνη Λέσβου [Mytiline, Lesvos]) (GR)

Bibl. Gymnas. (*Bibliotheca Gymnasii*, Γυμνασίου Βιβλιοθήκη [Gymnasium Library]), now Βιβλιοθήκη, Πρότυπο Πειραματικό Γενικό Λύκειο Μυτιλήνης του Πανεπιστημίου Αιγαίου (Library, Model experimental high school of Mytiline of the University of Aegean)

–

[0685]   1   II.40.

Papadopoulos-Kerameus 1888: 132.

[0686]   33   II.34, 80.

Papadopoulos-Kerameus 1888: 143.

Current shelfmark: 31 (Tsernoglou 1991: 356).

Iatrosofion dated 1774 (Karas 1994: 357-360).

Modena (IT)

Bibl. Estense (Biblioteca Estense [Estense Library], now Biblioteca Universitaria e Estense [University and Estense Library])

All manuscripts of the Biblioteca Estense collections mentioned by Diels are identified by their sequential number in Puntoni 1896, followed (except in [0701] and [0704]) by a shelfmark between parentheses made of three elements:

• a Roman numeral;

• a capital Latin letter;

• an Arabic numeral.

Neither of the two systems correspond to the current one, in which shelfmarks are made of four elements (separated by a period sign):

• a Greek minuscule letter (α in all cases here);

• a Latin capital letter;

• an Arabic numeral (between 1 and 9);

• a second Arabic numeral (between 3 and 28 here).

A table of concordance of the numbers in Puntoni 1896 and current shelfmarks is provided in Puliatti 1965.

[0687]   **18 (III A 4)**   II.67.

Puntoni 1896: 392.

Current shelfmark: α.U.9.18.

[0688]   **54 (III B 2)**   I.38.

Puntoni 1896: 419-420.

Current shelfmark: α.U.9.3.

[0689]   **61 (III B 9)**   I.18, 56, 112, 117, 148; II.7, 79, 102, 106.

Puntoni 1896: 426-427.

Current shelfmark: α.U.9.4.

[0690]   **78 (II C 11)**   I.96.

Puntoni 1896: 437.

Current shelfmark: α.W.2.9.

[0691]   **85 (III C 6)**   I.44, 49. See also II.114 on the text referred to at I.49.

Puntoni 1896: 441-443.

Current shelfmark: α.Q.5.16.

[0692]   **97 (III C 18)**   I.61.

Puntoni 1896: 448.

Current shelfmark: α.U.9.23.

[0693]   **107 (II D 8)**   I.96.

Puntoni 1896: 453.

Current shelfmark: α.P.5.18.

[0694]   **109 (II D 10)**   I.60, 71 (2), 83, 93; II.9, 22.

Puntoni 1896: 453-454.

Current shelfmark: α.P.5.20.

[0695]   **115 (II D 16)**   I.40, 128; II.28, 30, 32 (2), 33, 102.

Puntoni 1896: 458.

Current shelfmark: α.P.5.17.

[0696]   **135 (II E 2)**   II.9, 106.

Puntoni 1896: 470-471.

Current shelfmark: α.T.8.5.

[0697]   **145 (II E 12)**   II.9 (2), 22.

Puntoni 1896: 478-479.

Current shelfmark: α.V.7.17.

[0698]   **151 (II E 18)**   I.148.

Puntoni 1896: 481-482.

Current shelfmark: α.V.7.18.

[0699]   **174 (II F 9)**   II.82 (2).
                                    Puntoni 1896: 494.
                                    Current shelfmark: α.V.7.6.

[0700]   **175 (II F 10)**   I.65.
                                    Puntoni 1896: 494.
                                    Current shelfmark: α.V.7.4.

[0701]   **191**   I.38.
                                    Puntoni 1896: 501.
                                    Current shelfmark: α.N.8.8.

[0702]   **210 (III G 6)**   I.111; II.9 (2), 22.
                                    Puntoni 1896: 508.
                                    Current shelfmark: α.V.6.12.

[0703]   **211 (III G 7)**   I.104.
                                    Puntoni 1896: 508.
                                    Current shelfmark: α.G.3.11.

[0704]   **213**   I.73.
                                    Puntoni 1896: 509-510.
                                    Current shelfmark: α.G.3.12.
                                    See [0705]

[0705]   **213 (III G 9)**   I.22, 77, 82, 85, 95 (2), 100, 109.
                                    Same as [0704].

[0706]   **216 (II H 1)**   I.96, 133.
                                    Puntoni 1896: 511-512.
                                    Current shelfmark: α.O.4.9.

[0707]   **217 (II H 2)**   I.76, 100.
                                    Puntoni 1896: 512.
                                    Current shelfmark: α.O.4.7.

[0708]   **218 (II H 3)**   I.28, 81, 89.
                                    Puntoni 1896: 512.
                                    Current shelfmark: α.O.4.6.

[0709]   **219 (II H 4)**   I.68.
                                    Puntoni 1896: 512.
                                    Current shelfmark: α.O.4.11.

[0710]   **220 (II H 5)**   I.4, 20, 23 (2), 24 (2), 25, 26 (2), 27, 29, 33, 34, 35.
                                    Puntoni 1896: 512-513.
                                    Current shelfmark: α.O.4.8.

[0711]   **226 (II H 11)**   I.66, 87 (2), 88 (2), 115.
                                    Puntoni 1896: 514.
                                    Current shelfmark: α.O.4.12.

[0712]   **227 (II H 12)** I.11 (2), 22, 24, 25, 27 (2), 28, 29-30, 30 (2), 31 (2), 34.

Puntoni 1896: 514.

Current shelfmark: α.O.4.14.

[0713]   **233 (III H 5)** I.10, 11, 13, 19, 21, 28, 29.

Puntoni 1896: 516.

Current shelfmark: α.T.1.12.

[0714]   **237 (III G 18)** I.69, 70, 78 (2), 79, 80, 84, 103, 107, 130.

Puntoni 1896: 518.

Current shelfmark: α.W.3.12.

[0715]   **240 (III F 17)** I.101; II.67; N.34

Puntoni 1896: 519-520.

Current shelfmark: α.J.6.28.

Biblioteca Universitaria e Estense (University and Estense Library)

–

α.G.3.11	See [0703].
α.G.3.12	See [0704] and [0705].
α.J.6.28	See [0715].
α.N.8.8	See [0701].
α.O.4.6	See [0708].
α.O.4.7	See [0707].
α.O.4.8	See [0710].
α.O.4.9	See [0706]
α.O.4.11	See [0709].
α.O.4.12	See [0711].
α.O.4.14	See [0712].
α.P.5.17	See [0695].
α.P.5.18	See [0693].
α.P.5.20	See [0694].
α.Q.5.16	See [0691].
α.T.1.12	See [0713].
α.T.8.5	See [0696].
α.T.8.12	(f. 144r-v [?]) *Hippocratis quaedam.*
	Puntoni 1896: 475-478, no. 144.
α.T.8.20	Johannes Zacharias Actuarius: (ff. 2r et seq.) *De differentia urinarum*; (ff. 17r et seq.) *De urinarum indiciis libri II*; (ff. 42v et seq.) *De urinarum causis libri II*; (ff. 80r et seq.) *De praevidentia ex urinis libri II.*
	Puntoni 1896: 474, no. 141.

α.T.9.2	(ff. 68r et seq.) Nicander, *Theriaca*.
	Puntoni 1896: 405-406, no. 39.
α.T.9.21	(ff. 32v et seq.) Aristoteles, *De insomniis*.
	Puntoni 1896: 436, no. 76; Wartelle 1963: 75, no. 1038 (76 [II.C.9]).
α.U.4.9	See [0706].
α.U.5.14	(ff. 108r et seq.) Gregorius Nyssenus, *De hominis opificio*.
	Puntoni 1896: 434, no. 72.
α.U.9.3	See [0688].
α.U.9.4	See [0689].
α.U.9.18	See [0687].
α.U.9.23	See [0692].
α.V.6.12	See [0702].
α.V.7.4	See [0700].
α.V.7.6	See [0699].
α.V.7.17	See [0697].
α.V.7.18	See [0698].
α.W.2.9	See [0690].
α.W.3.12	See [0714].

Montpellier (FR)

Bibliothèque de l'école [de médecine] (Medical School Library)

–

[0716]   **v. Montfaucon, II.1199**   II.89.

This manuscript without shelfmark is listed under Rufus, *De corporis humani appellationibus*. The reference is to Montfaucon 1739: 2.119, where a mention "Rufi Ephesii Medici opera" appears.

The item appears in a list entitled as follows in Montfaucon 1739: 2.1198:

In codice Colbertino 2145. post catalogum Bibliothecae Cardinalis Bessarionis, quam Senatui Veneto dedit, recensentur codices Graeci Bibliothecae D. Guillelmi Pellicerii olim Episcopi Monspeliensis, qui etiam nunc in Bibliotheca Episcopi Monspeliensis esse putantur, quos hic quam brevissime potero recensebo ... habetur etiam in cod. Colb. 2276.

This catalogue is reproduced in Montfaucon 1739: 2.1198-1202.

The present manuscript did not pertain to the library of Montpellier School of Medicine contrary to Diels, but to the collection of Montpellier Bishop Guillaume Pellicier (ca. 1490-1568). It is now in Berlin, SBB-PKB, Phillipps 1536 (= [0132]).

Moskau (Москва [Moscow]) (RU)

Synodialbibl. (Synodialbibliothek [Synodal Library]), now Государственный Исторический Музей (ГИМ), Синодальная библиотека Московского Патриархата (Gosudarstvennyi Istoricheskii Muzei (GIM), Sinodal'naia Biblioteka Moskovskoi Patriarchii [State Historical Museum (GIM), Synodal Library of Moscow Patriarchate])

Mosquens. (*Mosquenses*)

All these manuscripts are now in the Manuscript Department of the State Historical Museum (MDSHM), Gosudarstvennyi Istoricheskii Muzei (GIM) (State Historical Museum), Synodal collection.

Except in [0717]-[0721], which are listed without shelfmark, Diels' catalogue refers to three different catalogues of this collection (listed below in chronological order of publication):

- in [0723], Matthaei 1805;
- in [0722], [0725] and [0726], Savva 1858;
- in all others, Vladimir 1894.

The shelfmarks now in use are those in Savva 1858.

In [0717]-[0720] the identification is imprecise, and in [0721] it refers to a mention in a publication.

[0717]   –   II.43.

This is a copy of the *Cyranides*.

Information is insufficient to allow for any further identification.

[0718]   ?   II.71.

This manuscript without any element of identification is listed under Oribasius, *Medicae collectiones ad Iulianum*.

Information is insufficient to allow for any further identification.

[0719]   [?]   I.110.

This is a copy of Galenus, *Linguarum s. dictionum exoletarum Hippocratis explicatio*.

This manuscript is now Jena, Thüringer Universitäts- und Landesbibliothek, Ms. G.B. f. 31 (see above, p. 91) (on this identification, see Perilli 2011: 179-185).

[0720]   **[complures]**   I.58.

Several manuscripts of Galenus, *Opera varia*, are referred to, without shelfmark or other information allowing for identification. The Galen manuscripts in the Synodal collection are the following:

- 51 (= [0731]);
- 283 (= [0733]);
- 507 (= [0734]).

[0721]   **vgl. Bussemaker *a. a. O.* p. 75**   II.20.

The reference to Bussemaker is to "Poët. de re phys. et medica rell." This is the edition of the Greek text of the *Fragmenta poematum rem naturalem vel medicinam spectantium* in a volume containing several Greek didactic poems under the general title *Poetae bucolici et didactici* published by Firmin Didot (Paris), 1862 (see pp. 71-134 in that volume for the fragments of natural history poems).

The manuscript referred to here by Bussemaker 1862: 75, is listed among the copies of the *Praecepta salubria* attributed to Asclepiades, Dioscorides, or Oribasius, and first edited by Christian Gottfried Gruner (1744-1815) in 1782.

This codex is the current *Mosquensis* Sinod. 292 (the number 279 in Perilli 2011: 184, comes from Matthaei 1805: 1.179-183). It is a 17th-century manuscript.

Vladimir 1894: 357-360, no. 260.

See [0724] and [0726].

[0722]   **51**   I.60.

This number refers to Savva 1858 and corresponds to no. 52 in Matthaei 1805 as specified in [0723].

Same as [0731]. Also [0723].

[0723]   **52** (*so!*) = **464** N.29.

Reference is made to I.60, that is, to the manuscript with shelfmark 51 (= [0722]). The number 52 quoted here comes from Matthaei 1805: 1.54, and the number 464 from Vladimir 1890: 701-703.

Same as [0731].

[0724]   **260**   I.72; II.74; N.31.

On N.31 referring to I.72, the catalogue specifies that "292 [*ist*] *identisch mit* Mosq. 260".

Vladimir 1894: 357-360, no. 260.

Current shelfmark is Sinod. 292. It is a *iatrosofion* dated 1630 (Karas 1994: 349, 375, 391).

See also [0721] and [0726].

[0725]   **283**   I.60; N.29.

At N.29 this item is identified as 283 = 466 (that is, 283 Savva 1858 = 466 Vladimir 1894).

Same as [0733].

[0726]   **292**   I.72; N.31.

According to N.31 this item is no. 260 (= [0724]) (that is, 292 Savva 1858 = 260 Vladimir 1894).

See also [0721] and [0724].

[0727]   **395**   I.77.

Vladimir 1894: 595-597, no. 395; Karas 1994: 349.

Current shelfmark: Sinod. 303.

16th/17th-century miscellaneous manuscript with iatrosofic texts (Karas 1994: 349).

[0728]   **436**   II.91.

Vladimir 1894: 662-664, no. 436.

Current shelfmark: Sinod. 298.

[0729]   **439**   I.40, 41.

Vladimir 1894: 667-671, no. 439.

Current shelfmark: Sinod. 426.

[0730]   **446**   II.11.

Vladimir 1894: 684-685, no. 446.

Current shelfmark: Sinod. 1.

[0731]   **464**   I.60, 87 (2), 88, 88-89, 92, 93, 111; II.106; N.29.

Vladimir 1894: 701-703, no. 464.

Current shelfmark: Sinod. 51.

Also [0722] and [0723], and possibly [0720].

[0732]   **465**   I.71 (2), 102.

Vladimir 1894: 703, no. 465.

Current shelfmark: Sinod. 282.

[0733]   **466**   I.60, 61, 63, 64, 65, 70, 71 (2), 79, 86, 92, 93, 96, 103, 108; II.48, 50, 96; N.29.

Vladimir 1894: 703-705, no. 466.

Current shelfmark: Sinod. 283.

Same as [0725].

See possibly [0720].

[0734]   **467**   I.73, 74 (2).

Vladimir 1894: 705, no. 467.

Current shelfmark: Sinod. 507.

See possibly [0720].

[0735]   **468**   I.100; II.7, 41.

Vladimir 1894: 706, no. 468.

Current shelfmark: Sinod. 508.

[0736]   **477**   II.34.

Vladimir 1894: 710, no. 477.

Current shelfmark: Sinod. 506.

17th-century *iatrosofion* (Karas 1994: 356).

[0737]   **498**   II.71.

Vladimir 1894: 719, no. 498.

Current shelfmark: Sinod. 187.

[0738]   **499**   II.72.

Vladimir 1894: 719-720, no. 499.

Current shelfmark: Sinod. 188.

Москва (Moskva [Moscow]) (RU)

Государственный Исторический Музей (ГИМ), Синодальная Библиотека Московского Патриархата (Gosudarstvennyi Istoricheskii Muzei (GIM), Sinodal'naia Biblioteka Moskovskoi Patriarchii [State Historical Museum [GIM], Synodal Library of Moscow Patriarchate])

Shelfmarks are those in Savva 1858 and descriptions those in Vladimir 1894. For a table of concordance of the shelfmarks in the two works, see Vladimir 1894: 857-878.

Синод. (Sinod.)

1   See [0730].

18   (ff. 71r-111r) Gregorius Nyssenus, *De hominis opificio*.
            Vladimir 1894: 123, no. 126.

20   (f. 314) Palimpsest: Paulus Aegineta, *Epitome medica*.
            Vladimir 1894: 122-123, no. 125; Heiberg 1921: VI.

51   See [0731].
            Also [0722] and [0723]. Possibly [0720].

52   (ff. 144v et seq.) Gregorius Nazianzenus, *De humana natura*.
            Vladimir 1894: 158-160, no. 156; Domiter 1999: 21.

125   (ff. 189r-191v) Gregorius Nyssenus, *De hominis opificio*.
            Vladimir 1894: 74-75, no. 81.

161   (ff. 1 and 3) Palimpsest: Paulus Aegineta, *Epitome medica*.
            Vladimir 1894: 569-571, no. 379; Heiberg 1921: VI.

174   (ff. 1-2) Palimpsest: Paulus Aegineta, *Epitome medica*.
            Vladimir 1894: 582, no. 387; Heiberg 1919: 276; Heiberg 1921: VI; Fonkič 2000: 169-170.
            See also Paris, Bibliothèque nationale, *Supplementum graecum* 1156 (= [1391]), ff. 24-25.
            See [0930] and [0935].

187   See [0737].

188   See [0738].

238   (ff. 110v et seq.) Nicephorus Gregoras, *Scholia in Synesii de insomniis*.
            Vladimir 1894: 699-700, no. 462.

251   (ff. 96r-148r) Gregorius Nyssenus, *De hominis opificio.*

        Vladimir 1894: 127-128, no. 132.

259   (ff. 258r et seq.) Nicephorus Blemmydes, *De phlebotomia.*

        Vladimir 1894: 636-638, no. 423.

282   See [0732].

283   See [0725] and [0733]. Possibly [0720].

292   See [0721]. Also [0724] and [0726].

298   See [0728].

314   (ff. 143r et seq.) Epiphanius, *De duodecim gemmis.*

        Vladimir 1894: 471-473, no. 325.

315   (ff. 1r-15r) Leo medicus, *Compendium artis medicae.*

        Vladimir 1894: 672-676, no. 441.

        This manuscript is identified as Moscow, GIM Sinod. gr. 441 in Zipser 2004: 395.

316   (f. 436r) Lucas, *Sales.*

        Vladimir 1894: 695-697, no. 459.

326   (ff. 27r et seq.) Nicephorus Gregoras, *Scholia in Synesii de insomniis.*

        Vladimir 1894: 693, no. 455.

339   (ff. 174r et seq.) Epiphanius, *De duodecim gemmis.*

        Vladimir 1894: 633-634, no. 420.

386   (ff. 238r-250r) Basilius Caesariensis, *De hominis opificio.*

        Vladimir 1894: 129-131, no. 134.

410   *Remedia varia.*

        Vladimir 1894: 716, no. 490.

415   Hermes Trismegistus: (ff. 63r et seq.) *Ad Asclepium de plantis septem astrorum*; (ff. 65v et seq.) *Aliae plantae*; (ff. 72v et seq.) *Ad Asclepium discipulum, de plantis 12 zodiacalium signorum.*

        Vladimir 1894: 725-726, no. 509; *CCAG* XII (Šangin) 1936: 74-76.

426   See [0729].

507   See [0734]. Possibly [0720].

508   See [0735].

509   (ff. 8v et seq.) Epiphanius, *De duodecim gemmis.*

        Vladimir 1894: 329-331, no. 247, where it is identified as Savva 309. However, in the table at p. 877 in Vladimir 1894, the same item is identified as Savva 509.

Научная Библиотека Московского Государственного Университета Имени М. В. Ломоносова (МГУ) (Nauchnaia Biblioteka Moskovskogo Gosudarstvennogo Universiteta Imeni M. V. Lomonosova [MGU], Research Library, M. V. Lomonosov Moscow State University [MSU])

гр. (gr.)

1   This item was Paris, Bibliothèque nationale, Coislin 229 (= [0940]).

Fonkič 2006: 13-36.

Российский Государственный Архив Древних Актов (РГАДА) (Rossiiskii Gosudarsdarstvennyi Arkhiv Drevnikh Aktov [RGADA], Russian State Archive of Ancient Documents [RGADA])

фонда 181: Рукописный отдел библиотеки МГАМИД (Fonda 181: Rukopisnyi otdel biblioteki MGAMID, Collection 181: Manuscript Department Library MGAMID)

описи 14 (Греческие, голландские и грузинские рукописи) (opisi 14 [Grecheskie, gollandskie i gruzinskie rukopisi], Inventory 14 [Greek, Dutch and Georgian Manuscripts])

1270   (ff. 1r-2v) Epiphanius, *De mensuris et ponderibus*.

Фонда 1607: Дрезденские рукописные книги (Коллекция греческих рукописей) (Fonda 1607: Drezdenskie rukopisnye knigi [Kollektsiya grecheskikh rukopisei], Collection 1607: Dresden manuscripts [A collection of Greek manuscripts)

Da. 01   See [0223].

Tyurina 2012: 25 no. 26.

This codex is identified as *Dresdensis* Da 1 in Boudon 2002: 198n110, and Petit 2009: LXXXIII.

Da. 05   See [0224].

Tyurina 2012: 45 no. 20.

Da. 24   Nicander, *Theriaka* et *Alexipharmaka* cum scholiis.

Schnorr von Carolsfeld 1882 (1979): 289.

According to von Gebhardt 1898: 545 and 552, this item might be a part of a Moscow manuscript broken by Christian Friedrich Matthaei (1744-1811) and divided into several pieces now preserved in different libraries.

Whatever its provenance, this item was sold by Matthaei to Dresden Library (Ebert 1822: 246, no. 24). In 1947 it was returned to Russia (Schnorr von Carolsfed 1979: 289). The manuscript is identified as Pak. N 1791-K in Geymonat 1974: 18; Ikonomakos 2002: 1, and 2002/2: 28*; and Jacques 2002: CLIV (with previous shelfmark *Dresdensis* N D a 24), and 2007: CXLI.

Tyurina 2012: 44 no. 8.

München (Munich) (DE)

    Bayerische Staatsbibliothek (BSB) (Bavarian State Library)

      See below **Hof- und Staatsbibliothek** (Court and State Library)

    Bibl. August. (*Bibliotheca Augustea* [Augustean Library])

      -

[0739]   **542**   II.44.

                This item containing Hermes Trismegistus, *De succis plantarum*, is actually *Monacensis graecus* 542, on which see below and also [0764].

    Hof- und Staatsbibliothek (Court and State Library), now Bayerische Staatsbibliothek (BSB) (Bavarian State Library)

      Monac. (*Monacenses*)

      All München (*Monacenses*) items are now identified as "Cod. graec." followed by the number (in Arabic numerals) they have in Hardt 1806-1812.

[0740]   **- (*vgl.* Bussemaker *a. a. O.* p. 75)**   II.20.

      This manuscript without shelfmark in Diel's catalogue is listed among the copies of Asclepiades, *Praecepta salubria*.

      The reference to Bussemaker is to "Poët. de re phys. et medica rell.". This is actually the edition of the Greek text of the *Fragmenta poematum rem naturalem vel medicinam spectantium* in a volume containing several Greek didactic poems under the general title *Poetae bucolici et didactici* published by Firmin Didot (Paris), 1862. The *fragmenta* published by Bussemaker 1862 can be found at pp. 71-134.

      The manuscript referred to here is mentioned in the *Praefatio* by Bussemaker 1862: 74-75; see p. 75. It was used by Berger 1807 to publish the 25 first verses of the *Praecepta salubria* ascribed to Asclepiades. In Berger's *Praefatio* (p. 1001) the manuscript is identified as "cod. ms. 336. bibliothecae regiae Bavaricae".

      Although no Asclepiades is listed in the index of Hardt 1806-1812: 5.475, the text can be found in codex *Monacensis graecus* 336, f. 206 (Hardt 1806-1812: 2.328-336; especially 334-335), as Choulant 1841: 66 noticed.

[0741]   **[-]**   I.149.

      This codex listed without shelfmark is supposed to contain a *Compendium ex. Gal.*

      Although no *Monacensis* manuscript seems to contain a text with this title, codex *Monacensis graecus* 551 (= [0772]) may be the intended reference. It contains from f. 296r a text *De alimentorum facultate* "è Galeno ... compositum" and, from f. 336r, another text identified as "Synopticum iatrosophium ... Galeni" (on both texts, see Hardt 1806-1812: 5.402-403).

      On this manuscript, see Hardt 1806-1812: 5.378-404.

[0742]   **[Hardt I p. 448]**   II.81.

      The text referred to (Paulus Nicaeensis, *De cognitione et curatione variorum morborum*) as being contained in this manuscript listed without identifier, appears in Cod. graec. 72 (= [0748]) described in Hardt 1806-1812: 1.444-449.

      10   (pp. 274-279) Nicephorus Gregoras, *Praefatio explicationis in Synesii librum de insomniis*.

                Tiftixoglu 2004: 71-82.

	21	(f. 324r) Gregorius Nyssenus, *De hominis opificio* (frg., paraphrasis).
		Tiftixoglu 2004: 117-122.
[0743]	**29**	II.67, 71.
		Tiftixoglu 2004: 179-185.
		Current shelfmark: Cod. graec. 29.
[0744]	**39**	I.76, 126 (zu streichen; see N.38), 134, 135; II.63; N.31-32, 38, 39 (2), 58.
		Tiftixoglu 2004: 235-240.
		Current shelfmark: Cod. graec. 39.
[0745]	**69**	II.79, 109, 110.
		Molin Pradel 2013: 120-122.
		Current shelfmark: Cod. graec. 69.
[0746]	**70**	II.17, 18 (2), 28.
		Molin Pradel 2013: 123-129.
		Current shelfmark: Cod. graec. 70.
[0747]	**71**	I.4, 5, 8, 10 (2), 11 (3), 12, 13, 18 (2), 19, 20 (3), 21 (2), 22 (2), 23 (3), 24 (3), 25 (2), 26 (2), 27 (2), 28 (2), 29 (2), 30 (3), 31 (3), 32 (3), 33 (3), 34 (3), 35 (3), 38, 46, 48, 110; II.37, 93; N.36.
		Molin Pradel 2013: 129-139.
		Current shelfmark: Cod. graec. 71.
[0748]	**72**	I.40, 46; II.17, 18 (2), 19, 37, 58, 72.
		Molin Pradel 2013: 140-145.
		Current shelfmark: Cod. graec. 72.
		Also [0742].
	85	(ff. 215v-237v) Synesius Cyrenensis, *De insomniis*, cum Nicephori Gregorae commentario.
		Molin Pradel 2013: 199-207.
	87/III	(ff. 353r-385v) Nicephorus Gregoras, *Scholia in Synesii de insomniis*.
		Molin Pradel 2013: 210-214 for the whole manuscript; 212 for this component.
[0749]	**100**	II.67.
		Molin Pradel 2013: 270-279.
		Current shelfmark: Cod. graec. 100.
[0750]	**105**	I.112; II.41, 44; N.36, 51.
		Molin Pradel 2013: 303-312.
		Current shelfmark: Cod. graec. 105.

[0751]	**109**	I.72, 101, 111; N.31, 34, 36.
		Molin Pradel 2013: 325-326.
		Current shelfmark: Cod. graec. 109.
	121	(f. 514r-v) Hippocrates, *Epistulae*, 1.
		Hajdú 2003: 83-89.
	151	(ff. 114r-123v) Michael Ephesius, *Commentarius in Aristotelis de insomniis*.
		Hajdú 2003: 228-232.
	192	(ff. 111-166v.) Gregorius Nyssenus, *De hominis opificio*.
		Hajdú 2012: 67-70.
	206/I	(ff. 1r-34r) Gregorius Nyssenus, *De hominis opificio*.
		Hajdú 2012: 151-154 for the whole manuscript; 151 for this component.
	225/IV	(ff. 262v-281v.) Nicephorus Blemmydes, *De corpore*.
		Hajdú 2012: 238-246 for the whole manuscript; 241 for this component.
[0752]	**227**	II.26.
		Hajdú 2012: 259-260.
		Current shelfmark: Cod. graec. 227.
[0753]	**231**	I.104; N.35.
		Hajdú 2012: 274-275.
		Current shelfmark: Cod. graec. 231.
	234/II	(f. 10r) Galenus, *De historia philosophica* (frg.).
		Hajdú 2012: 280-287 for the whole manuscript; 280 for this component.
	234/X	(f. 167v) Aristoteles, *Problemata* (frg.).
		Wartelle 1963: 82, no. 1123; Hajdú 2012: 280-287 for the whole manuscript; 283 for this component.
	234/XII	(ff. 179r-185r) Aristoteles, *Problemata* (frg.)
		Wartelle 1963: 82, no. 1123; Hajdú 2012: 280-287 for the whole manuscript; 284 for this component.
	235/IX	(f. 225r) Aristoteles, *Problemata* (frg.).
		Hajdú 2012: 287-297 for the whole manuscript; 292 for this component.
[0754]	**236**	I.93; II.30; N.34, 48, 49 (2).
		Hajdú 2012: 297-298.
		Current shelfmark: Cod. graec. 236.
	240	(ff. 65r-109v) Gregorius Nyssenus, *De hominis opificio*.
		Hajdú 2012: 307-308.

256/II   (f. 305v) Gregorius Nyssenus, *De hominis opificio* (frg.).

Hajdú 2012: 363-378 for the whole manuscript; 366-372 for this component.

[0755]   **276**   I.44, 130.

Hardt 1806-1812: 3.149-161.

Current shelfmark: Cod. graec. 276.

[0756]   **278**   I.130; N.39.

While I.130 lists this manuscript among the copies of Galenus, *Prognosticon*, N.39 states that this item should be deleted ("zu streichen"). Indeed, Cod. graec. 278 does not contain the Galenic text (see Hardt 1806-1812: 3.165-166).

[0757]   **287**   I.13, 49; II.87; N.51. See also II.114 on the text referred to at I.49.

Hardt 1806-1812: 3.198-210.

Current shelfmark: Cod. graec. 287.

[0758]   **288**   II.41, 52; N.54.

Hardt 1806-1812: 3.211-212.

Current shelfmark: Cod. graec. 288.

291   Nemesius Emesenus, *De natura hominis*.

Hardt 1806-1812: 3.215 (where the text is identified as Gregorius Nyssenus, *De anima*); Morani 1981: 58-59.

Cod. graec. 291.

[0759]   **308**   II.94.

Hardt 1806-1812: 3.245-250.

Current shelfmark: Cod. graec. 308.

336   See [0740].

350   Aretaeus, *De acutorum et diuturnorum morborum causis et signis libri VII*.

Hardt 1806-1812: 4.7-9.

[0760]   **362**   II.109.

Hardt 1806-1812: 4.50-56.

Current shelfmark: Cod. graec. 362.

384   (ff. 12r et seq.) Symeon Seth, *De alimentorum facultatibus*; (ff. 21r et seq. [?]) Galenus, *De diebus criticis* (frg.); (ff. 22r et seq.) Hippocrates, *Differentiae de phlebotomia*; (ff. 26r et seq.) Hippocrates, *Aphorismi*.

Hardt 1806-1812: 4.188-197.

387   Synesius Cyrenensis, *De insomniis*.

Hardt 1806-1812: 4.200.

389   Dioscorides, *De simplicibus medicinis*.

Hardt 1806-1812: 4.202-203.

	392	(ff. 11r et seq. [?]) *Emplastrum Petri et Pauli*.
		Hardt 1806-1812: 4.206-210.
[0761]	**401**	N.53.
		Hardt 1806-1812: 4.244-246.
		Current shelfmark: Cod. graec. 401.
[0762]	**419**	II.67; N.59.
		Hardt 1806-1812: 4.300-305.
		Current shelfmark: Cod. graec. 419.
	461	(ff. 81 et seq.) Synesius Cyrenensis, *De insomniis*.
		Hardt 1806-1812: 4.432-435.
[0763]	**469**	I.95, 96, 102, 111; II.88 (2), 90, 91; N.34, 35, 36, 37, 64, 65.
		Hardt 1806-1812: 4.451-454.
		Current shelfmark: Cod. graec. 469.
	476	(ff. 34r et seq.) Synesius Cyrenensis, *De insomniis*.
		Hardt 1806-1812: 5.6-19.
	481	(ff. 166r et seq.) Synesius Cyrenensis, *De insomniis* cum Nicephori Gregorae interpretatione; (ff. 182r et seq.) Hippocrates, *Epistulae*.
		Hardt 1806-1812: 5.27-35.
[0764]	**484 (542) (?)**	II.33.
		The manuscript is referred to as containing Dioscorides, *Liber agens de experientia medica ... ordine literarum digestus*.
		The *Monacensis gr.* 484 does not contain such text (Hardt 1806-1812: 5.46-51). This is a mistake (probably a misreading) for 489 (below).
		There is also some confusion with cod. graec. 542 (see p. 156), which contains the version of the same text that circulated under the name of Stephanus Atheniensis.
	489	(ff. 1r et seq.) Dioscorides, *Liber agens de experientia medica ... ordine literarum digestus*; (ff. 13r et seq.) Paulus Aegineta, *Epitome medica*.
		Hardt 1806-1812: 5.68-71; Savvinidou 2006: 347n1, 351-352.
		See [0764] and also 542 below.
	490	(ff. 54r et seq.) Hippocrates, *Epistulae*; (ff. 412r et seq.) Synesius Cyrenensis, *De insomniis*.
		Hardt 1806-1812: 5.71-142.
[0765]	**494**	I.46.
		Hardt 1806-1812: 5.148-151.
		Current shelfmark: Cod. graec. 494.
[0766]	**498**	II.94.
		Hardt 1806-1812: 5.180-200.
		Current shelfmark: Cod. graec. 498.

	506	(ff. Av, Dr-v) Synesius Cyrenensis, *De insomniis*.
		Hardt 1806-1812: 5.225-228.
[0767]	**511**	II.66.
		Hardt 1806-1812: 5.257-260.
		Current shelfmark: Cod. graec. 511.
	512	(ff. 25r et seq.) Nemesius Emesenus, *De natura hominis*.
		Hardt 1806-1812: 5.260-261; Morani 1981: 58-59.
[0768]	**514**	II.107.

This is a copy of Timotheus Gazaeus, *De animalibus quadrupedis physicisque eorum facultatibus*.

The identification of the manuscript (reproduced in Bodenheimer and Rabinowitz 1949: 14) is incorrect: Cod. gr. 514 contains Plato's works (Hardt 1806-1812: 5.262-269). Timotheus' work is in Cod. graec. 564 (below).

[0769]	**521**	N.48.
		Hardt 1806-1812: 5.280-282.
		Current shelfmark: Cod. graec. 521.
[0770]	**525**	I.13, 136.
		Hardt 1806-1812: 5.299-316.
		Current shelfmark: Cod. graec. 525.
	529	(ff. 1r et seq.) *Opusculum medicum*.
		Hardt 1806-1812: 5.318-329.
[0771]	**536**	II.67.
		Hardt 1806-1812: 5.338-341.
		Current shelfmark: Cod. graec. 536.
	542	(ff. 1r et seq.) *Capitula medica* (e.g. *De noscendo pulsu*; Galenus, *De succedaneis*; Diocles, *Ad Antigonum regem epistula de tuenda valetudine*); (ff. 10 et seq.) Symeon Seth, *De alimentorum facultatibus* (frg.) et Paulus Aegineta, *De purgantibus medicamentis*; (ff. 19 et seq.) *Opusculum medicum*; (ff. 50 et seq.) Stephanus Atheniensis, *De simplicium medicinarum et herbarum cura*; (ff. 57 et seq.) *Simile opusculum physico-medicum*; (ff. 67 et seq.) *Herbae zodiaci*.
		Hardt 1806-1812: 5.355-357.

In Diels'catalogue II.33 about **484 (542?)** (= [0764]), the two manuscripts are confused (besides the fact that **484** is a mistake for 489). This is probably because these two manuscripts contain different versions of the same text. While *Cod. graec.* 489 contains the version attributed to Dioscorides, *Cod. graec.* 542 contains the version ascribed to Stephanus Atheniensis (for the latter see Savvinidou 2006: 351).

[0772]   **551**   N.38, 39, 56.

Hardt 1806-1812: 5.378-404.

Current shelfmark: Cod. graec. 551.

Possibly [0741].

[0773]   **562**   II.67.

Hardt 1806-1812: 5.424-426.

Cod. graec. 562.

564   See [0768]. Hardt 1805-1812: 5.426-434.

566   (ff. 55 et seq.) *De signis ponderum et misurarum.*

Hardt 1806-1812: 5.436-438.

570   (ff. 90r et seq.) Gregorius Nyssenus, *De hominis opificio.*

Hardt 1806-1812: 5.440-444.

[0774]   **583 (olim Uffenbachianus)**   N.58.

The mention "olim Uffenbachianus" is not part of the shelfmark of the manuscript, but it refers to the collection assembled by Zacharias Konrad von Uffenbach (1683-1734) (exlibris in the manuscript).

The manuscript was no. XVI in Uffenbach's collection (Majus 1720: 537).

This is a 1656 copy of the 1545 printed edition of Melampus, *Ex palpitationibus divinatio*, by the Dutch scholar Hermannus Venius (Herman van der Veen)

Berger 2014: 60-61.

Current shelfmark: Cod. graec. 583.

633   (ff. 1r-97r) Symeon Seth, *De alimentorum facultatibus*; (ff. 99r-172r) Aetius Amidenus, *Libri medicinales* (frg.).

Tinnefeld 1988: 322 (without mention of the provenance); Berger 2014: 240-244.

Formerly [0216]. Also [0218].

lat.

[0775]   **807**   I.149.

Catalogus Bibliothecae Monacensis 1892: 197.

Late 15th-century *Collectanea et excerpta* (in Greek) by Petrus Crinitus (Pietro del Riccio Baldi [1474-1507]).

Current shelfmark: Clm 807.

Μυτιλήνη Λέσβου (Mytilene, Lesvos) (GR)

Βιβλιοθήκη, Πρότυπο Πειραματικό Γενικό Λύκειο Μυτιλήνης του Πανεπιστημίου Αιγαίου (Library, Model experimental high school of Mytiline of the University of the Aegean)

1   See [0685].

Napoli (Naples) (IT)

Biblioteca dei Gerolamini (Gerolamini Library)

See below **Neapel**, **Bibl. dei Gerolamini** (Gerolamini Library) (see below, p. 163)

Biblioteca Nazionale Vittorio Emanuele III (National Library Vittorio Emanuele III)

olim Vindobonenses graeci

These manuscripts were sent to Vienna in 1718, and returned to Italy in 1919 (see Mioni 1912: VII and n12).

1	Dioscorides, *De materia medica*.
	Mioni 1992: 3-9.
	Same as [1832].
18	(ff. 39r-44v) Nicephorus Gregoras, *Scholia in Synesii de insomniis*; (f. 50v) Aetius Amidenus, *De podagra*.
	Mioni 1992: 28-30.

olim Vindobonensis latinus

2	This manuscript is made of two parts (ff. 1-75 and 76-159), the first of which is palimpsest.

Scriptio superior:

- (ff. 1-42) *Miscellanea patristica*;
- (ff. 42-75) *Miscellanea grammaticalia*.

Scriptio inferior: (ff. 57-59, 61-62, 65-66, 68-70) Dioscorides, *De materia medica*; Galenus, *De theriaca ad Pamphilianum* et *De compositione medicamentorum per genera*; *Pharmacologia*.

De Paolis1996; Harlfinger, Brunschön and Vasiloudi 2006: 145, 150-151.

Same as [1764].

graeci

II A 12	(f. 148v) *De ponderibus*.
	Mioni 1992: 49-53.
II A 18	(ff. 91r-168r) Gregorius Nyssenus, *De hominis opificio*.
	Pernot 1979: 475; Mioni 1992: 59-61.
II A 24	(ff. 75v et seq.) Gregorius Nazianzenus, *De humana natura*.
	Mioni 1992: 68-70.
II B 25	(f. 100r) Splenius, *De generatione hominis*.
	Mioni 1992: 132-135.
II B 29	(ff. 119r-122r) Epiphanius, *De mensuris et ponderibus*.
	Mioni 1992: 139-147.

II B 30	(ff. 383r-429r) Meletius, *De natura hominis*.
	Mioni 1992: 147-150.
II C 9	(f. 199v) Hippocrates, *Aphorismi* (frg.).
	Mioni 1992: 171.
II C 32	(ff. 44r-45v) Gregorius Nyssenus, *De hominis opificio* (frg.); (ff. 351r-365r) Hippocrates, *Excerpta* (inter alia *Aphorismi*, on which see [0777] and [0782]); (f. 365r-v Galenus, *De methodo medendi* (frg.).
	Mioni 1992: 206-220; Formentin 1997: 212.
	Formerly [0790].
II C 33	(ff. 7v-8r) Splenius, *De generatione hominis*; (f. 471r) *Phlebotomia*.
	Pernot 1979: 478; Mioni 1992: 221-239; Formentin 1997: 209.
	See [0782]. Also [0777] and [0778].
	[0782] is identified as 91 (II C 33). This is incorrect, as the intended manuscript is actually II C 32.
II C 34	(ff. 22v-25r) *De natura mundi et hominis*.
	Mioni 1992: 239-246.
II C 37	(f. 381v) *De theriaca*.
	Mioni 1992: 254-262.
II D 4	(ff. 113v-114v) Nicephorus Constantinopolitanus Patriarcha, *Oneirocriticon*.
	Formentin 1995: 5-10.
II D 50	(ff. 53v-120r) Artemidorus, *Oneirocriticon*.
	Formentin 1995: 53-54.
II F 23	(f. IIr) *Praeceptiones medicae*.
	Formentin 1995: 145-147.
II F 30	See [0783].
	Formentin 1995: 153-154; Formentin 1997: 212-213.
III A 15	Hippocrates, *Epistulae*.
	Cyrillus 1832: 211.
III AA 14 bis	Formerly [0791].
	Napolitano, Nardelli and Tartaglia 1977: 26-27; Formentin 1997: 213-214.
III B 9	(ff. 415r et seq.) Synesius Cyrenensis, *De insomniis*.
	Cyrillus 1832: 311-312 (for the manuscript) and 435-436 (for the text).
III C 2	See [0779].

| III D 15 | See [0780] and [0784]. |
| | Pernot 1979: 493. |

III D 17 *Alchimia*, including (ff. 82r et seq.) Democritus, *De sympathicis et antipathicis*.

Cyrillus 1832: 390-394; *CMAG* II (Zuretti et al.) 1927: 217-224.

See [0776].

III D 18 *Alchimia*, including (ff. 1r et seq.) Democritus, *De physicis et mysticis* (frg.).

Cyrillus 1832: 394-396; *CMAG* II (Zuretti et al.) 1927: 225-230.

III D 20 See [0785].

Cyrillus 1832: 397; Formentin 1997: 213.

Formerly [0792].

Contrary to Petit 2010: 146, who stated that this manuscript is lost or cannot be found, the manuscript is present in the collections of the Biblioteca Nazionale in Naples.

III D 21 See [0781] and [0786].

Cyrillus 1832: 398; Pernot 1979: 493.

III D 22 See [0787].

Cyrillus 1832: 399; Pernot 1979: 493; Formentin 1997: 210.

III D 23 See [0788].

Cyrillus 1832: 400-416; Formentin 1997: 215-216.

III D 24 *Geoponica*.

Cyrillus 1832: 417.

III D 25 *Geoponica*.

Cyrillus 1832: 417-418; Pernot 1979: 493.

III D 26 Diodorus, *De ponderibus et mensuris*.

Cyrillus 1832: 418.

III D 36 (ff. 171r et seq.) Aristoteles, *Problemata*.

Cyrillus 1832: 427-428; Wartelle 1963: 86, no. 1186.

III E 19 (ff. 59r et seq.) Synesius, *De insomniis*.

Cyrillus 1832: 452-455.

III E 34 Achmet, *Oneirocriticon*.

Cyrillus 1832: 469-470.

Fondo Brancacciano

Branc. III D 4 Soranus, *De ponderibus et mensuris*.

Napolitano, Nardelli and Tartaglia 1977: 30.

Neapel (Napoli [Naples]) (IT)

Biblioteca Borbonica (Borbonica Library)

"Biblioteca Borbonica" (Bourbon Library)–actually "Biblioteca Reale Borbonica" (Royal Bourbon Library)–is the name given in 1816 to the "Real Biblioteca" (Royal Library) of Naples. The library was founded in 1804, under the King of Two-Sicilies Ferdinand I de Bourbon (or "di Borbone") (reign 1816-1825). After the unification of Italy, it became the National Library in 1860. In 1922, the library was moved to the royal palace under king Vittorio Emanuele III (1869-1947; reign 1900-1946) and became the Biblioteca Nazionale Vittorio Emanuele III (Vittorio Emanuele III National Library). It kept this name after Italy transitioned from a monarchy to a republic in 1946.

Except for [0776], the identifier of which is incorrect, the shelfmarks provided by Diels are of two types:

- in [0777]-[0781] current shelfmark;
- in [0782]-[0788] sequential number in Cyrillus 1832 (followed by the current shelfmark between parentheses).

Three items are listed according these two systems as if they were different manuscripts:

- [0777] (= [0778]) = [0782];
- [0780] = [0784];
- [0781] = [0786].

On all these manuscripts see pp. 158-160, under Napoli, Biblioteca Nazionale, sub *graeci*, under the current shelfmark.

Neapolit. (*Neapolitani*)

[0776]   **I 17**   N.60.

This is a copy of Nepualius, *De sympathicis et antipathicis*.

The number I 17 does not correspond to any current shelfmark of Greek manuscript at the Biblioteca Nazionale in Napoli. It is not a reference to Cyrillus 1832: tome 1, manuscript no. 17 (= pp. 43-46) which contains St. Athanasius, or tome 1, p. 17. Furthermore, no text by Nepualius appears in the index of Cyrillus 1832: 473-486, Mioni 1992: 281-321, or Formentin 1995: 209-223.

The information seems to be a mistake, possibly for III D 17, which contains (ff. 82r et seq.) Democritus, *De sympathicis et antipathicis*. The texts of Nepualius and Democritus have been transmitted together in some manuscripts and sometimes mixed up in scholarly literature.

On III D 17, see Cyrillus 1832: 390-394, and above, p. 160.

[0777]   **II C 33**   II.94.

Mioni 1992: 221-229; Formentin 1997: 209.

According to Magdelaine 1994: 88n1, II C 33 does not exist. Actually, II C 33 does exist; however, the codex that contains a fragment of Hippocrates, *Aphorismi*, is not II C 33, but II C 32 (see p. 159).

On II C 33, see also [0778] and [0782].

[0778]   **II C 33 (olim 34)**   II.82.

Same as [0777].

The mention "olim 34" is not an old shelfmark, but probably refers to the fact that this manuscript is erroneously described under the shelfmark II C 34 in Cyrillus 1832: 7-20 as Mioni 1992: 239 mentioned in the bibliography on II C 33, about Cyrillus 1832: 7-20.

[0779]   **III C 2 (260)**   I.44.

Cyrillus 1832: 341-344 (for the manuscripts and its other texts) and *ibid.* 416 (for the text here); Formentin 1997: 214-215.

[0780]   **III D 15**   N.30, 31, 41.

Cyrillus 1832: 388-389; Formentin 1997: 208-209.

Same as [0784].

[0781]   **III D 21**   N.45.

Cyrillus 1832: 398;

Formentin 1997: 210.

Same as [0786].

[0782]   **91 (II C 33)**   I.13, 35.

According to Diels' catalogue, this is a copy of Hippocrates, *Aphorismi* and *Praecepta*.

The number 91 is the sequential number in Cyrillus 1832: 5-6. The current shelfmark is II.C.33.

However, the codex that contains the Hippocratic texts (frg.) is not II C 33, but is instead II C 32. See Biblioteca Nazionale Vittorio Emanuele III (National Library Vittorio Emanuele III), *graeci*, II C 32 and II C 33 (see above p. 159).

Same as [0777].

[0783]   **187 (II F 30)**   I.38.

Current shelfmark: II F 30 (see above, p. 159).

[0784]   **229 (III D 15)**   I.63; N.30.

Current shelfmark: III D 15 (its number in Cyrillus 1832 is not 229, but 299).

Same as [0780].

[0785]   **304 III D 20**   I.96; II.71.

Current shelfmark: III D 20 (see above, p. 160).

Formerly [0792].

[0786]   **305 III D 21**   II.17, 18 (2), 19.

Current shelfmark: III D 21 (see above, p. 160).

Same as [0781].

[0787]   **306 III D 22**   II.77.

Current shelfmark: III D 22 (see above, p. 160).

[0788]   **307 III D 23**   II.32, 65, 110.

Current shelfmark: III D 23 (see above, p. 160).

Bibl. dei Gerolamini (Biblioteca dei Gerolamini [Gerolamini Library]), now Biblioteca statale oratoriana del Monumento nazionale dei Gerolamini, Napoli (State Oratorian Library of Gerolaminis' National Monument, Naples). See also **Bibl. Oratoriana** below.

[0789]   **XXII.1**   I.38, 44, 46, 64, 128; II.7, 28, 63.

The identifier XXII.1 is an incorrect form of the actual shelfmark of this manuscript: Pil. XXII. n°. I (Mandarini 1897: 263-265).

Same as [0793] and [0794].

Martini 1896 (1967): 397-415.

Bibl. di S. Giovanni di Carbonara (Biblioteca di S. Giovanni di Carbonara [St. John Library at Carbonara])

The three manuscripts listed as "Bibl. di S. Giovanni di Carbonara" belonged to the library of St. John's monastery in Naples, in the Carbonara neighborhood. In 1792, a royal decree transformed the library into a royal library. In 1800, its holdings were transferred to the Royal Library ("Libreria reale"), which became the National Library (Biblioteca Nazionale) in 1860, officially the Vittorio Emanuele III National Library (Biblioteca Nazionale Vittorio Emanuele III). See Gutiérrez 1966; Mioni 1992: VI-VIII, and Formentin 1995: XXII-XXVIII. For the medical manuscripts specifically, see Formentin 1997: 207-208 and 212-214.

Numbers in Diels' catalogue are not the shelfmarks of the manuscripts, but the sequential numbers they have received in the list compiled by Gaetano d'Ancora (1751-1816) and published in Fabricius, ed. Harles 1796: 796-800.

[0790]   **15**   I.56; II.47.

Current shelfmark: Napoli, Biblioteca Nazionale, II C 32 (see p. 159).

Formentin 1997: 208, 212.

[0791]   **27**   I.38.

Current shelfmark: Napoli, Biblioteca Nazionale, III AA 14bis (see p. 159).

Formentin 1997: 298, 213-214.

[0792]   **42**   II.71.

Current shelfmark: Napoli, Biblioteca Nazionale, III D 20 (see p. 160).

Formentin 1997: 208, 213.

Same as [0785].

Bibl. Oratoriana (Biblioteca Oratoriana [Oratorian Library]), now Biblioteca statale oratoriana del Monumento nazionale dei Gerolamini, Napoli (State Oratorian Library of Gerolaminis' National Monument). This library is the same as the **Bibl. dei Gerolamini** (see p. 163).

The number 152 in both [0793] and [0794] is not a shelfmark, but is instead a sequential number in Mandarini 1897: 263-265.

[0793]   **152**   I.44, 131, 133, 134.

Current shelfmark is Pil. XXII. n°. I (Mandarini 1897: 263-265).

As Formentin 1997: 207 noticed, this item is the same as [0789].

Same as [0794] and [0789].

[0794]   **152 (Pil. XXII no. 1)**   II.28, 63.

Current shelfmark is Pil. XXII n°. I (Mandarini 1897: 263-265).

Same as [0793] and [0789].

Nea-Ephesos (Νέα Ἔφεσος, former Ottoman Empire, now Selçuk [TR])

Bibl. Ephes. (*Bibliotheca Ephesiana* [Ephesian Library], actually Βιβλιοθήκη τῆς Ἀστικῆς Σχολῆς [Library of the City School])

[0795]   -   N.43.

This reference to a manuscript without shelfmark is to a codex of Aetius Amidenus, *Libri medicinales*, mentioned in Zervos 1905 (with 1906 as a year of publication listed in Diels' catalogue).

At p. 258, Zervos mentions a 19th-century manuscript of Aetius Amidenus, *Libri medicinales*, books 9-16, which he discovered in 1903 in the library of the local City School (Ἀστικὴ Σχολή).

No information is available about this manuscript, its state of preservation, or its current location.

Nelahozeves (CZ)

Lobkowiczká Knihovna (Lobkowicz Library)

VI Fc 37   See [1410] and [1411].

Olivier and Monégier du Sorbier 1983: 109-113.

VI Fe 4   (pp. 425-440, 457-859) Cassianus Bassus, *De re rustica eclogae.*
Olivier and Monégier du Sorbier 1983: 133-136.

New Haven, CT (US)

Yale University, Beinecke Rare Book and Manuscript Library

-

MS 234   *Scholia ad Galeni, De naturalibus facultatibus, De locis affectis, De elementis secundum Hippocratem.*
Shailor 1984: 338-341.
Formerly Cheltenham, Phillipps Collection, 890.

MS 606   Cassianus Bassus, *Geoponica.*
Sotheby's 1977: 86, lot 4982.
Formerly Cheltenham, Phillipps Collection, 6762.

MS 1121   Galen, *De temperamentis, De naturalibus facultatibus, De inaequali intemperie, De bono habitu, De difficultate respirartionis, Ad Glauconem de medendi methodo, De alimentorum facultatibus.*
Christie's 2006: 35-36 lot 22.
Former [0215].

Yale University, Harvey Cushing/John Hay Whitney Medical Library

-

Manuscript 31 vault   Former [0213].
Faye and Bond 1962: 61, no. 31.

Manuscript 32 vault   Former [1855].
Faye and Bond 1962: 61, no. 32.

Manuscript 33 vault   Former [0214].
Faye and Bond 1962: 61, no. 33.

Manuscript 34 vault   Former [0217].
Faye and Bond 1962: 61, no. 34.

Manuscript 35 vault   *Efodia.*
This codex was previously Zaragoza, Cabildo de la Santa Iglesia Mayor del Pilar, 327 (= 25-60 at La Seo; Olivier 1976: 56).
Graux, ed. Martin 1892: 211-212, no. 327; Faye and Bond 1962: 61, no. 35.

Manuscript 36 vault   *Efodia.*
This manuscript was previously Cheltenham, Phillipps Collection, 21595.
Faye and Bond 1962: 61, no.36.

Manuscript 37 vault   Galenus, *De antidotis*; *De theriaca ad Pisonem*.

Faye and Bond 1962: 61, no. 37.

Manuscript 50 vault   Former [1856].

Faye and Bond 1962: 63, no. 50.

New York, NY (US)

Morgan Library

MS M.

397   (ff. 8r-21v) *Physiologus*.

Kavrus-Hoffmann 2008: 101-112.

652   Former [0219].

Faye and Bond 1962: 352; Kavrus-Hoffmann 2008/2: 212-230.

[Norfolk] (GB)

-

-

[0796]   **[nr. 3189]**   I.13.

This item is listed among the copies of Hippocrates, *Aphorismi* in Greek.

The same information appears in Ackermann 1825: LXVI, where the manuscript is quoted among the Latin codices of the work, without brackets.

Number 3189 is not a shelfmark but a sequential number in a catalogue published in *C.M.A.* 1697: 2.1.74-84, entitled as follows (*ibid.*: 2.1.74):

Bibliothecae Norfolcianae in Collegio Greshamensi apud Londinum catalogus

Number 3189 (*ibid.*: 2.1.80) contains the following according to *C.M.A.*:

Psalmi Davidis, cum Precum Formulis ...

Number 3189 in Diels' catalogue probably is a mistake for 3184 in *C.M.A.* 1697: 2.1.80, which contains the following:

3184. 285 Gothofridi Flores Medicae, cum Commentario.

Bartholomaei Practica Medica.

De Pulsibus.

Hippocratis Aphorismi.

Evax de Lapidibus.

Recepta Medicinalia.

This is a Latin manuscript, which was not at Norfolk, but in London, Gresham College, to which Henry Howard (1628-1684), 6th Duke of Norfolk, donated his family's library collection in the late 17th century (Burgon 1839: 2.518-519).

This manuscript cannot be traced in the current state of research (it is not mentioned in Kibre 1985 or Magdelaine 1994).

Охрид (Ohrid) (MK)

Националниот музей (Natsionalniot Muzeyi [National Museum])

-

72   (pp. 108-294) Gregorius Nyssenus, *De hominis opificio*.
Mošin 1961: 224, no. 67; Morani 1981: 217-219.

Orléans (FR)

Bibl. communale (Bibliothèque communale [Municipal Library]), now Médiathèque (Media Center)

-

[0797]   **1032**   II.47.

This is a copy of Hermes Trismegistus, *Excerpta varia*.

This is a 17th-century collection of fragments from alchemical treatises including (pp. 121 et seq.) Hermes Trismegistus, *Tabula smaragdina* .

Catalogue général des manuscrits 1904: 589-590.

Oxford (GB)

[Ashmol.] (*Ashmoleani*)

These manuscripts were in the Ashmolean Museum (or *Bibliotheca Ashmoliana*) from which they were transferred to the Bodleian Library in 1860 (Morgan 1973: 159). Numbers in Diels' catalogue are not shelfmarks, but sequential numbers in *C.M.A.* 1697: 1.1.

-

[0798]   **[ms. Angl. 7638]**   I.122.

This manuscript contains Galenus, *De XII portis*.

Number 7638 appears in *C.M.A.* 1697: 1.1.339 in a catalogue of manuscripts collected by Elias Ashmole (1617-1692) and preserved in the *Bibliotheca Ashmoliana* (*ibid.*: 315-356 for the catalogue). The content of this item is described as follows:

7638. Alberti Magni Mineralium Libri quattuor.

Quadripartitum Hermetis, p. 50.

Ars fusoria ac tinctoria Gemmarum, p. 64.

Ptolemaei liber de Lapidibus pretiosis, p. 64.

Galeni liber de 12. portis, p. 68. Membr. fol. 1471.

It is a Latin manuscript, now Bodleian Library, MS. Ashmole 1471.

Black 1845: 1280-1286.

Also [0799].

[0799]   **[ms. Angl. 7787]**   I.122.

This manuscript contains Galenus, *De XII portis*.

Number 7787 appears in *C.M.A.* 1697: 1.1.342 in the same list as [0798], among the *Medici Lat[ini]* of the *Ashmoleani* (see *ibid.*: 1.1.341) and is described as follows:

7787. Galeni liber de 12 portis, Membr. 1471. p. 68.

This description is the same as that of item 5 in [0798]. It thus is highly probable that this entry duplicates no. 7638 in *C.M.A.* 1697: 1.1.339, and that this manuscript is the same as [0798].

Bibl. Aedis Christi (*Bibliotheca Aedis Christi* [Aedes Christi Library]), now Christ Church Library.

Shelfmark of manuscripts is "Christ Church MS. gr." followed by the numbers below.

[0800]   **34**   I.56, 149.

Kitchin 1867: 20.

45   (ff. 115r-194r) Gregorius Nyssenus, *De hominis opificio*.

Kitchin 1867: 23.

47   (ff. 180 et seq.) Gregorius Nazanzienus, *De quattuor elementis e quibus homo factus est*.

Kitchin 1867: 23-24.

[0801]   **81**   II.17, 18 (2), 19.

Kitchin 1867: 30.

Bibl. Bodleiana (*Bibliotheca Bodleiana*), now Bodleian Library

These manuscripts are identified in different ways in Diels' catalogue, including:

- [0804]-[0808] and [0839] are numbered according to their sequential number in different parts of *C.M.A.* 1697 introduced by "cat. mss. Angl."
- [0842]-[0845] are identified by their sequential number in *C.M.A.* 1697, without any reference to *C.M.A.*;
- [0840] and [0846]-[0848] include the current shelfmark introduced by "nunc";
- [0841] is identified by its current shelfmark, followed, between parentheses, by its sequential number in *C.M.A.* 1697.

For a concordance between *C.M.A.* 1697 sequential numbers and the current shelfmarks, see Madan and Craster 1922.

In each collection, items in Diels' catalogue are numbered in different ways, identified in the introduction to each collection.

[0802]   **- (Puschm. I p. 90)**   II.12.

This manuscript without a collection name or shelfmark is a copy of Alexander Trallianus, *Therapeutica*.

Reference is to Puschmann 1878-1879: 1.90, where a manuscript of the Bodleian library is mentioned without further identification.

This is ms. Oxford, Bodleian Library, MS. D'Orville 34.

Madan 1897: 45-46, no. 16912.

17th/18th-century scholarly manuscript.

[0803]   *e 19 [31.528]*   II.30 (listed in entry "**Edschmiadzin**").

Current shelfmark: MS. Gr. class. e. 19.

This is a set of photos of a fragment of a manuscript (Dioscorides, *De materia medica*) in the codex now identified as Yerevan, Matenadaran, arm. M 141 (see p. 372).

Madan and Craster 1924: 62, no. 31528.

[0804]   **[cat. mss. Angl. 1355]** I.61.

This item contains Galenus, *Ars medica*.

Number 1355 appears in *C.M.A.* 1697: 1.1.71, in the list of the manuscripts that " illustrissimus dominus Guilielmus Laudus" donated to the Bodleian Library" (*ibid.*: 1.1.46-76 for the list). This item is described as follows:

1355.15. Hippocrates Aphorismi, & Prognostica.

2. Theophilus de Urinis.

3. Philaretus de Pulsu.

4. Galeni Techne, etc.

The same information as in Diels' catalogue (without brackets) appears in Ackermann 1821: CXV, no. 50 ctd. (about Galenus, *Ars medica*), where this manuscript is listed among the Greek manuscripts of the work.

The same number also appears in Ackermann 1825: XLVII (Hippocrates, *Prognosticon*, where this item is listed among the Greek manuscripts of the work), and LXV (Hippocrates, *Aphorismi*, where the codex it listed among the Latin manuscripts of the work).

It is not a Greek manuscript (none of the following authors mention it: Alexanderson 1963 or Jouanna 2013 for the *Prognosticon*; Magdelaine 1994 for the *Aphorismi*; Boudon 2002: 197-200 for Galenus, *Ars medica*), but a Latin one (Kibre 1985: 45 [*Aphorismi*] and 206 [*Prognostica*]).

Current shelfmark: Bodleian Library, MS. Laud Lat. 65 (see also Boudon 2002: 197n109 ctd.).

Hunt 1953: 26, no. 1355, and Madan and Craster 1922: 58 (for the concordance between *C.M.A.* 1697 and the current shelfmark); Coxe 1858: 30 (catalogue).

Same as [0845].

[0805]   **[cat. mss. Angl. 1552]** I.61.

This item is referenced as a copy of Galenus, *Ars medica* in Greek.

Number 1552 appears in *C.M.A.* 1697: 1.1.74, in the same list as [0804]. It does not contain any medical text, but works by St. Augustinus (= Laud. Misc. 125; Hunt 1953: 26, no. 1552, for the concordance of *C.M.A.* 1697 and the current shelfmark; Coxe 1858: 128 for a description). This manuscript is not listed in Boudon 2002: 197-200.

The information (without brackets) comes from Ackermann 1821: CXV, no. 50 ctd. ("In bibl. Bodlei. cat. Mss. Angl. no., 1552"), where this item is listed among the Greek manuscripts of Galenus, *Ars medica*.

This probably is a mistake for 1252 in *C.M.A.* 1697, where no. 1252 is described as follows (1.1.68-69):

1252. 87. Johannitii Isagoge ad Galeni Technen.

2. Hippocratis Aphorismi et Prognostica.

3. Theophilus de Urinis.

4. Philaretus de Pulsibus.

5. Galeni Techne.

6. Constantini Monachi [...]

7. Aegidii Poema de Urinis. It. de Pulsibus cum Commentario.

It is a Latin manuscript (it is not mentioned in Boudon 2002: 197-200 for Galenus, *Ars medica*, or in Magdelaine 1994 for Hippocrates, *Aphorismi*; instead, it is listed in Kibre 1985: 8-9 [*Acutorum Regimen*], 45 [*Aphorismi*]).

Current shelfmark: Bodleian Library, MS. Lat. 106 (*pace* Boudon 2002: 197n109 ctd., who mentions that this item of Diels' catalogue is Misc. 125).

Hunt 1953: 26, no. 1252 (concordance of *C.M.A.* 1697 and current shelfmark); Madan and Craster 1922: 54: Coxe 1858: 48-49 (catalogue).

Also [0843] and probably [0844].

[0806]   **[Cat. mss. Angl. n. 2062]**   I.117.

This item contains Galenus, *Lexicon botanicum*.

The number 2062 appears in *C.M.A.* 1697: 1.1.107, in a catalogue of manuscripts "ex dono Viri perillustris et Fundatoris munificentissimi Thomae Bodleii." (*ibid.*: 1.1.89-156). It is described as follows (1.1.107):

2062.1. Several Medicines, most by natural means, some by Charmes with an Herbal proceeding alphabetically in respect of the Latine names.

The Virtues of Herbs, which are Hot or Cold, and for how many things they are good; after Plato, Galen, and Hippocrates.

A Physical Tract of the Conception, Birth, etc. of Man.

De Morbis Mulierum, etc.

This is neither a Greek nor a Latin manuscript, but an English one (see Madan and Craster 1922: 190-191).

Current shelfmark: Bodleian Library, MS. Bodl. 483.

[0807]   **[2753]**   I.5.

This item is listed among the manuscripts of Hippocrates, *Prognosticon*.

Number 2753 appears in *C.M.A.* 1697: 1.1.147 (in the same list as [0806]), where its contents is identified as follows:

2753.11. Joannitii Isagoge ad Microtechnum Galeni.

2. Hippocratis Aphorismi et Prognostica.

3. Lib. Urinarum à voce Theophili.

4. Philareti Lib. de negotio Pulsuum.

5. Lib. qui inscribitur Galeni Techna.

6. Diaetae Universales et particulares, per Mag. Isaac.

7. Ejusdem lib. Urinarum.

8. Constantini Africani lib. de Stomacho.

9. Ejusdem de regendorum sanorum ratione liber. Imperf.

This is a Latin manuscript (Alexanderson 1963 does not mention it [*Pronosticon*]; see, instead, Kibre 1985: 44-45 [*Aphorismi*]).

This manuscript is Bodleian Library, MS. Auct. F. 5. 30.

See Madan and Craster 1922: 528-529, no. 2753.

Information in Diels' catalogue comes from Ackermann 1825: XLVII (without brackets), where the codex is listed among the "CODICES MSS" without specification of language.

[0808]   **[bibl. Brit. n. 3500]**   I.135.

This item is a copy of Galenus, *De chirurgia*.

Number 3500 appears in *C.M.A.* 1697: 1.1.169 in a list of manuscripts "benefactorum variorum" (*ibid.*: 1.1.168-186). The treatise of Galenus, *De chirurgia*, is described as follows (*ibid.*: 1.1.169, no. 5 in manuscript 3500, which contains 11 different medical Latin treatises):

Galeni Chirurgia, sive Capitula varia ex Operibus ejus Collecta.

This is a Latin ms. Current shelfmark: Bodleian Library, MS. e Mus. 19.

Madan, Craster and Denholm-Young 1937: 659-661.

Auct. (*Auctarium* [Additional collection])

[0809]   **F. Inf. II 3**   I.13, 18 (2).

Madan, Craster and Denholm-Young 1937: 1002, no. 5304.

Current shelfmark: MS. Marshall 72 (formerly MS. Auct. F. inf. 2. 3).

See [0810] and [0854].

See Magdelaine 1994: 88 n1.

[0810]   **T II 3**   I.5, 56.

This manuscript is listed among the copies of Hippocrates, *Prognosticon* (I.5) and Hippocratic *Excerpta* (I.56).

The current manuscript Auct. T. 2. 3 contains Euthymius Zigabenus (see Coxe 1853: 758, Misc. 203; Hunt 1953: 433, no. 20587. Also Alexanderson 1963: 69).

The item referred to here seems to be Auct. F. inf. 2. 3 (= [0809]) (current shelfmark: *Marshall 72*), which does indeed contain Hippocrates, *Prognosticon* (Diels, I.5; see Alexanderson 1963: 78-79 [*Marshall* 72]), and three other Hippocratic treatises that might have been incorrectly identified as *Excerpta* (Diels, I.56) (see Alexanderson 1963: 78-79, *Marshall 72*).

Same as [0809]. Also [0854].

[0811]   **T II 10**   I.38.

Madan 1897: 434, no. 20613.

Current shelfmark: MS. Auct. T. 2. 10.

Also [0857].

Baroccian. (*Barocciani*; Francesco Barozzi [1537-1604] and his nephew Iacopo Barozzi [1562-1617])

The manuscripts of this collections are now identified as "MS. Barocci" followed by a number in Arabic numerals (e.g. 10 in Diels = MS. Barocci 10).

[0812]   **10**   I.41.

Coxe 1853: 15-18.

34   Gregorius Nazianzenus, *De humana natura*.

Coxe 1853: 53; Domiter 1999: 22.

[0813]   **50**   II.4, 107.

Coxe 1853: 70-78.

[0814]   **51**   I.38.

Coxe 1853: 78-79.

54   Cassianus Bassus, *Geoponica*.

Coxe 1853: 80.

70   (ff. 379r et seq.) Petosiris, *Prognosticon sive epistula ad Nechepsum*.

Coxe 1853: 111-113.

[0815]   **76**   I.5.

Coxe 1853: 128-138.

[0816]   **82**   II.67.

Coxe 1853: 142.

84   (f. 174r) *Remedium magicum contra morsum animalis rabidi*.

Coxe 1853: 143-144.

87   (ff. 2r et seq.) Aristoteles, *Problemata* (frg.); (f. 33v) Imago Iohannis Argyropuli medici.

Coxe 1853: 151-152; Wartelle 1963: 89, no. 1226.

[0817]   **88**   I.44 (2), 121, 128, 130, 131; II.6, 20 (2), 21, 34, 47, 57, 75, 77, 81.

Coxe 1853: 152-153.

Probably also [0818].

[0818]   **[88]**   I.126.

This item contains Galenus, *De morbis Excerpta*.

No text explicitly entitled in that way appears in Ms. *Baroccianus* 88 (see Coxe 1853: 152-153). However, this text might correspond to item no. 4 in *Baroccianus* 88 according to Coxe's description (col. 153):

Fasciculus morborum et remediorum in capita DCCVIII. distributus.

If so, this item might be the same as [0817].

[0819]	**94**	II.67.
		Coxe 1853: 159-160.
	95	(ff. 223r et seq.) Epiphanius, *Physiologus*.
		Coxe 1853: 160-163.
	96	(ff. 28r et seq.) Gregorius Nazianzenus, *De humana natura*.
		Coxe 1853: 163-168; Domiter 1999: 22.
	108	(ff. 104r et seq.) Gregorius Nyssenus, *De fabrica corporis humani*.
		Coxe 1853: 176-178.
[0820]	**111**	II.98.
		Coxe 1853: 181-185.
	129	(ff. 148v et seq.) Epiphanius, *De duodecim gemmis*.
		Coxe 1853: 209-210.
[0821]	**131**	I.47, 56, 72, 78, 88, 110, 126; II.9 (2), 63, 75.
		Coxe 1853: 211-230.
	139	(ff. 195r et seq.) Synesius Cyrenensis, *De insomniis*.
		Coxe 1853: 240-241.
	144	(ff. 98v-174) Gregorius Nyssenus, *De hominis opificio*.
		Coxe 1853: 247.
	145	(ff. 171r et seq.) Aristoteles, *Problemata* (frg.).
		Coxe 1853: 247-251; Wartelle 1963: 90, no. 1231.
[0822]	**150**	I.41, 133; II.11, 17, 21, 33, 34, 38, 41, 49 (2), 56, 58 (2), 60, 69, 74, 80, 85, 86, 99, 100; N.67.
		Coxe 1853: 262-264.
	164	*Varia veterinaria et medica*.
		Coxe 1853: 278.
[0823]	**171**	II.69.
		Coxe 1853: 285-286.
[0824]	**173**	II.66.
		Coxe 1853: 288-292.
[0825]	**204**	I.4, 5, 8, 10, 11 (3), 12, 13, 18 (2), 19, 20 (3), 21 (2), 22 (2), 23 (2), 24 (3), 25 (2), 26 (2), 27 (3), 28 (2), 29 (2), 30 (3), 31 (2), 33 (2), 34 (3), 35 (2), 38, 66, 110; II.37, 93, 104.
		Coxe 1853: 358-361.

[0826]   **216**   II.33.

Coxe 1853: 376-383.

219   (ff. 178r-180v, 166r-174v, 181r) Synesius Cyrenensis, *De insomniis*.

Coxe 1853: 385-387.

[0827]   **220**   I.84; II.43.

Coxe 1853: 387.

[0828]   **224**   I.43, 134; II.8, 28, 58, 71, 77, 80.

Coxe 1853: 390-392.

Also [0829].

228   (ff. 65r et seq.) Gregorius Nyssenus, *De hominis opificio*.

Coxe 1853: 393-394.

[0829]   **264**   I.76.

This manuscript is listed among the copies of Galenus, *De alimentorum facultatibus libri III*.

The Barocci collection contains 244 numbers (Madan and Craster 1922: 3).

This text appears in Barocci 224 (= [0828]), no. 15 (= ff. 51v et seq. [frg.]). The present information seems to result from confusion with this codex.

[0830]   **2304**   II.109.

This item is listed among the copies of Ioannes Zacharias Actuarius, *De spiritu animali libri II*.

No Barocci manuscript has a 2304 shelfmark. The number probably refers to *C.M.A.* 1697, which contains three items with shelfmark 2304:

- 1.1.119 (in the same catalogue as [0806]): this manuscript contains *Distinctiones super Psalterium. De quantitate Syllabarum tractatus Metricus & Prosaicus*;

- 1.2.168 (in the catalogue entitled [*ibid.*: 1.2.164] "Librorum manuscriptorum In Bibliotheca Publica celeberrimae Academiae Cantabrigiensis catalogus" [*ibid.*: 1.2.164-173, for the catalogue]): this item contains *Summa Richardi and the Historia Bruti. Pr.Britannia insularum optima ...*;

- 2.1.77 (in the catalogue entitled [*ibid.*: 2.1.71] "Librorum manuscriptorum Collegii S, Mariae Magdalenae in Oxonia catalogus" [*ibid.*: 2.1.71-78, for the catalogue): this manuscript contains *Quodlibeta Doctoris Joannis Duns, sive Scoti*.

The text cited by Diels here appears in [0872], now MS. Roe 15 (which is number 261.15 in *C.M.A.* 1697: 1.136).

The origin of this number 2304 is unknown. See Madan and Craster 1922: 299-300.

Alternatively, this item might have been confused with *Parisinus graecus* 2304 (= [1252]), which does contain (ff. 114 et seq.) Actuarius, *De spiritu animali libri II* (Omont 1886-1888: 2.233; Costomiris 1897: 428-430) and does not appear in Diels' list for this text (II.109).

Canonician. (*Canoniciani*, Matteo Luigi Canònici [1727-1805])

The manuscripts of this collection are now identified as "MS. Canon. Gr." followed by a number in Arabic numerals (e.g. 1 in Diels = MS. Canon. Gr. 1).

[0831]	**1**	I.40, 47, 125, 130; II.7.
		Coxe 1854: 1-4.
[0832]	**44**	I.84, 85.
		Coxe 1854: 50-51.
[0833]	**56**	II.67.
		Coxe 1854: 63-65.
[0834]	**109**	II.6; N.43.
		Coxe 1854: 99.

Clarkian. (*Clarkiani*, William N. Clarke [1799-1855])

	11	(ff. 110r et seq.) Epiphanius, *De duodecim gemmis*.
		Madan 1897: 301, no. 18373 (does not specifically identify the text).
[0835]	**16 (18378)**	I.41, 113, 133.
		18378 is not a shelfmark, but the sequential number of the manuscript in Hunt 1953: 15, and Madan 1897 (below).
		Madan 1897: 302, no. 18378.
		Current shelfmark: MS. E. D. Clarke 16.

Ger. Langbainii Advers. (*Gerardi Langbainii Adversaria*, Gerard Langbaine [1609-1658])

[0836]	**2**	I.41.
		Coxe 1853: 877-878.
		Current shelfmark: MS. Langbaine 2.

Is. Casauboni Advers. (*Isacii Casauboni Adversaria*, Isaac Casaubon [1559-1614])

[0837]	**4**	I.72.
		Coxe 1853: 824-825.
		Current shelfmark: MS. Casaubon 4.
[0838]	27	II.34.
		Coxe 1853: 839-840.
		Current shelfmark: MS. Casaubon 27.

Laudian. (*Laudiani*, William Laud [1573-1645], Archbishop of Canterbury)

Identification of these manuscripts in Diels' catalogue is made in five different ways:

- in [0839] and [0842]-[0845], sequential numbers in *C.M.A.* 1697: 1.1.46-76;
- in [0849], shelfmark (capital Latin letter C followed by a number in Arabic numerals) followed, between parentheses, by the sequential number in *C.M.A.* 1697: *ibid.*;

- in [0841], current shelfmark followed, between parentheses, by the sequential number in *C.M.A.* 1697: *ibid.*;
- in [0846]-[0848], shelfmark in *C.M.A.* 1697: *ibid.*, followed by the current shelfmark (introduced by "nunc") and the sequential number in *C.M.A.* 1697: *ibid.*;
- in [0840], a part of the shelfmark (the Arabic number without the C letter) according to *C.M.A.* 1697: *ibid.*, followed by the current shelfmark and the sequential number in *C.M.A.* 1697.

[0839]   **[cat. ms. Angl. N. 877]**   I.133.

This manuscript is listed as a copy of Galenus, *Remedia*.

The reference is to *C.M.A.*1697: 1.1.60.

This is a Latin manuscript containing according to *C.M.A.* 1697 "Galeni Fragmenta quaedam p. 289" (actually: "Ex Galeni libro de situ regionum et temporum constitutione: et aliis operibus. fol. 289" [Coxe 1858: 445]).

Madan and Craster 1922: 37, no. 877 (concordance *C.M.A.* 1697 and current shelfmark); Coxe 1858: 444-445 (catalogue).

Current shelfmark: MS. Laud Misc. 617.

[0840]   **58 (nunc 59; Bodl. 708)**   I.128; II.20, 88.

This manuscript is identified in the same way in Daremberg 1879: XII.

Current shelfmark: MS. Laud Gr. 59.

[0841]   **62 (Bodl. 747)**   II.110.

Current shelfmark: MS. Laud Gr. 62.

[0842]   **[1013]**   I.5, 13.

This codex is listed among the copies of Hippocrates, *Prognosticon* (I.5) and *Aphorismi* (I.13).

The reference is to *C.M.A.* 1697: 1.1.63, reproduced (without brackets) in Ackermann 1825: XLVII (*Prognosticon*, where the manuscript is listed among "CODICES MSS" without specification of language), and LXV (*Aphorismi*, where it is listed among the Latin codices of the work).

This is a Latin manuscript (neither Alexanderson 1963 nor Magdelaine 1994 mention it; Kibre 1985 lists it: 45 [*Aphorismi*] and 202 [*Prognostica*]).

Hunt 1953: 24, no. 1013, and Madan and Craster 1922: 43, no. 1013 (concordance *C.M.A.* 1697 and current shelfmark); Coxe 1858: 200-202 (catalogue).

Current shelfmark: MS. Laud Misc. 237.

[0843]   **[1252]**   I.13.

This item is listed among the copies of Hippocrates, *Aphorismi*.

The reference is to *C.M.A.* 1697: 1.1.68-69, followed by Ackermann 1825: LXV (where the codex is listed without brackets, among the Latin codices of the work).

This is not a Greek manuscript (it does not appear in Magdelaine 1994), but a Latin one, now MS. Laud Lat. 106 (see Kibre 1985: 45).

Hunt 1953: 26, no. 1252, and Madan and Craster 1922: 54, no. 1252 (concordance *C.M.A.* 1697 and current shelfmark); Coxe 1858: 48-49 (catalogue).

See [0805]. Probably also [0844].

[0844]   **[1257]**   I.5.

This manuscript appears in the list of the copies of Hippocrates, *Prognosticon*.

The number 1257 in *C.M.A.* 1697: 1.1.69 (reproduced in Ackermann 1825: XLVII, without brackets among the "CODICES MSS" without specification of language), corresponding to current MS. Laud Lat. 43 (Hunt 1953: 25, no. 1257, and Madan and Craster 1922: 54, no. 1257), does not contain medical text (Kibre 1985 does not mention it), but it does contain the *Epistles* and the *Apocalypse* (Coxe 1858: 20).

There probably has been confusion between 1257 and 1252. If so, 1257 is the same as [0843], that is, Laud. Lat. 106.

Alexanderson 1963 does not mention this *Laudianus* Lat. 106, but Kibre 1985: 206 does.

See [0843].

[0845]   **[1355]**   I.5, 13.

This manuscript is listed among the codices containing Hippocrates, *Prognosticon* (I.5) and *Aphorismi* (I.13).

The reference is to *C.M.A.* 1697: 1.1.71 (reproduced in Ackermann 1825: XLVII [*Prognosticon*] among the "CODICES MSS" without specification of language, and LXV [*Aphorismi*] among the Latin codices of the text; in both cases, without brackets).

This is not a Greek manuscript (neither Alexanderson 1963 nor Magdelaine 1994 mention it), but a Latin one, now MS. Laud Lat. 65 (Kibre 1985: 45 [*Aphorismi*], 206 [*Progonosticon*] referring to Diels' catalogue in the latter case).

Hunt 1953: 26, no. 1355, and Madan and Craster 1922: 58, no. 1355 (for the concordance of *C.M.A.* 1697 and the current shelfmark); Coxe 1858: 30 (catalogue).

Same as [0804].

[0846]   **C 54 (nunc 56; Bodl. 706)**   I.92.

                                                    Current shelfmark: MS. Laud Gr. 56.

[0847]   **C 55 (nunc 57; Bodl. 707)**   I.87, 88 (2), 89.

                                                    Current shelfmark: MS. Laud Gr. 57.

[0848]   **C 57 (nunc 58, Bodl. 709)**   I.63, 64, 65, 83-84, 85, 89, 91, 115.

                                                    Current shelfmark: MS. Laud Gr. 58.

[0849]   **C 60 (Bodl. 749)**   II.6.

                                                    Current shelfmark: MS. Laud Gr. 60.

Miscell. (*Miscellanei*)

[0850]   -   II.28.

Coxe 1853: 712, no. 155.

This copy of Diocles, *Ad Antigonum regem epistula de tuenda valetudine* without any identification is current MS. Rawl. G. 94.

[0851]   **20**   I.70, 131; II.21, 40.

Coxe 1853: 630-631.

Current shelfmark: MS. Auct. E. 1. 6.

[0852]   **69**   II.67.

Coxe 1853: 655.

Current shelfmark: MS. Auct. E. 5. 4.

[0853]   **130**   I.26, 77-78; II.99.

Coxe 1853: 696.

Current shelfmark: MS. Auct. F. inf. 2. 1.

[0854]   **132**   I.5, 13, 18 (2), 77.

Coxe 1853: 697.

Current shelfmark: MS. Marshall 72.

Same as [0809].

Also [0810].

[0855]   **162**   II.67.

Coxe 1853: 714-715.

Current shelfmark: MS. Rawl. G. 122.

[0856]   189   II.6.

Coxe 1853: 742-752.

Current shelfmark: MS. Auct. T. 1. 11.

[0857]   **210**   I.38.

Coxe 1853: 767.

Current shelfmark: MS. Auct. T. 2. 10.

Same as [0811].

[0858]   **211**   II.36.

Coxe 1853: 767-770.

Current shelfmark: MS. Auct. T. 2. 11.

Also [0859].

[0859]   **211 (Auct. T II 11)**   N.50.

Same as [0858].

[0860]   212   II.36.

Coxe 1853: 770.

Current shelfmark: MS. Auct. T. 2. 12.

Also [0861].

[0861]   **212 (Auct. T II 12)**   N.50.

Same as [0860].

[0862]   **241**   II.79.

Coxe 1853: 788-789.

Current shelfmark: MS. Auct. T. 4. 3.

Formerly [1738].

Also [0863].

[0863]   **241. Auct. T IV 3**   II.109.

Same as [0862].

[0864]   **278**   II.49, 68.

Coxe 1853: 818-819.

Current shelfmark: MS. Auct. T. 5. 16.

Orvillian. (*Orvilliani*, Jacques Philippe D'Orville [1696-1751])

Shelfmarks in Diels' catalogue are those in the *Codices D'Orvilliani* 1806 by [Thomas Gaisford] (1779-1855). The manuscripts of this collection are now identified as "Ms. D'Orville" followed by a number in Arabic numerals.

[0865]   **X 1. 1. 3**   I.101, 110, 111; II.37, 71.

Codices D'Orvilliani 1806: 2.

Current shelfmark: MS. D'Orville 3.

[0866]   **X 1. 4. 3**   II.67.

Codices D'Orvilliani 1806: 21.

Current shelfmark: MS. D'Orville 105.

[0867]   **X 1. 4. 29**   I.49.

Codices D'Orvilliani 1806: 28-29.

Copy by Isaac Vossius (1618-1689) (see *Codices D'Orvilliani* 1806: 29, no. 11 "Ex Ms. Hadriani Junii Hornani Medici descripsit Is. Vossius").

Current shelfmark: MS. D'Orville 131.

[0868]   **X 2. 6. 2 (= 432)**   II.67.

Codices D'Orvilliani 1806: 55.

Printed edition of Nemesius Emesenus, *De natura hominis*, Oxford, 1671, with handwritten collation of manuscripts by Jacques Philippe D'Orville (see *Codices D'Orvilliani* 1806: 55 "cum Var. Lect. MSS. J. P. D'Orvillii").

Current shelfmark: MS. D'Orville 432.

Roe. (Sir Thomas Roe [1580 or 1581-1644])

[0869]   **14**   II.6, 38.

Coxe 1853: 466-467.

Current shelfmark: MS. Roe 14.

See [0870], [0871] and [0874].

[0870]   **14 (260)**   I.41.

Number 260 is not a shelfmark, but a sequential number in *C.M.A.* 1697: 1.1.36, in a catalogue entitled (*ibid.*: 35 for the title, and 35-38 for the catalogue):

Librorum Manuscriptorum Bibliothecae Bodleianae Classis Secunda. Codices Graeci XXVI. Hebraicus I. Arabicus I. & Latinus I. Ex Dono Viri Illustris Thomae Roe Militis.

See also Madan and Craster 1922: 11.

Same as [0869]. Also [0871] and [0874].

[0871]   **14 (Bodl. 260)**   II.63, 104.

Same as [0869]. Also [0870] and [0874].

[0872]   **15 (Bodl. 261)**   I.125; II.10, 63, 102 (2), 109 (2), 110.

On number 261, see *C.M.A.* 1697: 1.1.36, in the same catalogue as [0869]. Also Madan and Craster 1922: 11.

Coxe 1853: 468-469.

Current shelfmark: MS. Roe 15.

Also [0873].

[0873]   **15 (Bodl. 260 [261 bei Ackermann])**   I.128.

This is a copy of the text identified as Galenus, *De urinis*.

Reference is to Ackermann 1821: CLXIV, no. 117, with the following description:

Urinarum divisio Galeni est in bibl. Bodl. no. 261.

Ackermann's reference is to *C.M.A.* 1697: 1.1.36, where no. 261 includes:

Galeni urinarum divisio 89 b. Οὖρον λευκὸν μὴ ἔχοντα ὑπόστασιν.

Same as [0872].

[0874]   **XIV (260)**   I.13, 34-35.

Same as [0869]. Also [0870] and [0871].

17   (ff. 206v et seq.) Epiphanius, *De duodecim gemmis*.

Coxe 1853: 470-471.

Bodleian Library

Auctarium

E. 1. 6   See [0851].

E. 5. 4   See [0852].

F. 4. 15   Manuel Philes, *De animalium proprietate*.

Coxe 1853: 686, Misc. 114.

F. 6. 1   (f. 318r-v) Aristoteles, *Problemata* (frg.).

                 Madan and Craster 1922: 95-96, no. 1882.

F. inf. 2. 1   See [0853].

T. 1. 11   See [0856].

T. 2. 10   See [0811] and [0857].

T. 2. 11   See [0858] and [0859].

T. 2. 12   See [0860] and [0861].

T. 2. 16   (ff. 1 et seq.) Gregorius Nyssenus, *De hominis opificio*.

                 Coxe 1853: 773, Misc. 216.

T. 4. 3   See [0862], [0863] and [1738].

T. 4. 24   (ff. 432r et seq.) Aristoteles, *De insomniis*.

                 Coxe 1853: 808-809, Misc. 262; Wartelle 1963: 92, no. 1257.

T. 5. 16   See [0864].

T. 5. 18   *Index Graeco-Latinus in Hippocratis opera.*

                 Coxe 1853: 819 (Misc. 280).

Barocci

See **Bibl. Bodleiana, Baroccian.** (see above, pp. 172-174).

Canon. Gr.

See **Bibl. Bodleiana, Canonician.** (see above, p. 175).

Casaubon

See **Bibl. Bodleiana, Is. Casauboni Advers.** (see above, p. 175).

E.D. Clarke

See **Bibl. Bodleiana, Clarkian.** (see above, p. 175).

Holkham

Gr. 71   (ff. 219r et seq.) Nicephorus Blemmydes, *De corpore*.

                 Barbour 1960: 605.

Gr. 92   See [0403]. Also [0886] and [0903].

                 Barbour 1960: 609.

Gr. 106   See [0406].

                 Barbour 1960: 611.

Gr. 107   (ff. 10r et seq.) Nemesius Emesenus, *De natura hominis* (frg.).

                 Barbour 1960: 612.

Gr. 108   See [0404]. Also [0901].

                 Barbour 1960: 612.

Gr. 110   (f. 214v) Hippocrates, *Aphorismi* (frg.).

                 CCAG IX.2 (Weinstock) 1953: 65-77 (especially 76); Barbour
                 1960: 612; Magdelaine 1994: 203.

Gr. 112   See [0405].

Barbour 1960: 612-613.

Langbaine

See **Bibl. Bodleiana, Ger. Langbainii Advers**.

Laud Gr.

56   See [0846].

Coxe 1853: 538.

57   See [0847].

Coxe 1853: 538-539.

58   See [0848].

Coxe 1853: 539.

59   See [0840].

Coxe 1853: 539-541.

60   See [0849].

Coxe 1853: 541.

61   (ff. 52r-89v) Psellus, *De cibariorum facultate, utilitate et noxia*.

Coxe 1853; 541-542.

62   See [0841].

Coxe 1853: 542.

Marshall

72   See [0809] and [0810].

D'Orville

3   See [0865].

Madan 1897: 38, no. 16881.

105   See [0866].

Madan 1897: 62, no. 16983.

110   *Cyranides*.

Madan 1897: 63-64, no. 16988.

Rawlinson

G. 94   See [0850].

G. 122   See [0855].

Roe

14   See [0869]-[0871] and [0874].

15   See [0872] and [0873]. Possibly [0830]

Selden

Selden Supra 15   (ff. 69v et seq) Petrus Zyphomust, *Narratio physiologica*.

Coxe 1853: 592, no. 14.

Christ Church Library

See p. 168, **Bibl. Aedis Christi**.

[**Coll. Merton.**] (*Collegium Mertonense*) now Merton College

The numbers in Diels' catalogue are not shelfmarks, but rather sequential numbers in the list of manuscripts "Collegii Mertonensis in Oxonia" in *C.M.A.* 1697: 1.2.12-24. These numbers are used in Ackermann 1821 and 1825 (without brackets).

[0875]

[**685**]   I.63, 91.

This item is referenced among the copies of Galenus, *De elementis secundum Hippocratem* (I.63), and *De diebus decretoriis Libri III* (I.91).

Number 685 appears in *C.M.A.* 1697: 1.2.20 (where *De diebus decretoriis* is identified as "Ejusd. [i. e. Galeni] de diebus Criticis"), followed by Ackermann 1821 (without brackets):

- LXXV, no. 8: *De elementis secundum Hippocratem*, where the manuscript is listed among the *codices graeci*;
- CVII, no. 42: *De diebus decretoriis*, where the manuscript is identified as "*latinus* no. 685".

This is a Latin manuscript, which is mentioned in Ackermann 1821 in reference to other Galenic texts, and it is identified there as a Latin codex:

- LXXVII, no. 9 ctd.: *De temperamentis*, where it is listed among the copies of the *versio latina* of the work;
- XCIX, no. 31 ctd.: *De locis adfectis*, where it is among the *Latini [codices]* of the work;
- CVIII, no. 43: *De crisibus*, where the manuscript is among the *latini*.

It is Merton College Library, 218.

Thomson 2009: 156.

[0876]

[**687**]   I.5, 13.

This is a copy of Hippocrates, *Prognosticon* (I.5) and *Aphorismi* (I.13).

Reference is to *C.M.A.* 1697: 1.2.20 (followed by Ackermann 1825: XLVII [*Prognosticon*] among the "CODICES MSS" without specification of language, and LXV [*Aphorismi*] among the Latin codices of the treatise; in both cases without brackets).

This is not a Greek manuscript (neither Alexanderson 1963 nor Magdelaine 1994 list it), but a Latin one.

It is Merton College Library, 220.

Thomson 2009: 158-159.

[0877]

[**688**]   I.5, 13.

This is Hippocrates, *Prognosticon* (I.5) and *Aphorismi* (I.13).

The reference is to *C.M.A.* 1697: 1.2.20 (followed by Ackermann 1825: XLVII [*Prognosticon*] among the "CODICES MSS" without specification of language, and LXV [*Aphorismi*], among the Latin codices of the treatise, in both cases without brackets).

This is not a Greek manuscript (neither Alexanderson 1963 nor Magdelaine 1994 mention it), but a Latin one.

It is Merton College Library, 221.

Thomson 2009: 159-160.

[0878]   **[689]**   I.5, 13.

This is a manuscript of Hippocrates, *Prognosticon* (I.5) and *Aphorismi* (I.13).

The reference is to *C.M.A.* 1697: 1.2.20 (followed by Ackermann 1825: XLVII [*Prognosticon*], among the "CODICES MSS" without specification of language, and LXV [*Aphorismi*], among the Latin codices of the work, in both cases without brackets).

This is not a Greek manuscript but a Latin one (neither Alexanderson 1963 nor Magdelaine 1994 list it).

It is Merton College Library, 222.

Thomson 2009: 160-161.

[0879]   **[722]**   I.13.

This is a copy of Hippocrates, *Aphorismi*.

The reference is to *C.M.A.* 1697: 1.2.22, followed by Ackermann 1825: LXV, without brackets.

This is not a Greek, but a Latin manuscript (Ackermann lists it among the Latin copies of the work, and Magdelaine 1994 does not mention it).

It is Merton College Library, 255.

Thomson 2009: 196-197.

[0880]   **[729]**   I.49.

This is a manuscript of Hippocrates, *De remediis*.

Reference is to *C.M.A.* 1697: 1.2.22 listing the following text:

Liber Hippocratis de Solutivis, & Signis mortalibus.

Similar information is found in Ackermann 1825: CXXXVIII, no. 26, about a text entitled περὶ φαρμάκων *De purgantibus* (without brackets).

This is a Latin manuscript.

It is Merton College Library, 262.

Thomson 2009: 202, where the text of ff. 249r-251v is identified as [Hippocrates], *Capsula eburnea*.

[Coll. Novi] (*Collegii Novi*) now New College.

Numbers provided by Diels are not shelfmarks, but are instead sequential numbers in *C.M.A.* 1697: 1.2.31-38, in a list of manuscripts of "Collegii Novi", among the "Libri Medicine" (*ibid.*: 34-35).

[0881]   **[1130]**   I.13.

This is a copy of Hippocrates, *Aphorismi*. The same information (without brackets) appears in Ackermann 1825: LXVI.

Number 1130 is from *C.M.A.* 1697: 1.2.34.

This is not a Greek manuscript (Ackermann lists it among the Latin copies of the *Aphorismi*, and Magdelaine 1994 does not mention it), but rather a Latin one (see Kibre 1985: 45 [*Aphorismi*], in addition to 9 [*Acutorum regimen*], and 206 [*Prognostica*]).

This is Oxford, New College Library, MS 166.

Coxe 1852: 1.7.63-64.

[0882]   **[1134]**   I.13.

This is Hippocrates, *Aphorismi*.

Number 1134 is from *C.M.A.* 1697: 1.2.35, followed by Ackermann 1825: LXVI (without brackets).

This is not a Greek manuscript, but a Latin one (Ackermann lists it among the Latin copies of the *Aphorismi*, and Magdelaine 1994 does not mention it; see Kibre 1985: 56 [*Aphorismi*], as well as 14 [*Acutorum regimen*], and 210 [*Prognostica*]).

This is Oxford, New College Library, MS 170.

Coxe 1852: 1.7.66.

Same as [0195].

Corpus Christi College

-

113   (ff. 1r et seq.) Aristoteles, *Problemata*.

Coxe 1852: 2.3.39; Wartelle 1963: 94, no. 1283.

[Eccl. Wigorn.] (*Ecclesia Wigornensis*) now Worcester Cathedral, Worcester (GB)

The manuscripts identified as Oxford, *Ecclesia Wigornensis*, are not at Oxford, but rather at Worcester, at the Worcester Cathedral Library. This may have resulted from confusion about the library of Worcester College at Oxford (on which see Morgan 1973) and that of Worcester Cathedral (for its catalogue, see Thomson 2001).

The numbers in Diels' catalogue are not shelfmarks, but rather sequential numbers in the list of manuscripts "Ecclesiae Cathedralis apud Wigorniam" published in *C.M.A.* 1697: 2.1.16-22.

[0883] appears in Ackermann 1821, and [0884] and [0885] in Ackermann 1825, in all cases without brackets.

-

[0883]   **[745]**   I.97-98.

This item is listed among the copies of Galenus, *De compositione medicamentorum secundum locos libri X*. It is mentioned by Ackermann 1821: CXXIV, no. 54 ctd., among the "Codices mss. graeci" that contain the treatise (*ibid.*, CXXIII-CXXV, no. 54, about this treatise, and CXXIV for the manuscripts):

Et inter codd. Mss. cathedr. eccles. Wigorniensis n. 745.

Number 745 is described as follows *C.M.A.* 1697: 2.1.18:

745. 70. Theoricae Constantini montis Cassin. libri 10.

Galeni libri 5. de Simplicium Medicam. compositione.

De Complexionibus.

This is a Latin manuscript. Ackermann 1821: LXXVII, no. 9 ctd., mentions it for *De temperamentis* among the copies of the *versio latina* of that work.

It probably corresponds to Worcester, Worcester Cathedral Library, Q.96, containing (ff. 7r-58r) Galenus, *De simplici medicina*.

Thomson 2001: 182-183.

[0884]   **[768]**   I.13.

This manuscript is listed among the copies of Hippocrates, *Aphorismi*.

In Ackermann 1825: LXV, a manuscript of the *Aphorismi* is identified as "In Wigorn. no. 768" (without brackets).

The number 768 appears in *C.M.A.* 1697: 2.1.18 in the same list as [0883]. It does not contain medical texts, but instead contains "Sermones ex iisdem (i.e. Jo. Chrysostomo, Hieronymo, Augustino, Leone, Maximo, Fulgentio, Gregorio, Beda, Rabano et aliis) a Pascha ad Aventum".

This may result from confusion with [0885] numbered 760.85 in *C.M.A.* 1697: 2.1.18, and containing among others Hippocrates, *Aphorismi* (below).

This is a Latin manuscript (Ackermann 1825: LXV, lists it among the Latin copies of the work; Magdelaine 1994 does not mention it).

This item probably corresponds to Worcester, Worcester Cathedral Library, F.85, ff. 10v-21v.

Thomson 2001: 54.

See [0885].

[0885]   **[1760]**   I.5.

This manuscript is listed among the copies of Hippocrates, *Prognosticon*.

The manuscripts of Worcester Library are numbered 676-924 in *C.M.A.* 1697: 2.1.16-22.

The number 1760 appears in Ackermann 1825: XLVII ("in ecclesia Wigorn. no. 1760", without brackets), where the manuscript is listed among "CODICES MSS" without specification of language.

This number might be a mistake for 760 (listed in *C.M.A.* 1697: 2.1.18), whose contents are identified as follows in *C.M.A.* 1697:

760. 85. Isagoge Joannitii ad legendos Galeni libros Prognosticorum.

Ejusdem libri Aphorismorum Hippocratis in 7 particulis.

Liber Prognosticorum Hippocratis.

Liber Urinarum Theophili.

Liber Philareti de Pulsibus.

Liber Galeni de corporibus, causis, signis, sanis, aegris, neutris.

Liber de Diaeta.

De 4 Complexionibus.

De generibus Cibariorum.

Liber Constantini de Febribus.

Liber Urinarum Isaac.

Liber Aegidii de Urinis, et Pulsibus.

This is a Latin manuscript (Alexanderson 1963 does not list it), and it probably corresponds to Worcester, Worcester Cathedral Library, F.85, ff. 21v-27r.

Thomson 2001: 54.

Probably same as [0884].

New College Library

-

MS 226   (ff. 30r et seq.) Aristoteles, *De insomniis*.

Coxe 1852: 1.7.83; Wartelle 1963: 95, no. 1289.

Padova (Padua) (IT)

Biblioteca civica (City Library)

-

644   Iohannes Zacharias Actuarius, *Methodus medendi*.

Mioni 1965: 1.237-238. Also Formentin 1978: 25.

Biblioteca del Seminario Vescovile (Episcopal Seminary Library)

-

194   Mioni 1965: 1.244-246.

Formerly [0889].

Also [0898].

Padua (Padova [Padua]) (IT)

In Diels' catalogue, all references to manuscripts in Padua are taken from the volume *Bibliothecae patavinae manuscriptae publicae et privatae ...* by Giacomo Filippo Tomasini (1597-1654) published in 1639 (listed in Diels I.XVI among the sources of the catalogue).

Except for [0886], [0889] = [0898], [0890], [0894] = [0899], [0901]-[0903], [0903, second part], and possibly also [0887], the current location of these manuscripts is not known.

[Bibl. Canonicor. Lateranens.] (*Bibliotheca Canonicorum Lateranensium* [Library of Canons Regular of the Lateran])

[0886]   [-]   I.28; N.26.

This manuscript without shelfmark is listed among the copies of Hippocrates, *De genitura*.

N.26 lists, without additional information, a manuscript identified as **Padua, S. Joann. in Viridario** (= Bibliotheca S. Joannis in Viridario, on the manuscripts of which see [0901]-[0903]) and identifies it as Holkham 282.

The manuscripts referred to at I.28 and N.26 are the same, as "Bibliotheca Canonicorum Lateranensium" and the "Bibliotheca S. Joannis in Viridario" are two different names of the same institution (see Formentin 1978: 18-20).

In Tomasini 1639: 21, col. 2, item 6, a manuscript of Hippocrates is listed in the collection of San Giovanni a Viridario (in the section *Primus Ordo Librorum ad dextrum Latus, pluteus XVII*). *De genitura* is not specifically mentioned, as the description of the content gives only some major titles followed by "aliaque opera".

A reference to this manuscript (without any element of identification) appears as follows in Ackermann 1825: CLVII, no. 43 (without brackets):

"In Patavina Canonicorum Lateranensium bibliotheca".

Manuscript Holkham 282 (= [0403]) is now at Oxford, Bodleian Library (see p. 181), together with the whole Holkham collection. Its current shelfmark is Hokham Gr. 92 (above, p. 181).

On this manuscript, see also [0903].

[Bibl. Cathedr.] *(Bibliotheca Cathedralis* [Cathedral Library])

[0887]   **[P 129]**   II.17, 18 (2), 19; N.45.

This is a manuscript of Aretaeus, *De causis et signis acutorum morborum* and *De causis et signis diuturnorum morborum*.

According to N.45 (followed by Formentin 1978: 25-26, herself followed by Cutolo 2012: 27n24), the number **P 129** is not the shelfmark of this manuscript, but the page number in Tomasini 1639.

As N.45 rightly stresses, this copy of Aretaeus was not in the Padua Cathedral library (the volumes of which are listed in Tomasini 1639: 3-8), but in Tomasini's own collection (the holdings of which are listed *ibid.*: 126-136).

This item is identified as follows in Tomasini 1639: 129, col. 2, item 2:

Aretaeus Cappadox Medicus de Diuturnis & Acutis affectibus. Cui deest principium Lib. 1 de acutorum causis & signis usque ad Cap. VI reliqua totius operis integra sunt ...

As N.45 already mentions, this information (without the brackets) goes back to "Kühn 1828: XV" (that is, to Kühn's edition of Aretaeus), who took it from Montfaucon I.489 (actually Montfaucon 1739: 1.489).

Montfaucon 1739: 1.485-490 provides selected information from Tomasini 1639 in the section "Bibliothecae Patavinae" (Montfaucon 1739: 1.485: "Selecta ex Bibliothecis Patavinis cura J. Philippi Thomasini cusis."). References to Tomasini 1639 in Montfaucon 1739 are to a page number preceded by the letter "P." (for "pagina"):

P. 126. Ex Museo Philippi Thomasini.

Medicinae libri.

...

P. 129. Aretaeus Cappadox de diuturnis & acutis morbis.

Kühn reproduced Montfaucon's information, explicitly stating that he did not know whether this is a Greek manuscript (*nescio an Grece*).

In Diels' catalogue, all references to the manuscript identified as **[Bibl. Cathedr.]**, **[P 129]** are followed by a reference to a manuscript identified as **Bibl. Tomasini**, as if these were two different manuscripts. However, both designations refer to the same manuscript.

The present item is listed also in Diels' catalogue under Tomasini's name (see [0904]).

According to Formentin 1978: 25-26, the current location of this manuscript is unknown. The editions of Kühn 1828: XV, and Hude 1958: VII-X do not identify this manuscript.

The text in the manuscript according to Tomasini (i. e. with the lacuna of Chapters 1-5 in Book I) corresponds to the text of the following manuscripts according to Hude 1958: VIII-IX (listed below with their provenance when known):

- *Harleianus* 6326 (= [0553]), purchased in a 1695 auction (McKendrick 1999: 210);
- *Ambrosianus* B 157 sup. (= [0612]), from the Pinelli collection (Martini and Bassi 1906: 172);
- *Parisinus* 2186 (= [1111]) (Omont 1886-1888: 2.211);
- *Parisinus* 2334 (= [1279]), from Roger de Gaignières (d. 1715) (Omont 1886-1888: 2.242).

Currently, it is not known if the present item corresponds to any of these four manuscripts, if it is another codex, or if it is lost.

Also [0904].

Bibl. Joann. Rhodii (*Bibliotheca Joannis Rhodii* [Johann Rhodius' Library])

The Danish Johann Rhodius (1587-1659), who moved to Italy and was the Praefectus of Padua Botanical Garden, owned a collection of manuscripts.

Diels' catalogue lists manuscripts containing works by Dioscorides, Galen, Hippocrates, Oribasius, and Stephanus Atheniensis under Rhodius' name.

As Formentin 1978: 26-27 already noticed, information about these items in Diels' catalogue was taken from Tomasini 1639: 136-141, where several manuscripts are listed.

I reproduce below the list according to Tomasini (with reference to the mentions of the manuscripts in Diels' catalogue). Manuscripts are listed below according to the alphabetical order of the author of the text or texts they contain. The titles correspond to those in Diels' catalogue.

All these manuscripts are considered lost in Diels' catalogue (*Verbleib unbekannt*), which is not necessarily the case (see [0889] = [0898], [0890] and [0894] = [0899]). A note in N.24 mentions that, according to Emil Jacobs (1868-1940), Rhodius' manuscripts could be in the Library of Padua Chapter. According to Formentin 1978: 27, Rhodius' manuscripts that were not acquired by Copenhagen Library or left in Padua were destroyed in a fire in 1670.

[0888]   -   II.30.

This is a copy of Dioscorides, *De materia medica*. In Tomasini 1639: 138, col. 2, item 6, it is identified as *Dioscorides Graecè 4 c.* Although this item may be the same as [0889], it may also be a different codex, in which Dioscorides' text was not alphabetized. Furthermore, the size of the present item (4°) does not suggest it can be identical to the following, of a larger size (*f.* = folio).

[0889]   -   II.29, 33.

The references II.29 and 33 are to Dioscorides, *Opera varia* and *Alphabetum empiricum*, respectively. These two references in Diels' catalogue (to which [0898] needs to be added) are probably to the same item. Tomasini 1639: 138, col. 2, item 9, mentions only one item: *Dioscorides, & Stephanus Atheniensis de Pharmacis ordine literarum. Graecè. f. c.*

This item corresponds to present manuscript Padova, Biblioteca del Seminario, 194 (see p. 187), which is a large-size volume and contains an alphabetical version of Dioscorides' text with illustrations.

The attribution to Stephanus Atheniensis (on which see [0898]) reflects confusion with the so-called *Alphabetum empiricum* ascribed to either Dioscorides or Stephanus Atheniensis in both the manuscript tradition and, consequently, modern scholarship. This does not contradict the identification with the Padua manuscript.

See also Formentin 1978: 92, and Savvinidou 2006.

[0890]   -   I.61.

This manuscript is a copy of Galenus, *Ars medica*.

In Tomasini 1639: 139, col. 1, item 7, it is identified as *Galeni Ars Medica. Grec. fol. & 8. c. Diversa a vulgatis.*

It is now København, Det Kongelige Bibliotek, e don. var., 42, 4° (= [0448]) mentioned on the same page in Diels' catalogue (see also Boudon 2002: 198n109 ctd.).

[0891]   -   I.66, 68.

This is a copy of Galenus, *De anatomicis administrationibus* (I.66) and *De usu partium* (I.68).

This codex is identifed in Tomasini 1639: 139, col. 1, item 8 as follows:

Galenus de Administratione Anatomica, Gr. f. c. de Usu Partium.

On the basis of this identification, it seems that these two Galenic works were found in the same manuscript.

The present location of this manuscript is unknown (see also Garofalo 1986: XIIn38).

[0892]   -   I.89.

This is a copy of Galenus, *Synopsis de pulsibus*.

Tomasini 1639: 139, col. 1, item 9, identifies it as *Eiusdem* [i.e. *Galeni*] *Synopsis de Pulsibus.*

No information is available on the present location of this manuscript.

[0893]   -   I.63, 64, 85, 96, 98 (2), 104, 119, 134.

Based on Tomasini 1639 (below), the following Galenic works were found in the same manuscript (references to Diels' catalogue follow the titles):

- *De compositione medicamentorum per genera* (I.98);
- *De compositione medicamentorum secundum locos* (I.98);
- *De simplicium medicamentorum temperamentis et facultatibus* (I.96);
- *De locis affectis* (I.85);
- *In Hippocratis epidemias commentarium* (I.104);
- *De partibus philosophiae* (I.134);
- *De consuetudinibus* (I.119);
- *De facultatibus naturalibus* (I.65);
- *De elementis secundum Hippocratem* (I.63);
- *De temperamentis* (I.64).

An item containing all these works appears in Tomasini 1639: 139, col. 1, item 10:

Idem [i. e. *Galeni*] *de Simplicium facultatibus. Compositione Medicamentorum. Liber mutilus. Locis affectis. in 2 Lib. Epidem. Hippocrat. de Philosophia. de Moribus. De Potentiis Naturalibus. Elementis secundùm Hippocratem. Temperamentis Gr. f. c.*

Discrepancies in the titles of the works (*de Simplicium facultatibus, de Philosophia, de Moribus,* and *De potentiis Naturalibus* in Tomasini corresponding to *De simplicium medicamentorum temperamentis et facultatibus, De partibus philosophiae, De consuetudinibus,* and *De facultatibus naturalibus,* respectively, in Diels) result from different usages. The second item in the codex according to Tomasini (*Compositione Medicamentorum. Liber mutilus*) can correspond to both *De compositione medicamentorum per genera* and *De compositione medicamentorum secundum locos.*

The current location of this manuscript is not known.

[0894]   -   I.93.

This is a manuscript of Galenus, *Ad Glauconem.*

In Tomasini 1639: 139, col. 1, item 11, it is described as follows:

Idem [i. e. *Galeni*] *de Arte Curativa ad Glauconem. Gr. f. c.*

According to Dickson 1990, this is København, Det Kongelige Bibliotek, e don. var. 29, 2° (= [0451]).

May be the same as [0899].

[0895]   -   I.13.

This copy of Hippocrates, *Aphorismi* is identified in Tomasini 1639: 139, col. 1, item 21, as follows:

Hippocratis Aphorismi. Gr. 8. c.

A reference to this manuscript appears in Ackermann 1825: LXV.

The current location of this codex is unknown. See Formentin 1978: 43, and Magdelaine 1994: 88n1.

[0896]   -   I.10, 19.

This is a copy of Hippocrates, *De morbis popularibus I et III*, and *II et IV-VII*.

In Tomasini 1639: 139, col. 1, item 22, this manuscript is described as *[Hippocratis] Epidemia. Gr. f. c.*

The current location of this manuscript is unknown.

[0897]   -   II.70.

This is a copy of Oribasius, *Opera*.

In Tomasini 1639: 140, col. 1, item 19, this item is identified as *Oribasius. Mutilus. f. c.*

The current location of this manuscript is unknown.

[0898]   -   II.97.

This is Stephanus Atheniensis, *De remediis alphabetice* (Tomasini 1639: 138, col. 2, item 9)

Same as [0889].

[0899]   -   II.97.

This codex contains Stephanus Atheniensis, *In Galeni de methodo medendi*.

In Tomasini 1639: 137, col. 1, item 23, it is described as follows:

Stephanus Atheniensis in Galenum de Arte Curat. ad Glauconem. Graece f. ch.

Björk 1938: 140, hypothesizes that this manuscript might be the codex of København, Det Kongelige Bibliotek, e don. var. 29, 2° (= [0451]). See also Petit 2006: 183n38 ctd., who confirms that the manuscript of København belonged to Johannes Rhodius.

See [0894].

Bibl. Marci Mantuae (*Bibliotheca Marci Mantuae* [Marco Mantua's Library])

[0900]   -   II.30.

This item is a copy of Dioscorides, *De materia medica*.

Information comes from Tomasini 1639: 102-103, listing the volumes in the collection of Marcus Mantua Benavidius (i.e. Marco Mantova Benavides [1489-1582]).

The Dioscorides codex is described as follows (*ibid.*: 103, col. 2, item 4):

Dioscorides Liber Primus de materia Medica Graecè f. ch.

According to Formentin 1978: 26, it is now lost.

Bibl. S. Joann. in Viridario (*Bibliotheca Sancti Joannis in Viridario* [St. John in Viridario Library])

[0901]   **ad dextr. plut. 16**   II.6; N.43.

This copy of Aetius Amidenus, *Libri medicinales*, appears in Tomasini 1639: 20, col. 2, *sub* XVI, item 3, among the holdings of the library of San Giovanni in Viridario.

While in II.6 the manuscript is considered lost (*Verbleib unbekannt*), in N.43 (followed by Formentin 1978: 20) it is identified as Holkham 283 (= [0404]). Since then, the Holkham collection has been moved to Oxford, Bodleian Library (above, p. 89). The current shelfmark of this manuscript is Holkham Gr. 108 (see above, p. 181).

[0902]   **ad dextr. plut. XVI**   II.70.

This is a copy of Oribasius, *Opera*, which is listed by Tomasini 1639: 20, col. 2, *sub* XVI, item 2, among the volumes of the library of San Giovanni in Viridario.

Whereas this volume was not located in Diels' catalogue (*Verbleib unbekannt*), it is now *Venetus Marcianus, Appendix graeca* V.1 (coll. 834) (= [1710]), as Formentin 1978: 19-20 noticed.

[0903]   **ad dextr. plut. XVII**   I.3, 5, 13, 21, 30; II.77; N. 25 (3), 26 (3).

This volume contains the following collection of works (listed in alphabetical order of title; references to Diels' catalogue follow the titles):

- Hippocrates, *Aphorismi* (I.13);
- Hippocrates, *De genitura* (N.26);
- Hippocrates, *De natura hominis* (I.21);
- Hippocrates *De virginum morbis* (I.30);
- Hippocrates, *Opera varia* (I.3);
- Hippocrates, *Prognosticum* (I.5);
- Paulus Aegineta, *Epitome medica* (II.77).

Mention of a codex of "S. Joannis in viridario Patav." appears in Ackermann 1825: LXV (*Aphorismi*), with a reference to "Montf. I. p. 485."

The reference is to Montfaucon 1739: 1.485, where the following can be read:

"Bibliothecae Patavinae. Selecta ex Bibliothecis Patavinis cura J. Philippi Thomasini cusis ... In Bibliotheca S. Joannis in Viridario ... P. 20 ... Libri Graeci ... P. 21 ... Pauli Aeginetae opera ... Hippocratis Aphorismi ...".

The reference to Tomasini in Montfaucon is to Tomasini 1639: 12, col. 2, *sub* XVII ctd, item 9, where a volume of Hippocrates is described as follows among the holdings of San Giovanni in Viridario:

Hippocratis Aphorismi, Prognostica, liber de Natura humana, de Virginibus. aliaq[ue] opera.

While in Diels' catalogue I.3, 5, 13, 21, 30, and II.77, this item is considered missing (*Verbleib unbekannt*), in N. 25 (3) and 26 (3) (referring to I.3, 5, 13, 21, 30) it is identified as Holkham 282 (= [0403]). The item does not appear on I.12 contrary to N.25 (where Holkham 282 is referenced, instead).

This identification has been further confirmed by Formentin 1978: 19, followed by Magdelaine 1994: 88n1 for Hippocrates, *Aphorismi*, and Jouanna the 2002: 62n4, *sub* 1 for Hippocrates, *De natura hominis*.

See also [0886].

The Holkham collection is now at Oxford, Bodleian Library, and the present item is manuscript Holkham Gr. 92 (see p. 181).

The case of Paul of Aegina, *Epitomae* is different (see Tomasini 1639: 21, col. 1, *sub* XVII, item 2). The Holkham manuscript does not contain the work (above). The copy of St. John in the Viridario Library must be considered lost or missing, unless it corresponds to another manuscript. Whereas Köhler and Milchsack 1913: 34-35, link this item with the current manuscript 47 Gud.

graec. fol. of Wolfenbüttel library (= [1842]-[1843]), Heiberg 1919: 271, estimates that it corresponds to the current *Venetus Marcianus, Appendix graeca* V.1 (coll. 834) (= [1710]).

Bibl. Tomasini (*Bibliotheca Tomasini*, Giacomo Filippo Tomasini [1597-1654] [Tomasini's Library])

[0904]   -   II.17, 18 (2), 19.

This copy of Aretaeus, *De causis et signis acutorum morborum* et *De causis et signis diuturnorum morborum* is the same as [0887].

Palermo (IT)

Biblioteca nazionale (National Library), now Biblioteca centrale della Regione siciliana "Alberto Bombace" ("Alberto Bombace" Central Library of Sicily Region)

               -

[0905]   **IV H 8**   II.9.

                              Martini 1893: 88-90.

[0906]   **XIII C 3**   I.13, 42, 123, 128; II.6, 55, 98, 102, 110.

                              Martini 1893: 109-119.

Biblioteca centrale della Regione siciliana "Alberto Bombace" ("Alberto Bombace" Central Library of Sicily Region)

       Fondi antichi (Ancient Collections)

       IV.H.8   See [0905].

       XIII.C.3   See [0906].

Paris (FR)

[Bib. Regia] (*Bibliotheca Regia* [Royal Library]), now Bibliothèque nationale de France (National Library of France)

[0907]   **2 Parisini regii bei Migne**   N.46.

[0908]   According to Diels' catalogue, these two manuscripts contain S. Basilius, *Ad Eustathium medicum.* A reference is made to "Migne, patrol. gr. 32, p. 684 ff. Ep. 189" (= Migne 1857: 683/684-695/696 [columns, not pages as in Diels]).

This is *Letter 189* of S. Basilius (= *Clavis Patrum Graecorum* 2900 for the whole collection of *Letters*), edited by Courtonne 1961: 132-141. According to Courtonne 1957: xxii, the Maurists responsible for the 1730 edition (reproduced by Migne 1857: 683/684-695/696, and cited by Diels) consulted two manuscripts *Regii*:

- 2293, which is now Paris, Bibliothèque nationale de France, *graecus* 506 (on which see Fedwick 1993: 23-26);

- 2897, which is now Paris, Bibliothèque nationale de France, *graecus* 971 (on which see Fedwick 1993: 133-134).

The *Letter* is addressed to a certain *Eustathius medicus* (in the *Bibliotheca Basiliana Universalis* by Fedwick 1993: XVI, the *Letter* is identified as *EustArc*

2/189, that is, Basilius' *Letter 189*, being the second addressed to *Eustathius archiater*). This letter is of dubious authenticity and may be by Gregorius Nyssenus (= *Ad Eustathium de sancta trinitate* [= *Clavis Patrum Graecorum* 3137]; edition by Mueller 1958: 1-16).

This is a theological text not medical in nature. It was probably included in Diels' catalogue because of its recipient's medical profession.

[0909]   **[120 ap. Montf. II 902]**   I.103.

This is a copy of Galenus, *in Hippocratis de humoribus librum commentarii III*.

The same information (without brackets) appears in Ackermann 1821: CLXXVII, no. 5: "in B. R. Paris. n. 120. Montf. II. p. 902".

The reference is to Montfaucon 1739: 2.902, manuscript no. CXX of the *Bibliotheca regia Parisiensis*, where the contents of the manuscript are identified as follows:

Cod. CXX. in charta.

1. περὶ μέτρων.

2. περὶ μέτρων πάλιν, eadem manu.

3. Alia manu recentiore sed elegantissima [*sic!*], Galeni εἰς τὸ περὶ χυμῶν Ἱπποκράτους ἢ περὶ καιρῶν.

From the description of its contents, this manuscript seems to correspond to codex *Coislinianus* 163 (= [0937]; Devreesse 1945: 146-147), copied by Andreas Darmarios whose hand may have been described as "recentior" and "elegantissima".

The description of the manuscript in Montfaucon 1715 (= *Bibliotheca Coisliniana*), Pars prima, page 222, no. CLXIII, is more precise and confirms the identification of this item. The mention of two works περὶ μέτρων in Montfaucon 1739 (above) does not appear in either Montfaucon 1715 (above) or Devreesse 1945 (above), and seems to be a mistake in Montfaucon 1739 (above).

On Coislin 163, see Devreesse 1945: 146-147.

Same as [0937].

[0910]   **[349]**   II.58.

This is a manuscript of Lucas, *Compositio salsi intinctus*.

The current codex *Parisinus graecus* 349 does not contain this text, but it does contain an *Euchologium* followed by some other short texts (Omont 1886-1888: 1.36).

None of the manuscripts with shelfmark 349 in the several inventories and catalogues of the "Bib. Regia" (that is, the *Bibliotheca Regia* in Paris), contain Lucas, *Sales* (on these inventories and catalogues, see Balayé 1988: 59 [Rigault 1622], 67 [Dupuy 1645], 100-101 [Clément 1682], 226 [printed catalogue 1740]):

• 1622, 1st catalogue by Rigault: 349 (380) Demosthenis opera (Omont 1909: 42);

• 1622, 1st catalogue by Rigault (revised by Dupuy): 349 Josephus contra Manetonem et alios stoicos, latine (Omont 1909: 38, in parte inferiori paginae in nota (1) ad numerum 340);

- 1622, 2nd catalogue by Rigault: 349 Consuetidunes et leges Angliae (Omont 1909: 279);

- 1645, inventory by Pierre and Jacques Dupuy: 349. Innocentii IV. Pontificis apparatus (Omont 1910: 21);

- 1682, catalogue by Clément: Missale sancti Basilii, cophtice et arabice (Omont 1910: 184);

- 1740, printed catalogue: CCCXLIX Codex chartaceus, ex Oriente in Bibliothecam regiam illatus. Ibi continetur liber precum ad usum Ecclesiae Graecae. Initium & finis desiderantur (*Bibliotheca Regia* 1740: 49).

According to Omont 1898: 126, *sub nomine* Lucas evangelista, *sub titulo* Excerpta medica, the only copies of this text at the Bibliothèque nationale de France, are *graecus* 2510 (= [1294]), where the text appears in the medical collection of ff. 125r-132r (Omont 1886-1888: 2.275), and *Supplementum graecum* 1188 (see p. 261), which contains the text on f. 3v (Astruc and Concasty 1960: 357-358).

The codex *Supplementum graecum* 1188 comes from the collection of Emmanuel Miller (1812-1886) and entered the Bibliothèque nationale sometimes after Miller's death in 1886, but before 1897 (Omont 1897: V).

It might be significant that manuscript *graecus* 2510 was no. 3495 in the *Bibliotheca Regia* (Omont 1886-1888: 2.275; Omont 1898: LXXXI, *sub numero* 3495; Omont 1921: 93, *sub numero* 3495). On this basis, number 349 in Diels' catalogue might be an incorrect reproduction of this old number. However, the reference to f. 156 would not be correct, since the manuscript contains 142 folios. Perhaps this is an additional transcription mistake for 126r, that is, a folio in the section of the manuscript that Omont 1868-1888: 2.275, identifies as "Remedia varia" that includes the text of Lucas, *Sales*.

The manuscript does not appear in Montfaucon 1739: 2.742, in the catalogue of the *Bibliotheca Regia Parisiensis ... Bibliothecae Regiae Manuscripti Codices* (*ibid.* 2.710-921 for the whole catalogue, and 725-743 for the Greek manuscripts), because the content of numbers 3492-3500 has been summarized as follows:

In sequentibus codicibus (= 3492-3500) Iatrica, seu medicinalia multa.

Possibly same as [1294].

Bibl. de la ville de Paris (Bibliothèque de la ville de Paris [Library of the city of Paris])

The two manuscripts listed under **Bibl. de la ville de Paris** were incorrectly identified. The numbers used to identify them appear in Omont, *Inventaire sommaire des manuscrits grecs de la Bibliothèque nationale et des autres bibliothèques de Paris et des Départments*, tome 3 (1888), pp. 347-358 (= Omont 1886-1888: 3.347-358), in a section entitled "Manuscrits grecs des bibliothèques de Paris autres que la Bibliothèque nationale". According to this catalogue, they were preserved in the following two libraries in Paris:

- Bibliothèque Mazarine ([0911]);
- Bibliothèque de la Faculté de médecine ([0912]).

The numbers used to identify these items in Diels' catalogue (12 and 58, respectively) are not shelfmarks, but instead are sequential numbers in Omont 1886-1888: 3.347-356 (and also in Omont 1883 and 1884 for [0911]).

The two manuscripts are listed a second time in Diels' catalogue under the name of the libraries where they are actually preserved, but with different numbers (see [0924] and [0922], respectively).

[0911]   **12**   II.33.

According to Diels' catalogue, this is a copy of Dioscorides, *Metaphrasis in Nicandri Theriaca et Alexipharmaca*.

Number 12 appears in Omont 1883: 120, no. 12 (1235); Omont 1884: 310, no. 12 (1235); and Omont 1886-1888: 3.349, no. 12 (1235). On this basis, it appears that the text is incorrectly identified in Diels' catalogue: it is not a paraphrasis of Nicander, but is instead Pseudo-Dioscorides, *Alexipharmaca* and *Theriaca*.

Current location and shelfmark: Paris, Bibliothèque Mazarine, 4461 (= [0924]).

[0912]   **58**   II.6, 8.

This copy of Aetius is now Paris, Bibliothèque Interuniversitaire de Santé-BIU Santé MS 2105 (= [0922]).

Omont 1886-1888: 3.355-356, no. 58 [76], and also Omont 1883: 123, no. 50 (76).

Bibl. de Paris (Bibliothèque de Paris [Paris Library])

The three manuscripts listed under **Bibl. de Paris** have been incorrectly identified in Diels' catalogue. The numbers used to identify them appear in Omont, *Inventaire sommaire des manuscrits grecs de la Bibliothèque nationale et des autres bibliothèques de Paris et des Départements*, tome 3 (1888), pp. 347-358 (= Omont 1886-1888: 3.347-358), in a section entitled "Manuscrits grecs des bibliothèques de Paris autres que la Bibliothèque nationale". According to this catalogue, they were preserved in the following three libraries in Paris:

- Bibliothèque Mazarine ([0913]);
- Bibliothèque Sainte-Geneviève ([0914]);
- Bibliothèque de la Faculté de médecine ([0915]).

The numbers used to identify these items in Diels' catalogue (4, 42 and 57 respectively) are not shelfmarks but sequential numbers in Omont 1886-1888: 3.347-358 (and also in Omont 1883 and 1884 for [0913]). Based on its contents, number [0915] appears to be listed several more times in Diels' catalogue under the name of the library where it is actually preserved, but under different identifications:

- **14 (ol. Bibl. de Paris 57)** in [0921];
- **14** in [0920];
- **nr. ?** in [0919];
- without number in [0916]-[0918].

[0913]   **4**   I.38.

This copy of Hippocrates, *Epistulae*, is Paris, Bibliothèque Mazarine, 4454 (see below, p. 200).

Omont 1883: 119, no. 4 (611. A); Omont 1884: 398, no. 4; Omont 1886-1888: 3.347-348, no. 4 [611 A].

[0914]   **42**   II.67.

This copy of Nemesius Emesenus, *De natura hominis* (frg.) is Paris, Bibliothèque Sainte-Geneviève, 3394 (see p. 262).

Omont 1886-1888: 3.353, no. 42 [Ao. 2 *bis*, in-fol.]. Also Omont 1883: 122, no. 39 (2 bis); 1884: 316, no. 3 (2 *bis*).

[0915]   **57**   II.71.

This manuscript of Oribasius, *Medicae collectiones ad Iulianum*, L. XVVIII, is Paris, Bibliothèque Interuniversitaire de Santé MS 44 (= [0921]).

Omont 1886-1888: 3.355, no. 57 [14].

Bibl. Facult. Med. (Bibliothèque de la Faculté de Médecine [Medical School Library]), now Bibliothèque Interuniversitaire de Santé-BIU Santé (Interuniversity Health Library-BIU Santé)

According to the list of catalogues consulted to compile Diels, these manuscripts are identified on the basis of Omont 1883. Numbers used to identify them are not the sequential numbers in this article, but the numbers between brackets following this sequential number.

In [0916]-[0919] no number is provided (either the sequential number in Omont 1883 or another).

In [0921] and [0923], a reference to **Bibl. de Paris** is provided with a number (57 and 59, respectively), which is, in fact, the sequential number of these two manuscripts in Omont 1886-1888: 3.355 and 356, respectively.

[0916]   -   II.15.

This is a copy of Apollonius Citiensis, *Commentarius in Hippocratis de articulis* listed without shelfmark but with a reference to "Dietz, Schol. in Hipp. et Gal. I pref. p. XI" (= Dietz 1834).

It may correspond to the text present in [0921], ff. 18r et seq.

Also [0917]-[0920].

[0917]   -   II.74.

This copy of Oribasius, *De fracturis fragmenta* listed without shelfmark probably corresponds to the text found in [0921], ff. 18r et seq.

Also [0916] and [0918]-[0920].

[0918]   -   II.109.

This is copy of "Anon. [fort. Actuar.] de urinis" listed without shelfmark probably correspond to thext contained in [0921], fr. 12r et seq.

Also [0916]-[0917] and [0919]-[0920].

[0919]   **nr. ?**   I.150.

This copy of *Indices in Galenum* listed without shelfmark may be the index contained in [0921], ff. 1r et seq., identified as *Hippocratis lexicon* in Omont 1883: 123, no. 49 (14), and Omont 1886-1888: 3.355, no. 57 [14]. See also [0920].

Also [0916]-[0918].

[0920]   **14**   I.57, 103.

This manuscript containing *Lexicon Hippocratis* (I.57) and Galenus, *In Hippocratis de humoribus librum commentarii II* (I.103) is [0921].

Also [0916]-[0919].

[0921]   **14 (ol. Bibl. de Paris 57)**   II.74, 89.

This is a copy of Oribasius, *De fracturis fragmenta* (II.74), and Rufus, *De corporis humani appellationibus* (II.89).

Omont 1883: 123, no. 49 (14); Omont 1886-1888: 3.355, no. 57 [14]; Boinet 1908: 12-13, no. 31 (44); *Catalogue général des manuscrits* 1909: 226, no. 31 (44); Richard 1958: 187, no. 31 (44); Olivier 1995: 642, no. 31 (44).

This seems to be a scholarly copy by the botanist and physician Paul de Reneaulme (ca. 1560-1624).

Current shelfmark: MS 44.

See [0916]-[0920].

[0922]   **76**   II.6.

This copy of Aetius is now MS 2105.

Omont 1883: 123, no. 50 (76); Omont 1886-1888: 3.355-356, no. 58 [76]; Boinet 1908: 32, no. 147 (2105); *Catalogue général des manuscrits* 1909: 246, no. 147 (2105); Richard 1958: 187, no. 147 (2105); Olivier 1995: 642, no. 147 (2105).

This is a 17th-century codex by René Moreau (1587-1656), professor at Paris Faculty of Medicine and its Dean between 1630 and 1632.

Same as [0912].

[0923]   **145 (ol. Bibl. de Paris 59)**   II.71.

The identification "ol. Bibl. de Paris 59" refers to Omont 1883: 356, no. 59 [145], and Omont 1886-1888: 3.356, no. 59 [145].

Also Boinet 1908: 50, no. 231 (5112); *Catalogue général des manuscrits* 1909: 264, no. 231 (5112); Richard 1958: 187, 231 (5112); Olivier 1995: 642, 231 (5112).

It is a 19th-century handwritten copy of *Parisinus graecus* 2188 (= [1113]).

Current shelfmark: MS 5112.

Bibl. Mazarine (Bibliothèque Mazarine [Mazarine Library])

-

[0924]   **4461**   II.33.

Molinier 1890: 355.

See also [0911].

Bibliothèque Mazarine (Mazarine Library)

-

4453   (pp. 143 et seq.) Synesius Cyrenensis, *De insomniis*.

Molinier 1890: 353.

4454   Molinier 1890: 353-354.

See [0913].

4461   See [0924] and also [0911].

Bibl. Nationale (Bibliothèque nationale [National Library]), now Bibliothèque nationale de France (National Library of France)

Coislin. (*Coisliniani*)

[0925]   **Coislin.**   N.46.

According to Diels' catalogue, this manuscript listed without shelfmark contains S. Basilius, *Ad Eustathium medicum*. A reference is made to "Migne, patrol. gr. 32, p. 684 ff. Ep. 189" (= Migne 1857: 683/684-695/696 [columns, but not pages as in Diels]).

This is *Letter 189* of S. Basilius (= *Clavis Patrum Graecorum* 2900 for the whole collection of *Letters*), edited by Courtonne 1961: 132-141.

According to Courtonne 1957: xxii, the Maurists responsible for the 1730 edition (reproduced by Migne 1857: 683/684-695/696, and cited by Diels) consulted the manuscript Paris, Bibliothèque nationale de France, *Coislinianus* 237 (on which see Fedwick 1993: 103-107; also Devreesse 1945: 216-217).

The letter is addressed to a certain *Eustathius medicus* (in the *Bibliotheca Basiliana Universalis* by Fedwick 1993: XVI, it is identified as *EustArc 2/189*, that is, Basilius' *Letter 189*, being the second addressed to *Eustathius archiater*). This letter is of dubious authenticity and may be by Gregorius Nyssenus (= *Ad Eustathium de sancta trinitate* [= *Clavis Patrum Graecorum* 3137]; edition by Mueller 1958: 1-16).

This is a theological text not medical in nature. It was probably included in Diels' catalogue because of its recipient's medical profession.

[0926]   **[ap. Montf. II 447]**   I.64, 65.

This manuscript without shelfmark in Diels' catalogue is listed as a copy of Galenus, *De temperamentis* (I.64) and *De facultatibus naturalibus* (I.65).

The same information (also without shelfmark, but with the reference to Montfaucon, though without brackets) appears in Ackermann 1821: LXXVII, no. 9 ctd. (*De temperamentis*), and LXXXI, no. 14 ctd. (*De facultatibus naturalibus*).

The reference to Montfaucon is to *Bibliotheca Coisliniana* (1715), Pars Secunda, p. 447, no. CCCXXXIV.

Though incomplete, the information in Montfaucon allows for an identification of this item as *Coislinianus* 334 (= [0949]) (on which, see Devreesse 1945: 317-318).

Identification of the content of the manuscript in Diels' catalogue is not correct as the manuscript does not contain Galen, but Actuarius (using Galen).

Also [0927].

[0927]   **[ap. Montf. II 447] (Es ist wohl Coislin. 335)**   I.128.

This manuscript without shelfmark is listed among the copies of Galenus, *De urinis*.

The same information (including the reference to Montfaucon, but without the identification as Coislin 335 or the brackets) appears in Ackermann 1821: CLXV, no. 119.

There might be some confusion about this manuscript. The reference to Montfaucon is to *Bibliotheca Coisliniana* (1715), Pars Secunda, p. 447, where a *De urinis* by Galen is mentioned. However, this text is contained in codex no. CCCXXXIV (= 334). Nevertheless, a *De urinis* is mentioned in Montfaucon 1715, codex CCCXXXV (= 335). However, it appears on p. 448 and is considered anonymous (this text is not listed in Devreesse 1945: 318-320, particularly 320).

The identification of this item as Coislin 335 (= [0950]) is probably inexact. *Coislinianus* 334 (= [0949]) contains a summary of Galenus, *De urinis* (ff. 10r-18r) in addition to two others *De urinis* (ff. 215r-281v [Actuarius] and 346r-355v [anonymous]).

Devreesse 1945: 317-318.

Same as [0926] and [0949].

[0928]   **[ap. Montf. II 448]**   I.96.

This manuscript without shelfmark is listed among the copies of Galenus, *De simplicium medicamentorum temperamentis et facultatibus libri XI*.

The information (without brackets) comes from Ackermann 1821: CXIII, no. 49 ctd. (adding that the manuscript contains only *excerpta*).

Diels' reference is to Montfaucon, *Bibliotheca Coisliniana* (1715), Pars Secunda, where manuscript CCCXXXV (= 335) is described on pp. 447-449. In Montfaucon's catalogue (p. 448), the text is identified as follows:

Fol. 21. Excerpta passim ἀτάκτως ex Galeni libris de simplicium medicamentorum facultatibus.

On the basis of this description, this manuscript can be identified as current *Coislinianus* 335 (= [0950]) (on which Devreesse 1945: 318-320), which contains (ff. 21r-60r) a *iatrosofion* under Galen's name and not *De simplicium medicamentorum temperamentis et facultatibus* (the manuscript is not listed in Petit 2010: 146).

Same as [0950] and [0929], but not [0927]. Also [0951].

[0929]   **[ap. Montfauc. II 448] I.126.**

According to Diels' catalogue, this codex listed without shelfmark contains a text identified as Galenus, *De morbis Excerpta*, and also "Exc. ex Hipp. Gal. Meletio". A supplementary information identifies this manuscript as follows: "*Wohl* Coislin. 335; *vgl. unter* Iatrosofia".

A mention of this manuscript (including the reference to "Coislin. Montfauc. in bibl. Coislin. part. II. p. 448" as in Diels' catalogue) appears (without brackets) in Ackermann 1825: CLXXVIII, *sub titulo* Excerpta de morbis ex Hippocrate, Galeno et Meletio.

The reference is to Montfaucon, *Bibliotheca Coisliniana* (1715), Pars Secunda, where the manuscript is described on pp. 447-449. On p. 448, Montfaucon lists a text identified as follows:

Fol. 75. Excerpta de morbis ex Hippocrate, Galeno, & Meletio.

This is *Coislinianus* 335 (Devreesse 1945: 318-320), in which a *iatrosofion* by Galenus, Hippocrates, and Meletius can be found on ff. 75r-150r.

Same as [0950] and [0928], but not [0927]. Also [0951].

[0930]   **8**   II.77; N.62.

The ff. 1 and 283 (palimpsest) come from the same manuscript as f. I of *Coislinianus* 123 (= [0935]).

Devreesse 1945: 7-8.

The palimpsested ff. 24-25 of Paris, *Supplementum graecum* 1156 (= [1391]) and 1-2 of Москва (Moskva), Государственный Исторический Музей (ГИМ), Синодальная Библиотека Московского Патриархата (Gosudarstvennyi Istoricheskii Muzei (GIM), Sinodal'naia Biblioteka Moskovskoi Patriarkhii [State Historical Museum [GIM], Synodal Library of Moscow Patriarchate]), Sinod. 174 (387 Vlad.) (see above, p. 148), do not come from the same manuscript contrary to Heiberg 1919: 276, Devreesse 1945: 7-8 (about *Coislinianus* 8) and 117-118 (about *Coislinianus* 123), and Astruc and Concasty 1960: 320 (about Paris, *Supplementum graecum* 1156).

Omont 1897: 13, already noted the different origin of the palimpsested folios of *Supplementum graecum* 1156 and *Coislinianus* 8 (although he did not distinguish f. 23 and ff. 24-25 in the *Supplementum graecum* 1156).

Recently, Fonkič 2000: 170n7, discusses all of these manuscripts.

12   (f. 8r) *Remedia.*

Devreesse 1945: 10.

56   (ff. 84r-87v) Gregorius Nazianzenus, *De humana natura.*

Devreesse 1945: 52-53; Domiter 1999: 21.

[0931]   **78**   II.52.

Devreesse 1945: 68-69.

[0932]	**79**	II.52.
		Devreesse 1945: 69-70.
	114	(ff. 256r-261v) Johannes Chrysostomus, *De adversa valetudine et medicis*.
		Devreesse 1945: 105-106.
[0933]	**115**	II.67.

This manuscript is listed among the copies of Nemesius Emesenus, *De natura hominis* (frg.).

Codex *Coislinianus* 115 contains Anastasius Sinaiticus, *Quaestiones*, which include fragments from Nemesius (Morani 1981: 122).

Devreesse 1945: 106-107.

[0934]	**120**	II.67.

This manuscript is listed among the copies of Nemesius Emesenus, *De natura hominis* (frg.).

Codex *Coislinianus* 120 contains Anastasius Sinaiticus, *Quaestiones*, which include fragments from Nemesius (Morani 1981: 122).

Devreesse 1945: 109-111.

[0935]	**123**	N.62.

The f. I (palimpsest, containing Paul of Aegina) comes from the same manuscript as ff. 1 and 283 of *Coislinianus* 8 (= [0930]).

Devreesse 1945: 117-118.

The palimpsested ff. 24-25 of Paris, *Supplementum graecum* 1156 (= [1391]) and 1-2 of Москва (Moskva), Государственный Исторический Музей (ГИМ), Синодальная Библиотека Московского Патриархата (Gosudarstvennyi Istoricheskii Muzei (GIM), Sinodal'naia Biblioteka Moskovskoi Patriarkhii [State Historical Museum [GIM], Synodal Library of Moscow Patriarchate]), Sinod. 174 (387 Vlad.) (see p. 148) come from a different manuscript contrary to Heiberg 1919: 276, Devreesse 1945: 7-8 (about *Coislinianus* 8) and 117-118 (about *Coislinianus* 123), and Astruc and Concasty 1960: 320 (about Paris, *Supplementum graecum* 1156).

Omont 1897: 13 already noted the different origin of the palimpsested folios of *Supplementum graecum* 1156 and *Coislinianus* 8 (although he did not distinguish f. 23 and ff. 24-25 in *Supplementum graecum* 1156).

Recently, see Fonkič 2000: 170n7, discusses all of these manuscripts.

[0936]	**158**	II.41, 43, 56.
		Devreesse 1945: 142-143.
[0937]	**163**	I.103.
		Devreesse 1945: 146-147.
		See [0909].
[0938]	**168**	II.77.
		Devreesse 1945: 150.

| | 173 | (ff. 3r-29v) Synesius Cyrenensis, *De insomniis* cum Nicephori Gregorae commentario. |

173   (ff. 3r-29v) Synesius Cyrenensis, *De insomniis* cum Nicephori Gregorae commentario.

Devreesse 1945: 154-155.

224   (f. 14r-v) Epiphanius, *De ponderibus et mensuris* (sub titulo *Explicatio nominum ebraicorum*) (frg.) et *De adamanta gemma*.

Devreesse 1945: 204-206 (especially 205).

[0939]   **228**   I.101; II.40.

Devreesse 1945: 207-208.

[0940]   **229**   II.40.

This manuscript contains Gregorius Nyssenus, *De hominis opificio*.

Montfaucon 1715: 2.292.

According to Devreesse 1945: 209, it is missing ("aujourd'hui disparu") from the collections of the Bibliothèque nationale de France.

It is now in Москва, Научная Библиотека Московского Государственного Университета Имени М. В. Ломоносова (МГУ), гр., 1 (Moskva, Nauchnaia Biblioteka Moskovskogo Gosudarstrennogo] Universiteta Imeni M. V. Lomonosova [MGU], Research Library, Lomonosov Moscow State University [MSU]), gr., 1) (see above, p. 150).

233   (ff. 151v-153r) Basilius Caesariensis, *Quaestio de medicis*.

Devreesse 1945: 212-213.

234   (f. 129r-v) Basilius Caesariensis, *Quaestio de medicis*.

Devreesse 1945: 213-214.

[0941]   **235**   II.40.

Devreesse 1945: 214-215.

249   (ff. 48v-60v) Synesius Cyrenensis, *De insomniis*.

Devreesse 1945: 228-229.

[0942]   **259**   II.67.

This manuscript is listed among the copies of Nemesius Emesenus, *De natura hominis* (frg.).

This manuscript does not contain Nemesius' treatise, but works by Anastasius Sinaiticus and Ioannes Chrysostomus (Devreesse 1945: 237), which include fragments from Nemesius (Morani 1981: 121-122).

[0943]   **294**   II.67.

Devreesse 1945: 275-276, and Morani 1981: 28, for Nemesius Emesenus, *De natura hominis*.

[0944]   **300**   I.123.

This manuscript is listed among the copies of Galenus, *Iatrosofion*.

This codex has been described by Montfaucon 1715: 2.416. Although it does not contain any text explicitly identified as a *iatrosofion*, it has some *medicinalia* at the end of the volume ("In fine aliquot praecepta medicinalia") and could very well be the item referred to here.

According to Devreesse 1945: 285, the manuscript is in Leningrad.

Actually the manuscript is now in Санкт-Петербург, Российская национальная библиотека (РНБ), Собрание греческих рукописей, 116 (Sankt-Petersburg, Rossiiskaia natsional'naia biblioteka [RNB], Sobranie grecheskie rukopisei, 116 [Saint-Petersburg, National Library of Russia [NLR], Greek manuscripts, 116]) (see below, p. 311).

Also [1407].

[0945]   **321**   I.41.

Devreesse 1945: 308-309.

Also [0946].

[0946]   **[321 (?)]**   I.41.

The information about the Pseudo-Hippocratic *Epistula ad Ptolemaeum regem de sanitate tuenda* appears in Ackermann 1825: CLXXIV, *sub titulo*, with a reference to "Montfauc. in biblioth. Coislin. part. II. p. 444", but without brackets or question mark.

Reference is to Montfaucon 1715, Pars Secunda, p. 444, manuscript CCCXXI (= 321) described as containing Hippocrates, *Epistula ad Ptolemaeum* at f. 115.

This text can be found in *Coislinianus* 321, ff. 115r-116r (see Devreesse 1945: 308-309).

Same as [0945].

[0947]   **332**   II.9 (2).

Devreesse 1945: 316.

[0948]   **333**   I.68.

Devreesse 1945: 316-317.

[0949]   **334**   I.80, 130; II.109, 110.

Devreesse 1945: 317-318.

See [0926] and [0927].

[0950]   **335**   I.42, 114, 117, 123, 133, 136, 149; II.15, 25, 28, 64, 79, 91.

Devreesse 1945: 318-320.

See [0928]-[0929] and also [0951].

[0951]   **[335]**   I.28.

This is a copy of Hippocrates, *De genitura*.

The same information appears in Ackermann 1825: CLVII, no. 43 (without brackets), with the following addition:

Codices Mss. exstant in bibl. Coisliniana nr. 335 Montfaucon in biblioth. Coisliniana part. II. pag. 448.

In Montfaucon 1715: 2.448 (on manuscript CCCXXXV [= 335]) described *ibid.* 447-449), a text entitled as follows is listed:

Fol. 34. vers. Excerpta ex Hippocrate περὶ τῆς γονῆς καὶ κατασκευῆς τοῦ ἀνθρώπου. Quae secunda portio liber est editus a Cornario Basileae anno 1558. sub titulo, Hippocratis de hominis structura.

Diels' reference here is probably to this text, which seems to be included in the *iatrosofion* under Galen's name in *Coislinianus* 335, ff. 21r-60r (see Devreesse 1945: 319, no. VII, about the text, and 318-320 about the manuscript), unless this is a reference to the text of f. 68v identified as follows in Devreesse 1945: 319, no. VIII.3: "de quibusdam feminarum morbis".

Probably same as [0950].

[0952]	**336**	I.72.
		Devreesse 1945: 321.
	346	(ff. 293r-294r) *Lexicon botanicum.*
		Devreesse 1945: 330-331; Touwaide 1999: 217, 227.
[0953]	**384**	II.63.
		Devreesse 1945: 366-367.
[0954]	**387**	II.98.
		Devreesse 1945: 368-370.
[0955]	**[1018 (?)]**	I.13.

This manuscript is listed among the copies of Hippocrates, *Aphorismi.*

A similar reference (without brackets or question mark) appears in Ackermann 1825: LXVI: "In bibl. Coislin. S. German. n. 1018", where this codex is listed among the "Latini [codices]" of the *Aphorismi* (see p. LXV for the mention of Latin manuscripts).

This item appears in Montfaucon 1739: 2.1113, no. 1018, and is described as follows:

1018. Hippocratis Heraclidae filii, hujus nominis secundi, Aphorismi

It is listed among the holdings of the *Bibliotheca Coisliniana San-Germanensis.*

This is a Latin manuscript, *Coislinianus latinus* 1018. It does not appear in Magdelaine 1994.

Imprimés

[0956]	**Rés. Te 138.27**	I.117; II.33.
		Omont 1886-1888: 3.343.
		Humanist copy.

Parisin. (*Parisini*)

[0957]	**36**	I.5, 13, 25, 49; II.29, 80.
		Omont 1886-1888: 1.6; *CMAG* I (Lebègue) 1924: 210-211.
		Also [1332].
	39	Gregorius Nazianzenus, *De humana natura.*
		Omont 1886-1888: 1.7 (does not specifically identify the text); Mossay 1981: 41; Domiter 1999: 21.
	390	(ff. 71r et seq.) Epiphanius, *Physiologus* (frg.).
		Omont 1886-1888: 1.40.

[0958]	**396**	I.5, 32; II.28, 49.
		Omont 1886-1888: 1.41-42; 3.393.
[0959]	**476**	II.40.
		Omont 1886-1888: 1.53-54.
[0960]	**478**	II.21.
		Omont 1886-1888: 1.54.
[0961]	**479**	II.40.
		Omont 1886-1888: 1.54.
[0962]	**500**	II.21.
		Omont 1886-1888: 1.62.
[0963]	**503**	II.40.
		Omont 1886-1888: 1.63-64.
[0964]	**777 A**	II.40.
		Omont 1886-1888: 1.144.
[0965]	**825**	II.67, 101.
		Omont 1886-1888: 1.155.
[0966]	**826**	II.67.
		Omont 1886-1888: 1.155.
[0967]	**827**	II.67.
		Omont 1886-1888: 1.155.
[0968]	**827 A**	II.67.
		Omont 1886-1888: 1.155.
	830	(ff. 66r et seq.) Synesius Cyrenensis, *De insomniis*, cum Nichephori Gregorae praefatione et commentariis.
		Omont 1886-1888: 1.156.
	831	(ff. 31v et seq.) Synesius Cyrenensis, *De insomniis*, cum Nicephori Gregorae commentariis.
		Omont 1886-1888: 1.156.
[0969]	**834**	II.35.
		Omont 1886-1888: 1.156-157.
[0970]	**835**	N.50.
		Omont 1886-1888: 1.157.
	854	Nemesius Emesenus, *De natura humanis* (frg.).
		Omont 1886-1888: 1.159-160; 3.394.
[0971]	**912**	II.21, 52.
		Omont 1886-1888: 1.172-173.
	924	(ff. 23v-36r) Nemesius Emesenus, *De natura hominis* (frg.).
		Omont 1886-1888: 1.177 (where the text is not listed); Morani 1981: 28.

[0972]	**940**	II.40.
		Omont 1886-1888: 1.180.
[0973]	**956**	II.40.
		Omont 1886-1888: 1.184.
[0974]	**968**	II.40.
		Omont 1886-1888: 1.187-188.
[0975]	**985**	I.43, 68, 80; II.49, 98.
		Omont 1886-1888: 1.195-196.
	990	Gregorius Nazianzenus, *De humana natura*.
		Omont 1886-1888: 1.198 (does not mention the text); Domiter 1999: 22.
	992	Gregorius Nazianzenus, *De humana natura*.
		Omont 1886-1888: 1.198 (does not mention the text); Domiter 1999: 22.
[0976]	**993**	II.106.
		Omont 1886-1888: 1.198.
	995	Gregorius Nazianzenus, *De humana natura*.
		Omont 1886-1888: 1.198 (does not mention the text); Domiter 1999: 22.
[0977]	**1000**	II.52.
		Omont 1886-1888: 1.199-200.
[0978]	**1007**	II.40.
		Omont 1886-1888: 1.201.
[0979]	**1009**	II.40.
		Omont 1886-1888: 1.201.
[0980]	**1010**	II.40, 99.
		Omont 1886-1888: 1.201-202.
	1038	(ff. 67r et seq.) Synesius Cyrenensis, *De insomniis*.
		Omont 1886-1888: 1.208-209.
	1039	(ff. 153v et seq.) Synesius Cyrenensis, *De insomniis*.
		Omont 1886-1888: 1.209.
	1040	(ff. 130v et seq.) Synesius Cyrenensis, *De insomniis*.
		Omont 1886-1888: 1.209.
	1042	(ff. 1-15) Synesius Cyrenensis, *De insomniis*.
		Omont 1886-1888: 1.209.
	1043	(ff. 133v-150r) Aetius Amidenus, *Libri medicinales* (frg.); (ff. 151v-154r) [Galenus], fragmenta.
		Omont 1886-1888: 1.209-210 (does not list the texts); *CCAG* VIII.3 (Boudreaux) 1912: 4-5.

[0981]   **1044**   II.67.

                              Omont 1886-1888: 1.210.

[0982]   **1045**   II.67.

                              Omont 1886-1888: 1.210; *CCAG* VIII.3 (Boudreaux)
                              1912: 6-7.

[0983]   **1046**   II.67.

                              Omont 1886-1888: 1.210.

[0984]   **1053**   II.40.

                              Omont 1886-1888: 1.211-212.

[0985]   **[1097 (?)]**   I.63.

This item is listed among the manuscripts of Galenus, *De elementis secundum Hippocratem*. The same information appears in Ackermann 1821: LXXV, no. 8, without brackets or question mark.

This treatise does not appear in *Parisinus graecus* 1097 (Omont 1886-1888: 1.219 for the description of the content of this manuscript; also Ihm 2002: 237, 238, who does not mention this *Parisinus*).

There must have been some confusion. According to Omont 1898: 67 *sub nomine* Galenus, *De elementis secundum Hippocratem*, the treatise is contained instead in the *Parisini graeci* 1883 (= [1014]), 2267 (= [1207]) and 2317 (= [1264]), and also *Supplementum graecum* 634 (= [1362]).

According to Diels' catalogue, it is in the *Parisini graeci* 1883 and 2317, and *Supplementum graecum* 634. According to Omont's catalogue, these three manuscripts contain the following works:

* *Hippocratis et Galeni excerpta de quattuor elementis* (*graecus* 1883; Omont 1886-1888: 2.158);

* *Galeni excerpta de quattuor elementis* (*graecus* 2317; Omont 1886-1888: 2.238);

* Galenus, *De elementis* (*Supplementum graecum* 634; Omont 1886-1888: 3.287).

The *Parisinus* 2267 (= [1207]) not mentioned by Diels, contains Galenus, *De elementis secundum Hippocratem*, according to Omont 1886-1888: 2.226-227. It is not listed by Ihm 2002: 238, who mentions, instead, the *Parisinus* 2147 (= [1058]), not included by Omont 1898: 67 *sub nomine* Galenus, *De elementis secundum Hippocratem*.

There seems to have been much confusion about these manuscripts, the source of which in Ackermann 1821 (from which Diels' catalogue most likely took the information) cannot be explained.

                1220   (ff. 67r et 205r) Gregorius Nazianzenus, *De humana natura*.

                              Omont 1886-1888: 1.270-271, with no precise identification
                              of the text; Domiter 1999: 22.

[0986]   **1247**   II.40.

                              Omont 1886-1888: 1.276.

[0987]	**1268**	II.9, 67.
		Omont 1886-1888: 1.282.
[0988]	**1277**	II.40.
		Omont 1886-1888: 1.284-285.
	1289	(f. 283) *De corporis humani appellationibus.*
		Omont 1886-1888: 1.288-289; Björck 1938: 144.
[0989]	**1297**	I.13.
		Omont 1886-1888: 1.292.
		Probably same as [1394].
[0990]	**1310**	I.126; II.94.
		Omont 1886-1888: 1.295-297.
[0991]	**1327**	I.38.
		Omont 1886-1888: 2.8-10.
[0992]	**1346**	II.94.
		Omont 1886-1888: 2.19.
	1356	(ff. A + 340 and 341 + B) Gregorius Nyssenus, *De hominis opificio* (frg.).
		Astruc 1985 for this fragment, and Omont 1886-1888: 2.22-23 for the manuscript.
[0993]	**1389**	II.25.
		Omont 1886-1888: 2.35-36.
[0994]	**1405**	II.44.
		Omont 1886-1888: 2.38.
[0995]	**1438**	I.101.
		Omont 1886-1888: 2.42.
[0996]	**[1444 (?)]**	I.11.

This manuscript is listed among the copies of Hippocrates, *De articulis*.

The same information (without brackets or question mark) appears in Ackermann 1825: CXXII, no. 8.

The codex *Parisinus graecus* 1444 does not contain this text, but rather Hermias Sozomenus, *Ecclesiastica historia*, and Evagrius Scholasticus, *Ecclesiastica historia* (Omont 1886-1888: 2.43).

This is probably a mistake for one of the *Parisini* containing the work according to Omont 1898: 89 *sub nomine* Hippocrates:

- 2140 (= 1041]);
- 2141 (= [1043]);
- 2142 (= [1045]);

- 2143 (= [1048]);
- 2144 (= [1051]);
- 2145 (= [1053]);
- 2146 (= [1055]);
- 2255 (= [1190]),

to which 1868 (= [1013]) should be added.

Codex *graecus* 2144, ff. 44v-71 (= [1051]) may be the most probable.

[0997]	**1542**	II.40.
		Omont 1886-1888: 2.85; *CMAG* I (Lebègue) 1924: 215-221.
[0998]	**1603**	II.34, 67.
		Omont 1886-1888: 2.102-103.
[0999]	**1630**	I.40, 41, 113, 130; II.9, 14, 59, 64, 102 (2).
		Omont 1886-1888: 2.109-112.
[1000]	**1631**	II.28.
		Omont 1886-1888: 2.112-113.
[1001]	**1644**	I.61.
		Omont 1886-1888: 2.115.
[1002]	**[1667 (?)]**	I.46.

This manuscript is listed among the copies of Hippocrates, *De febribus*.

The same information (without brackets or question mark) appears in Ackermann 1825: CLXXVI, *sub titulo*, who cites this manuscript and also *Parisinus graecus* 1885 (= [1018]) for this treatise.

The *Parisinus* 1667 (on which Omont 1886-1888: 2.118) does not contain this text, which, among the *Parisini graeci*, appears only in codex 1884, ff. 92v-95v (= [1015]) according to Omont 1898: 89 *sub nomine* Hippocrates.

There seems to have been some confusion between the *Parisini* 1667 and 1884, and, secondarily, also between 1884 and 1885 in Ackermann (above), that cannot be explained.

[1003]	**1739**	II.67.
		Omont 1886-1888: 2.132-133.
[1004]	**1760**	I.38.
		Omont 1886-1888: 2.136.
[1005]	**1766**	II.94.
		Omont 1886-1888: 2.137-138.
	1782	(ff. 111r et seq.) Epiphanius, *De duodecim gemmis*.
		Omont 1886-1888: 2.142.
[1006]	**1788**	II.94.
		Omont 1886-1888: 2.143-144.

[1007]   **[1819 (?) = 1849 (?)]**   I.66.

This manuscript is listed among the copies of Galenus, *De anatomicis administrationibus*.

The same information appears in Ackermann 1821: LXXXIII, no. 16 ctd. (without brackets or question marks, but with the identification as *Parisinus* 1849).

Whereas *Parisinus graecus* 1819 does not contain the treatise (Omont 1886-1888: 2.149), *Parisinus* 1849 (= [1011]), does at ff. 9r-95r (Omont 1886-1888: 2.152; Garofalo 1986: IX; see also *ibid.*: XIIn38).

Same as [1011].

[1008]   **1831**   I.149.

Omont 1886-1888: 2.150.

[1009]   **1848**   II.10.

Omont 1886-1888: 2.152.

[1010]   **[1848 ?]**   I.13.

This manuscript is thought to be a copy of Hippocrates, *Aphorismi*, which is not the case (it is not listed in Magdelaine 1994).

This codex is listed (without brackets or question mark) among the copies of the *Aphorismi* in Ackermann 1825: LXIV.

It seems to have been confused with 1884 (= [1015]), which contains (ff. 158r-331r) Galenus, *In Hippocratis Aphorismos commentarius*, and is listed in Magdelaine 1994: 226.

[1011]   **1849**   I.11 (3), 66, 69, 106, 108 (2).

Omont 1886-1888: 2.152.

See [1007].

1859   (ff. 236r et seq.) Aristoteles, *De insomniis*.

Omont 1886-1888: 2.153-154; Wartelle 1963: 99, no. 1344.

1861   (ff. 78r et seq.) Aristoteles, *De insomniis*.

Omont 1886-1888: 2.154; Wartelle 1963: 99, no. 1346.

[1012]   **1865**   I.149; II.10, 80.

Omont 1886-1888: 2.155.

[1013]   **1868**   I.4, 11, 18, 21 (2), 22, 28, 29; II.37.

Omont 1886-1888: 2.155-156.

[1014]   **1883**   I.5, 13, 46, 60, 61, 63, 76, 80, 114, 131; II.6, 9, 71, 74, 104; N.32, 43.

Omont 1886-1888: 2.158.

[1015]   **1884**   I.5, 13, 46, 105; II.9, 40.

Omont 1886-1888: 2.158.

See [1002] and [1016]-[1019].

Possibly also [1010].

[1016]   **[1884]**   I.38.

According to Omont 1886-1888: 2.158, this manuscript does not contain Hippocrates, *Epistulae*, but only (f. 95v) *eiusdem* (i.e. Hippocratis), *Epistola ad Ptolemaeum, regem Aegypti.*

Same as [1015].

[1017]   **[1884 (?)]**   I.41.

The text referred to in Diels' catalogue (Hippocrates, *Epistula ad Ptolemaeum regem de sanitate tuenda*) is mentioned in Ackermann 1825: CLXXIV, *sub titulo* (without brackets or question mark).

It appears in *Parisinus graecus* 1884, ff. 95v-96v (Omont 1886-1888: 2.158).

Same as [1015].

[1018]   **[1885]**   I.38.

Contrary to Diels' catalogue, the *Epistulae* attributed to Hippocrates are not in this manuscript, which contains, according to Omont 1886-1888: 2.158: (ff. 1r et seq.) Herennius, *Commentarius in Aristotelis Metaphysica*, and (ff. 59r et seq.) Proclus Diadochus, *Elementa theologica.*

This may be a mistake for *Parisinus graecus* 1884 (= [1015]).

The *Parisini* 1884 and 1885 seem to have been confused also with *Parisinus* 1667 (= [1002]).

Also [1019].

[1019]   **[1885 (?)]**   I.46.

This manuscript is listed among the copies of Hippocrates, *De febribus.*

The same information (without brackets or question mark) appears in Ackermann 1825: CLXXVI, *sub titulo.*

This manuscript does not contain the text, contrary to Diels' catalogue (Omont 1886-1888: 2.158).

This may be a mistake for *Parisinus graecus* 1884, ff. 92v-95v, which, according to Omont 1898: 89, *sub nomine* Hippocrates, *sub titulo*, is the only copy of this work in the collections of the Bibliothèque nationale de France.

On the manuscript, see Omont 1886-1888: 2.158.

Same as [1015].

[1020]   **1893**   II.9.

Omont 1886-1888: 2.159-160.

1918   (ff. 144r et seq.) Aristoteles, *Problemata.*

Omont 1886-1888: 2.163; Wartelle 1963: 103, no. 1404.

1934   (ff. 385r et seq.) Theodorus Metochita, *De insomniis.*

Omont 1886-1888: 2.166-167.

	1935	(ff. 14v et seq.) Theodorus Metochita, *De insomniis*.
		Omont 1886-1888: 2.167.
[1021]	**1943**	II.22.
		Omont 1886-1888: 2.168.
[1022]	**1949**	I.80.
		Omont 1886-1888: 2.169.
[1023]	**1991**	I.112-113, 135; II.44, 47, 77, 82, 111; N.69.
		Omont 1886-1888: 2.175.
[1024]	**1995**	I.43.
		Omont 1886-1888: 2.176.
[1025]	**2027**	II.35.
		Omont 1886-1888: 2.181.
[1026]	**2028**	II.9.
		Omont 1886-1888: 2.181.
[1027]	**[2030 (?)]**	I.20, 33.

This item is thought to contain Hippocrates, *Praesagiorum Libri II*, but it does not (see Omont 1886-1888: 2.181).

The information comes from Ackermann 1825: LVIII (without brackets or question mark).

This may be a mistake for 2330 (= [1274]), where *Praesagiorum libri I* and *II* can be found.

	2035	(ff. 39v et seq.) Aristoteles, *De insomniis*.
		Omont 1886-1888: 2.182; Wartelle 1963: 109, no. 1466.
	2036	(ff. 1r et seq.) Aristoteles, *Problemata*.
		Omont 1886-1888: 2.182; Wartelle 1963: 109, no. 1467.
[1028]	**2037**	N.58 (2).
		Omont 1886-1888: 2.182.
[1029]	**2047**	I.18, 40; II.77, 106.
		Omont 1886-1888: 2.183-184.
[1030]	**2047 A**	II.9, 22, 63.
		Omont 1886-1888: 2.184.
[1031]	**2048**	II.9.
		Omont 1886-1888: 2.184.
[1032]	**2077**	II.67.
		Omont 1886-1888: 2.189-190.
[1033]	**2091**	I.43, 125.
		Omont 1886-1888: 2.192-193; 3.396.

[1034]   **2098**   II.109.

Omont 1886-1888: 2.194.

[1035]   **[2113 (?)]**   I.101.

This manuscript is listed among the copies of Galenus, *Introductio sive medicus*.

The same information appears in Ackermann 1821: CXLVIII, no. 83 (without brackets or question mark).

The *Parisinus* 2113 contains Aristoteles, *Ethicorum ad Nicomachum libri X*, and not the Galenic treatise (Omont 1886-1888: 2.196; Wartelle 1963: 112, no. 1510).

This seems to be a mistake for *Parisinus* 2153 (= [1069]), ff. 1r-12v, which contains this work (see Omont 1886-1888: 2.205; Petit 2009: LXXXII-LXXXIII, where the *Parisinus* 2113 does not appear, whereas 2153 does. However, Petit 2009: LXXXII n125 does not include the *Parisinus* 2113 among the manuscripts erroneously mentioned by Diels as containing the work).

Same as [1069].

[1036]   **2118**   N.58.

Omont 1886-1888: 2.197.

[1037]   **[2123 (?)]**   I.98.

This manuscript is listed among the copies of Galenus, *De compositione medicamentorum secundum locos*.

The same information appears in Ackermann 1821: CXXVIV, no. 54 ctd. (without brackets or question mark).

The *Parisinus* 2123 contains Epictetus, *Enchiridion* (Omont 1886-1888: 2.197).

This seems to be a confusion with *Parisinus graecus* 2173 (= [1097]), where Galen's treatise can be found (ff. 71r-319v) (Omont 1886-1888: 2.209).

[1038]   **[2137 (?)]**   I.88.

The treatise by Galenus, *De causis pulsuum* is not present in this manuscript (Omont 1886-1888: 2.199) contrary to Diels' catalogue.

The information, which is present in Ackermann 1821: CV, no. 40 ctd. (without brackets or question mark), may result from confusion with *Parisinus* 2167 (= [1088]), which does contain this text, at ff. 343r-387r (Omont 1886-1888: 2.208-209).

[1039]   **2139**   II.44 (2), 76, 82 (2).

Omont 1886-1888: 2.199.

Also [1040].

[1040] **[2139 (?)]**   I.113.

The text referred to here is Galenus, *Prognostica de decubitu ex mathematica scientia.*

This reference probably corresponds to *Galeni praenotiones astrologicae, a tempore decubitus, de morbi exitu*, actually contained in *Parisinus graecus* 2139 (= [1039]), ff. 23 et seq., according to Omont 1886-1888: 2.199.

See also *CCAG* VIII.3 (Boudreaux) 1912: 12-13.

Same as [1039].

[1041] **2140**   I.4, 5, 8, 10, 11 (3), 12, 13, 18 (2), 19, 20 (3), 21 (2), 22, 23 (2), 24 (3), 25 (2), 26 (2), 27 (3), 28 (2), 29 (2), 30 (3), 31 (2), 33 (2), 34 (2), 35 (3), 38, 110; II.93.

Omont 1886-1888: 2.199-200.

Also [1042] and [1057].

[1042] **[2140]**   I.22.

This is a copy of Hippocrates, *De salubri diaeta*, a text following (or: included in, according to modern authors) *De natura hominis* (see Jouanna 2002: 19-38).

According to Omont 1886-1888: 2.199-200, the *Parisinus* 2140 (= [1041]) contains (ff. 22v et seq.) *De natura hominis* (see also Jouanna 2002: 61, 71-72).

Same as [1041].

For this text, see also the following *Parisini*:

- 2141 (= [1043]);
- 2142 (= [1045]);
- 2143 (= [1048]);
- 2144 (= [1051]);
- 2145 (= [1053]);
- 2146 (= [1055]);
- 2147 (= [1058]);
- 2253 (= [1184]);
- 2255 (= [1190]).

[1043] **2141**   I.4, 5, 8, 10, 11 (3), 12, 13, 18 (2), 19, 20 (3), 21 (2), 22, 23 (2), 24 (3), 25 (2), 26 (2), 27 (3), 28 (2), 29 (2), 30 (3), 31 (2), 33 (2), 34 (2), 35 (3), 38, 110; II.37, 93.

Omont 1886-1888: 2.200-201.

Also [1044].

[1044] **[2141]**   I.22.

This is a copy of Hippocrates, *De salubri diaeta* (on this treatise, see [1042]).

According to Omont 1886-1888: 2.200-201, the *Parisinis* 2141 (= [1043]) contains (ff. 20r et seq.) *De natura hominis* (see also Jouanna 2002: 61).

Same as [1043].

[1045]   **2142**   I.1, 4, 5, 8, 10, 11 (3), 12, 13, 18 (2), 19, 20 (3), 21 (2), 22, 23, 24 (3), 25 (2), 26 (2), 27 (3), 28 (2), 29 (2), 30 (3), 31, 32, 33 (2), 34 (2), 35 (2), 38, 110; II.37, 93.

Omont 1886-1888: 2.201.

Also [1046] and [1168].

[1046]   **[2142]**   I.22, 31.

This is Hippocrates, *De salubri diaeta* (I.22) (on which see [1042]), and *De exsectione foetus*, *De exsectione pueri* (I.31).

The same information appears in Ackermann 1825: CXXVI, no. 13 (*De exsectione foetus*), without brackets, however.

According to Omont 1886-1888: 2.201, the *Parisinus* 2142 (= [1045]) contains (ff. 28r et seq.) *De natura hominis* (which includes *De salubri diaeta* on which see [1042]; see also Jouanna 2002: 61, 85-86) and *De exsectione infantis* (ff. 441r et seq.).

Same as [1045].

[1047]   **[2142 (?)]**   I.23 (2), 35.

According to Diels' catalogue, this is a copy of three Hippocratic works:

• *De affectionibus* (I.23);

• *De locis in homine* (I.23);

• *Praeceptiones* (I.35).

The same information (without brackets or question mark) appears in Ackermann 1825: CXXVIII, no. 15 ctd. (*De affectionibus*), CLIII, no. 37 ctd. (*De locis in homine*), and CLXVII, no. 51 (*Praeceptiones*).

De affectionibus is not contained in *Parisinus graecus* 2142 (= [1045]; Omont 1886-1888: 2.201), but in the *Parisini* 2140-2141 (= [1041] and [1043]), 2143-2145 (= [1048], [1051] and [1053]) and 2148 (= [1061]).

Similarly, *De locis in homine* is not in *Parisinus* 2142, but in *Parisinus* 2146 (= [1055]), ff. 228v et seq. (Joly 1978: 33, and also Omont 1886-1888: 2.204, where it is entitled *De partibus corporis humani*).

Parisinus 2142 (= [1045]) contains (ff. 292v et seq.) *Praenotiones*, and (ff. 442 et seq.) *Praedictorum libri II* (Omont 1886-1888: 2.201). According to Diels I.35, *Praeceptiones* appears in *Parisini* 2140-2141 (= [1041] and [1043]), 2143-2145 (= [1048], [1051] and [1053]), and 2255 (= [1190]).

The manuscript referred to here cannot be identified, as there seem to have been several mistakes over its identification.

[1048]   **2143**   I.4, 5, 8, 10, 11 (3), 12, 13, 18 (2), 19, 20 (3), 21, 22, 23 (2), 24 (3), 25 (2), 26 (2), 27 (3), 28 (2), 29 (2), 30 (3), 31 (2), 33 (2), 34 (2), 35 (3), 38, 110; II.37, 93.

Omont 1886-1888: 2.201-202.

See also [1049] and [1050], and possibly [1062].

[1049]

[2143]   I.22.

This is Hippocrates, *De salubri diaeta* (on this treatise, see [1042]).

Although Omont 1886-1888: 2.201-202, does not list this text among those in the *Parisinus* 2143, it can be found in the manuscript, at ff. 136r-155v (Jouanna 2002: 61, 82-83).

Same as [1048].

[1050]

[2143 (?)]   I.21.

This is a copy of Hippocrates, *De arte*.

Although Omont 1886-1888: 2.201-202, does not list the treatise in the description of *Parisinus* 2143, it can be found in this manuscript at ff. 12v-15v (Jouanna 1988: 193).

Same as [1048].

[1051]

2144   I.4, 5, 8, 10, 11 (3), 12, 13, 18 (2), 19, 20 (3), 21 (2), 22, 23 (2), 24 (3), 25 (2), 26 (2), 27 (3), 28 (3), 29 (2), 30 (3), 31 (2), 33 (2), 34 (2), 35 (3), 38, 110; II.37, 93, 111.

Omont 1886-1888: 2.202-203.

Also [1052] and possibly [1071].

[1052]

[2144]   I.22.

This is a copy of Hippocrates, *De salubri diaeta* (on this treatise, see [1042]).

According to Omont 1886-1888: 2.202-203, *Parisinus* 2144 (= [1051]) contains (ff. 29r et seq.) *De natura hominis* (see also Jouanna 2002: 61, 82-83).

Same as [1051].

[1053]

2145   I.4, 5, 8, 10, 11 (3), 12, 13, 18 (2), 19, 20 (3), 21, 22, 23 (2), 24 (3), 25 (2), 26 (2), 27 (3), 28 (2), 29 (2), 30 (3), 31 (2), 33 (2), 34 (2), 35 (3), 38, 110; II.37, 93.

Omont 1886-1888: 2.203-204.

Also [1054], [1297], [1298] and [1299], and possibly [1071].

[1054]

[2145]   I.22.

This is a copy of Hippocrates, *De salubri diaeta* (on this text, see [1042]).

Although Omont 1886-1888: 2.203-204, does not include this text in the description of the manuscript, *Parisinus* 2145 does contain it at ff. 217r-247v (see Byl 1977; Jouanna 2002: 61).

Same as [1053].

[1055]

2146   I.4, 5, 8, 10 (2), 11 (3), 13, 18 (2), 19, 21, 27 (2), 28 (2), 29, 30 (3), 31 (3), 32 (3), 33, 34, 35, 38, 40.

Omont 1886-1888: 2.204.

Also [1056], [1057] and [1300].

[1056]

[2146]   I.22, 30.

This is a copy of Hippocrates, *De salubri diaeta* (I.22) and *De sterilibus* (I.30).

The same information (without brackets) appears in Ackermann 1825: CXXXVI, no. 22 ctd. (*De sterilibus*).

According to Omont 1886-1888: 2.204, *Parisinus* 2146 (= [1055]) contains. at ff. 179v et seq. *De natura hominis* (in which *De salubri diaeta* is included; see [1042] and also Jouanna 2002: 61) and, at ff. 241v et seq., *De morbis mulierum libri III* (= *De sterilibus*).

Same as [1055].

[1057]   **[2146 (?)]**   I.23, 34, 35.

According to Diels' catalogue, this item contains the following three Hippocratic works (references to Diels' catalogue follow the titles):

- *De locis in homine* (I.23);
- *De visu* (I.34);
- *De iudicationibus* (I.35).

According to Omont 1886-1888: 2.204, only *De locis in homine* appears in *Parisinus* 2146 (ff. 228v et seq., under the title *De partibus corporis humani*) (also Joly 1978: 33).

For the other two texts, there is some confusion:

- *De visu* is contained, among others, in *Parisinus* 2140 (= [1041]), ff. 171v et seq. (Omont 1886-1888: 2.199-200). This may be the intended reference;
- *De iudicationibus* (= *De crisibus*), which is not contained in *Parisinus* 2146, may have been confused with *De diebus criticis* (= *De diebus iudicatoriis*), which is in *Parisinus* 2146, at ff. 321 et seq. (Omont 1886-1888: 2.203-204). The manuscript *Parisinus* 2146 (= [1055]) appears in the list of the witnesses of *De diebus iudicatoriis* in Diels' catalogue (I.35).

The information about *De visu* may come from Ackermann 1825: CXXX, no. 17 ctd. (without brackets or question mark).

[1058]   **2147**   I.13, 21, 22, 28, 29, 150; II.98.

Omont 1886-1888: 2.204.

See also [1059] and [1060].

[1059]   **[2147]**   I.22.

This is a copy of Hippocrates, *De salubri diaeta* (on this text, see [1042]).

While Omont 1886-1888: 2.204, does not list this text in *Parisinus* 2147, the manuscript does contain, at ff. 6r-23r, *De natura hominis* (in which *De salubri diaeta* is included; see [1042]). See Jouanna 2002: 62, 89-90.

Same as [1058].

[1060]   **[2147 (?)]**   I.28.

This is a copy of Hippocrates, *De genitura*.

The same information appears in Ackermann 1825: CLIX, no. 44 ctd. (without brackets or question mark).

While Omont 1886-1888: 2.204, lists this manuscript as containing, at ff. 1r et seq., *De natura pueri* identified as "Hippocratis, vel Polybii, *liber de natura pueri*", in fact the manuscript contains extracts from both *De genitura* and *De natura pueri* (Giorgianni 2006: 82).

Same as [1058].

[1061]	**2148**	I.8, 18 (2), 21, 23 (2), 24, 25 (2), 26, 27, 29, 33, 39, 68, 96; II.37.
		Omont 1886-1888: 2.204.
[1062]	**[2148]**	I.13, 24 (2), 26, 34, 35.

This manuscript is listed among the copies of the following six Hippocratic treatises (listed here in the order of Diels' catalogue; references to Diels' catalogue follow the titles):

- *Aphorismi* (I.13);
- *De haemorroïdibus* (I.24);
- *De morbo sacro* (I.24);
- *De insomniis* (I.26);
- *De visu* (I.34);
- *De diebus iudicatoriis* (I.35).

None of these works appears in the *Parisinus graecus* 2148 according to Omont 1886-1888: 2.204 (description of manuscript) and Omont 1898: 89-90, *sub nomine* Hippocrates (see also Magdelaine 1994 for the *Aphorismi*, for example).

Similar information about the *Aphorismi* appears in Ackermann 1825: LXIV.

Assuming that all these works were in the same manuscript, the shelfmark 2148 probably results from a mistake, possibly for *Parisinus graecus* 2143 (= [1048]), which contains all the treatises mentioned here (see Omont 1886-1888: 2.201-202):

- (ff. 71v-76v) *De morbo sacro*;
- (ff. 155v-158) *De insomniis*;
- (ff. 158-159) *De visu*;
- (ff. 159-160v) *De diebus decretoriis*;
- (ff. 160v-169) *Aphorismi*;
- (ff. 314-315) *De haemorroidibus*.

Same as [1048].

[1063]	**2149**	I.13, 56, 115, 149; II.37, 69, 74, 77, 104.
		Omont 1886-1888: 2.204-205.
		Also [1064].
[1064]	**2149 (?)**	I.24.

This manuscript contains Hippocrates, *De ulceribus*. It is mentioned in Littré 1839-1861: 6.398.

Although the text is not listed in Omont 1886-1888: 2.204-205, it is present in the manuscript (f. 176v), though only as a fragment (Duminil 1998: 26).

Same as [1063].

[1065]	**2150**	I.13; II.26.
		Omont 1886-1888: 2.205.
[1066]	**2151**	I.117; II.33, 37, 71, 89 (2), 97.
		Omont 1886-1888: 2.205.

[1067]   **[2151 (?)]**   I.111.

This manuscript is listed among the copies of Galenus, *Definitiones medicae*.

The same information (without brackets or question mark) appears in Ackermann 1821: CLIX, no. 102.

According to Omont 1886-1888: 2.205, this manuscript does not contain this text.

This seems to be a mistake. According to Omont 1898: 67 *sub nomine* Galenus, *sub titulo*, *Definitiones medicae* are contained only in the following *Parisini graeci*:

- 2167 (= [1088]);
- 2175 (= [1099]);
- 2282 (= [1229]).

The manuscript referred to here cannot be identified.

[1068]   **2152**   II.66, 91.

Omont 1886-1888: 2.205.

[1069]   **2153**   I.88, 101, 118; II.7, 79 (2), 80, 92, 109 (2), 110.

Omont 1886-1888: 2.205; 3.396.

See [1035] and [1078].

[1070]   **2154**   I.68; II.62; N.58.

Omont 1886-1888: 2.206.

[1071]   **[2154]**   I.13.

Hippocrates, *Aphorismi* is not in *Parisinus graecus* 2154 (see Omont 1886-1888: 2.206; it is not listed in Magdelaine 1994: 88-90).

This manuscript is listed among the copies of the *Aphorismi* in Ackermann 1825: LXIV (without brackets).

The incorrect information here could refer to two different *Parisini* that contain the work:

- 2144 (= [1051]), ff. 188r-208r (Omont 1886-1888: 2.202-203; Magdelaine 1994: 89);
- 2145 (= [1053]), ff. 255r-268v (Omont 1886-1888: 2.203-204; Magdelaine 1994: 89).

[1072]   **2155**   I.33, 68, 80, 89, 98, 131, 149; II.40, 101.

Omont 1886-1888: 2.206.

[1073]   **2156**   I.80, 96, 98, 101, 111, 126.

Omont 1886-1888: 2.206.

[1074]   **[2156 (?)]**   I.93.

This manuscript does not contain Galenus, *Ad Glauconem de medendi methodo* (see Omont 1886-1888: 2.206), contrary to Diels' catalogue and Ackermann 1821: CXXIX, no. 57 (without brackets or question mark).

Omont 1898: 67 *sub nomine* Galenus, *sub titulo*, lists the manuscript among the copies of the work, although he does not mention the work in the description of the content of the manuscript.

This seems to be a mistake (misreading) for any other *Parisinus* containing Galen's treatise, possibly 2166 (= [1087]), ff. 1r-34v (Omont 1886-1888: 2.208).

[1075]   **2157**   I.78, 79 (2), 80, 85, 92, 93, 96.

Omont 1886-1888: 2.206-207.

Possibly [1100].

[1076]   **[2157 (?)]**   I.80, 87, 88, 89.

This codex is considered to contain four Galenic treatises (listed here in the order of Diels' catalogue; references to Diels' catalogue follow the titles):

- *De differentiis febrium* (I.80);
- *De pulsuum differentiis* (I.87);
- *De dignoscendis pulsibus* (I.88);
- *De praesagitione ex pulsibus* (I.89).

According to Omont 1886-1888: 2.206-207, *Parisinus* 2157 (= [1075]) does not contain any of these treatises. All of them appear, instead, in the *Parisinus graecus* 2167 (= [1088]) (see Omont 1886-1888: 2. 208-209):

- (ff. 188r et seq.) *De differentiis febrium*;
- (ff. 287r et seq.) *De pulsuum differentiis*;
- (ff. 303r et seq.) *De dignoscendis pulsibus*;
- (ff. 387r et seq.) *De praesagitione ex pulsibus*.

The mistake may come from Ackermann 1821 (where there are no brackets and question mark, however):

- CI, no. 2 ctd. (*De febrium differentiis*);
- CV, no. 40 (the corpus of sphygmological treatises).

See Gundert 2009: 33-34.

[1077]   **2158**   I.80, 96, 98, 101, 111, 126.

Omont 1886-1888: 2.207.

[1078]   **[2158 (?)]**   I.88.

This codex is listed among the copies of Galenus, *De dignoscendis pulsibus*.

The same information appears in Ackermann 1821: CV, no. 40 ctd. (without brackets or question mark).

According to Omont 1886-1888: 2.207, this *Parisinus* (= [1077]) does not contain the Galenic treatise.

This could result from confusion with *Parisinus* 2153 (= [1069]), which contains the treatise at ff. 81r et seq. (Omont 1886-1888: 2.205).

Possibly same as [1069].

[1079]	**2159**	I.96.
		Omont 1886-1888: 2.207.
[1080]	**2160**	I.92, 101.
		Omont 1886-1888: 2.207.
		Possibly [1092].
[1081]	**[2160 (?)]**	I.96.

This manuscript does not contain Galenus, *De simplicium medicamentorum temperamentis et facultatibus*, contrary to Diels' catalogue and to Ackermann 1821: CXII, no. 49 (without brackets or question mark), but it contains Galenus, *De medendi methodo* and *Introductio* (Omont 1886-1888: 2.207, and Petit 2010: 146).

This is a mistake, possibly for 2260 (= [1198]), which contains the work at ff. 196r et seq. (Omont 1886-1888: 2.225-226).

[1082]	**2161**	I.13, 85, 87, 88 (2), 89, 105.
		Omont 1886-1888: 2.207.
		See possibly [1221].
[1083]	**2162**	I.92.
		Omont 1886-1888: 2.207.
		See possibly [1201].
[1084]	**2163**	I.61.
		Omont 1886-1888: 2.207.
[1085]	**2164**	I.59, 67 (2), 68, 69, 70, 74 (2), 76, 77, 83, 98, 99 (2), 106, 110, 111, 133; N.36.
		Omont 1886-1888: 2.207-208.
		Possibly [1089] and [1092], and also [1308].
[1086]	**2165**	I.10, 19, 68, 70, 78, 79, 80, 82, 84, 95 (2), 102, 104, 109, 112, 113.
		Omont 1886-1888: 2.208.
[1087]	**2166**	I.20, 73, 82, 84, 93, 95, 103.
		Omont 1886-1888: 2.208.
		See possibly [1074].
[1088]	**2167**	I.76, 78, 79, 80, 87, 88 (2), 89, 101, 111, 130.
		Omont 1886-1888: 2.208-209.
		See [1038] and [1076]. Possibly [1221].

[1089]   **[2167 (?)]**   I.98.

This manuscript is listed as a copy of Galenus, *De compositione medicamentorum secundum locos*.

The information comes from Ackermann 1821: CXXIV, no. 54 ctd. (without brackets or question mark).

According to Omont 1886-1888: 2.208-209, this *Parisinus* does not contain such a text.

This is a mistake for one of the *Parisini* that contain the treatise, possibly 2164 (= [1085]), ff. 259r et seq. (Omont 1886-1888: 2.207-208).

[1090]   **2168**   I.5, 13, 103, 105, 107.

Omont 1886-1888: 2.209.

[1091]   **2169**   I.61, 78, 79 (2), 80, 92.

Omont 1886-1888: 2.209.

[1092]   **[2169 (?)]**   I.59, 101.

This item is listed among the copies of Galenus, *Quod optimus medicus sit etiam philosophus* (I.59), and *Introductio sive medicus* (I.101).

Contrary to Diels' catalogue, *Parisinus* 2169 (= [1091]) does not contain such treatises (Omont 1886-1888: 2.209).

The treatise *Quod optimus medicus sit etiam philosophus*, is not listed in Boudon-Millot 2007: 251 (see also *ibid.*, n32 where Boudon points out the mistake in Diels' catalogue).

As for the *Introductio*, the manuscript is not listed in Petit 2009: LXXXII-LXXXIII (who does not mention this *Parisinus* on p. LXXXII, n125, where she points out the manuscripts erroneously listed in Diels as containing the *Introductio*).

More than one manuscript may have been confused. At the Bibliothèque nationale de France, *Quod optimus medicus sit etiam philosophus* seems to appear only in *Parisinus graecus* 2164 (= [1085]) according to Omont 1898: 67, *sub nomine* Galenus, *sub titulo* (see also Boudon-Millot 2007: 251). This *Parisinus* is probably the one mistakenly referred to here for this treatise. The mistake is present in Ackermann 1821: LXXI, no. 5 (without brackets or question mark, however).

The *Introductio* can be found in several of the manuscripts in Paris (Omont 1898: 67, *sub nomine* Galenus, *sub titulo*; see also Petit 2009: LXXXII-LXXXIII), except in manuscript 2164. The mistake may result from a misreading of 2160 (= [1080]), which contains the text at ff. 220r-247r (Petit 2009: LXXXVIII). It comes from Ackermann 1821: CXLVIII, no. 83 (without brackets or question mark).

[1093]   **2170**   I.82, 96.

Omont 1886-1888: 2.209.

Also [1094].

[1094]   **[2170 (?)]**   I.81, 82.

This manuscript is listed among the copies of Galenus, *De totius morbi temporibus* (I.81) and *De typis* (I.82).

This information comes from Ackermann 1821: CLI, no. 91, and CLI-CLII, no. 92 (*De totius morbi temporibus* and *De typis*, respectively), in both case without brackets or question mark.

According to Omont 1886-1888: 2.209, *De totius morbi temporibus* is not contained in *Parisinus* 2170, but rather in 2270 (= [1212]), at ff. 71r-84v.

De typis does not appear in the codex either. This text has been confused with *Adversus eos qui de typis scripserunt*, actually present in *Parisinus graecus* 2170 (= [1093]) (ff. 248r et seq.) and correctly listed in Diels' catalogue (I.82).

[1095]   **2171**   I.92, 101.

Omont 1886-1888: 2.209.

[1096]   **2172**   I.75.

Omont 1886-1888: 2.209.

[1097]   **2173**   I.76, 98.

Omont 1886-1888: 2.209.

Also [1037].

[1098]   **2174**   I.10, 104.

Omont 1886-1888: 2.209.

[1099]   **2175**   I.101, 111.

Omont 1886-1888: 2.209.

[1100]   **[2175 (?)]**   I.61.

This manuscript is listed among the copies of Galenus, *Ars medica*.

Contrary to Diels' catalogue and to Ackermann 1821: CXV, no. 50 ctd. (without brackets or question mark), the *Parisinus* 2175 (= [1099]) does not contain this treatise (see Omont 1886-1888: 2.209, and also Boudon 2002: 197n109).

The manuscript listed here must be one of the several copies of the work in the collections of the Bibliothèque nationale de France (see Omont 1898: 66, *sub nomine* Galenus, *sub titulo*, and Boudon 2002: 197-200), perhaps *graecus* 2157 (= [1075]), which contains, at f. 424v, a fragment of the treatise (Omont 1886-1888: 2.206-207; Boudon 2002: 200).

[1101]   **2176**   I.134.

Omont 1886-1888: 2.210; *CMAG* I (Lebègue) 1924: 131.

[1102]   **2177**   I.103; II.37, 72.

Omont 1886-1888: 2.210.

[1103]   **2178**   I.13, 44, 80, 126, 131; II.13, 80, 106.

Omont 1886-1888: 2.210.

[1104]	**2179**	II.30.
		Omont 1886-1888: 2.210.
[1105]	**2180**	II.30, 45 (2).
		Omont 1886-1888: 2.210-211; *CMAG* I (Lebègue) 1924: 221.
[1106]	**2181**	II.33, 97.
		Omont 1886-1888: 2.211.
[1107]	**2182**	II.30, 32 (2), 33.
		Omont 1886-1888: 2.211.
[1108]	**2183**	I.122; II.25, 29, 30, 32 (2), 33, 86.
		Omont 1886-1888: 2.211.
[1109]	**2184**	II.30, 32 (2), 33, 101.
		Omont 1886-1888: 2.211.
[1110]	**2185**	II.29, 30, 32 (2), 33.
		Omont 1886-1888: 2.211.
[1111]	**2186**	II.17, 18 (2), 19.
		Omont 1886-1888: 2.211.
		See [0887] and [0904].
[1112]	**2187**	II.17, 18 (2), 19.
		Omont 1886-1888: 2.211-212.
[1113]	**2188**	II.71.
		Omont 1886-1888: 2.212.
[1114]	**2189**	II.71.
		Omont 1886-1888: 2.212.
[1115]	**2190**	II.71.
		Omont 1886-1888: 2.212.
[1116]	**2191**	II.6, 8, 77.
		Omont 1886-1888: 2.212.
[1117]	**2192**	II.6, 8, 77; N.43.
		Omont 1886-1888: 2.212.
[1118]	**2193**	II.6, 8, 90; N.65.
		Omont 1886-1888: 2.212.
[1119]	**2194**	II.6, 24, 38; N.51, 63.
		Omont 1886-1888: 2.212; 3.397.
[1120]	**2195**	I.99; II.6.
		Omont 1886-1888: 2.213.
[1121]	**2196**	II.6; N.43.
		Omont 1886-1888: 2.213.

[1122]	**2197**	II.6.
		Omont 1886-1888: 2.213.
[1123]	**2198**	II.6.
		Omont 1886-1888: 2.213.
[1124]	**2199**	II.6.
		Omont 1886-1888: 2.213.
[1125]	2200	II.11.
		Omont 1886-1888: 2.213.
[1126]	**2201**	II.11.
		Omont 1886-1888: 2.213.
[1127]	2202	II.11, 17, 18 (2), 19.
		Omont 1886-1888: 2.213.
[1128]	2203	II.11.
		Omont 1886-1888: 2.213.
[1129]	2204	II.11, 77, 102.
		Omont 1886-1888: 2.214; 3.397.
[1130]	2205	II.77.
		Omont 1886-1888: 2.214.
[1131]	2206	II.17.
		Omont 1886-1888: 2.214.
[1132]	2207	I.86; II.77.
		Omont 1886-1888: 2.214.
[1133]	2208	II.3, 74, 77.
		Omont 1886-1888: 2.214.
[1134]	[2208 (?)]	I.114.

This manuscript (= [1133]) is thought to contain Galenus, *De succedaneis*, which is not the case (Omont 1886-1888: 2.214).

The same information (without brackets or question mark) appears in Ackermann 1821: CLXX, no. 138: "... excerpta ex eod. n. 2208 ....".

Number 2208 could be a misreading of 2238 (= [1165]) (Omont 1886-1888: 2.219), since this manuscript contains the treatise at ff. 593r et seq.

[1135]	**2209**	II.77.
		Omont 1886-1888: 2.214.
[1136]	2210	I.121, 149; II.26, 50, 76, 77.
		Omont 1886-1888: 2.214.
[1137]	**2211**	II.77.
		Omont 1886-1888: 2.214.
[1138]	**2212**	II.77.
		Omont 1886-1888: 2.214.

[1139]	**2213**	II.77.
		Omont 1886-1888: 2.214.
[1140]	**2214**	II.77.
		Omont 1886-1888: 2.214.
[1141]	**2215**	II.77.
		Omont 1886-1888: 2.215.
[1142]	**2216**	II.77.
		Omont 1886-1888: 2.215.
[1143]	**2217**	II.3, 77-78.
		Omont 1886-1888: 2.215.
[1144]	**2218**	II.75, 98.
		Omont 1886-1888: 2.215.
[1145]	**2219**	I.5, 13, 67, 105, 109; II.101.
		Omont 1886-1888: 2.215; 3.397.
[1146]	**2220**	II.17, 18, 89, 96, 99, 101, 102.
		Omont 1886-1888: 2.215.
[1147]	**2222**	I.13; II.63, 97, 104.
		Omont 1886-1888: 2.216.
[1148]	**2223**	I.13; II.63, 97, 104.
		Omont 1886-1888: 2.216.
[1149]	**2224**	I.13, 44, 125, 128; II.30, 32 (2), 52, 63, 69, 85.
		Omont 1886-1888: 2.216.
[1150]	**2225**	II.63, 67.
		Omont 1886-1888: 2.216.
[1151]	**2226**	II.63.
		Omont 1886-1888: 2.217.
[1152]	**2227**	II.63.
		Omont 1886-1888: 2.217.
[1153]	**2228**	I.5, 13, 103, 112, 128, 129; II.6, 34, 36, 75, 83, 92, 98, 104, 106.
		Omont 1886-1888: 2.217; 3.397.
		See also [1319].
[1154]	**2229**	I.5, 10, 13, 40, 89, 131; II.28, 96, 99, 101, 102.
		Omont 1886-1888: 2.217-218.
		Also [1155].

[1155]   **[2229 (?)]**   I.19, 41.

This item is listed among the copies of Hippocrates, *De morbis popularibus II, IV-VII* (fragm.) (I.19) and *Epistula ad Ptolemaeum regem de sanitate tuenda* (I.41).

The manuscript is mentioned in Ackermann 1825: CLXXIV (*Epistula ad Ptolemaeum regem de sanitate tuenda*) (without brackets or question mark).

According to Omont 1886-1888: 2.217-218, the *Parisinus* 2229 (= [1154]) does not contain *De morbis popularibus*, whereas it has the *Epistula, sub nomine* Hippocratis, vel Dioclis (f. 25r) (see also *CCAG* VIII. 1 [Cumont] 1929: 8).

The manuscript referred to as containing *De morbis popularibus* cannot be identified (for the list of the manuscripts of *Epidemiae* V and VI, see Jouanna and Grmek 2000: XC-XCII).

[1156]   **2230**   I.118; II.6, 9; N.37.

Omont 1886-1888: 2.218.

Also [1157].

[1157]   **[2230]**   I.126, 133.

According to Diels' catalogue, this is a copy of Galenus, *De morbis excerpta* (I.126) and *Remedia* (I.133).

While no text explicitly identified as such appears in *Parisinus* 2230 according to Omont 1886-1888: 2.218, the two references in Diels' catalogue may refer to the following texts contained in the manuscript:

- ff. 120r et seq., *Galeni liber de diaeta et morbis curandis* (Omont, *ibid.* on this text, see Costomiris 1889: 375-365, 377);

- ff. 37r et seq., *Collectio ex Galeni libro de simplicum medicamentorum* (see Costomiris 1889: 377).

Same as [1156].

2231   (ff. 1r et seq.) Symeon Seth, *De alimentorum facultatibus*.

Omont 1886-1888: 2.218.

[1158]   **2232**   I.92; II.109 (2).

Omont 1886-1888: 2.218.

[1159]   **[2232]**   I.26.

This manuscript is listed among the copies of Hippocrates, *De morbis II* and *III*.

According to Omont 1886-1888: 2.218, the *Parisinus* 2232 does not contain these works.

The manuscript referred to here must be one of the other *Parisini* that do contain the works (see Omont 1898: 90, *sub nomine* Hippocrates, *sub titulo*), possibly 2332 (= [1276]) listed in Littré 1839-1861: 7.6 (*De morbis II*) and 7.115 (*De morbis III*).

The description of this manuscript in Omont 1886-1888: 2.243 mentions "Hippocratis variorum librorum excerpta".

The identification of this item as *Parisinus* 2332 is all the more probable because in Diels' catalogue, number 2232 (*falso pro* 2332) is listed between 2255 and 2545, and probably results from a typo.

[1160]	**2233**	II.110.
		Omont 1886-1888: 2.218.
[1161]	**2234**	II.18, 19, 109.
		Omont 1886-1888: 2.219.
[1162]	**2235**	II.110.
		Omont 1886-1888: 2.219.
[1163]	**2236**	II.41, 52, 111.
		Omont 1886-1888: 2.219; 3.397.
[1164]	**2237**	I.149; II.6, 7, 69, 71, 74.
		Omont 1886-1888: 2.219.
[1165]	**2238**	I.114; II.33, 69.
		Omont 1886-1888: 2.219.
		Possibly [1134].
[1166]	**2239**	II.20.
		Omont 1886-1888: 2.219.
[1167]	**2240**	I.41, 75; II.8, 23, 64, 65, 74, 79, 91; N.59.
		Omont 1886-1888: 2.219-220.
		Also [1313].
	2241	Isaac Israelita, *Viaticorum metaphrasis e Constantis Memphitae ore excerpta* (= *Efodia*).
		Omont 1886-1888: 2.220.
[1168]	**[2242 (?)]**	I.30.

This manuscript is listed as a copy of Hippocrates, *De mulierum affectibus*. The same information (without brackets or question mark) appears in Ackermann 1825: CXXXIV, no. 19 ctd.

The codex *Parisinus graecus* 2242 does not contain such a work (Omont 1886-1888: 2.220), but it does contain Georgius Sanginatus, consul Romanorum et comes, *Liber de pulsibus*.

This may be a mistake for 2142 (= [1045]), which does contain the treatise at ff. 351r et seq. (Omont 1886-1888: 2.201).

[1169]	**2243**	II.33, 69, 74; N.53 (2).
		Omont 1886-1888: 2.220.
[1170]	**2244**	II.28, 57.
		Omont 1886-1888: 2.220-221.
[1171]	**[2245 (?)]**	I. 107.

This manuscript is thought to contain Galenus, *De fasciis*.

The *Parisinus* 2245 does not contain such a text, but it does contain "Hippiatricum, ex variis auctoribus ...; De ponderibus et mensuris in rebus *hippiatricis*; *Orneosophium* ...", according to Omont 1886-1888: 2.221).

This information, which appears in Ackermann 1821: CLVII, no. 100 (without brackets or question mark), cannot be explained.

According to Omont 1898: 67, *sub nomine* Galenus, *sub titulo*, the only manuscript in the collections of the Bibliothèque nationale de France containing this work is *Parisinus graecus* 2383 (= [1284]).

Perhaps this is a mistake (misreading) for *Parisinus graecus* 2247 (= [1173]), ff. 237r-251r, or 2248 (= [1176]), ff. 324v-339v, both of which contain the treatise *De fasciis* by Soranus (Ilberg 1927: XII, and Marchetti 2010: 87-88 and 95-87 for the *Parisini* 2247 and 2248 respectively).

[1172]   **2246**   I.80, 89, 91, 101.

              Omont 1886-1888: 2.221.

[1173]   **2247**   I.10, 11 (3), 12, 49, 106; II.15, 37, 71, 89.

              Omont 1886-1888: 2.221.

              See also [1171], [1174] and [1175].

[1174]   **[2247]**   I.34.

This item is a copy of Hippocrates, *De ossium natura*.

Although Omont 1886-1888: 2.221 does not mention this text, the *Parisinus* 2247 does contain it (see Duminil 1998: 118, and Marchetti 2010: 87-88).

Same as [1173].

[1175]   **[2247 (?)]**   I.107.

According to Diels' catalogue, this is a copy of Galenus, *De fasciis*.

The same information appears in Ackermann 1821: CLVII, no. 100 (without brackets or question mark).

The *Parisinus* 2247 does not contain such work (Omont 1886-1888: 2.221), which, according to Omont 1898: 67, *sub nomine* Galenus, *sub titulo*, is contained, among the manuscripts of the Bibliothèque nationale de France, only in *Parisinus* 2383 (= [1284]).

However, the *Parisinus graecus* 2247 contains, at ff. 237r-251r, a treatise *De fasciis* by Soranus (Ilberg 1927: XII; Marchetti 2010: 87-88).

Same as [1173].

[1176]   **2248**   I.10, 11 (3), 12, 106; II.15, 37, 71, 89.

              Omont 1886-1888: 2.221.

              Also [1171], [1177] and [1178].

[1177]   **2248 (?)**   I.107.

This manuscript is thought to contain Galenus, *De fasciis*, which is not the case (see Omont 1886-1888: 2.221).

According to Omont 1898: 67, *sub nomine* Galenus, *sub titulo*, among the manuscripts of the Bibliothèque nationale de France, this treatise is contained, only in *Parisinus* 2383 (= [1284]).

However, *Parisinus* 2248 (= [1176]) contains (ff. 324v-339v) *De fasciis* by Soranus, which might be the intended reference (Ilberg 1927: XII; Marchetti 2010: 85-87).

See Ihm 2002: 64-65, no. 13, 179, no. 192, 251, no. 300.

[1178]   **[2248]**   I.34.

This is a copy of Hippocrates, *De ossium natura.*

Although this text is not listed in Omont 1886-1888: 2.221, the *Parisinus* 2248 does contain this work at ff. 128r-134r (Duminil 1998: 118; Marchetti 2010: 85-87).

Same as [1176].

[1179]   **2249**   II.111, 112 (3).

Omont 1886-1888: 2.221-222; *CMAG* I (Lebègue) 1924: 101-115.

[1180]   **[2250]**   I.13.

This manuscript is listed among the copies of Hippocrates, *Aphorismi.*

The codex is listed in Ackermann 1825: LXIV (without brackets).

Contrary to Diel's catalogue and to Ackermann, this codex does not contain the Hippocratic work (see Omont 1886-1888: 2.222, and *CMAG* I [Lebègue] 1924: 115-117; the manuscript does not appear in Magdelaine 1994: 88-90).

This is probably a mistake (misreading), possibly for one of the following three *Parisini*:

- 2256 (= [1193]), ff. 9r-23r (Omont 1886-1888: 2.224-225; Magdelaine 1994: 89);

- 2258 (= [1196]), ff. 1r-32r (Omont 1886-1888: 2.225; Magdelaine 1994: 89);

- 2259 (= [1197]), ff. 1r-56v (Omont 1886-1888: 2.225; Magdelaine 1994: 89).

[1181]   **2251**   II.112.

Omont 1886-1888: 2.222; *CMAG* I (Lebègue) 1924: 117-125.

[1182]   **2252**   II.111, 112.

Omont 1886-1888: 2.222-223; *CMAG* I (Lebègue) 1924: 125-129.

[1183]   **[2252 (?)]**   I.111.

This manuscript is listed among the copies of Galenus, *Definitiones medicae.*

According to Omont 1886-1888: 2.222-223, this codex contains a wide range of alchemical treatises.

This information, which appears in Ackermann 1821: CLIX, no. 102 (without brackets or question mark), probably results from a misreading of the shelfmark of another of the *Parisini* that contain this work, possibly 2282 (= [1229]), ff. 53v et seq. (Omont 1886-1888: 2.229).

| [1184] | **2253** | I.4, 5, 8, 10, 20, 21 (2), 22 (2), 23, 33, 38, 40, 68; II.113. |

Omont 1886-1888: 2.223; 3.397.

Formerly [1736].

Also [1185] and [1186].

| [1185] | **[2253]** | I.22. |

This codex is listed among the copies of Hippocrates, *De salubri diaeta* (on this treatise, see [1042]).

According to Omont 1886-1888: 2.223, the *Parisinus* 2253 contains (ff. 81r et seq.) *De natura hominis* in which the text is included (see [1042]; see also Jouanna 2002: 61, 64-66).

Same as [1184].

| [1186] | **[2253 (?)]** | I.20, 33. |

This item is listed among the copies of Hippocrates, *Praesagiorum liber I* (I.20) and *Liber II* (I.33).

The same information appears in Ackermann 1825: LVIII (without brackets or question mark).

According to Omont 1886-1888: 2.223, this text is not in this manuscript which contains some Hippocratic treatises (*Praenotiones, De alimento, De victu in morbis acutis, De humoribus, De humidorum usu, De arte, De natura hominis, De flatibus, De partibus corporis humani, De veteri medicina, De morbis popularibus*), in addition to Thessalus, *Oratio ad Athenienses*, and Galenus, *De usu partium*.

Unless there is confusion with *Praenotiones,* which can be read in *Parisinus* 2253 (= [1184]), ff. 1r et seq. (*ibid.*), this seems to be a mistake for any other *Parisinus* containing *Praesagiorum libri II* (see Omont 1898: 90, *sub nomine* Hippocrates, *sub titulo*), possibly 2254 (= [1187]), ff. 207v et seq. (Omont 1886-1888: 2.223-224).

| [1187] | **2254** | I.8, 11 (2), 12, 19, 20 (2), 21, 22, 24 (2), 25, 27 (2), 28, 30 (3), 31 (2), 33, 34, 38, 57; II.37. |

Omont 1886-1888: 2.223-224.

See [1185]. Possibly also [1186].

| [1188] | **[2254]** | I.4, 5. |

This manuscript is listed among the copies of the Hippocratic treatises *De aëre, aquis et locis* (I.4) and *Prognosticon* (I.5).

The codex is listed (without brackets) in Ackermann 1825: XLVIII (*Prognosticon*) and CIII (*De aere, aquis et locis*).

Neither work appears in this manuscript (Omont 1886-1888: 2.223-224; Diller 1932: 9; Diller 1970: 7, and Jouanna 1996: 83-84 do not mention it for *De aëre, aquis et locis*, and Alexanderson 1963 does not either for *Prognosticon*).

The manuscript referred to here may be *Parisinus* 2255 (= [1190]), which contains both works (see Omont 1886-1888: 2.224; also Diller 1932: 9; Diller

1970: 7, and Jouanna 1996: 84 for *De aëre, aquis et locis*, and Alexanderson 1963: 82-83 for *Prognosticon*).

[1189]   **[2254 (?)]**   I.10, 12, 18 (2), 20, 21, 22, 23 (3), 24, 25, 26 (2), 27, 28, 29 (2), 31, 32 (3), 33, 34, 35 (4).

This manuscript appears in the list of codices containing the following Hippocratic treatises (alphabetical order of titles; references to Diels' catalogue follow the titles): *De affectionibus* (I.23); *De anatome* (I.31); *De arte* (I.21); *De articulis* (I.12); *De capitis vulneribus* (I.10); *De carnibus* (I.32); *De corde* (I.33); *De decenti ornatu* (I.35); *De dentitione* (I.32); *De diebus iudicatoriis* (I.35); *De genitura* (I.28); *De glandulis* (I.32); *De humoribus* (I.20); *De humidorum usu* (I.22); *De insomniis* (I.26); *De internis affectionibus* (I.27); *De iudicationibus* (I.35); *De locis in homine* (I.23); *De morbis I* (I.23); *De morbis II & III* (I.26); *De morbis IV* (I.29); *De natura pueri* (I.29); *De ulceribus* (I.24); *De victus ratione I-III* (I.25); *De visu* (I.34); *Iusiurandum* (I.18); *Lex* (I.18); *Praeceptiones* (I.35).

Except for *De internis affectionibus, Parisinus* 2254 is listed (without brackets or question mark) in Ackermann 1825 among the manuscripts of the following treatises: *De affectionibus*: CXXVIII, no. 15 ctd.; *De anatome*: CXXVII, no. 14 ctd.; *De arte*: CLXIX, no. 53; *De articulis*: CXXII, no. 8; *De capitis vulneribus*: CVI, no. XXIV ctd.; *De carnibus*: CLV, no. 40; *De corde*: CLVI, no. 41; *De decenti ornatu*: CLXVI, no. 50; *De dentitione*: CXLI, no. 31; *De diebus iudicatoriis*: CXVIII, no. 5; *De genitura*: CLVII, no. 43; *De glandulis*: CXLI, no. 30; *De humoribus*: CXVI, no. 3 ctd.; *De humidorum usu*: CXL, no. 28 ctd.; *De insomniis*: CXLIV, no. 33; *De iudicationibus*: CXVII, no. 4; *De locis in homine*: CLIII, no. 37 ctd.; *De morbis I, De morbis II & III* and *De morbis IV*: CXXXIII, no. 18 ctd.; *De natura pueri*: CLIX, no. 44; *De ulceribus*: CXXIV, no. 10 ctd.; *De victus ratione I-III*: CXLIII, no. 32 ctd.; *De visu*: CXXX, no. 17 ctd.; *Iusiurandum*: CLXII, no. 47 ctd.; *Lex.*: CLXV, no. 48 ctd.; *Praeceptiones*: CLXVII, no. 51.

The manuscript Paris *graecus* 2254 does not contain any of these works, which are contained, instead, in *Parisinus graecus* 2255 (= [1190]) mentioned in Diels' catalogue for the following treatises (Omont 1886-1888: 2. 224, some with a variant title) (references to Diels' catalogue follow the titles):

(ff. 265v et seq.) *De affectionibus* (see I.23); (ff. 369v et seq.) *De anatome* (see I.31); (ff. 57r et seq.) *De arte* (see I.21); (ff. 449v et seq.) *De articulis* (see I.12); (ff. 389v et seq.) *De capitis vulneribus* (see I.10); (ff. 367v et sq.) *De carnibus* (see I.32); (ff. 370r et seq.) *De corde* (see I.33); (ff. 86v et seq.) *De decenti ornatu* (under the title *De medici decoro*) (see I.35); (ff. 369v et seq.) *De dentitione* (under the title *De dentibus*) (see I.32); (ff. 363r et seq.) *De diebus iudicatoriis* (under the title *De diebus criticis*) (I.35); (ff. 101r et seq.) *De genitura* (see I.28); (ff. 371r et seq.) *De glandulis* (see I.32); (ff. 165r et seq.) *De humoribus* (see I.20); (ff. 378v et seq.) *De humidorum usu* (see I.22); (ff. 356v et seq.) *De insomniis* (see I.26); (ff. 281v et seq.) *De internis affectionibus* (see I.27); (ff. 379v et seq.) *De iudicationibus* (under the title *De crisibus*) (I.35); (ff. 371v et seq.) *De locis in homine* (under the title *De partibus corporis humani*) (see I.23); (ff. 191r et seq.) *De morbis I* -IV(see I.23 [I], 26 [II-III] and 29 [IV]); (ff. 104v et seq.) *De natura pueri* (see I.29); (ff. 173v et seq.) *De ulceribus* (see I.24); (ff. 316r et seq.) *De victus ratione I-III* (under the title *De diaeta libri III*) (see I.25);

(ff. 361v et seq.) *De visu* (see I.34); (f. 55) *Iusiurandum* (see I.18); (f. 56) *Lex* (see I.18); (ff. 83r et seq.) *Praeceptiones* (under the title *Praecepta*) (see I.35).

Same as [1190].

[1190]   **2255**   I.4 (2), 5, 8, 10, 11, 12, 13, 18 (2), 20, 21 (2), 22, 23 (2), 24 (2), 25, 26 (2), 27, 28, 29 (2), 31, 32 (3), 33(2), 34 (2), 35 (2), 38, 40, 57, 110; II.37, 93.

Omont 1886-1888: 2.224.

Also [1188], [1189], [1191], and [1192].

[1191]   **[2255]**   I.22.

This is a copy of Hippocrates, *De salubri diaeta* (on this treatise, see [1042]).

According to Omont 1886-1888: 2.224, *Parisinus* 2255 (= [1190]) contains (ff. 90r et seq.) *De natura hominis* in which *De salubri diaeta* is included (Jouanna 2002: 61).

Same as [1190].

[1192]   **[2255 (?)]**   I.23, 35.

This manuscript is referred to for Hippocrates, *De locis in homine* (I.23) and *De decenti ornatu* (I.35).

This manuscript is mentioned in Littré 1839-1861: 6.274 for *De locis in homine*, and 9.224 for *De decenti ornatu* (without brackets or question mark in both cases).

In Omont 1886-1888: 2.224, these treatises appear under the following titles in the description of *Parisinus graecus* 2255: *De partibus corporis humani* (ff. 371v et seq.) and *De medici decoro* (ff. 86 v et seq.). These titles reproduce those of the catalogue of the *Bibliotheca Regia* 1740: 2.471-472, no. MMCCLV (= 2255).

Same as [1190].

[1193]   **2256**   I.5, 13, 28, 30, 117; II.6, 7, 43, 45 (3), 68, 109 (2), 110.

Omont 1886-1888: 2.224-225; *CMAG* I (Lebègue) 1924: 164-176.

Also [1206], and possibly [1180].

[1194]   **2257**   I.5, 13, 105, 107; II.63, 101, 102.

Omont 1886-1888: 2.225.

Also [1331].

[1195]   **[2257 (?)]**   I.31.

This manuscript is listed among the copies of Hippocrates, *De exsectione foetus. De exsectione pueri.*

The same information (without brackets or question mark) appears in Ackermann 1825: CXXVI, no. 13.

This manuscript does not contain this work, but it does contain the following works (listed here in the order of the folios according to Omont 1886-1888: 2.225): (ff. 1r et seq.) Hippocrates, *Aphorismi* et *Galeni commentarius in eosdem*; (ff. 129r et seq.) Galenus, *Commentarius in Hippocratis Praenotiones*; (ff. 230v et seq.) *De balnei utilitate*; (ff. 231r et seq,) Gregorius Thaumaturgus, *De anima*; (ff. 239r et seq.) Meletius, *De natura hominis*; (ff. 327v et seq.) Aristoteles, *De mundo*; (ff. 345r et seq.) Theophilus, *De urinis*; (ff. 359v et seq.) *Liber de pulsibus*; (ff. 363v et seq.) Theophilus, *De pulsibus*.

This could be a mistake (misreading) for *Parisinus* 2254 (= [1187]), where *De exsectione foetus. De exsectione pueri* can be found.

[1196]	**2258**	I.13.
		Omont 1886-1888: 2.225.
		Possibly [1180].
[1197]	**2259**	I.13.
		Omont 1886-1888: 2.225.
		Possibly [1180].
[1198]	**2260**	I.13, 41, 80, 86, 93, 128, 133; II.30, 60, 96, 99, 109, 110; II.20.
		Omont 1886-1888: 2.225-226.
		See also [1081] and [1227]. Possibly [1213].
[1199]	**2261**	II.71, 89.
		Omont 1886-1888: 2.226.
[1200]	**2262**	II.71, 89.
		Omont 1886-1888: 2.226.
[1201]	**[2262 (?)]**	I.92.

This manuscript is listed among the copies of Galenus, *Methodi medendi libri XIV*.

The same information appears in Ackermann 1821: CXXVI, no. 56 (without brackets or question mark).

According to Omont 1886-1888: 2.226, this manuscript does not contain the treatise. The reference here is a mistake (misreading), probably for 2162 (= [1083]), which actually contains the treatise on ff. 1 et seq., and appears among the copies of the treatise in Diels' catalogue.

[1202]	**2263**	II.71, 89.
		Omont 1886-1888: 2.226.
[1203]	**2264**	II.89.
		Omont 1886-1888: 2.226.
[1204]	**2265**	I.61, 93.
		Omont 1886-1888: 2.226.
[1205]	**2266**	I.5, 13, 105, 107.
		Omont 1886-1888: 2.226.
[1206]	**[2266 (?)]**	I.20, 33.

This item is listed among the copies of Hippocrates, *Praesagiorum libri II*.

The information comes from Ackermann 1825: LVIII (without brackets or question mark).

The *Parisinus graecus* 2266 (= [1205]) does not contain the Hippocratic treatise, but it does contain, at ff. 1r et seq., Galenus, *In Hippocratis praenotiones commentariorum libri III* (Omont 1886-1888: 2.226).

The present information may also result from a mistake (misreading) for another *Parisinus* containing the work, possibly 2256 (= [1193]), ff. 23r et seq. (Omont 1886-1888: 2.224-225). It might be significant that 2256 is not listed in Diels I.20 or I.33.

[1207]	**2267**	I.63, 64, 65, 77, 80; II.98.
		Omont 1886-1888: 2.226-227.
[1208]	**2268**	I.13, 105.
		Omont 1886-1888: 2.227.
[1209]	**2269**	I.5, 44, 49, 68, 73, 78, 80, 81, 82, 83, 93, 95, 96, 109, 112 (2), 128, 129, 130, 134; II.75.
		Omont 1886-1888: 2.227.
		Also [1211]. Possibly [1210] and [1216].
[1210]	**[2269]**	I.56.

This item is a copy of Hippocrates, *Excerpta* not better identified.

The same information is found in Ackermann 1825: CLXXVIII, *sub titulo* Alia excerpta ex Hippocrate.

According to Omont 1886-1888: 2.227, this manuscript (= [1209]) contains (f. 94r et seq.) *excerpta de urinis*, and (f. 126r et seq.) *excerpta de eodem* (*scilicet de venae sectione*) attributed to Hippocrates (*et alii*). This may correspond to the text referred to in Diels' catalogue.

Possibly same as [1209].

[1211]	**[2269 (?)]**	I.20, 33, 82, 113.

The texts referred to here are (listed here in the order of Diels' catalogue; references to Diels' catalogue follow the titles):

• Hippocrates, *Praesagiorum liber I* and *II* (I.20 and 33);

• Galenus, *De typis* (I.82);

• *De urinis ex Hippocrate, Galeno aliisque quibusdam* (I.113).

According to Omont 1886-1888: 2.227, the *Parisinus* 2269 (= [1209]) does not contain Hippocrates, *Praesagia*, but rather (in the order of the folios according to Omont): (ff. 68r et seq.) Hippocrates, *Praenotiones*; (ff. 94r et seq.) *Hippocratis, etc. excerpta de urinis*; (ff. 128r et seq.) *Galeni liber II. de praesagitione ex urinis*.

De typis is not contained in the manuscript. The mistake comes from Ackermann 1821: CLI-CLII, no. 92 (without brackets or question mark) and cannot be explained.

[1212]   **2270**   I.61, 68, 73, 81, 82, 96, 101, 118, 129; II.6, 109.

Omont 1886-1888: 2.227; 3.397.

Also [1094] and possibly [1216].

[1213]   **[2270 (?)]**   I.93.

This codex is listed among the copies of Galenus, *Ad Glauconem de medendi methodo*, althought this treatise does not seem to be contained in the *Parisinus* 2270 (= [1212]) (Omont 1886-1888: 2.227).

This information comes from Ackermann 1821: CXXIX, no. 57 (without brackets or question mark).

According to Omont 1898: 67, *sub nomine* Galenus, *sub titulo*, the work appears, instead, in the following *Parisini graeci*:

- 2156 (= [1073]);
- 2157 (= [1075]);
- 2158 (= [1077]);
- 2166 (= [1087]);
- 2260 (= [1198]);
- 2265 (= [1204]);
- 2269 (= [1209]);
- 2304 (= [1252]);
- 2308 (= [1257]).

The manuscript referred to here has been confused with one these items, possibly with 2260 (= [1198]).

[1214]   **2271**   I.61, 68, 73, 81, 82, 96, 101.

Omont 1886-1888: 2.227.

Possibly [1216].

[1215]   **2272**   I.80, 89, 91.

Omont 1886-1888: 2.228.

See [1216].

[1216]   **[2272 (?)]**   I.81, 82.

This codex is listed among the copies of Galenus, *De totius morbi temporibus* (I.81) and *De typis* (I.82).

The information on both works comes from Ackermann 1821: CLI (*De totius morbi temporibus*) and CLI-CLII (*De typis*) (without brackets or question mark in both references).

De totius morbi temporibus is not in *Parisinus graecus* 2272 (= [1215]) (see Omont 1886-1888: 2.228).

This item has probably been confused with one of the two *Parisini* that contain it according to Omont 1898: 68, *sub nomine* Galenus, *sub titulo*:

- 2269 (= [1209]), ff. 183r et seq. (Omont 1886-1888: 2.227);
- 2270 (= [1212]), ff. 71r et seq. (*ibid.*).

The text referred to here may also have been confused with *De morborum temporibus* contained in *Parisinus* 2271 (= [1214]), at ff. 75r et seq. (Omont 1886-1888: 2.227), unless it is an incorrect reference to *De crisibus* contained in *Parisinus* 2272 (= [1215]) (ff. 41r et seq.) (Omont 1886-1888: 2.228).

De typis is not contained in the manuscript either. This mistake, which also appears in Ackermann 1821 (above), results from some confusion that cannot be explained. It might be significant, however, that both treatises are mentioned on the same page in Ackermann 1821.

[1217]   **2273**   I.61.

Omont 1886-1888: 2.228.

[1218]   **2274**   I.92.

Omont 1886-1888: 2.228.

[1219]   **2275**   II.24, 100, 115.

Omont 1886-1888: 2.228; *CMAG* I (Lebègue) 1924: 68-82.

[1220]   **2276**   I.78, 80, 86, 101, 102; II.17, 83, 98.

Omont 1886-1888: 2.228.

Possibly [1221].

[1221]   **[2276 (?)]**   I.87, 88 (2), 89.

Four sphygmological treatises by Galen are referred to here (listed below in the order of Diels' catalogue; references to Diels' catalogue follow the titles):

- *De pulsuum differentiis* (I.87);
- *De causis pulsuum* (I.88);
- *De dignoscendis pulsibus* (I.88);
- *De praesagitione ex pulsibus* (I.89).

Similar information appears in Ackermann 1821: CV, no. 40 ctd. (without brackets or question mark, however).

None of Galen's sphygmological treatises are contained in *Parisinus* 2276 (= [1220]), according to Omont 1886-1888: 2.228.

Nevertheless, this *Parisinus* contains, according to Omont, *ibid.*, a letter by Galen on the topic of sphygmology (*Ad Teuthram epistola de pulsibus* [ff. 199r et seq.]), which may have created confusion, unless the manuscript referred to here is either *Parisini* 2161 (= [1082]) or 2167 (= [1088]), both of which contain Galen's sphygmological corpus.

[1222]   **2277**   I.61, 74.

Omont 1886-1888: 2.228-229.

Probably [1224].

[1223]   **2278**   I.13, 69, 105.

Omont 1886-1888: 2.229.

[1224]   **[2278 (?)]**   I.61, 74.

This item is listed among the copies of Galenus, *Ars medica* (I.61) and *De placitis Hippocratis et Platonis* (I.74).

The same information appears in Ackermann 1821: CXV, no. 50 ctd. (*Ars medica*), and XCII, no. 26 ctd. (*De placitis Hippocratis et Platonis*) without brackets or question mark in both cases.

Neither work appears in *Parisinus* 2278 (= [1223]) (see Omont 1886-1888: 2.229; for *Ars medica*, see also Boudon 2002: 197n109, where the author mentions that the manuscript does not contain the text contrary to Diels' catalogue; and for *De placitis Hippocratis et Platonis*, see De Lacy 2005, who does not mention this manuscript).

The manuscript referred to here has been confused with another one, probably with *Parisinus* 2277 (= [1222]), which contains both texts (Omont 1886-1888: 2.228-229, Boudon 2002: 199, and De Lacy 2005: 28-29).

[1225]   **2279**   I.70, 96.

Omont 1886-1888: 2.229.

[1226]   **2280**   I.92, 101.

Omont 1886-1888: 2.229.

[1227]   **[2280 (?)]**   I.96.

This manuscript (= [1226]) does not contain Galenus, *De simplicium medicamentorum temperamentis et facultatibus* (Omont 1886-1888: 2.229; see also Petit 2010: 146).

The number 2280 results probably from a misreading of number 2260 (*Parisinus graecus* 2260 = [1198]).

Diels' information comes from Ackermann 1821: CXII, no. 49 (without square bracket and question mark).

[1228]   **2281**   I.68.

Omont 1886-1888: 2.229.

[1229]   **2282**   I.101, 111.

Omont 1886-1888: 2.229.

Possibly [1183].

[1230]   **2283**   I.60, 63, 64, 68, 71 (2), 73, 74, 75, 78, 79 (2), 80 (2), 81, 82, 83, 84, 89, 91, 92, 109, 112, 130.

Omont 1886-1888: 2.229.

[1231]   **2284**   I.80.

Omont 1886-1888: 2.229.

[1232]   **2285**   I.61.

Omont 1886-1888: 2.229; 3.397.

[1233]   **2286**   I, 133; II.17, 20, 25, 29, 33, 34, 54, 55 (2), 68, 70, 107; N.55 (2), 60, 68.

Omont 1886-1888: 2.229-230; *CMAG* I (Lebègue) 1924: 180-191.

[1234]	**2287**	I.24, 110; II.30.
		Omont 1886-1888: 2.230.
[1235]	**[2287 (?)]**	I.11.

This item is a copy of Hippocrates, *De officina medici.*

The same information (without brackets or question mark) appears in Ackermann 1825: CXIX, no. 6 ctd.

According to Omont 1886-1888: 2.230, this manuscript does not contain the text.

This is a mistake for one of the other *Parisini* containing this work (Omont 1898: 90, *sub nomine* Hippocrates, *sub titulo*): 2141-2146 (= [1043], [1045], [1048], [1051] and [1055]), or 2254-2255 (= [1187] and [1190], respectively).

The manuscript referred to here cannot be identified.

[1236]	**2288**	II.17, 18 (2), 19, 88.
		Omont 1886-1888: 2.230.
[1237]	**2289**	II.17, 18 (2).
		Omont 1886-1888: 2.230-231.
[1238]	**2290**	II.108.
		Omont 1886-1888: 2.231.
[1239]	**2291**	II.108.
		Omont 1886-1888: 2.231.
[1240]	**2292**	II.70.
		Omont 1886-1888: 2.231.
[1241]	**2293**	II.78.
		Omont 1886-1888: 2.231.
[1242]	**2294**	I.41, 44, 114, 128, 133; II.34, 78, 80.
		Omont 1886-1888: 2.231; 3.397.
[1243]	**2295**	II.67, 76.
		Omont 1886-1888: 2.231.
[1244]	**2296**	I.13; II.96, 104.
		Omont 1886-1888: 2.232; 3.397.
[1245]	**2297**	II.101.
		Omont 1886-1888: 2.232.
[1246]	**2298**	II.99.
		Omont 1886-1888: 2.232.
[1247]	**2299**	II.21, 62, 63 (2), 67.
		Omont 1886-1888: 2.232.
[1248]	**2300**	II.63.
		Omont 1886-1888: 2.232.

| [1249] | **2301** | I.40; II.28. |

Omont 1886-1888: 2.232.

Also [1250].

| [1250] | **[2301 (?)]** | I.40. |

This manuscript is listed among the copies of Hippocrates, *Ad Ptolemaeum regem epistula de hominis fabrica,*

According to Omont 1886-1888: 2.232, this manuscript contains (ff. 124r et seq.) Hippocratis, *Ad Ptolemaeum regem* [Dioclis, *Ad Antigonum*] *epistola* [*sic*].

Same as [1249].

| | 2302 | (ff. 1r et seq.) Symeon Seth, *De alimentorum facultatibus.* |

Omont 1886-1888: 2.232.

| [1251] | **2303** | N.59. |

Referring to *Excerpta varia* (actually, *de urinis*) by Meletius (the manuscripts of which are listed at II.64), Diels mentions that this text is attested in some manuscripts under the name of Nicophorus [*sic*] Blemmydes and in others under the name of Maximus Planudes.

Since no indication of folio is provided in Diels' catalogue, the text referred to seems to be (ff. 87r et seq.) Nicephorus Blemmydes, *Poema de urinis*, on the basis of Omont 1886-1888: 2.232-233.

On *Parisinus* 2303, see also Omont 1886-1888: 3.397, where the texts *De alimentis* (ff. 91r et seq.) and *De variis morborum generibus* (ff. 110v et seq.) considered anonymous by Id., 2.232-233, are attributed to Theophanes Nonnus in Diels' catalogue.

| [1252] | **2304** | I.44, 93; II.109 (2), 110. |

Omont 1886-1888: 2.233.

Possibly [0830].

| [1253] | **[2304 (?)]** | I.61, 101. |

This item is listed among the codices of Galenus, *Ars medica* (I.61) and *Introductio sive medicus* (I.101).

The information (without brackets or question mark) comes from Ackermann 1821: CXV, no. 50 (*Ars medica*), and CXLIX, no. 83 (*Introductio*).

This manuscript does not contain these texts (Omont 1886-1888: 2. 233; for *Ars medica*, see also Boudon 2002: 197n109, and, for *Introductio*, Petit 2009: LXXXII-LXXIII, who does not mention the manuscript, without including it, however, at n125, among the items erroneously listed in Diels' catalogue).

This is a mistake (misreading), possibly for 2307 (= [1256]), which contains both works (Boudon 2002: 200; Petit 2009: LXXXIII).

| [1254] | **2305** | II.109 (2), 110. |

Omont 1886-1888: 2.233.

| [1255] | **2306** | I.61, 101; II.102 (2), 109 (2). |

Omont 1886-1888: 2.233.

[1256]	**2307**	I.61, 101; II.65, 102 (2), 109 (2), 110 (2).
		Omont 1886-1888: 2.233-234.
		See also [1253].
[1257]	**2308**	I.44, 93, 113, 120; II.102, 109 (2); N.37 (2).
		Omont 1886-1888: 2.234.
[1258]	**2309**	I.128.
		Omont 1886-1888: 2.234.
	2310	*Viaticum peregrinantium a Constantino Rhegino graece versum* (= *Efodia*).
		Omont 1886-1888: 2.234.
	2311	*Viaticum peregrinantium a Constantino Rhegino graece versum* (= *Efodia*).
		Omont 1886-1888: 2.234.
[1259]	**2312**	I.114.
		Omont 1886-1888: 2.234.
[1260]	**2313**	I.133; II.34, 80.
		Omont 1886-1888: 2.234-235.
[1261]	**2314**	II.14, 49.
		Omont 1886-1888: 2.235; 3.397; *CMAG* I (Lebègue) 1924: 130.
[1262]	**2315**	I.40, 89, 113, 114; II.51, 64, 65, 69, 79; N.59.
		Omont 1886-1888: 2.235-236.
		See below *Vaticanus graecus* 109 (see p. 287).
[1263]	**2316**	I.5, 13, 21, 43, 47, 78, 113, 125; II.13, 40, 54, 60, 80, 102.
		Omont 1886-1888: 2.236-237; 3.397.
[1264]	**2317**	I.21, 63-64, 131, 136.
		Omont 1886-1888: 2.238.
[1265]	**2318**	I.114; II.79.
		Omont 1886-1888: 2.238.
		Possibly [1266].
[1266]	**[2319 (?)]**	I.114.

Contrary to Diels' catalogue, the *Parisinus* 2319 does not contain Galenus, *De succedaneis* (see Omont 1886-1888: 2.238).

This information, which comes from Ackermann 1821: CLXX, no. 138 (without brackets or question mark), is probably a mistake (misreading) for 2318 (= [1265]), the text of which is identified as follows in Omont's catalogue (*ibid.*):

Pauli Aeginetae fragmentum, ex Galeno, de succedaneis (ff. 72r et seq.).

[1267]	**2320**	I.28, 43, 44, 49, 117, 121, 131, 132, 134; II.20, 24, 80.
		Omont 1886-1888: 2.238; *CMAG* I (Lebègue) 1924: 211-215.
[1268]	**2321**	II.71, 89.
		Omont 1886-1888: 2.239; 3.397.
[1269]	**2324**	I.123; II.36, 48, 60.
		Omont 1886-1888: 2.239.
[1270]	**2325**	II.100, 112 (2), 115.
		Omont 1886-1888: 2.239; *CMAG* I (Lebègue) 1924: 1-17.
[1271]	**2326**	II.115.
		Omont 1886-1888: 2.239; *CMAG* I (Lebègue) 1924: 82-85.
[1272]	**2327**	II.24, 43, 100, 111, 112 (2), 115 (2).
		Omont 1886-1888: 2.240-241; *CMAG* I (Lebègue) 1924: 17-62; *CMAG* II (Zuretti et al.) 1927: 341-358; *CMAG* IV (Goldschmidt) 1932: 399-432.
[1273]	**2329**	II.112 (2).
		Omont 1886-1888: 2.241-242; *CMAG* I (Lebègue) 1924: 85-101.
[1274]	**2330**	I.5, 13, 28, 44, 49, 128.
		Omont 1886-1888: 2.242.
		Possibly [1027].
[1275]	**2331**	II.88, 90.
		Omont 1886-1888: 2.242.
[1276]	**2332**	I.4, 5, 8, 64, 73, 78, 79 (2), 80, 85, 89 (2), 91, 100, 102, 105, 119, 131; II.60.
		Omont 1886-1888: 2.242.
		Also [1277], and probably [1159].
[1277]	**[2332]**	I.10, 11, 12 (2), 19, 20 (3), 21, 22, 23 (2), 24 (3), 25 (2), 26, 27 (2), 28, 29 (2), 30 (2), 31 (2), 33 (2), 34 (2), 35 (3), 38, 61, 64.

According to Omont 1886-1888: 2.242, the manuscript *Parisinus* 2332 (= [1276]) contains *Hippocratis variorum librorum excerpta* (ff. 204r et seq.). These excerpts probably account for the several references here. See also Gundert 2009: 24-25.

[1278]	**2333**	I.61.
		Omont 1886-1888: 2.242.
[1279]	**2334**	II.17, 18 (2), 19.
		Omont 1886-1888: 2.242.
		Possibly [0887] and [0904].

[1280]   **2335**   II.72.

Omont 1886-1888: 2.242.

[1281]   **2336**   II.55.

Omont 1886-1888: 2.243.

[1282]   **2337**   II.34, 74, 80.

Omont 1886-1888: 2.243.

[1283]   **2381**   II.3, 9.

Omont 1886-1888: 2.250.

[1284]   **2383**   I.107, 129, 150.

Omont 1886-1888: 2.250; 3.397.

See [1171], [1175], and [1177].

2403   (ff. 99v-114r) Nicander, *Theriaca*; (ff. 114r-114v) Nicander, *Alexipharmaca*, vv. 1-29.

Omont 1886-1888: 2.253-254.

[1285]   **2408**   II.61, 74.

Omont 1886-1888: 2.254-255; *CMAG* I (Lebègue) 1924: 226.

[1286]   **2419**   I.42, 43; II.43, 45, 75.

Omont 1886-1888: 2.256-257; *CMAG* I (Lebègue) 1924: 125-156; *CMAG* III (Anderson et al.) 1924: 76-77.

2421   (ff. 1r et seq.) Astrampsychus, *Epistula ad Ptolomaeum regem*.

Omont 1886-1888: 2.258.

[1287]   **2422**   II.107.

Omont 1886-1888: 2.258.

2424   (ff. 226r et seq.) Astrampsychus, *Epistula ad Ptolomaeum regem*.

Omont 1886-1888: 2.258-259.

[1288]   **2426**   II.35, 44, 82 (2), 87, 88.

Omont 1886-1888: 2.259.

[1289]   **2428**   II.67.

Omont 1886-1888: 2.260.

2438   (ff. 109 et seq.) Hero, *Geoponica*.

Omont 1886-1888: 2.261-262.

2465   (ff. 160v et seq.) Synesius Cyrenensis, *De insomniis*.

Omont 1886-1888: 2.266.

2474   (f. 1) Hero, *Geoponica* (frg.).

Omont 1886-1888: 2.267.

[1290]	**2494**	I.130.
		Omont 1886-1888: 2.270-271.
[1291]	**2502**	II.43, 45 (3).
		Omont 1886-1888: 2.273; *CMAG* I (Lebègue) 1924: 192-205.
[1292]	**2506**	N.53.
		Omont 1886-1888: 2.273.
[1293]	**2509**	II.35.
		Omont 1886-1888: 2.274-275; *CMAG* I (Lebègue) 1924: 131-132.
[1294]	**2510**	I.42, 48, 114, 121, 133, 149; II.34, 58, 71, 74, 80, 106.
		Omont 1886-1888: 2.275; *CMAG* I (Lebègue) 1924: 205-208.
		See [0910].
	2511	(ff. 7r et seq.) Achmet, *Oneirocriticon*; (ff. 19r et seq.) Nicephorus Constantinopolitanus Patriarcha, *Oneirocriticon*; (ff. 26r et seq.) *Anonymi oneirocriticon ex lunae diebus*; (ff. 27r et seq.) *Oneirocriticon aliud* (alphabeticum).
		Omont 1886-1888: 2.275-276.
	2526	(ff. 34r et seq.) Manuel Philes, *De animalium proprietate*.
		Omont 1886-1888: 2.278.
[1295]	**2537**	II.43, 56.
		Omont 1886-1888: 2.280; *CMAG* I (Lebègue) 1924: 135-152.
	2538	Achmet, *Oneirocriticon*.
		Omont 1886-1888: 2.280.
[1296]	**2540**	II.10.
		Omont 1886-1888: 2.280.
[1297]	**2545 (? = 2145 ? cf. Kühn 1.1)**	I.5.

This manuscript is listed among the copies of Hippocrates, *Prognosticon*.

The *Parisinus* 2545 does not contain Hippocratic treatises, but instead it contains Theodorus Gaza, *Grammatica* (Omont 1886-1888: 3.1). Alexanderson 1963 does not include this *Parisinus* in the list of the manuscripts containing the work.

As Diels' catalogue suggested (though with question marks), the information here refers to 2145 (= [1053]), where the *Prognosticon* can be found (ff. 268v-277v). See Alexanderson 1963: 81.

The reference is to Kühn: 1825-1827, volume 1, i.e., to the *Historia literaria Hippocratis* by Ackermann in Kühn 1825-1827: 1.I-CCVI.

While the volume number is correct, the page number does not correspond to any mention of a manuscript of Hippocrates, *Prognosticon*. The treatise is discussed on pp. XLVI-LV, with a list of its Greek manuscripts on pp. XLVII-XLVIII, where the *Parisinus graecus* 2545 can be found (p. XLVII), without brackets or question mark.

In Omont's catalogue (below) the treatise is entitled *Praenotiones* as in the ancient catalogue of the *Bibliotheca Regia* 1740: 2.452-453 (see 452, MMCXLV [= 2145], no. 19, for the title).

The *Parisinus* 2145 appears in Diels I.5 among the copies of the *Prognosticon*.

See Omont 1886-1888: 2.203-204, and Alexanderson 1963: 81.

Same as [1053].

[1298]   **[2545 (?) = 2145 ?]**   I.4, 11 (2), 12, 13.

The codex *Parisimus* 2545 appears in the list of the manuscripts containing the following five Hippocratic treatises (listed here in the order of Diels' catalogue; references to Diels' catalogue follow the titles):

- *De prisca medicina* (I.4)
- *De fracturis* (I.11);
- *De officina medici* (I.11);
- *De articulis* (I.13);
- *Aphorismi* (I.13).

The manuscript is quoted by Ackermann 1825 (without brackets, question marks or the possible correspondence with *Parisinus* 2145) among the manuscripts of these treatises (same order as above):

- *De prisca medicina*: CLVIII, no. 52;
- *De fracturis* (*De fractis* in Ackermann): CXXI, no. 7 ctd.;
- *De officina medici*: CXIX, no. 6 ctd.;
- *De articulis*: CXXII, no. 8;
- *Aphorismi*: LXIV.

The *Parisinus* 2545 does not contain these works, but instead it contains Theodorus Gaza, *Grammatica* (Omont 1886-1888: 3.1).

The manuscript referred to here is *Parisinus* 2145 (Omont 1886-1888: 2. 203-204) (= [1053]) as Diels' catalogue suggested, though with question marks.

[1299]   **[2545 (? = 2145?)]**   I.8, 18 (2), 20 (3), 21(2), 22, 23, 24, 25, 26 (2), 29(2), 30(2), 31(2), 33(2), 34 (2), 35 (3).

The manuscript *Parisinus* 2545 is thought to contain the following 22 Hippocratic treatises (order of citations in Diels' catalogue; references to Diels' catalogue follow the titles): *De diaeta (regimine) acutorum* (I.8); *Iusurandum* (I.18); *Lex* (I.18); *De humoribus* (I.20); *Praesagiorum liber I* (I.20); *Coa praesagia* (I.20); *De arte* (I.21); *De natura hominis* (I.21); *De flatibus* (I.22); *De morbis I* (I.23); *De morbo sacro* (I.24); *De victus ratione I-III* (I.25); *De insomniis* (I.26); *De morbis II et III* (I.26); *De natura pueri* (I.29); *De morbis liber IV* (I.29); *De sterilibus* (I.30); *De virginum morbis* (I.30); *De superfoetatione* (I.31); *De exsectione foetus* (I.31); *Praesagiorum liber II* (I.33); *De alimento* (I.33); *De visu* (I.34); *De ossium natura* (I.34); *De decenti ornatu* (I.35); *Praeceptiones* (I.35); *De diebus iudicatoriis* (I.35).

It is listed in Ackermann 1825 (without brackets, question marks or the possible correspondence with *Parisinus* 2145) among the manuscripts of these treatises (same order as above): *De diaeta (regimine) acutorum*: XCIX; *Iusurandum*: CLXII, no. 47 ctd.; *Lex*: CLXV, no. 48 ctd.; *De humoribus*: CXVI, no. 3 ctd.; *Praesagiorum liber I*: LVIII; *Coa praesagia*: CXIV, no. 2 ctd.; *De arte*: CLXIX, no. 53; *De natura hominis*: CXLVII, no. 34 ctd.; *De flatibus*: CXL, no. 29; *De morbis I*: CXXXIII, no. 18 ctd.; *De morbo sacro*: CXXXVII, no. 24 ctd.; *De victus ratione I-III*: CXLIII, no. 32 ctd.; *De insomniis*: CXLIV, no. 33; *De morbis II et III*: CXXXIII, no. 18 ctd.; *De natura pueri*: CLIX, no. 44 ctd.; *De morbis liber IV*: CXXXIII, no. 18 ctd.; *De sterilibus*: CXXXVI, no. 22 ctd.; *De virginum morbis*: CXXXV, no. 20 ctd.; *De superfoetatione*: CXXXVI, no. 23; *De exsectione foetus*: CXXVI, no. 13; *Praesagiorum liber II*: LVIII; *De alimento*: CL, no. 35 ctd.; *De visu*: CXXX, no. 17 ctd.; *De ossium natura*: CLIV, no. 38 ctd.; *De decenti ornatu*: CLXVI, no. 50; *Praeceptiones*: CLXVII, no. 51; *De diebus iudicatoriis*: CXVIII, no. 5.

None of these works appears in *Parisinus* 2545, which contains Theodorus Gaza, *Grammatica* (Omont 1886-1888: 3.1).

As Diels' catalogue suggested (though with a question mark), these texts can be found in *Parisinus* 2145 (= [1053]) (Omont 1886-1888: 2. 203-204).

[1300]   **[2546 (? = 2146 ?)]**   I.27, 28.

This manuscript is listed among the copies of Hippocrates, *De septimestri partu* (I.27) and *De octimestri partu* (I.28).

The *Parisinus* 2546 is listed in Ackermann 1825: CLX, no. 46, among the manuscripts of *De octimestri partu* (without brackets, question marks or the possible correspondence with *Parisinus* 2146).

The manuscript does not contain these two works, but instead it contains grammatical works, and *Excerpta e canonibus SS. Apostolorum et conciliorum, SS. Basilii et Joannis Chrysostomi* (Omont 1886-1888: 3.2).

The two Hippocratic treatises can be found instead in the following *Parisini*:

- 2140 (= [1041]; Omont 1886-1888: 2.199-200);
- 2141 (= [1043]; *ibid.*: 2. 200-201);
- 2142 (= [1045]; *ibid.*: 2. 201);
- 2143 (= [1048]; *ibid.*: 2.201-202);
- 2144 (= [1051]; *ibid.*: 2.202-203);
- 2145 (= [1053]; *ibid.*: 2.203-204);
- 2146 (= [1055]; *ibid.*: 2.204);
- 2254 (= [1187]; *ibid.*: 2.223-224).

It is probable that the present reference is to *Parisinus* 2146 (= [1055]) as Diels' catalogue indicates, though with question marks. See Grensemann 1968: 14.

[1301]   **[2548 (?)]**   I.30.

This codex is listed among the copies of Hippocrates, *De mulierum affectibus*.

The same information (without brackets or question mark) appears in Ackermann 1825: CXXXIV, no. 19 ctd.

This manuscript does not contain the work (Omont 1886-1888: 3.2), which appears, instead, in the *Parisini* 2140-2146 (= [1041], [1043], [1045], [1048], [1051], [1053], [1055]) and in 2254 (= [1187]).

The manuscript referred to here cannot be identified.

	2582	(ff. 85 et seq.) *Lexicon botanicum.*

Omont 1886-1888: 3.8; Touwaide 1999: 215, 227.

[1302]	**2596**	I.13, 18; II.93.

Omont 1886-1888: 3.10.

[1303]	**2614**	II.37.

Omont 1886-1888: 3.13.

[1304]	**2615**	II.37, 59.

Omont 1886-1888: 3.13.

	2629	(ff. 99r et seq.) Synesius Cyrenensis, *De insomniis*, cum Nicephori Gregorae commentario.

Omont 1886-1888: 3.15-16.

[1305]	**2633**	II.61.

Omont 1886-1888: 3.16.

	2650	(ff. 153r et seq.) Symeon Seth, *De alimentorum facultatibus*; (ff. 201r et seq.) *Anonymi de re medica tractatus*; (ff. 205r et seq.) *Praecepta medica secundum menses.*

Omont 1886-1888: 3.18.

[1306]	**2651**	II.37.

Omont 1886-1888: 3.19.

[1307]	**2652**	I.38.

Omont 1886-1888: 3.19.

[1308]	**2664**	I.99.

This manuscript is listed among the copies of Galenus, *De antidotis libri II.*

According to Omont 1886-1888: 3.22, *Parisinus* 2664 contains an anonymous lexicon.

This manuscript may have been confused with another of the *Parisini* containing Galen's work (see Omont 1898: 66, *sub nomine* Galenus, *sub titulo*), possibly 2164 (= [1085]), which is listed in Ackermann 1821: CXLVII, no. 81.

It might be significant that *Parisinus* 2164 is not listed in Diels I.99 among the manuscripts of *De antidotis.*

[1309]	**2665**	II.36; N.50.

Omont 1886-1888: 3.22.

[1310]   **2671**   I.41.

Omont 1886-1888: 3.23-24; 3.397.

Also [1311].

[1311]   **[2671 (?)]**   I.13.

This codex does not contain Hippocrates, *Aphorismi* with Theophilus'
commentary (Omont 1886-1888: 3.23-24; it is not listed in Magdelaine 1994:
274-277), but instead it contains the *Aphorismi* (Ead.: 1.89) with some glosses
(Ead.: 1.126n2). These glosses are not Theophilus' commentary (Ead., contrary
to Ihm 2002: 213-216, no. 257 [especially 215]).

Same as [1310].

[1312]   **[2682 (?)]**   II.17, 18 (2), 19.

This item is supposed to be a copy of Aretaeus.

Parisinus 2682 contains the *Ilias* with some other related texts (Omont 1886-
1888: 3.25).

The shelfmark here is probably a mistake for that of one of the *Parisini* that
actually contain Aretaeus and cannot be identified. See Hude 1958: VII-X:

- 2186 (= [1111]; Omont 1886-1888: 2.211);
- 2187 (= [1112]; *ibid.*: 2.211-212),;
- 2202 (= [1127]; *ibid.*: 2.213);
- 2220 (= [1146]; *ibid.*: 2.215);
- 2288 (= [1236]; *ibid.*: 2.230);
- 2289 (= [1237]; *ibid.*: 2.230-231);
- 2334 (= [1279]; *ibid.*: 2.242).

[1313]   **[2699 (?)]**   I.41.

This codex is supposed to contain Hippocrates, *Epistula ad Ptolemaeum regem
de sanitate tuenda*.

Manuscrit *Parisinus* 2699 contains *Eustathii Thessalonicensis commentarius in
Homeri Iliadis libros XIV-XIX* (Omont 1886-1888: 3.27).

Number 2699 appears in the catalogue of the *Bibliotheca Regia* published
by Montfaucon 1739: 2.724-743. Its description (*ibid.*: 2.735) includes
"Hippocratis, vel Alexandri Medici Epistola de Diaeta".

According to Omont 1898: LXXII, number 2699 in the *Bibliotheca Regia*
corresponds to current 2240 (= [1167]), which contains the Hippocratic letter
and is mentioned in Diels' catalogue in the same paragraph as the present item.

Same as [1167].

[1314]   **2720**   II.36; N.44.

Omont 1886-1888: 3.29-30.

[1315]   **2726**   II.8.

Omont 1886-1888: 3.31.

	2728	(ff. 120r-136r) Nicander, *Theriaca*; (ff. 136r-146v) Nicander, *Alexipharmaca*.
		Omont 1886-1888: 3.32.
[1316]	**2731**	II.36; N.44.
		Omont 1886-1888: 3.32.
	2737	(ff. 76r et seq.) Manuel Philes, *De animalium proprietate*.
		Omont 1886-1888: 3.33.
[1317]	**2755**	I.38.
		Omont 1886-1888: 3.35-36.
[1318]	**2760**	I.111.
		Omont 1886-1888: 3.36.
[1319]	**[2828 (? = 2228 ?)]** I.5.	

This is supposed to be Hippocrates, *Prognosticon*.

The same information (without brackets, question mark or the possible equivalence with *Parisinus* 2228) appears in Ackermann 1825: XLVIII, with the mention "quo usus est Bosquillon (in praef. laud. p. 18)".

The reference is to the edition (Paris, 1784) of Hippocrates, *Aphorismi et Praenotionum liber* by Edouard-François-Marie Bosquillon (1744-1814). The citation is not correct, however. At 18n1, Bosquillon refers to manuscript 2228 which contains, according to him, Galen's commentary on the Hippocratic *Praenotiones*.

Codex *Parisinus* 2828 does not contain the Hippocratic treatise, but works by Aristophanes (Omont 1886-1888: 3.46).

Codex 2228 (= [1153]), meanwhile, does not contain the Hippocratic *Prognosticon* (it is not listed in Alexanderson 1963), but Galen's commentary on it (ff. 66 et seq.) as Bosquillon rightly stated (see Omont 1886-1888: 2.217).

The *Parisinus* 2228 is listed in Diels' catalogue (I.103) among the copies of Galen's commentary on the Hippocratic *Prognosticon*.

Same as [1153].

[1320]	**2830**	I.86; II.36; N.44.
		Omont 1886-1888: 3.46.
	2842	(f. 30v) *De corporis humani appellationibus*.
		Omont 1886-1888: 3.48; Björck 1938; 144.
[1321]	**2847**	I.56; II, 7, 28.
		Omont 1886-1888: 3.49.
	2871	(ff. 1r et seq.) Manuel Philes, *De animalium proprietate*.
		Omont 1886-1888: 3.52.
	2872	(ff. 125r et seq.) Epiphanius, *De duodecim gemmis*.
		Omont 1886-1888: 3.52.

	2875	Gregorius Nazianzenus, *De humana natura*.
		Omont 1886-1888: 3.53 (does not specifically mention the text); Domiter 1999: 21.
[1322]	**2894**	I.40; II.57, 94.
		Omont 1886-1888: 3.56; *CMAG* I (Lebègue) 1924: 208-210.
	2988	(ff. 58r et seq.) Synesius Cyrenensis, *De insomniis*.
		Omont 1886-1888: 3.80.
	2992	(ff. 239v et seq) *De mensuris, ponderibus et eorum notis*.
		Omont 1886-1888: 3.82-83.
[1323]	**3023**	II.94.
		Omont 1886-1888: 3.94.
	3025	(ff. 25v et seq.) Epiphanius, *De duodecim gemmis*.
		Omont 1886-1888: 3.94-95.
	3031	(ff. 47r et seq.) *Tractatus physicus de corpore*; *Excerpta de anima et re medica*.
		Omont 1886-1888: 3.96.
[1324]	**3035**	I.89, 110, 113, 131.
		Omont 1886-1888: 3.96-97.
[1325]	**3044**	II.9.
		Omont 1886-1888: 3.98-99.
[1326]	**3047**	I.38.
		Omont 1886-1888: 3.99.
[1327]	**3050**	I.38.
		Omont 1886-1888: 3.100.
[1328]	**3052**	I.38.
		Omont 1886-1888: 3.100.
[1329]	**3076**	II.17, 74.
		Omont 1886-1888: 3.104.
	3095	(ff. 81 et 93) Apollonius Citiensis, *Commentarium in Hippocratis librum de articulis* (frg.).
		Omont 1886-1888: 3.106-107.
[1330]	**3099**	II.71.
		Omont 1886-1888: 3.107.
[1331]	**[3140 (?)]**	I.13.
		According to Diels' catalogue, this is a copy of Hippocrates, *Aphorismi*.
		The same information (without brackets or question mark) appears in Ackermann 1825: LXIV (with a reference to "Montf. II. p. 739" [= Montfaucon 1739: 2.739]).

The *graecus* series of the Bibliothèque nationale de France currently contains 3117 items.

As the reference to Montfaucon 1739: 2.739 in Ackermann 1825 reveals, no. 3140 ("Hippocratis Aphorismi, cum Scholiis & alia opuscula") is the shelfmark of the manuscript in the *Bibliotheca Regia*.

According to the table of concordance provided in Omont 1898: LXXVII, the number 3140 of the *Bibliotheca Regia* corresponds to the current 2257 (= [1194]), which contains the *Aphorismi* and is mentioned in the same paragraph as the present item in Diels' catalogue.

Same as [1194].

[1332]   **[3170 (?)]   I.5.**

This is supposed to be copy of Hippocrates, *Prognosticon*.

The same information (without brackets or question mark) appears in Ackermann 1825: XLVIII.

It is incorrect, since the *Parisinus graecus* series contains 3117 manuscripts.

Number 3170 was a shelfmark in the *Bibliotheca regia* (see Montfaucon 1739: 2.740, no. 3170: "Hippocratis prognostica, & alia variorum opuscula medica"), which, according to Omont 1898: LXXVII, corresponds to current *Parisinus graecus* 36 (= [0957]). This manuscript contains Hippocrates, *Prognosticon* and is mentioned in the same paragraph of Diels' catalogue as the present item.

Same as [0957].

Suppl. (*Supplementum graecum*)

[1333]	**2**	I.103.
		Astruc, Concasty et al. 2003: 18-19.
[1334]	**3**	II.34.
		Astruc, Concasty et al. 2003: 19-22.
		Manuscript dated 1616, copied by the botanist and physician Paul de Reneaulme (ca. 1560-1624).
	28	(f. I) *Notae medicae.*
		Astruc, Concasty et al. 2003: 72-82 (see 82, *sub* "Annotations").
[1335]	**35**	I.60, 70, 72, 73, 74, 81 (2), 83, 95, 96, 99 (3), 110, 111 (2), 112, 113.
		Astruc, Concasty et al. 2003: 94-96.
	47	(ff. 78r-110v) Synesius Cyrenensis, *De insomniis.*
		Astruc, Concasty et al. 2003: 116-117.
[1336]	**49**	II.63.
		Astruc, Concasty et al. 2003: 119-120.
	57	*Efodia.*
		Astruc, Concasty et al. 2003: 129-131.

[1337]	**64**	I.13; II.104.

The Hippocratic *Aphorismi* (I.13) and the commentary by Theophilus (II.104) form *Parisinus Supplementum graecum* 64/XVI.

For manuscript 64, see also below 64/XIV, 64/XV and 64/XVI.

Astruc, Concasty et al. 2003: 150-151.

	64/XIV	Symeon Seth, *De alimentorum facultatibus*.

Astruc, Concasty et al. 2003: 148-149.

	64/XV	(ff. 151v-205f) *De simplicibus medicinis*; (f. 206r-v) *Medica varia*.

Astruc, Concasty et al. 2003: 149-150.

	64/XVI	See [1337].
	67	(f. 233r) *Menologium aegrotantium*.

Astruc, Concasty et al. 2003: 159-165 (see 164, *sub* "Annotations").

[1338]	**84**	II.63.

Astruc, Concasty et al. 2003: 198-200.

[1339]	**86**	II.67.

Astruc, Concasty et al. 2003: 200-201.

	139	(f. 158r, ll. 1-14) *De planta molu*.

Astruc, Concasty et al. 2003: 300-302.

[1340]	**148**	II.67.

Astruc, Concasty et al. 2003: 343-344.

[1341]	**165**	I.40; II.11.

Omont 1886-1888: 3.227.

[1342]	**194**	II.67.

Omont 1886-1888: 3.230.

	204	(ff. 259r et seq.) Aristoteles, *Problemata*.

Omont 1886-1888: 3.231; Wartelle 1963: 117, no. 1580.

[1343]	**205**	I.38.

Omont 1886-1888: 3.231.

	223	(ff. 1r et seq.) Manuel Philes, *De animalium proprietate*.

Omont 1886-1888: 3.235.

	247	(ff. 2r-27v) Nicander, *Theriaca*; (ff. 29r-46v) Nicander, *Alexipharmaca*.

Omont 1886-1888: 3.238.

[1344]	**263**	II.56.

Omont 1886-1888: 3.240.

The text referred to here (*Liber kerastonis*) is in fact a work in Latin: it is the translation by Gerard of Cremona (d. 1187) of the Arabic *Kitâb al-qarastun* (*Book on beam balance*) by Thâbit ibn Qurra (836-901 AD) (ed. and trans. Moody and Clagett 1952: 88-117; on Thâbit, see Rosenfeld and Grigorian 1976).

This manuscript is now latin 10260 (Delisle 1863: 67; Björnbo 1911: 139-140; Lejeune 1956: 43*).

For the old shelfmark, see f. Ar: "Cod. gr. Suppl. Nr. 263".

[1345]	**270**	II.15.
		Omont 1886-1888: 3.241-242.
		17th-century manuscript.
[1346]	**292**	I.149.
		Omont 1886-1888: 3.244-245.
		Collectanea by Ismaël Bouillaud (1605-1694).
[1347]	**338**	II.18.
		Omont 1886-1888: 3.250.
[1348]	**341**	II.40.
		Omont 1886-1888: 3.251-252.
[1349]	**352**	I.41.
		Omont 1886-1888: 3.252-253.
[1350]	**445**	II.17, 18 (2), 19.
		Omont 1886-1888: 3.262.
		19th-century collation of manuscripts by Minoïde Mynas (see also Cutolo 2012: 27).
[1351]	**446**	I.5, 13, 41, 80, 86, 89, 93, 111, 113 (2), 128, 130, 151; II.57, 71, 74, 78, 82, 98; N.56.
		Omont 1886-1888: 3.262; 3.398 (where the text contained at ff. 35v et seq. [*Remedia pro morbis oculorum*] is attributed to Oribasius).
		Same as [1783].
[1352]	**447**	I.13, 22, 101, 105.
		Omont 1886-1888: 3.262-263.
		Same as [1798].
	452	(ff. 22v et seq.) *Geoponica*.
		Omont 1886-1888: 3.264.
[1353]	**493**	II.30, 34.
		Omont 1886-1888: 3.269.
		19th-century collation of the Athos copy (Lavrae) of Dioscorides, *De materia medica*, Ω 75 (= [0082]) by Minoïde Mynas.
[1354]	**494**	II.78.
		Omont 1886-1888: 3.269.

[1355]	**496**	I.42, 61.
		Omont 1886-1888: 3.270.
		17th-century *iatrosofion*.
	542	Galenus, *Ars medica*.
		Omont 1886-1888: 3.275.
		See also Petit 2002: 196n109, and 200.
[1356]	**608**	I.18.
		Omont 1886-1888: 3.283.
[1357]	**629**	I.89, 131; II.59, 88, 89, 93, 99, 101, 102 (2), 106.
		Omont 1886-1888: 3.287.
[1358]	**630**	II.6.
		Omont 1886-1888: 3.287.
[1359]	**631**	II.6.
		Omont 1886-1888: 3.287.
[1360]	**632**	II.6.
		Omont 1886-1888: 3.287.
[1361]	**633**	II.17.
		Omont 1886-1888: 3.287.
		19th-century collations of manuscripts by Minoïde Mynas (see also Cutolo 2012: 27).
[1362]	**634**	I.60, 61, 64 (2), 67, 76, 77, 83, 92, 93, 113, 119, 125, 128, 133, 150.
		Omont 1886-1888: 3.287.
[1363]	**635**	I.119, 120; N.32.
		Omont 1886-1888: 3.287-288.
[1364]	**636**	I.100; II.37, 48.
		Omont 1886-1888: 3.288.
		17th-century manuscript.
[1365]	**637**	I.41; II.7, 55, 63, 90, 102 (2).
		Omont 1886-1888: 3.288.
		Possibly [1373].
[1366]	**638**	II.53.
		Omont 1886-1888: 3.288.
[1367]	**639**	II.107.
		Omont 1886-1888: 3.288.
		19th-century *iatrosofion*.
[1368]	**640**	II.67.
		Omont 1886-1888: 3.288.
		18th-century manuscript.

[1369]	**641**	II.67.
		Omont 1886-1888: 3.288.
		18th-century *iatrosofion*.
[1370]	**652**	II.44.
		Omont 1886-1888: 3.290.
[1371]	**654**	II.65.
		Omont 1886-1888: 3.290-291.
		Manuscript by Minoide Mynas.
	659	(f. 125r) *Lexicon botanicum.*
		Omont 1886-1888: 3.291-292; Touwaide 1999: 217, 227.
	660	(ff. 79v et seq.) Synesius Cyrenensis, *De insomniis.*
		Omont 1886-1888: 3.292.
[1372]	**662**	II.61.
		Omont 1886-1888: 3.292-293.
[1373]	**675**	I.41.

According to Diels' catalogue, this item contains (f. 83) Hippocrates, *Sententiae de vita et morte.*

According to Omont 1886-1888: 3.294-295, this text does not appear in the manuscript which contains a great variety of non-medical texts (including 19th-century catalogues of manuscripts in the libraries of Mount Athos by Minoïde Mynas).

In the Index of Omont 1898: 90, *sub nomine* Hippocrates, *sub titulo*, this work is contained in *Supplementum* 637 (= [1365]), where such text appears, at f. 65r according to Omont 1886-1888: 3. 288. This *Supplementum* 637 is listed in Diels I.41.

Probably same as [1365].

	676	(ff. 105r et seq.) *Onomatopoeia partium corporis humani, cum duobus figuris.*
		Omont 1886-1888: 3.295.
[1374]	**681**	I.117.
		Omont 1886-1888: 3.297.
[1375]	**682**	I.13, 114; II.26.
		Omont 1886-1888: 3.297.
[1376]	**683**	I.149; II.7, 60, 74.
		Omont 1886-1888: 3.298.
[1377]	**684**	I.42, 100, 123.
		Omont 1886-1888: 3.298-299; 3.397; *CMAG* I (Lebègue) 1924: 133.

[1378]   **688**   II.93.

Omont 1886-1888: 3.299-300.

690   (ff. 123v et seq.) *Oneirocritica.*

Omont 1886-1888: 3.300-302.

[1379]   **702**   II.67.

Omont 1886-1888: 3.303.

[1380]   **727**   I.67, 120.

Omont 1886-1888: 3.305.

Manuscript by Minoide Mynas.

[1381]   **728 (Minas IZ)**   I.47.

This manuscript is listed among the copies of Hippocrates, *Ad Galenum discipulum liber de pulsibus et de temperamentis corporis humani*, whereas it does not contain this text. It is a copy of the catalogue of manuscripts owned by Minoïde Mynas (Omont 1886-1888: 3.305).

A note following the mention of this manuscript in Diels' catalogue refers to "Costomiris Revue des ét. gr. II [1889] p. 353". There, Costomiris provides the following information:

Ce traité pseudonyme (i.e. Hippocrates, *Ad Galenum discipulum liber* ...) existe dans un des mss. de M. Minas [*sic*], qui ne se trouve pas à la Bibliothèque nationale. Il est désigné ainsi: ms. IZ, du XIVe siècle, en papier in-12 (catalogue des mss. de M. Minas, suppl. gr. 728, f° 28).

A manuscript listed in codex Paris, *Supplementum graecum* 728, f. 28r, corresponds to Costomiris' description. Interestingly enough, it is numbered IZ (= 17). The list of its contents includes (f. 28r, l. 20) the text mentioned in Diels' catalogue:

IZ Manuscrit in 12 cartaceus [*sic*] du 14eme siècle contenant

...

14°Ἱπποκράτους πρὸς Γαληνὸν περὶ σφυγμῶν καὶ κράσεων

...

Diel's catalogue misinterprets Costomiris' information, because it gives a reference to f. 28 as if it were the beginning of the text of Hippocrates, *Ad Galenum discipulum liber* ..., in the Paris manuscript, whereas it is the reference to the folio where Mynas' manuscript is listed in the catalogue of his collection that Mynas himself compiled (which is the manuscript *Supplementum graecum* 728).

A modern handwritten note in the margin of the *Supplementum graecum* 728 identifies manuscript IZ as *Supplementum graecum* 1254 (= [1397]). This manuscript contains the Pseudo-Hippocratic text listed here. It is included among the witnesses of this piece at the same page as the present one in Diels' catalogue.

Same as [1397] and [1382].

[1382]   **754 (Minas)**   I.47.

This manuscript is identified as a copy of Hippocrates, *Ad Galenum discipulum liber de pulsibus et de temperamentis corporis humani*, which is not the case (Omont 1886-1888: 3.307).

A supplementary note following the mention of this manuscript in Diels' catalogue refers to "Costomiris Revue des ét. gr. II [1889] p. 353" as in [1381].

There, Costomiris mentions the following:

Un autre exemplaire de ce traité existe au Mont-Athos, dans un ms. du couvent Iberon, en papier, in-12, entre autres traités non médicaux (Minas [*sic*], suppl. grec de Paris 754, fol. 523), si ce n'est pas le même ms. emporté par Minas du Mont-Athos: les deux mss. cités par Minas contiennent tout à fait les mêmes traités. Mais peut-être y avait-il deux exemplaires semblables dans la Bibliothèque du couvent Iberon.

The manuscript *Supplementum graecum* 754 contains only 314 folios. The reference to f. 523 by Costomiris is thus incorrect. On f. 12r, ll. 22-24, under number IZ, the *Supplementum graecum* 754 contains the description of a manuscript which corresponds to that of [1381] in the Paris, *Supplementum graecum* 728, as Costomiris rightly mentions.

However, the manuscript number IZ in the *Supplementum graecum* 754 is not listed in the catalogue of the Iviron library contained in codex Paris, *Supplementum graecum* 754, ff. 37r-106v (title f. 37r, ll, 1-3: "Catalogue des manuscrits de la bibliotheque [*sic*] du Couvent Ιβηρος [*sic*] le 13 juillet 1841"), but rather in a list of books that Minoïde Mynas stored in Thessalonica. See f. 11v, ll. 1-3 for the title of this list: «ouvrages et effets contenus dans la malle en peau que je laisse aussi dans le même magasin de Mrs Abbot frères à Salonique», and ff. 11v-12v, l. 17 for the whole list.

This manuscript is the same as [1381], and it is Paris, *Supplementum graecum* 1254 (= [1397]).

[1383]   **755**   II.23.

Omont 1886-1888: 3.307-308.

Manuscript by Minoïde Mynas.

[1384]   **764**   I.76, 93, 149; II.11.

Omont 1886-1888: 3.309; 3.399 (where the following text is mentioned: ff. 44r et seq.: Theophanes Nonnus, *Collectio medica*).

[1385]   **765**   I.67.

Omont 1886-1888: 3.309.

17th-century manuscript.

773   (ff. 237r et seq.) Epiphanius, *De duodecim gemmis*.

Omont 1886-1888: 3.310.

[1386]   **793**   I.150.

Omont 1886-1888: 3.311.

17th-century manuscript.

[1387]   **836**   II.10.

Omont 1886-1888: 3.315.

17th-century manuscript.

[1388]   **924**   II.80.

Astruc and Concasty 1960: 23-25.

[1389]   **1022**   II.100, 115.

Astruc and Concasty 1960: 104-105; *CMAG* I (Lebègue) 1924: 129.

1033   (ff. 4r-74v) Synesius Cyrenensis, *De insomniis*, cum Nicephorus Gregoras, *Scholia in Synesii De insomniis*.

Astruc and Concasty 1960: 130.

1090   (ff. 107r-111v) Gregorius Nazianzenus, *De humana natura*.

Astruc and Concasty 1960: 211-216; Domiter 1999: 22.

[1390]   **1098**   II.30.

Astruc and Concasty 1960: 228-229.

1146   (ff. 79r-80v) *Lexicon plantarum*.

Astruc and Concasty 1960: 294-296.

1148   (no. 26 = ff. 66r-73v, 114r-121v, 58r-65v, 98r-v) Galenus, *Prognostica de decubitu ex mathematica scientia*; (no. 27 = f. 98 v, l. 11-99v) *De decubitu ex mathematica scientia*; (no. 32 = ff. 88r-89v) *Geoponica* (frg.); (no. 74 = ff. 166r-170r) *De neo-natorum vita*; (no. 83 = f. 182r) *De neonati sexo*; (no. 100 = ff. 206r-227r) *Cyranides* (frg.); (no. 101 = ff. 227r, l. 13-231v) *Remedia*.

Astruc and Concasty 1960: 296-308; *CCAG* VIII.3 (Boudreaux) 1912: 81-87; *CMAG* I (Lebègue) 1924: 221-224.

[1391]   **1156**   II.78; N.62.

(ff. 24-25) Palimpsest (Omont 1897: 13; Heiberg 1919: 276; Fonkič 2000: 170).

Astruc and Concasty 1960: 318-321.

See Москва (Moskva), Государственный Исторический Музей (ГИМ), Синодальная Библиотека Московского Патриархата (Gosudarstvennyi Istoricheskii Muzei (GIM), Sinodal'naia Biblioteka Moskovskoi Patriarkhii [State Historical Museum [GIM], Synodal Library of Moscow Patriarchate]), Sinod. 174 (387 Vlad.) (see p. 148).

The f. 23 of this manuscript–palimpsest and not distinguished by Omont 1897:13–, does not come from the same volume as ff. 24-25 and ff. 1-2 of the Moskva codex (Fonkič 2000: 170n7).

Contrary to Heiberg 1919: 276, Devreesse 1945: 7-8 and117-118 about Coislin 8 and 123, respectively, and Astruc and Concasty 1960: 320, the ff. 24-25 of this manuscript and 1-2 of the Moscow one do not come from the same codex as the palimpsested ones of the *Coisliniani* 8 and 123 (Fonkič 2000: 170n7).

	1188	(f. 3v) Lucas, *Sales.*
		Astruc and Concasty 1960: 357-358.
		See [0910].
[1392]	**1193**	I.99, 114; II.79.
		Astruc and Concasty 1960: 368-370.
[1393]	**1194**	I.56, 149.
		Astruc and Concasty 1960: 370-371.
[1394]	**1197**	II.30.

This item is listed as a copy of Dioscorides, *De materia medica.*

The manuscript *Parisinus, Supplementum graecum* 1197, does not contain this text, but Aphthonius and Hermogenes (Astruc and Concasty 1960: 372).

This is most likely a mistake for *graecus* 1297 (= [0989]) where Dioscorides' text appears.

[1395]	**1202**	I.149; II.17, 34, 60, 74, 80, 86, 92.
		Astruc and Concasty 1960: 375-380.
	1238/XIX	(ff. 127r-128v, 130r-131v, 129r-v, 132r-v) Nicomedes, *Lexicon.*
		Astruc and Concasty 1960: 416-435 for the whole manuscript and 434 for this text.
[1396]	**1240**	II.6.
		Astruc and Concasty 1960: 436-437.
		See below (p. 313) София (Sofia [BU]), Българска Академия на Науките (БАН), Научен Архив (НА) (Bulgarska Akademiia na Naukite [BAN], Nauchen Arkhiv [Bulgarian Academy of Sciences, Scientific Archives]), BAN гр (BAN gr.), 5.
[1397]	**1254**	I.47.
		Astruc and Concasty 1960: 486-491.
		Same as [1381] and [1382].
	1275	(ff. 74v-78r) Epiphanius, *De duodecim gemmis.*
		Astruc and Concasty 1960: 512-520.
	1284	(f. 1r-v) Paulus Aegineta, *Epitome medica* (frg.).
		Astruc and Concasty 1960: 533-543.
[1398]	**1297**	I.114; II.11, 79, 93.
		Astruc and Concasty 1960: 560-564.
	1327	(ff. 1r-35v) Symeon Seth, *De alimentorum facultatibus.*
		Astruc and Concasty 1960: 627-628.
	1328	Galenus, *Definitiones medicae.*
		Astruc and Concasty 1960: 628. In Karas 1994: 347, the manuscript is mistakenly identified as *graecus* 1328.
	1366	(ff. 67r-70r) Epiphanius, *Physiologus.*
		Astruc and Concasty 1960: 686-690.

Bibliothèque nationale de France (National Library of France)

See above **Bibl. Nationale.**

Bibliothèque Sainte-Geneviève (St. Geneviève Library)

-

3394	See [0914].
3401	Manuel Philes, *De animalium proprietate.*
	Omont 1886-1888: 3.353, no. 47 [Ao 37, in-4].

Collection particulière (Private collection)

-       This manuscript is [0220], part 3.

Institut français d'études byzantines (French Institute of Byzantine Studies)

-

IFEB 34   (ff. 129r-150r)   *Physiologus.*

Papadopoulos-Kerameus 1887: 8, no. 35; Stefou 2011: 9, 12-13; Bingeli et al. 2014: 58-60 (with table 11).

Parma (IT)

   Bibl. Palatina (Biblioteca Palatina [Palatine Library])

   Fondo De-Rossiano

[1399]   7   II.28.

                              Martini 1893: 198-200.

                              Current shelfmark: Ms. Parm. 3062.

   Biblioteca Palatina (Palatine Library)

   Ms. Parm.

      3062   See [1399].

                     Eleuteri 1993: 84-86.

Patmos (Πάτμος [Patmos]) (GR)

   Bibl. monast. St. Johann. Evang. (*Bibliotheca monasterii Sancti Johannis Evangelisti,* Βιβλιοθήκη τῆς Μονῆς τοῦ ῾Αγίου Ἀποστόλου καὶ Εὐαγγελίστου᾽Ιωάννου [Library of the Monastery of St. John the Evangelist]), now Ιερά Μονή Αγίου Ιωάννου του Θεολόγου [Monastery of St. John the Theologian)

      -

[1400]   -   II.67.

                  This is a copy of Nemesius Emesenus, *De natura hominis.*

                  It probably corresponds to current *Patmiacus* 202 (see p. 264).

                  See also [1402].

[1401]   -   N.43.

This item without any identifier does not seem to refer to any of Aetius manuscripts listed in Diels' volume II.

The note related to this unidentified *Patmiacus* specifies that this manuscript consists of only two folios (Book I), according to Skevos Zervos (1875-1966).

Although there is no precise indication in that sense in Diels' catalogue, this might be a reference to Zervos 1905: 262, where the author mentions that a manuscript of Aetios is made of 2 folios. The only Aetius manuscript in Patmos according to Sakkelion 1890: 333, is current *Patmiacus* 277 (= [1406]). However, this is not a two-folio codex.

Strangely enough, Zervos 1905: 261-262, does not make reference to Sakkelion 1890.

The item referred to here cannot be identified.

[1402]   **11 (bei Coxe, Mss. gr. of the Levant)   N.59.**

Refers to II.67 (= [1400]) where the copy of Nemesius Emesenus, *De natura hominis* is not identified by means of an exact number.

Besides the reference to Coxe 1858b: 62 (no. 11), Diels' catalogue provides a further information about the identification of this item: "vgl. no. λ′ bei Migne, Patrol. gr. 149, 1049". This is the catalogue of Patmos library published in Migne's *Patrologiae cursus completus, Series graeca posterior*, volume 149 (1865), cols. 1048-1052.

As stated in the title (cols. 1048-1049), this catalogue reproduces the publication by "May, Biblioth. nov. P.P., tom. VI" (= Mai 1853: 537-539). A historical explanation follows:

Confectus fuit hic Catalogus regnante Joanne Palaeologo, qui anno 1355 floruit; nec liber recentior occurrit.

This catalogue is contained in codex *Vaticanus latinus* 1205. Number λ′ (mentioned by Diels) contains (see cols. 1049-1050) Nemesius Emesenus, περὶ φύσεως ἀνθρώπου (*De natura hominis*).

It is probably the current *Patmiacus* 202 (see p. 264).

[1403]   **71 bei Coxe, Mss. gr of the Levant   N.62.**

Supplementary information about [1405].

Refers to Coxe 1858/2: 65 (no. 71).

Most probably same as current *Patmiacus* 208 (see p. 264).

[1404]   **ΚΓ   N.51.**

This is a copy of Gregorius Nyssenus, *De hominis opificio*.

The number **ΚΓ** mentioned in Diels is not a shelfmark, but a sequential number in the same catalogue as [1402], col. 1049.

Gregorius Nyssenus, *De hominis opificio* is not contained in the current *Patmiacus* 23 (= ΚΓ), but rather in the current *Patmiaci* 27 and 47 (below). The current Patmiacus 23 contains Basilius, *Orationes, Predicationes* and *Epistulae* (Kominis 1988: 57-59).

[1405]   **111**   II.78.

This is a copy of Paulus Aegineta, *Epitome medica*.

The current *Patmiacus* 111 contains works by Theodorus Studites (Sakellion 1890: 67).

The number 111 comes from Guérin 1856: 111, in the catalogue of the manuscripts of Patmos library (see 101-119 for the catalogue).

This manuscript of Paulus of Aegina described as "fort ancient" is most probably current *Patmiacus* 208 (below).

See [1403].

[1406]   **277**   II.6.

Sakkelion 1890: 143; Karas 1994: 338.

17th-century *iatrosofion*.

See [1401].

Πάτμος (Patmos) (GR)

Ιερά Μονή Αγίου Ιωάννου του Θεολόγου (Monastery of St. John the Theologian)

27   (ff. 85r-95r) Gregorius Nyssenus, *De hominis opificio*.
            Kominis 1988: 64-67.
            See [1404].

38   (f. Ir-v) Gregorius Nyssenus, *De hominis opificio* (frg.).
            Kominis 1988: 98-100.

47   (ff. 67v-121v) Gregorius Nyssenus, *De hominis opificio*.
            Kominis 1988: 120-122.
            See [1404].

202   Nemesius Emesenus, *De natura hominis*.
            Sakkelion 1890: 113; Morani 1981: 1-5.
            See [1400] and [1402].

208   Paulus Aegineta, *Epitome medica*.
            Sakkelion 1890: 116.
            See [1405] and also [1403].

263   (ff. 191r-193r) Epiphanius, *De mensuris et ponderibus*.
            Sakkelion 1890: 127-136.

378   no. 4: Nicephorus Blemmydes, *De corpore*.
            Sakkelion 1890: 171-172.

450   (no. 4) Epiphanius, *Physiologus*.
            Sakkelion 1890: 203-204.

Petersbourg (Санкт-Петербург [Saint-Petersburg]) (RU)

Kaiserl. öffentl. Bibl. (Kaiserliche öffentliche Bibliothek [Public Imperial Library]), now Российская Национальная Библиотека, Санкт-Петербург (Rossiskaia Natsional'naia Biblioteka, Sankt-Peterburg [National Library of Russia, Saint-Petersburg])

[1407]   **116**   I.123.

Muralt 1864: 67-68; *CCAG* XII (Šangin) 1936: 58-59, 169.

Same as [0944].

Current shelfmark: Греч. (Grech.) 116.

See below, p. 311, Санкт-Петербург (Sankt-Peterburg [Saint-Petersburg]).

[1408]   **164**   II.88, 89, 90.

Muralt 1864: 86.

This manuscript was originally among the holdings of the Załuski Library (Biblioteka Załuskich) in Warsaw. In 1794, it was brought to Saint-Petersburg with the whole collection of the library, and entered the Imperial Public Library. It was returned to Warsaw in 1924 and was burned in the World War II fire that destroyed the whole library in 1944.

Bleskina et al. 2013: 281, no. 3783 (for a catalogue of the manuscripts of the Załuski books shipped to Saint Petersburg and returned to Warsaw); Sideras 1977: 14-15n2 (for the history of the manuscript in the 20th century) and 75-76.

Philadelphia, PA (US)

University of Pennsylvania, Van Pelt-Dietrich Library, Kislak Center for Special Collections, Rare Books and Manuscripts

Medieval & Renaissance Manuscripts Collection

Misc. MSS, Paulus Aegineta, *Epitome medica* (frg.).

This is only one folio.

Zacour and Hirsch 1970: 91-92 (where this item is identified as Ms. Lea 475).

Pistoia (IT)

Biblioteca Capitolare Fabroniana (Fabroniana Capitular Library)

Ms 308   See [1409].

Mioni 1965: 2.348.

Pistoja (Pistoia) (IT)

Biblioteca Fabroniana (Fabroniana Library), now Biblioteca Capitolare Fabroniana (Fabroniana Capitular Library)

-

[1409]   **141 (308)**   I.13, 105, 107.

Number 141 is not a shelfmark, but the sequential number attributed to the manuscript in Zanelli 1890: 276.

The current shelfmark is Ms 308 (see above p. 265).

Provo, UT (US)

Brigham Young University, Lee Library

L. Tom Perry Special Collections

Vault 091 G13 1475   Formerly [0220], part 2.

Kraus 1978: no. 16.

Raudnitz (Roudnice) (CZ)

The collection of the Lobkowicz family, which dates back to Bohuslav Hasištensky z Lobkowic (1461-1510), was preserved since 1657 at the Lobkowicz castle in Roudnice, north of Prague. During World War II the castle was confiscated by the German troops in 1941. The library was evacuated and it was deposited at Prague University Library which was first renamed as the State Library of the Socialist Czech Republic in Prague (Statni Knihovna CSR), and then as the National Library of the Czech Republic in 1990 (Národní Knihovna České Republiky Praha), where it was identified as the Roudnice Lobkowicz Library collection (Roudnická lobkowiczká knihovna). In 1992, it was returned to the Lobkowicz family, and it is currently preserved at the Nelahozeves Castle (Zámek Nelahozeves), north of Prague, as the Lobkowicz Library (Lobkowiczká knihovna) (on which see above, pp. 164-165).

[1410]   -

-

11   II.6.

Passow 1825: VII note * ctd.

This manuscript listed without library and collection name was in the Lobkowicz Library at Roudnice. It is now at Nelahozeves (CZ), Lobkowiczká Knihovna, VI Fc 37 (see above, p. 164).

Also [1411].

Bibl. Ducis Lobcovic (*Bibliotheca Ducis Lobcovic* [Duke Lobkowicz's Library])

-

[1411]   **VI F c 37**   II.6.

Same as [1410].

Ravenna (IT)

Biblioteca Classens. (Biblioteca Classense [Classense Library])

-

[1412]   **70**   I.58.

                              Mioni 1965: 2.357.

                              Also [1413].

[1413]   **131 2 H**   I.61, 101.

                              131 2 H is an old shelfmark of [1412].

                              Current shelfmark is Ms. 70 (below).

                              Same as [1412].

Biblioteca Classense (Classense Library)

-

            Ms. 70   See [1412] and [1413].

[Reims] (FR)

[Bibl. S. Remig.] (*Bibliotheca Sancti Remigi* [St. Rémy Library], Bibliothèque du monastère de Saint-Rémy [St. Rémy monastery Library])

-

[1414]   **[548]**   I.21.

This is supposed to be a copy of Hippocrates, *De natura hominis*.

The same information (without brackets) is found in Ackermann 1825: CXLVII, no. 34 ctd., with a reference to "Montfauc. II. pag. 1289", that is, Montfaucon 1739: 2.1289, no. 548, in a catalogue (*ibid.*: 2.1288-1290) entitled (*ibid.*: 2.1288): "Ex catalogo Graecorum manuscript. Abbatiae S. Remigi Rhemensis".

This manuscript was destroyed in the fire that ravaged Saint Rémy abbey and library in January 1774 (Fleury and Paris 1837: 105-118; Poussin 1857: 251-260; Jadart 1902: 130-144).

Rhodope (Родопи [*Rodopi*], Ροδόπη [Rodopi], Rhodope Mountains, ex Ottoman Empire, now Bulgaria)

Bibl. Mon. Mpatskobou (*Bibliotheca Monasterii Mpatskobou* [Βιβλιοθήκη Μονῆς Μπατσκόβου] [Library of Batskobou Monastery])

-

[1415]   -   I.3.

This manuscript listed without collection name and shelfmark in Diels' catalogue is a copy of Hippocrates, *Opera varia*.

The source of this information is Papageorgios 1887 (see Diels I.XXIII). There, the identification of the manuscript is somewhat more precise (Papageorgios 1887: 116, 2nd paragraph on the page, item no. 2 [β´]):

Ἱπποκράτους ἐν παραφράσει

However short it may be, such a description indicates that this manuscript contained a post-Byzantine adaptation of works by Hippocrates in the way of *iatrosofia*.

Most manuscripts of Batskobou Monastery are currently in София, Българска Патриаршия, Църковно-исторически и архивен институт (ЦИАИ) (Sofia, Patriarchate of Bulgaria, Ecclesiastical Historical and Archival Institute) (see Getov 1997 and 2014). However, the present item does not seem to be in this collection. Its current location cannot be identified in the current state of research.

Rodosto (Ῥαιδεστός [Rodosto] in the former Ottoman Empire, now Tekirdag [TR])

Bibl. Episkopou (Βιβλιοθήκη Ἐπισκόπου [Episcopal Library])

[1416]   -   I.117.

This manuscript mentioned without collection name or shelfmark in Diels' catalogue is listed as a copy of Galen, *De demonstrationibus*.

Mention of this manuscript is accompanied by references to "Foerster de antiqu. et libris mss. Constantinopol. und Costomiris a. a. O. p. 383" (that is, Rev. des ét. gr. II).

The first reference is to Foerster 1877: 29, col. 1, l. 4-31, that is, the edition of one of the lists of manuscripts contained in codex *Vindobonensis, historicus graecus* 98, ff. 51r-54r. For a more recent edition of this list, see Papazoglou 1983: 403-409.

This list is about an unidentified collection in Raidestos (Rodosto, now Tekirdag in Turkey), which was considered to be the Episcopal Library.

The item referred to here is no. [140] identified as follows (Foerster 1877: 31, col. 1, l. 4):

γαληνοῦ περὶ ἀποδείξεων ἰατρῶν

See also Papazoglou 1983: 408, no. 140.

Diels' reference to Costomiris is to Costomiris 1889: 383, which refers to Foerster 1877: 31, and repeats the title of the work as above.

Although the Rodosto Episcopal Library and School Library contained some manuscripts (for a bibliography on these libraries and their holdings, see Olivier 1995: 778-779, *sub nomine* Tekirdağ, and, secondarily 281, *sub nomine* Eleuthéroupolis), they did not hold all the items in the list of manuscript *Vindobonensis, historicus graecus* 98 (see Papadopoulos-Kerameus 1886: 5), which is a forgery (Krumbacher 1897; Przychocki 1938; Maas 1938; Lauxtermann 2013: 275-276). See, however, Papazoglou 1983: 161-182.

Rom (Roma [Rome]) (IT)

-

Fonds Colonna (Fondo Colonna [Colonna Collection])

[1417]   **12**   II.89.

This manuscript mentioned without library name in Diel's catalogue appears among the copies of Rufus, *De corporis humani appellationibus*. It is the *Vaticanus Ottobonianus graecus* 235 (= [1456]).

The identification of this manuscript as "Fonds Colonna 12" most probably comes from Charles Daremberg (1817-1872), who first referred to it in 1850: 229, and 1850/2: 265, without any number however:

(1850: 229) ... J'ai fait un dépouillement scrupuleux des catalogues grecs ... des fonds ... *Ottobomins* [*sic*] ... j'ai collationné sur deux manuscrits le traité de Rufus, *Du nom des parties du corps humain* ...

(1850/2: 265) ... les manuscrits ... du fonds Colonna ... Un manuscrit du fonds Colonna contient des SCHOLIES sur une partie considérable du traité de Rufus: *Du nom des parties du corps humain* ... Le même manuscrit renferme encore plusieurs morceaux inédits que j'ai également copiés ...

Further on, Daremberg identified this manuscript with nr. 12 (1852: 5 = 1853: 125). This information was repeated in the edition of Rufus' works prepared by Daremberg and posthumously published by Charles-Emile Ruelle (1833-1912), with several statements (Daremberg 1879):

(XXXIII): ... Ms. de Rome. Fonds Colonna n° 12 ...

(XXV): ... Col. ms. de Rome, bibliothèque du Vatican, fonds Colonna n° 12 ....

(LIV): *Dénominations de la nature de l'homme.* — Dès 1852 , M. Daremberg signalait ce texte inédit dans les *Archives des missions* (t. III, p. 5). Il l'a tiré d'un ms. du Vatican (fonds palatin, n° 302, fol. 84 r°). puis collationné sur une copie du fonds Colonna, n° 12 ...

(237): SCHOLIES SUR LE TRAITÉ DU NOM DES PARTIES DU CORPS. I. SCHOLIES COLONNA. Ces scholies proviennent d'un manuscrit (bibliothèque du Vatican, fonds Colonna. n° 12) dont personne jusqu'ici n'a parlé; je les ai copiées en 1849; elles ont un grand intérêt, puisqu'elles nous fournissent plusieurs fragments inédits du livre de Soranus *Sur les noms des parties du corps* ...

Interestingly enough, the manuscript *Vaticanus Ottobonianus* 235 is also mentioned in Daremberg 1879, in the list of the copies of Rufus' treatise *Des noms du partie du corps* (Daremberg 1879: XXII-XXIV for the list of the manuscripts, and XXIII, nr. 5 for the *Ottobonianus* manuscript, and nr. 18 [same page] for the Colonna codex) and in the *Index siglorum* (pp. XXIV-XXV, for the list; XXV, *sub* "O", for the *Ottobonianus*; and, [same page], *sub* "Col. Ms. de Rome", for the Colonna codex).

The *Ottobonianus* manuscript is listed in Diels' catalogue among the copies of Rufus' treatise (II.89).

The identification of the manuscript as in Diels' catalogue refers to its first identified owner, Cardinal Ascanio Colonna (1560-1608), who owned a collection of Greek manuscripts in Rome. His library went through different hands between 1611 and 1748 (except some items identified as the *Columnenses* manuscripts at the Vatican Library [= *Vaticani graeci* 2162-2254] which had a different history [Lilla 2011: 605-606]). After Ascanio Columna's death it was sold to the Duke Giovanni Angelo d'Altemps (d. 1620) in 1611. The *Bibliotheca Altempsiana* (on which see Serrai 2008) was bought in 1690 by Pietro Ottoboni (1610-1691, who became Pope Alexander VIII in 1689). The collection was donated by the pope to his homonymous nephew Cardinal Pietro Ottoboni (1667-1740) (see Montfaucon 1739: 1.186 C 17-18 for the present item, in the list [1.183-1888] entitled [1.183] *In Bibliotheca Eminentissimi Cardinalis Ottoboni*). After the latter's death, the Ottoboni collection was bought by Pope Benedict XIV (1675; elected 1740; d. 1758) in 1748, and it entered the *Bibliotheca Vaticana*.

Bibl. Angelica (Biblioteca Angelica [Angelica Library])

In Diels' catalogue, identifiers of the manuscripts of this collection are made of two different elements:

- a number in Arabic numerals;
- a composite shelfmark between parentheses, made of a Latin capital letter, followed by two numbers in Arabic numerals separated by a period sign.

The second of Diels' identifiers goes back to the organization of the Angelica library in the 19th century (Piccolomini 1896: 27-29). These shelfmarks are no longer used. The shelfmarks currently used are the sequential numbers in the catalogue by Franchi de' Cavalieri and Muccio 1896 (Arabic numerals, which correspond to the identifiers in Diels' catalogue according to the first system above). These numbers are preceded by an abbreviation that distinguishes the different collections according to the language (here "gr." for Greek).

[1418]	**4 (C.4.16)**	I.39, 40, 46; II.15, 37, 58 (2), 81; N.56.
		Franchi de' Cavalieri and Muccio 1896: 34-35.
		Current shelfmark: Ang. gr. 4.
[1419]	**17 (C.5. 4)**	I.116, 133; II.44, 52, 58, 64, 74, 78, 80, 85, 102.
		Franchi de' Cavalieri and Muccio 1896: 44-49.
		Current shelfmark: Ang. gr. 17.
	29	(f. 179r) Nechepso et Petosiris, *De mense*.
		Franchi de' Cavalieri and Muccio 1896: 60-64 (the text is not mentioned); *CCAG* V.1 (Cumont and Boll) 1904: 4-57 (especially 55).
		Current shelfmark: Ang. gr. 29.
[1420]	**68 (C.2.7)**	II.79.
		Franchi de' Cavalieri and Muccio 1896: 119-120.
		Current shelfmark: Ang. gr. 68.

69	(ff. 72r et seq.) Gregorius Nyssenus, *De hominis opificio*.
	Franchi de' Cavalieri and Muccio 1896: 120-121.
	Current shelfmark: Ang. gr. 69.
78	Aristoteles, *Problemata*.
	Franchi de' Cavalieri and Muccio 1896: 125; Wartelle 1963: 149, no. 2021.
	Current shelfmark: Ang. gr. 78.
80 (C.1. 11)	I.13.
	Franchi de' Cavalieri and Muccio 1896: 126-127.
	Current shelfmark: Ang. gr. 80.
90	(ff. 207r et seq.) Basilius Caesariensis, *De hominis opificio*.
	Franchi de' Cavalieri and Muccio 1896: 134-137; Piccolomini 1898: 178.
	Current shelfmark: Ang. gr. 90.

[1421]

Bibl. Barberina (Biblioteca Barberiniana [Barberini Library])

The Barberini library in Rome, which dates back to Francesco Barberini (1597-1679), was purchased in 1902 by the Biblioteca Apostolica Vaticana, where it forms the Barberiniana collection (D'Aiuto 2011: 1.338-339).

For items [1422]-[1436], the shelfmarks used in Diels' catalogue are those given to the Barberini manuscripts by Sante Pieralisi (1802-1887) sometimes around mid 19th-century (Pieralisi n.d.). These shelfmarks are no longer used. The current ones were introduced on the occasion of the transfer of the Barberini collection to the Vatican Library. For a table of concordance of Pieralisi and current shelfmarks, see Canart and Peri 1970: 112-116.

For some items ([1423], [1426]-[1429] and [1434]), Diels' catalogue adds (with or without a "=" sign) a number in Arabic numerals between parentheses. These are the so-called "segnature antiche" (old shelfmarks) of the manuscripts which date back to the 18th century and can be found in the inventories of the collection in the manuscripts *Barberiniani latini* 3137-3139. A table of concordance is provided in Canart and Peri 1970: 108-112.

In [1437] and [1439] the old shelfmark is followed by Pieralisi's shelfmark.

For item [1438], Diels seems to use these old shelfmarks. However, this number (with the content mentioned in Diels' catalogue) does not correspond to any identifiable manuscript.

For two manuscripts, Diels uses both systems of shelfmarks as if the numbers attributed to these two manuscripts in each system referred to two different items:

[1423] and [1437];

[1429] and [1439].

For one manuscript ([1425]), Diels uses Pieralisi's shelfmark. In the next item ([1426]), he uses this shelfmark followed (between parentheses) by the previous one of the same item, as if [1425] and [1426] were two different manuscripts.

[1422]   **I 5**   I.4, 13.
Capocci 1958: 6-7.
Current selfmark: *Barberinianus graecus* 5.

[1423]   **I 11 (= 136)**   I.13.
Capocci 1958: 11-12.
Current shelfmark: *Barberinianus graecus* 11.
Also [1437].

[1424]   **I 17**   N.48.
Capocci 1958: 18-19.
Current shelfmark: *Barberinianus graecus* 17.

[1425]   **I 49**   II.7.
Capocci 1958: 52-53.
Current shelfmark: *Barberinianus graecus* 49.
Also [1426].

[1426]   **I 49 (= 359)**   II.92.
Same as [1425].

[1427]   **I 72 (440)**   II.81.

This is Perzoe, *Liber physiologicus ex India translatus et Chosroe regi Persarum traditus a Perzoe etc.*

This manuscript is now *Barberinianus graecus* 72 (see Capocci 1958: 79-80).

This is not a medical work, but the *incipit* of the Byzantine novel Στεφανίτης καὶ Ἰχνελατής (*Stefanitês and Ichnelatês*) (actually the Greek translation of the Arabic tales best known as كليلة و دمنة [*Kalila wa Dimna*] in the version published by Stark 1697 and identified as number II by Puntoni 1889: III-IV), as Mercati 1916: 211 (no. 10) noted. See Capocci 1958: 80:

Quae leguntur de codice nostro et de Perzoe τῷ σοφῷ apud H. Diels (*Handschriften d. ant. Ärzte*, II, p. 81) falsa sunt, v. etiam Ioh. Mercati in *Bessarione*, XXXII, 1916, p. 211.

This manuscript was used by Puntoni 1889 to publish version IV of the novel (see pp. V-VI, XII about the manuscript, and pp. 3-47 for the edition).

See also Sjöberg 1962: 42, and Condylis-Bassoukos 1997: XXVII (where the manuscript is identified as *Barberinianus* I 72).

[1428]   **I 80 (= 273)**   I.67, 121.
Capocci 1958: 99-100.
Current shelfmark: *Barberinianus graecus* 80.

[1429]   **I 91 (382)**   II.90.
Capocci 1958: 124-125.
Current shelfmark: *Barberinianus graecus* 91.
Probably also [1439].

[1430]	**I 118**	I.67; II.33, 71.
		Capocci 1958: 163-164.
		Current shelfmark: *Barberinianus graecus* 118.
[1431]	**I 127**	I.26, 39, 40, 56, 101, 113, 117, 118, 128, 131; II.10, 15, 28, 62, 76, 80, 87, 102 (2).
		Palimpsest (Canart 2004: 47).
		Scriptio inferior: unidentified text.
		Capocci 1958: 186-218.
		Current shelfmark: *Barberinianus graecus* 127.
		Possibly also [1438].
[1432]	**I 152**	I.121.
		Capocci 1958: 263-265.
		Current shelfmark: *Barberinianus graecus* 152, part III.
[1433]	**II 58**	II.32, 62; N.57.
		Mogenet 1989: 79-83.
		Current shelfmark: *Barberinianus graecus* 237, part IV.
[1434]	**III 63 (= 245)**	I.42, 123; II.57, 64.
		Current shelfmark: *Barberinianus graecus* 344. See above, p. 54.
[1435]	**V 18**	II.67.
		Current shelfmark: *Barberinianus graecus* 522. See above, p. 54.
[1436]	**VI 5**	II.67.
		Current shelfmark: *Barberinianus graecus* 566. See above, p. 54.
[1437]	**136 (= I 11)**	I.5.
		Same as [1423].
[1438]	**276**	I.3.

This manuscript is listed as a copy of Hippocrates, *Opera varia*.

The old shelfmark 276 corresponds to current *Barberinanus* 252 which contains Eunapius and Porphyrius (Mogenet 1989: 100-101).

In the *Barberini* collection, the following items contain Hippocratic works:

- 5 ([pp. 1-83] *Aphorismi*) (Capocci 1958: 6-7);
- 11 ([ff. 1v-46v] *Aphorismi*) (Capocci 1958: 11-12);
- 127 ([f. 250v] *De sterilibus* [frg.]; [ff. 313r-332v] *Hippocratis operum fragmenta*) (Capocci 1958: 186-218);
- 220 ([ff. I-II] *Aphorismi*) (Mogenet 1989: 161);
- 272 ([ff. 143, 142r, 143r, 144] *Prorrheticum*) (Mogenet 1989: 116-117, 166).

The item referred to here could be *Barberinianus graecus* 127 (= [1431]), if it were not for the inexplicable fact that it does not correspond to ancient number 276.

[1439]   **382 (I 91)**   II.88; N.64.

The old shelfmark 382 corresponds to four manuscripts (Canart and Peri 1970: 111, sub numero 382):

- 91 (= Pieralisi I.91);
- 92 (= Pieralisi I.92);
- 132v (= Pieralisi I.132);
- 404 (= Pieralisi III.404).

From the correspondence between old and Pieralisi's shelfmarks (I.91, rightly mentioned in Diels' catalogue) and the description of the content, it appears that it is *Barberinianus* 91.

Possibly same as [1429].

Bibl. Corsiniana (= Acc. d. Lincei) (Biblioteca Corsiniana, Accademia dei Lincei [Corsiniana Library, Lincei Academy])

-

[1440]   **14 (Rossi 358)**   II.29.

Pierleoni 1901: 475-476.

Number 14 is not a shelfmark, but the sequential number in Pierleoni's list.

Current shelfmark: *Corsin.* 43. D. 32 (Rossi 358).

Agati 2007: 105-108.

[1441]   **1410 (36. E. 26)**   N.26, 28 (2), 39 (2).

Current shelfmark: *Corsin.* 36. E. 26 (1410).

Agati 2007: 127-135.

[Bibl.] Passioneian. (*Bibliotheca Passioneiana* [Passionei Library])

-

[1442]   **2**   I.68.

This is a copy of Galenus, *De usu partium* in the collection of Cardinal Domenico Passionei (1682-1786) in Rome (on which, see Serrai 2004 and Sciarra 2009).

In 1788, this collection was acquired by the Biblioteca Angelica in Rome, where this manuscript had the shelfmark C.1.5. Whereas most of the Cardinal's collection is currently at the Angelica (on which see above, pp. 270-271), some items were taken from the collection during the years 1833-1836. The copy of Galenus, *De usu partium* was among them (Sciarra 2009: 275).

The manuscript later entered the collection owned by Giovanni Francesco de Rossi (1796-1854), which was donated to the Societas Jesu by his widow in 1855. The Jesuit collection was moved from Rome to Vienna (Austria) in 1877, and relocated in the *Collegium Societatis Jesu* in 1895 in Lainz (a town in the periphery of Vienna, which was absorbed into the city as a part of its 13th district in 1890/92). The Galen manuscript had the shelfmark XI.132 (see below, under [1742]). In 1921, however, the collection was moved back to Città del Vaticano, Biblioteca Apostolica Vaticana, where this copy of Galen is now codex Ross. 982 (see p. 55). On the history of the library, see Grafinger 1997.

The number 2 attributed to the codex in Diels' catalogue does not correspond to any shelfmark of the manuscript, but probably comes from Piccolomini 1898: 182, where the manuscript is listed as number 2 among the *codices graeci Bibliothecae Angelicae deperditi* (*ibid.*: 180-184). This number is repeated by Helmreich 1907-1909: 1.XII, who identified the manuscript as a *Vaticanus Passioneianus* (probably because of the imprecision in the location of the library in Diels' catalogue ["Rom"], as for the many *Vaticani* listed in the catalogue). However, Helmreich added that he *does not know what he should think about the codex* ("Quid de reliquis codicibus, quos H. Diels ... p. 68 commemorat, ... Vaticano Passioneiano 2 ... statuendum sit, nescio"), making it clear that he did not know its location at that time.

Bibl. St. Petri (*Bibliotheca Sancti Petri* [St. Peter's Library]), now Città del Vaticano, Biblioteca Apostolica Vaticana, Archivio di San Pietro (Vatican City, San Pietro Archive)

[1443]   **H 45**   I.58.

This manuscript is now Città del Vaticano, Biblioteca Apostolica Vaticana, Archivio di San Pietro H 45 (see p. 53).

Palimpsest.

Scriptio inferior: (inter alia) Galenus, *De crisibus*;

Scriptio superior: Galenus, *Methodus medendi*.

Canart 1966: 66-71 (especially 66-68); Canart 2004: 47; Harlfinger, Brunschön and Vasiloudi 2006: 145, 152-154.

Bibl. Vallicellana [*sic*] (Biblioteca Vallicelliana [Vallicelliana Library])

Apart from the first manuscript [1444], identifiers of the manuscripts in this library in Diel's catalogue are made of two elements:

• a number in Arabic numerals;
• another made of two components: a capital letter (Latin alphabet) followed by a number in Arabic numerals.

The first identifier is not a shelfmark, but the sequential number attributed to the manuscripts in Martini 1902: 1-200 (mentioned in the list of catalogues of manuscripts consulted to compile Diels' catalogue, I.XVII). Only the second identifier is a shelfmark. This shelfmark is still used in the present day.

[1444]   **- (Allatianus)** II.68.

This manuscript listed without collection name (except its identification as "Allatianus") or precise shelfmark appears among the copies of Nepualius, *De sympathicis et antipathicis*.

No manuscript in the *Appendix Allatiana* (that is, *notulae* by Leo Allatius [ca. 1586-1669]) at the Biblioteca Vallicelliana appears to contain a text under Nepualius' name. However, codex *Allatianus* VI (on which see Martini 1902: 201-202) contains notes by Allatius on a *De sympathicis et antipathicis* treatise attributed to Democritus. The two authors and their respective works have been transmitted together in several manuscripts and sometimes mixed up in modern scholarly literature.

[1445]   **15 (B 70)**   II.11.

                                     Martini 1902: 29-30.

                                     Current shelfmark: B 70.

[1446]   **21 (B 93)**   I.72.

                                     Martini 1902: 36.

                                     Current shelfmark: B 93.

[1447]   **78 (F 9)**   II.37.

                                     Martini 1902: 128-132.

                                     Current shelfmark: F 9.

[1448]   **106 (F 83)**   I.26.

                                     Martini 1902: 186-188.

                                     Current shelfmark: F 83.

Bibl. Vaticana (Biblioteca Vaticana [Vatican Library]), actually not in Rome as in Diel's catalogue, but at Città del Vaticano and identified as Biblioteca Apostolica Vaticana (Vatican City, Vatican Apostolic Library)

Ottobon. (*Ottoboniani graeci*)

                43   (ff. 48r-50r) Gregorius Nyssenus, *De hominis opificio*.

                                     Feron and Battaglini 1893: 31-32.

                60   (ff. 13r et seq.) Zozimus Panopolita, *De sacra divinaque arte auri et argenti faciendi.*

                                     Feron and Battaglini 1893: 39-41; *CMAG* II (Zuretti et al.) 1927: 69-70.

[1449]   **89**   II.11.

                                     Feron and Battaglini 1893: 55.

                                     Possibly [1512].

                112   (ff. 33v et seq.) Theophylactus Simocatta, *Quaestiones naturales*.

                                     Feron and Battaglini 1893: 65-66.

[1450]   **129**   II.71, 72.

                                     Feron and Battaglini 1893: 75.

[1451]   **145**   II.63.

                                     Feron and Battaglini 1893: 81.

[1452]   **150**   I.13.

                                     Feron and Battaglini 1893: 83-84.

                153   (ff. 34r et seq.) *Notulae duae de medicinis purgantibus*; (ff. 83r-91v) Theophylactus Simocatta, *Quaestiones naturales* (frg.); (ff. 213r et seq.) *Opus medicum.*

                                     Feron and Battaglini 1893: 86-87.

[1453]	**157 A**	I.13.
		Feron and Battaglini 1893: 89.
[1454]	**157 B**	I.5, 13.
		Feron and Battaglini 1893: 89-90.
	167	(ff. 1r et seq.) Gregorius Nyssenus, *De hominis opificio*.
		Feron and Battaglini 1893: 94-95.
	177	(f. 59 et seq.) *De medicina*.
		Feron and Battaglini 1893: 100.
[1455]	**192**	I.5; II.94.
		Feron and Battaglini 1893: 109-113.

According to Alexanderson 1963: 63, the manuscript does not contain Hippocrates, *Prognosticon*, contrary to Diels' catalogue (I.5). In effect, the text of ff. 16r-18v (*inc.*: εἰσὶ δὲ τὰ δώδεκα ζώδια ...) has been identified as Hippocratic in a note at the end (f. 18v: ἐκ τῆς ἱπποκράτους προγνωστικῆς), whereas it is a piece of Hermes Trismegistus' corpus (*CCAG* V.4 [Weinstock] 1940: 65).

	193	(ff. 113 et seq.) Johannes Damascenus, *De medicaminibus purgantibus*.
		Feron and Battaglini 1893: 113-114; *CMAG* II (Zuretti et al.) 1927: 2-7.
	205	(ff. 258r-266r) *Physiologus*.
		Feron and Battaglini 1893: 118-120.
[1456]	**235**	II.71, 89.
		Feron and Battaglini 1893: 135.
		Also [1417].
[1457]	**259**	II.36.
		Feron and Battaglini 1893: 146.
[1458]	**275**	II.67.
		Feron and Battaglini 1893: 153.
	300	(f. 1r et seq.) Demetrius Pepagomenus, *De podagra*.
		Feron and Battaglini 1893: 162.
[1459]	**311**	I.64, 65, 80, 111; II.6, 98, 100.
		Feron and Battaglini 1893: 166.
	320	(ff. 1r et seq.) *De partibus hominis*.
		Feron and Battaglini 1893: 169.
	327	(f. Ir) *Medicamina*.
		Feron and Battaglini 1893: 172.
	338	(ff. 39r-40r) Theophylactus Simocatta, *Quaestiones naturales*.
		Feron and Battaglini 1893: 176-177 (does not mention the text).

	339	(ff. 250v-254v) Nicephorus Blemmydes, *De urinis*.
		Feron and Battaglini 1893: 177-179.
	354	Epiphanius, *Physiologus*.
		Feron and Battaglini 1893: 183.
	418	(ff. 59r et seq.) Epiphanius, *De duodecim gemmis*.
		Feron and Battaglini 1893: 229-232.
[1460]	**441**	II.20.
		Feron and Battaglini 1893: 245-248.
	459	(ff. 272r-274v) Nemesius Emesenus, *De natura hominis* (frg.).
		Feron and Battaglini 1893: 255-257.
[1461]	**464**	II.67.
		Feron and Battaglini 1893: 258.

Palat. (*Palatini graeci*)

[1462]	**13**	II.94-95.
		Stevenson 1885: 7-8.
[1463]	**31**	I.96.
		Stevenson 1885: 17.
[1464]	**48**	II.30; N.45, 49 (2).
		Stevenson 1885: 25.
	51	(ff. 155 et seq.) Nicephorus Gregoras, *In Synesii de insomniis commentarius*.
		Stevenson 1885: 26.
[1465]	**54**	I.80, 85, 93, 98.
		Stevenson 1885: 28.
	59	(ff. 207v et seq.) Synesius Cyrenensis, *De insomniis*, cum Nicephori Gregorae exegesi et anonymi glossis inter lineas.
		Stevenson 1885: 29-31.
[1466]	**77**	II.30, 32 (2), 34, 68.
		Stevenson 1885: 40-41.
	90	Gregorius Nazianzenus, *De humana natura*.
		Stevenson 1885: 43-44 (does not mention the text); Domiter 1999: 22.
	102	(ff. 103 et seq.) Johannes Damascenus, *De medicamentis purgantibus*.
		Stevenson 1885: 50.
	109	*Geoponica*.
		Stevenson 1885: 52-53.

[1467]   **126**   I.56.

Stevenson 1885: 60.

[1468]   **128**   I.13, 61, 105.

Stevenson 1885: 60-61.

[1469]   **129**   I.56.

Stevenson 1885: 61-62.

[1470]   **132**   I.38.

Stevenson 1885: 63-64.

139   (ff. 61r et seq.) Nicander, *Theriaca*; (ff. 82r et seq.) Nicander, *Alexipharmaca*.

Stevenson 1885: 70-71.

[1471]   **143**   I.5, 13, 42, 44, 81, 110, 112, 113, 124, 133, 149.

Stevenson 1885: 74.

146   (foliis praeviis) *Remedium quoddam*; (f. 216r) *Herbae planetis subiectae quae vires habeant.*

Stevenson 1885: 75-80.

147   (ff. 49v et seq.) Synesius Cyrenensis, *De insomniis*; (ff. 76v et seq.) Nicephorus Gregoras, *In Synesii de insomniis commentarius.*

Stevenson 1885: 80.

[1472]   **155**   I.41.

Stevenson 1885: 83-84.

[1473]   **157**   I.80, 89, 91, 107, 130; N.35.

Stevenson 1885: 85.

See [1474].

164   (ff. 109 et seq.) Aristoteles, *Problemata.*

Stevenson 1885: 88; Wartelle 1963: 143, no. 1941.

[1474]   **173**   I.107.

This codex is identified as a copy (ff. 1r et seq.) of Galenus, *In Hippocratis prognosticum commentarii III*, which is not the case (Stevenson 1885: 91, according to whom the codex contains Plato).

This seems to be a mistake. If this is a *Palatinus*, it might be 157 (= [1473]), which contains (ff. 2r et seq.) the Galenic commentary on the Hippocratic *Prognosticon* and which is listed in Diels for this treatise. Most probably, however, it might be a *Reginensis*, all the more because *Reginensis* 173 (= [1495]) contains the work on ff. 1r et seq., and is not mentioned in Diels' catalogue for this treatise, whereas it is (rightly so) for other works.

[1475]   **192**   I.4, 5, 8, 10 (2), 11 (2), 12, 13, 18, 19, 21, 23 (2), 26, 27 (2), 28 (2), 29 (2), 30 (3), 31 (3), 32 (3), 33, 34, 35, 38, 44, 46, 48.

Stevenson 1885: 96-97.

[1476]   **199**   I.5, 13, 61, 76, 95, 96, 149; II.6, 9; N.25 (2), 29, 30, 32 (2), 36, 37, 41, 43, 60, 61, 65, 68.

Stevenson 1885: 99-101.

207   Cassianus Bassus, *Geoponica*.

Stevenson 1885: 105.

209   (f. 57v) *Lexici botanici fragmentum*; (f. 88r) *De tribus cerebri ventriculis*; (ff. 165v et seq.) *De scientia et de quinque generibus artis medicae*; (f. 263r) *Aphorismi physici*.

Stevenson 1885: 105-108.

[1477]   **226**   II.43.

Stevenson 1885: 120-122; *CMAG* II (Zuretti et al.) 1927: 326-329.

See [1511].

[1478]   **251**   I.68.

Stevenson 1885: 138.

256   (f. 390) *Ex libris iatricis capita quaedam necessaria et utilia*; (f. 390v) *Capita quaedam ex libris Geoponicis*.

Stevenson 1885: 139-141.

261   (f. dr) Strabo, *Medicina Indorum*.

Stevenson 1885: 143-144.

[1479]   **278**   I.105.

Stevenson 1885: 153-154.

[1480]   **279**   I.13, 89, 114, 125, 133, 134; II.7, 60, 80.

Stevenson 1885: 154-156.

See [1524].

[1481]   **295**   I.89, 126.

Stevenson 1885: 165.

296   (ff. 1r-290v) *Efodia*.

Stevenson 1885: 166.

[1482]   **297**   I.13, 48, 60, 111, 130, 149; II.75.

Stevenson 1885: 166-167.

[1483]   **302**   II.89.

Stevenson 1885: 170-171.

319   (ff. 31r et seq.) Daniel propheta, *Oneirocritica*; (ff. 48r et seq.) *Ecloga Oneirocriticae*.

Stevenson 1885: 184-186.

327   (ff. 64r-123r) Gregorius Nyssenus, *De hominis opificio*.

Stevenson 1885: 189-190.

[1484]   **328**   II.95.

Stevenson 1885: 190-192.

[1485]   **358**   II.7.

Stevenson 1885: 208-210.

[1486]   **363**   I.47.

Stevenson 1885: 216-222.

              365   (ff. 1r et seq.) Michael Psellus, *De lapidum virtutibus*; (ff. 17r et seq.) Cassianus Bassus, *Geoponica*.

Stevenson 1885: 228.

              367   (ff. 50r et seq.) Epiphanius, *Physiologus*.

Stevenson 1885: 229-235.

[1487]   **370**   II.67, 110.

Stevenson 1885: 238-239.

              374   (ff. 60r et seq.) Synesius Cyrenensis, *De insomniis* cum Nicephori Gregorae commentario.

Stevenson 1885: 240-242.

[1488]   **375**   II.71.

Stevenson 1885: 242.

[1489]   **385**   I.105; II.67.

Stevenson 1885: 247-248.

[1490]   **398**   I.38.

Stevenson 1885: 254-257.

[1491]   **400**   I.46, 48, 56, 80, 86, 130, 133, 134; II.32, 48, 49 (2), 63, 80; N.49 (2).

Stevenson 1885: 257-259.

              419   (f. 78v et seq.) Hippocrates, *Epistolae*.

Stevenson 1885: 271-272.

[1492]   **428**   I.57, 128, 150; II.10, 28.

Stevenson 1885: 277-278.

Reginenses graeci Pii II

              25   (ff 66r et seq.) Basilius Caesariensis, *De hominis origine*.

Stevenson 1888: 152.

              39   (ff. 227v et seq.) Epiphanius, *De duodecim gemmis*.

Stevenson 1888: 159-161.

              47   (ff. 74v et seq.) *De mensuris et ponderibus*.

Stevenson 1888: 164-166; *CCAG* V.4 (Weinstock) 1940: 106.

Reg. Suec. (*Reginae Suecorum* [Queen of Sweden]) (*Reginenses graeci*)

	46	(ff. 63v et seq.) Epiphanius, *De duodecim gemmis*.
		Stevenson 1888; 38-40.
	71	(ff. 52 et seq.) Synesius Cyrenensis, *De insomniis*; (ff. 82r et seq.) Epiphanius, *De duodecim gemmis*.
		Stevenson 1888: 58-59.
	124	(ff. 153v et seq.) Alexander Aphrodisiensis, *Problemata iatrica*.
		Stevenson 1888: 88-89.
[1493]	**154**	I.61, 72; N.31.
		Stevenson 1888: 107.
		Also [1517].
[1494]	**172**	I.98 (2), 115.
		Stevenson 1888: 116.
[1495]	**173**	I.75, 77, 99, 101 (2), 102; N.34 (2).
		Stevenson 1888: 116-117.
		Also [1474] and [1514].
[1496]	**174**	I.92; N.33.
		Stevenson 1888: 117.
[1497]	**175**	I.69, 70, 84, 103, 107; N.35.
		Stevenson 1888: 118.
		Possibly [1515].
[1498]	**176**	II.75, 78.
		Stevenson 1888: 118-119.
[1499]	**181**	I.40, 86, 113; II.110.
		Stevenson 1888: 121-123.
		Possibly [1558].
[1500]	**182**	I.13-14, 18, 22, 23, 25, 26, 28, 29 (2), 40, 44, 46, 47; II.53.
		Stevenson 1888: 123-125.
	183	(ff. 1 et seq.) Psellus, *De arte medica*.
		Stevenson 1888: 125.

Urbin. (*Urbinates graeci*)

	12	(ff. 29 et seq.) Gregorius Nyssenus, *De hominis opificio*.
		Stornajolo 1895: 19.
	37	(f. 15) *Formula* (*ratio conficiendi cuiusdam emplastri*).
		Stornajolo 1895: 43-45.
	50	(ff. 1 et seq.) Aristoteles, *Problemata*.
		Stornajolo 1895: 53; Wartelle 1963: 148, no. 2000.

	61	(f. 127v) *Scholium de aconito.*
		Stornajolo 1895: 66-68.
[1501]	**64**	I.5, 14, 18, 21, 22, 38, 49, 56, 104; II.76; N.35, 61.
		Stornajolo 1895: 70-76.
[1502]	**65**	I.105.
		Stornajolo 1895: 76-77.
[1503]	**66**	II.30, 32 (2), 33, 39 (3).
		Stornajolo 1895: 77-80.
[1504]	**67**	I.59, 96, 98, 100, 101, 103; N.54, 66.
		Stornajolo 1895: 80-84.
[1505]	**68**	I.4, 5, 8, 10, 11 (2), 12 (2), 14, 18 (2), 19, 20 (3), 21 (2), 22 (2), 23, 24 (3), 25 (2), 26 (2), 27 (3), 28 (2), 29 (2), 30 (3), 31 (2), 33 (2), 34 (2), 35 (3), 38, 48 (2), 110, 124; II.37, 93.
		Stornajolo 1895: 84-92.
[1506]	**69**	I.68.
		Stornajolo 1895: 92-93.
[1507]	**70**	I.73, 76, 94 (2), 95, 99, 114; II.7.
		Stornajolo 1895: 93-95.
	78	(ff. 93 et seq.) Psellus, *De lapidum proprietatibus.*
		Stornajolo 1895: 106-108.
	80	(f. 165v) *Ad Chiotem medicum.*
		Stornajolo 1895: 111-127.
	99	(ff. 24v et seq.) *Physicae causae.*
		Stornajolo 1895: 152-153.
	108	(ff. 122r et seq. et 124v et seq.) Theophrastus, *De sudoribus* et *De vertigine.*
		Stornajolo 1895: 166-168.
	120	(f. 270v) *Formula remedii.*
		Stornajolo 1895: 201-204.
	125	(f. 205r-v) Gregorius Nazianzenus, *De humana natura* (frg.).
		Stornajolo 1895: 217-227.
	129	(ff. 95r et seq.) Synesius Cyrenensis, *De insomniis.*
		Stornajolo 1895: 231-233.
	140	(ff. 187v-188r) *Remedia.*
		Stornajolo 1895: 259-266.
	145	(f. 84v-112v) Nicander, *Theriaca.*
		Stornajolo 1895: 280-281.

149   Manuel Philes, *De animalium proprietate*.

Stornajolo 1895: 284-285.

152   (f. 327v) *Remedia ad alopeciam*.

Stornajolo 1895: 293-299.

[1508]   **158**   II.80.

Stornajolo 1895: 304-305.

[1509]   **294**   II.80.

This item is supposed to contain of Paulus Aegineta, *Epitome medica*, 7.25 (*De succedaneis*), on f. 296.

The *Vaticani Urbinates graeci* collection contains 165 numbers.

The manuscript referred to here is not the *Vaticanus Urbinas graecus* 294, but most probably *Vaticanus graecus* 294 (= [1538]), which contains Paul of Aegina (on f. 296 as indicated in Diels).

Mercati and Franchi de' Cavalieri 1923: 412-415.

Same as [1538].

Vatic. (*Vaticani graeci*)

[1510]   **Vatic.**   N.46.

According to Diels' catalogue, this manuscript listed without shelfmark contains S. Basilius, *Ad Eustathium medicum*. A reference is made to "Migne, patrol. gr. 32, p. 684 ff. Ep. 189"(= Migne 1857: 683/684-695/696 [columns, but not pages as in Diels]).

This is *Letter 189* of S. Basilius (= *Clavis Patrum Graecorum* 2900 for the whole collection of *Letters*), edited by Courtonne 1961: 132-141. According to Courtonne 1957: xxii, the Maurists responsible for the 1730 edition (reproduced by Migne 1857: 683/684-695/696, cited by Diels) used the *Vaticanus graecus* 434 (on which see Fedwick 1993: 53-57).

The letter is addressed to a certain *Eustathius medicus* (in the *Bibliotheca Basiliana Universalis* by Fedwick 1993: XVI, it is identified as *EustArc 2/189*, that is, Basilius' *Letter 189*, being the second addressed to *Eustathius archiater*). This letter is of dubious authenticity and may be by Gregorius Nyssenus (= *Ad Eustathium de sancta trinitate* [= *Clavis Patrum Graecorum* 3137]; edition by Mueller 1958: 1-16).

This is a theological text not medical in nature. It was probably included in Diels' catalogue because of the medical profession of its recipient.

[1511]   [-]   II.41.

This manuscript listed without shelfmark is a copy of Harpocration, *De facultatibus naturalibus animalium et herbarum et lapidum*.

The only Vatican manuscript containing such text seems to be *Palatinus graecus* 226 (= [1477]) f. 194 (Stevenson 1885: 120-122).

Possibly same as [1477].

[1512]   **- (Puschm. I p. 89)**   II.12.

According to Diels' catalogue, this manuscript without precise identification is a copy of Alexander Trallianus, *Epistula de lumbricis*.

The reference is to Puschmann 1878-1879.

This item seems to be *Ottobonianus graecus* 89 (= [1449]).

Feron and Battaglini 1893: 55, which lists Alexander Trallianus, *Opera* without further precision.

[1513]   **? (Vgl. Daremb. I p. LVIII und 124)**   II.108.

This manuscript listed without shelfmark in Diels'catalogue is supposed to be a copy of Xenocrates, *De alimento ex aquatilibus*.

The reference is to Bussemaker and Daremberg, *Oeuvres d'Oribase*, tome 1 (1851). On p. LVIII, a Vatican manuscript is identified as follows:

Vᵃ. Ms. soi-disant du Vatican. Mêmes remarques que pour le précédent.

The previous manuscript referred to ("le précédent") is a manuscript of Paris cited at the same page, about which Bussemakers provides the following information:

Ms. ... qui n'existe plus ... Les variantes recueillies par un anonyme se trouvent dans les éditions de Franz et d'Ancora.

The editions referred to are those by Johann Georg Friedrich Franz (1737-1789) (Leipzig: Sommer, 1774 [with a second print in 1779]) and Gaetano d'Ancora (1751-1816) (Neapoli: regiis typis, 1794).

No further information is provided in Daremberg p. 124 (beginning of the edition of the text [Greek with French translation]), contrary to what Diels' reference to this page suggests.

Franz 1779: ff. *5v-[*6]r, provides the following information about the Vatican manuscript:

Casu quodam fortuito, nobis hanc curantibus editionem, in manus inciderunt variae lectiones a Viro quodam docto ad marginem editionis Gesneri ubi reliqua graeci textus verba, quae apud Gesneri desiderantur, erant adscripta, ex Codice Regio Parisiensi et Vaticano notatae ... de codice Vaticano simul Xenocratis libellum περὶ λίθων ... comprehendente, nihil nobis constat; nec praeter Labbei** relationem aliquid de eo reperire potuimus.

Note **: v. Labbei Bibl. Nou. MSS. p. 174 et 127.

The references are to Gessner, 1559 (on which see Wellisch 1975: 213, no. 28, and 1984: 87-88, no. 48), and Labbé 1653: 127-128 (without mention of a Vatican manuscript) and 174 (where Xenocratis, *De alimento ex aquatilibus* and *De lapidibus* are listed with the information "in Vaticana").

Variant readings of this Vatican manuscript are found in Franz 1779 in the footnotes *passim* (see for example, pp. 7, 8, 16, 19, 21, 23, 27, 29, 31, 32, 33, 34, 35, 36, 38, 40, 41, 53, 57, 62, 64, 69, 71, 73, 82, 83, 92, 93, 96, 97, 99, 101, 102 and 103).

d'Ancora 1794: VIII-IX, commented on Franz' s Vatican manuscript as follows:

... nimiam certe praestavit fidem variis lectionibus, quas invenisse dicit a viro quodam docto ad marginem editionis Gesneri adscriptas ex Mss. ... Vaticanae. Haud enim ignorabat Franzius neminem post Labbeum vidisse, aut memorasse Codicem Vaticanum, et ne nobis quidem ... de eo codice nullum indicium detegere fas fuit ...

d'Ancora nevertheless reproduces in the footnotes of his edition the variant readings cited by Franz as coming from the Vatican manuscript (see, for example, pp. 10, 25, 26, 29, 39, 40, 44, 45, 48, 49, 51, 71, 72, 78, 84, 87, 93, 98, 99, 107, 109, 114, 118, 120, 121, 122, 123, 125, 126, 128, 131, 132).

It is unclear whether this is a manuscript now lost (according to Daremberg cited in Diels), a mistake (possibly by Labbé), or a forgery (by Franz [?], possibly on the basis of a mistake in Labbé 1653: 174 [?]), as no manuscript of Xenocrates' text seems to be available or traceable at any point in time among the holdings of the Vatican Library.

In spite of d'Ancora, some 19th-century bibliographies and encyclopedias still mention that a manuscript of Xenocrates' work can be found in the Vatican Library (see for example, Hoffmann 1836: 771, and the *Penny cyclopedia* 1843: 620).

[1514]   **[apud Montfauc. p. 28]**   I.135.

This item listed without shelfmark is Galenus, *De hominis natura*.

The reference is to Montfaucon 1739: 1.28, where manuscripts of the Vatican Library are listed, specifically the manuscripts from Christina, Queen of Sweden (see Montfaucon 1739: 1.14 "Incipit Catalogus Manuscriptorum Codicum Bibliothecae Reginae Sueciae in Vaticana").

Montfaucon 1739: 1.28 lists one item containing the following:

649. Ejusdem (i.e. Galenus [see no. 648]) Prognosticon de diaeta in acutis, de Sanitate fruenda & de natura hominis.

Whereas the information in Diels' catalogue does not allow for any identification, the description provided by Montfaucon suggests that this manuscript is the current *Vaticanus Reginensis graecus* 173 (= [1495]) as its contents indicate (Stevenson 1888: 116-117):

- Galenus, *In Hippocratis Prognosticon commentariorum libri III*;
- Galenus, *De antidotis libri II*;
- Galenus, *In Hippocrates de diaeta in morbis acutis librum commentarii quattuor*;
- Galenus, *In librum Hippocratis de natura humana commentarii II*;
- Galenus, *In librum Hippocratis de victu salutari commentarius*;
- Galenus, *De sanitate tuenda*;
- [Galenus], *De ptisana*.

Same as [1495].

[1515]   **[ap. Montfaucon p. 34 (de motu animalium)]**   I.121.

According to Diels' catalogue, this is Galenus, *De animalibus*.

The reference is to Montfaucon 1739: 1.34, where manuscripts of the Vatican Library are listed, specifically the manuscripts from Christina, Queen of Sweden (see Montfaucon 1739: 1.14 "Incipit Catalogus Manuscriptorum Codicum Bibliothecae Reginae Sueciae in Vaticana").

Montfaucon 1739: 1.34 lists one item containing the following texts:

947. Galenus in prognostica Hipocratis [*sic*]. Item in Hippocratem de praedictionibus. Item de difficultate respirationis & motu animalium.

Based on this description, it appears that the item referred to here may be the *Vaticanus Reginensis graecus* 175 (= [1497]), which contains the following texts (Stevenson 1888: 118):

- Galenus, *In Hippocratis Prognosticon commentarii III*;

- Galenus, *In Hippocratis Prorrheticon commentarii III*;

- Galenus, *De difficili respiratione*;

- Galenus, *De respirationis causis*;

- Galenus, *De musculorum motu*.

The reference to Galenus, *De motu animalium* in Montfaucon 1739 is probably a mistake for Galenus, *De musculorum motu*. If so, Diels' information might be a further transformation of Montfaucon's incorrect title.

[1516]

12	II.89 (2), 91, 95.	
	Mercati and Franchi de' Cavalieri 1923: 7-10.	
15	(ff. 240r et seq.) Nicephorus Gregoras, *Explicatio in Synesii de insomniis*.	
	Mercati and Franchi de' Cavalieri 1923: 11-14; *CMAG* II (Zuretti et al.) 1927: 145.	
38	(ff. 187v et seq.) Rufus, *De corporis appellationibus*.	
	Mercati and Franchi de' Cavalieri 1923: 34-35.	
64	(ff. 121v et seq.) Synesius Cyrenensis, *De insomniis*.	
	Mercati and Franchi de' Cavalieri 1923: 58-60.	
91	(ff. 66r et seq.) Synesius Cyrenensis, *De insomniis*.	
	Mercati and Franchi de' Cavalieri 1923: 103-104.	
92	(ff. 146r et seq.) Synesius Cyrenensis, *De insomniis*.	
	Mercati and Franchi de' Cavalieri 1923: 104-105.	
94	(ff. 142r et seq.) Synesius Cyrenensis, *De insomniis*.	
	Mercati and Franchi de' Cavalieri 1923: 107.	
109	(ff. III-IV) Nicander, *Theriaca*, vv. 61-66, 71-117 and 122-139.	
	A bifolium from *Parisinus graecus* 2315 (= [1262]).	
	Mercati and Franchi de' Cavalieri 1923: 129-130 (on the manuscript) and XXV (Addenda ad cod. 109, p. 129, on Nicander's text).	

111   (ff. 298v et seq.) Iohannes Zacharias Actuarius, *De spiritu animali*.

Mercati and Franchi de' Cavalieri 1923: 132-133.

112   (ff. 13r et seq.) Hippocrates, *Epistulae*, 17.

Mercati and Franchi de' Cavalieri 1923: 134-136.

[1517]   **154**   I.72; N.31.

This is a copy of Galenus, *Quod animi mores*.

Information at I.72 is corrected at N.31 (with a reference to "Müller, Galeni Scripta minora II p. XXXIV" [= Müller 1891]).

Contrary to Müller, this item is not *Vaticanus graecus* 154 (which contains a *Chronicon usque ad Iustiniani imperium* ...; see Mercati and Franchi de' Cavalieri 1923: 176-177), but *Reginensis graecus* 154 (= [1493]) mentioned in Diels' catalogue for the same treatise.

[1518]   **178**   II.17.

Mercati and Franchi de' Cavalieri 1923: 204-206 *CMAG* II (Zuretti et al.) 1927: 145-146.

184   (f. IVr [?]) Hermes Trismegistus, *Iatromathematica*.

Mercati and Franchi de' Cavalieri 1923: 210-212.

191   (ff. 240v-248r) *Astrologica de vita et similia*.

Mercati and Franchi de' Cavalieri 1923: 220-227. Also *CCAG* V.2 (Kroll) 1906: 3-23 for the whole manuscript, and 14-15 for the text.

207   (f. 1r) *Remedia*; (f. 116v) *Remedium*; (f. 366v) *Nomina plantarum*.

Mercati and Franchi de' Cavalieri 1923: 249-254; Touwaide 1999: 215, 228.

211   (f. 160r) *Notulae medicae*.

Mercati and Franchi de' Cavalieri 1923: 264-269 (especially 268).

213   (f. 105v) *Remedia*.

Mercati and Franchi de' Cavalieri 1923: 275-277.

215   (ff. 1r et seq.) Hero, *Geoponica*; (ff. 24r et seq.) Cassianus Bassus, *Geoponica*.

Mercati and Franchi de' Cavalieri 1923: 278-279.

216   (ff. 10v, 12v-13r) Aetius Amidenus, *Libri medicinales*, 3.34; (ff. 41r et seq.) Cassianus Bassus, *Geoponica*.

Mercati and Franchi de' Cavalieri 1923: 279-282.

[1519]   **[216]**   I.22, 34.

This manuscript is supposed to contain the following two Hippocratic works:

- *De flatibus* (1.22)
- *De ossium natura* (1.34).

The same information appears in Ackermann 1825 (without brackets):

- CXL, no. 29 (*De flatibus*), with the following source "memorat Foësius in not. in libr. de ossium natura"
- CLIV, no. 38 ctd. (*De ossium natura*).

The current *Vaticanus graecus* 216 (above) does not contain these works, but rather (ff. 41r et seq.) the *Geoponica* (Mercati and Franchi de' Cavalieri 1923: 279-282).

The manuscript referred to here is probably *Vaticanus graecus* 278 (= [1523]) identified in Mercati and Franchi de' Cavalieri 1923: 369, as "olim 216", in which the two treatises can be read (Mercati and Franchi de' Cavalieri 1923: 369-372):

- (f. 520r et seq.) *De flatibus*;
- (ff. 542v et seq.) *De ossium natura*.

The *Vaticanus graecus* 278 is correctly listed among the manuscripts of these two treatises in Diels' catalogue.

223	(ff. 147r et seq.) Epiphanius, *De duodecim gemmis*.
	Mercati and Franchi de' Cavalieri 1923: 290-292.
224	(ff. 241v et seq.) Epiphanius, *De duodecim gemmis*; (f. 303v) *Remedia*.
	Mercati and Franchi de' Cavalieri 1923: 292-295.
246	(ff. 257r et seq.) Nicephorus Blemmydes, *De corpore*.
	Mercati and Franchi de' Cavalieri 1923: 319-324.
256	(ff. 422r et seq.) Nicephorus Blemmydes, *De corpore*.
	Mercati and Franchi de' Cavalieri 1923: 334-337.
260	(ff. 184r et seq.) Aristoteles, *De insomniis*.
	Mercati and Franchi de' Cavalieri 1923: 340-341; Wartelle 1963: 127, no. 1707.
261	(ff. 128 et seq.) Aristoteles, *De vaticinatione per somnum*.
	Mercati and Franchi de' Cavalieri 1923: 342-343; Wartelle 1963: 127, no. 1708.
264	(ff. 458r et seq. [?]) *Animi ne an corporis adfectiones sint peiores*.
	Mercati and Franchi de' Cavalieri 1923: 344-347.
267	(ff. 261r et seq.) Nicephorus Blemmydes, *De corpore*.
	Mercati and Franchi de' Cavalieri 1923: 351-352.

[1520]   **269**   I.115.

This manuscript is listed among the copies of Galenus, *De ponderibus et mensuris*.

The *Vaticanus graecus* 269 contains commentaries on Aristotelian works and Theocritus, *Syrinx* (Mercati and Franchi de' Cavalieri 1923: 353-356).

This is a mistake, most probably for *Vaticanus graecus* 296 (= 1540]), which contains on ff. 475 et seq. Galenus, *De succedaneis* and *De ponderibus et mensuris* (see Mercati and Franchi de' Cavalieri 1923: 416).

Probably the same as [1540].

[1521]	**276**	I.4, 5, 8, 10 (2), 11 (2), 12, 14, 18 (2), 19, 21, 23, 27 (2), 28 (2), 29, 30 (3), 31 (3), 32 (3), 33, 34, 38, 57.

Mercati and Franchi de' Cavalieri 1923: 362-365.

[1522]	277	I.4, 5, 8, 10, 11 (2), 12 (2), 14, 18 (2), 19, 20 (3), 21 (2), 22, 23 (2), 24 (3), 25 (2), 26 (2), 27 (3), 28 (2), 29 (2), 30 (3), 31 (2), 33 (2), 34 (2), 35 (3), 38, 57, 110; II.37, 93.

Mercati and Franchi de' Cavalieri 1923: 365-369.

[1523]	278	I.4, 5, 8, 10, 11 (2), 12 (2), 14, 18 (2), 19, 20 (3), 21 (2), 22, 23 (2), 24 (3), 25 (2), 26 (2), 27 (3), 28 (2), 29 (2), 30 (3), 31 (2), 33 (2), 34 (2), 35 (3), 38, 48; II.93.

Mercati and Franchi de' Cavalieri 1923: 369-372.

Also [1519].

[1524]	279	I.14, 105, 114, 117, 134; II.59, 60 (2), 80.

This item is listed among the copies of the following works (in the order they are cited in Diels' catalogue; references to Diels' catalogue follows the folio numbers):

- Hippocrates, *Aphorismi*, f. 95 (I.14);
- *Hippocratis Aphorismi et Galeni in eos commentarii VII*, f. 31 (I.105);
- Galenus, *De succedaneis*, f. 237 (I.114);
- Galenus, *Lexicon botanicum*, f. 237 (I.117);
- Galenus, *De venae sectione*, f. 213 (I.134);
- Magnus Emesenus, *Prognostica*, f. 280 (II.59);
- Magnus Emesenus, *De urinis ex ore Theophili*, f. 280 (II.60);
- Magnus Emesenus, *De febribus*, f. 280 (II.60);
- Paulus Aegineta, *Excerpta varia*, f. 214 (II.80).

In Diels' catalogue, this manuscript is considered lost ("Verbleib unbekannt" or "Hic codex deest"). At II.80, however, the information *Hic codex deest* is followed by the following: "Verwechslung mit Palat. 279?".

According to Stevenson 1885: 154-156, the *Vaticanus Palatinus graecus* 279 (= [1480]) contains some of the texts referred to here as being contained in the *Vaticanus graecus* 279 (titles are listed below according to the order of folios):

- (ff. 1r et seq.) Hippocrates, *Aphorismi*, et Galenus, *Commentarium*;
- (f. 212v) *De phlebotomia ex Galeno*;
- (f. 266r) *Ex Galeno, De succedaneis*;
- (f. 271r) *Lexicon botanicum*;
- (f. 280v) Magnus Emesenus, *De urinis*;
- (f. 312v) *De febrium diagnosi et curatione ex Aetii libris*.

On the basis of this comparison, it is by no means certain that the manuscript referred to here has been confused with the *Vaticanus graecus* 279, even though the *Vaticanus* has been moved into the *Palatina* collection for a certain period of time and was thought to be lost (Mercati and Franch de' Cavalieri 1923: 378, last paragraph on the *Vaticanus* 279). At any rate, the *Vaticanus graecus* 279 contains the texts listed in Diels' catalogue, and several others not listed, and thus needs to be taken into consideration.

On the *Vaticanus*, see Mercati and Franchi de' Cavalieri 1923: 372-378; on the *Palatinus*, see Stevenson 1885: 154-156.

Also [1557].

[1525]	**280**	I.14, 105, 113, 128; II.50, 60, 63, 88, 102.
		Mercati and Franchi de' Cavalieri 1923: 378-384.
[1526]	**281**	I.87, 88 (2), 89.
		Mercati and Franchi de' Cavalieri 1923: 384.
[1527]	**282**	I.64 (2), 65, 84, 89, 91; II.6, 55; N.30, 33, 55.
		Mercati and Franchi de' Cavalieri 1923: 384-391.
[1528]	**283**	I.5, 20, 33, 78, 83, 95, 105, 109, 112; II.75.
		Mercati and Franchi de' Cavalieri 1923: 391-393.
[1529]	**284**	II.30, 32, 34, 85; N.34, 43, 48, 49 (2), 64.
		Mercati and Franchi de' Cavalieri 1923: 393-394.
[1530]	**285**	I.47, 61, 68 (2), 73, 78, 80, 81 (2), 82, 96, 101; II.49, 98.
		Mercati and Franchi de' Cavalieri 1923: 395-400.
[1531]	**286**	II.17, 18 (2), 19.
		Mercati and Franchi de' Cavalieri 1923: 400-401.
[1532]	**287**	II.71.
		Mercati and Franchi de' Cavalieri 1923: 401-403.
[1533]	**288**	II.71.
		Mercati and Franchi de' Cavalieri 1923: 403.
[1534]	**289**	II.30; N.49 (2).
		Mercati and Franchi de' Cavalieri 1923: 403-405.
[1535]	**290**	II.32; N.49.
		Mercati and Franchi de' Cavalieri 1923: 405.
[1536]	**291**	II.88, 89; N.64.
		Mercati and Franchi de' Cavalieri 1923: 405-406.

292   (ff. 1r et seq.) Theophanus [Chrysobalantes], *De curatione morborum*; (ff. 68v et seq.) Theophanus [Chrysobalantes], *Synopsis remediorum*; (ff. 104r et seq.) Theophanus [Chrysobalantes], *De victus ratione*; (ff. 114r et seq.) Galenus, *De compositione medicamentorum secundum locos*, liber 8 (frg.); (ff. 117r et seq.) Galenus, *De urinis*; (f. 119r) *Alia expositio de urinis*; (ff. 119v et seq.) *De excrementis*; (ff. 120r et seq.) *Distinctiones de humano corpore*; (ff. 122r et seq.) Galenus,

De pulsibus; (f. 127r-v) Galenus, *De methodo medendi* 16.15; (ff. 128r et seq.) Meletius, *De natura hominis*; (ff. 179v et seq.) Galenus, *Introductio* (frg.); (f. 183v) *De hominis septem aetatibus*; (ff. 184r et seq.) *De olii preparatione*; (ff. 189r et seq.) Hippocrates, *Prognosticum* (frg.); (ff. 220r et seq.) *Formulae medicinarum xenonis*; (ff. 211 et seq.) Avicenna, *De urinis*; (ff. 233r et seq.) Mercurius, *De pulsibus*; (ff. 235r et seq.) Psellus, *De alimentorum facultatibus*; (ff. 279r et seq.) *De alimentis*.

Mercati and Franchi de' Cavalieri 1923: 406-409.

[1537]	**293**	I.41; II.55.

Mercati and Franchi de' Cavalieri 1923: 409-412.

[1538]	**294**	I.5, 8, 14, 117; II.80.

Mercati and Franchi de' Cavalieri 1923: 412-415.

Also [1509].

[1539]	**295**	II.15, 78.

Mercati and Franchi de' Cavalieri 1923: 415.

[1540]	**296**	I.114; II.78.

Mercati and Franchi de' Cavalieri 1923: 416.

Probably also [1520].

[1541]	**297**	II.6; N.43.

Mercati and Franchi de' Cavalieri 1923: 416-421; *CMAG* II (Zuretti et al.) 1927: 325-326.

[1542]	**298**	II.6, 8; N.43.

Mercati and Franchi de' Cavalieri 1923: 421-425.

[1543]	**299**	II.4 (2), 7, 26, 27, 33, 38, 42, 65, 68, 78, 109, 110; N.42 (2), 43, 56, 57, 59, 62.

Mercati and Franchi de' Cavalieri 1923: 425-430.

[1544]	**300**	I.91 II.20, 40.

Mercati and Franchi de' Cavalieri 1923: 430-437.

	305	(ff. 139r-170v) Nicander, *Theriaca cum glossis et scholiis*.

Mercati and Franchi de' Cavalieri 1923: 443-450.

	307	(f. 5r) *Excerpta medica varia*.

Mercati and Franchi de' Cavalieri 1923: 454-456.

	316	Palimpsest (Canart 2004: 50).

(f. IIIv) Fragmenta medica.

Scriptio inferior: Philo Iudaeus, *Opera*.

Mercati and Franchi de' Cavalieri 1923: 467-474.

	342	(ff. 274r-275r) *Quaestiones et responsiones diversae de homine*; (f. 280r) *De somniis*.

Devreesse 1937: 15-18.

	344	(f. 16r-v) Theophanes [Chrysobalantes], *De curatione morborum* (frg.).
		Devreesse 1937: 19-21.
	386	(f. 216v) Galenus, *De simplicium medicamentorum temperamentis et facultatibus*, liber 7 (frg.).
		Devreesse 1937: 81.
	405	(ff. 116r-203v) Gregorius Nyssenus, *De hominis opificio*.
		Devreesse 1937: 108-109.
	406	(ff. 103r-173v) Gregorius Nyssenus, *De hominis opificio*.
		Devreesse 1937: 109-110.
	407	(ff. 121r-199r) Gregorius Nyssenus, *De hominis opificio*.
		Devreesse 1937: 110-111.
	408	(ff. 92v-161v) Gregorius Nyssenus, *De hominis opificio*.
		Devreesse 1937: 111-112.
	413	(ff. 375v-413r) Gregorius Nyssenus, *De hominis opificio*.
		Devreesse 1937: 120-122.
[1545]	**423**	II.67.
		Devreesse 1937: 138-141.
[1546]	**429**	II.100, 109.
		Devreesse 1937: 149-151.
	435	(ff. 259r-266r) Synesius Cyrenensis, *De insomniis*.
		Devreesse 1937: 165-170.
	449	(ff. 1r-42r) Gregorius Nyssenus, *De hominis opificio*.
		Devreesse 1937: 199-200.
	482	(ff. 126v-130r) Gregorius Nazianzenus, *De humana natura*; (f. 145r) *De capitis morbis*.
		Devreesse 1937: 284-290; Domiter 1999: 22.
	483	(ff. 76v-103r) Nicephorus Blemmydes, *De corpore*.
		Devreesse 1937: 290-293.
	488	(f. 98r) Meletius, *De natura hominis* (frg.).
		Devreesse 1937: 301-304.
[1547]	**489**	II.67.
		Devreesse 1937: 304-305.
	491	(ff. 110r, 121r-v, 187r) Gregorius Nyssenus, *De hominis opificio* (frg.); (f. 114r) Nemesius Emesenus, *De natura hominis* (frg.).
		Devreesse 1937: 307-310.

495   Palimpsest.

Scriptio inferior: Aetius Amidenus, *Libri medicinales*; Paulus Aegineta, *Epitome medica*.

Scriptio superior: Johannes Damascenus, *Dialectica* (also below about f. 229r)

Canart 2004: 46; Harlfinger, Brunschön and Vasiloudi 2006: 145, 157-158.

Scriptio superior: (f. 229r) Gregorius Nyssenus, *De hominis opificio* (frg.).

Devreesse 1937: 316-321 (esp. 320).

497   (ff. 267r-268v) Gregorius Nazianzenus, *De humana natura*.

Devreesse 1937: 323-330; Domiter 1999: 22.

[1548]   **517**   II.108.

This manuscript appears among the copies of Ioannes Zacharias Actuarius, *Opera varia*.

According to Devreesse 1937: 372-373, it contains Iohannes Chrysostomus, *In Genesim Homiliae*.

In Diels' catalogue, reference is made to "Costomiris, Rev. des ét. gr. X p. 435" (that is, Costomiris 1897), where the following can be read:

Actuarius graecus ... 517 ... Bibliotheca Alexandri Petavii in Vaticana, dont la plus grande partie se trouve, à Rome, dans la Bibl. Reginae Sueciae in Vaticana

with a note referring to Montfaucon, Bibl. mss., p. 92, e.

The reference is to Montfaucon 1739, 1.92, where the following entry can be read:

Actuarius Graecus. 1191, 1194, 517.

This entry appears under "Anonymi" (*ibid.*) in the catalogue of the manuscripts once owned by Alexander Petau (d. 1672) entitled as follows (Montfaucon 1739: 1.61):

Catalogus alphabeticus Manuscriptorum Codicum qui extabant in Bibliotheca Alexandri Petavii, ac deinde divenditi in Sueciam sunt transportati, nunc autem plurimâ parte asservantur Romae in Bibliotheca Reginae Sueciae. 1660.

For the catalogue see Montfaucon 1739: 1.61-96 with *Addenda* at 1.96-97.

Alexander Petau has catalogued his own manuscripts (ed. de Meyïer 1947: 172-175). Three Actuarius entries are listed (de Meyïer 1947: 174, no. 151).

According to de Meyïer 1947: 174 note ad no. 151, one of them is current manuscript Glasgow, Hunterian Museum, U.5.11 (= [0387]). Another may be the copy of Actuarius in the collection of the Queen of Sweden Christina now at the Vatican Library (see [1499]). The Leiden library currently contains one copy of Actuarius: Voss. gr. F. 32 (= [0512]). However, this item does not seem to have been owned by either Alexander Petau or his father Paul (1568-1614). The third copy of Actuarius could be the present item 517, the location of which is unknown.

See [1567] and [1568].

	572	(f. 275r-v) *Remedium et preces.*
		Devreesse 1937: 462-469.
	573	(ff. 120r-213v) Achmet, *Oneirocriticon*; (f. 214r-v) *Oneirocriticon aliud.*
		Devreesse 1937: 469-477.
[1549]	**578**	II.75.
		Devreesse 1937: 486-490.
	579	(f. 198v) *Iatrica.*
		Devreesse 1937: 490-496.
	633	Palimpsest (Canart 2004: 46).
		Scriptio inferior: unidentified text.
		Scriptio superior: (f. 136v) Lucas, *Sales.*
		Devreesse 1950: 43-50.
	662	(ff. 221v-225v) Gregorius Nyssenus, *De hominis opificio* (frg.).
		Devreesse 1950: 98-105.
[1550]	**671**	II.54.
		Devreesse 1950: 117-122.
[1551]	**690**	I.41.
		Devreesse 1950: 154-160.
[1552]	**695**	I.135; II.35.
		Devreesse 1950: 169-172.
	698	(f. 101r-v) Epiphanius, *De duodecim gemmis.*
		Devreesse 1950: 174-176.
	703	(f. 293r-v) Epiphanius, *De duodecim gemmis.*
		Devreesse 1950: 181-186.
	728	(ff. 270v-311r) Gregorius Nyssenus, *De hominis opificio* (frg.).
		Devreesse 1950: 229-230.
	753	(f. 320r) Epiphanius, *De mensuris et ponderibus* (frg.).
		Devreesse 1950: 268-269.
	790	(ff. 57v-58v) *De insomniis*; (ff. 151r-156r) Epiphanius, *De mensuris et ponderibus.*
		Devreesse 1950: 307-314.
	847	(f. 272v) *Remedium*; (ff. 279v-281v) *Medica varia anonyma* (*Infirmorum habitus per singulos mensis dies*; *De phlebotomia*; *De urinis*; *Remedia*).
		Devreesse 1950: 405-407.

[1553]   **854**   II.95.

Devreesse 1950: 415-418.

[1554]   **855**   II.95.

Devreesse 1950: 418-419.

[1555]   **876**   I.41; II.74.

Schreiner 1988: 30-32.

905   (f. 1v) *Confectio medicinae kleidion.*

Schreiner 1988: 98-100.

914   (f. 187v) *Remedia in lunaticos.*

Schreiner 1988: 116-125; *CMAG* II (Zuretti et al.) 1927: 147-149.

927   (ff. 240v-259v) Synesius Cyrenensis, *De insomniis.*

Schreiner 1988: 162-165.

951   (pp. 205-207) Hermes Trismegistus, *Ad Asclepium de plantis duodecim zodiacis signorum.*

Devreesse 1965: 156, no. 47; 239, no. 39; 317 (paragraph between nos. 39 and 40).

[1556]   **952**   II.43.

This manuscript is listed as a copy of Hermes Trismegistus, *Canon.*

According to Allaci 1614-1630: 555-557, it contains the following:

(pp. 1 et seq.) Maximus Planudes, *De urinis;* (pp. 184 et seq.) *Medicinalia varia.*

See, however, *CCAG* V.4 (Weinstock) 1940: 8-12 (which records [p. 11] Hermes Trismegistus on f. 184v) and 118-120; *CCAG* VIII.2 (Ruelle) 1911: 166-171; *CMAG* II (Zuretti et al.) 1927: 149-152.

984   Palimpsest.

Scriptio superior: Flavius Josephus, *Antiquitates iudaicae* et *De bello iudaico.*

Scriptio media: Galenus, *De locis affectis.*

Scriptio infima: Hagiographico-homiletica.

Canart 2004: 46; Harlfinger, Brunschön and Vasiloudi 2006: 145, 155.

CMAG II (Zuretti et al.) 1927: 329-330; Turyn 1964: 149-150.

See also *Vaticanus graecus* 1882 (see p. 303).

[1557]   **1028**   I.92.

According to Diels' catalogue, this manuscript contains on f. Ir "Lib. X c. 10 vel exc. ex hoc capite" of Galenus, *Methodus medendi.*

However, according to Amati et al. 1800-1834: f. 21r-v, it contains Aristoteles, *De physica auscultatione* (also Wartelle 1963: 131, no. 1767). Nevertheless, according to Amati et al. 1800-1834: f. 21v, the codex includes the following:

Subiciuntur non numeratae chartae tres ... Galeni περὶ δυνάμεως τῶν τροφῶν ... et aliud περὶ ἐκτικῶν πυρετῶν.

A handwritten note pencilled by a modern hand in the manuscript in the upper margin of f. I' recto reads as follows:

Ff. I-III, quae e Vatic. 279 avolsa fuerant, in suum locum reposita sunt m. aprili an. 1918.

These folios are indeed in manuscript *Vaticanus graecus* 279 (= [1524]), as Mercati and Franchi de' Cavalieri 1923: 378 already mention.

[1558]   **1052**   II.108.

Whereas this codex is listed as a copy of *Opera varia* by Ioannes Zacharias Actuarius, it actually contains Theon Alexandrinus, *Commentarius in Ptolemaei expeditos canones*, and Isaac Argyrus, *Tabellae astronomicae novae*.

Amati et al. 1800-1834: f. 54r. Also Tihon 1992: 49.

In Diels' catalogue, reference is made to "Costomiris, Rev. des ét. gr. X p. 435". In Costomiris 1897, the paragraph on this manuscript reads as follows:

«1052. Actuarii opera Medica graeca. Item alia opera Medica quae Galeni esse videatur.» Il existe dans la Bibliotheca Reginae Sueciae in Vaticana.

This paragraph includes a footnote referring to "Montfaucon, Bibl. mss., p. 36, c.", that is, Montfaucon 1739: 1.36, where the description provided by Costomiris above does appear in the "Catalogus Manuscriptorum Codicum Bibliothecae Regiae Sueciae in Vaticana" (see Montfaucon 1739: 1.14 for the title; 1.14-61 for the catalogue; and 1.36 for the present item).

Number 1052 is not a shelfmark but a sequential number in Montfaucon's list of manuscripts of Queen Christina of Sweden in the Vaticana (Montfaucon 1739: 1.14-61).

The only codex of Actuarius in the collection of the Queen of Sweden seems to be the *Reginensis graecus* 181 (= [1499]) (see Stevenson 1888: 206 *sub nomine*).

[1559]   **1062**   II.104.

                                  Ihm 2002: 214.

[1560]   **1063**   I.78, 107, 109, 112; N.35.

                                  Palimpsest (Canart 2004: 46).

                                  Scriptio inferior: unidentified text.

                                  Fortuna 1997: 14-15; Ihm 2002: 113.

[1561]   **1064**   I.87, 88 (2), 89.

                                  Amati et al. 1800-1834: ff. 43v-44r.

[1562]   **1065**   I.41.

This manuscript appears in the list of the copies of Hippocrates, *Ad Ptolemaeum regem epistula.*

Its contents are not identified in Amati et al. 1800-1834, f. 44v, as the manuscript no longer was in the Vatican collections at that time ("desideratur"). Nevertheless, as a further note mentions, it has been returned to the Vatican library from Paris ("Parisiis redux").

CCAG V.4 (Weinstock) 1940: 14.

[1563]   **1066**   I.40, 96, 113; II.43; N.36, 52.

According to Diels' catalogue, this manuscript contains the following four texts (listed below according to the order of folios; references to Diels' catalogue follow the titles):

• Hippocrates, *Epistula de hominis fabrica*, f. 7v (I.40);

• Hermes Trismegistus, *Methodus*, f. 18 (II.43; cfr. v. N.52: f. 18v);

• Galenus, *Prognosticum*, f. 78 (I.113; cfr. N.36);

• Galenus, *De simplicium medicamentorum temperamentis et facultatibus*, ff. 168 and 169 (I.96).

According to Amati et al. 1800-1834, ff. 55v-46v, it contains these texts on ff. 7v, 18r, 78r and 169r, respectively, together with several others that are medical in nature.

CCAG V.1 (Cumont and Boll) 1904: 74-79; see also 239-240.

1085   (ff. 187v-191v) Hippocrates, *Epistulae.*

The contents of the manuscript are not listed in Amati et al. 1800-1834, f. 61v, as it was no longer in the library at that time ("Desideratur. Parisiis").

The manuscript has been returned to the Vatican Library since then, and does contain the text.

See Dilts et al. 1998: 43, no. 340 46.

[1564]   **1095**   I.41.

Amati et al. 1800-1834: 69r-70v.

[1565]   **1133**   I.49; II.37.

Amati et al. 1800-1834: 108r.

[1566]   **1174**   II.24, 27, 41, 95, 96, 100, 112; N.48.

Amati et al. 1800-1834: 157v-158v; Berthelot and Ruelle 1888: 191-193; Martelli 2011: 46-54.

[1567]   **1191**   II.108.

This manuscript is listed among the copies of Ioannes Zacharias Actuarius, *Opera varia.*

According to Amati et al. 1800-1834: 221v, it contains Theophylactus Bulgarus.

In Diels' catalogue, reference is made to "Costomiris, Rev. des ét. gr. X p. 435" (that is, Costomiris 1897), where the following can be read:

Actuarius graecus ... 1191 ... Bibliotheca Alexandri Petavii in Vaticana, dont la plus grande partie se trouve, à Rome, dans la Bibl. Reginae Sueciae in Vaticana

with a note referring to Montfaucon, Bibl. mss., p. 92, e.

The reference is to Montfaucon 1739, 1.92, where the following entry can be read:

Actuarius Graecus. 1191, 1194, 517.

This entry appears under "Anonymi" (*ibid.*) in the catalogue of the manuscripts once owned by Alexander Petau (d. 1672) entitled as follows (Montfaucon 1739: 1.61):

Catalogus alphabeticus Manuscriptorum Codicum qui extabant in Bibliotheca Alexandri Petavii, ac deinde divenditi in Sueciam sunt transportati, nunc autem plurimâ parte asservantur Romae in Bibliotheca Reginae Sueciae. 1660.

For the catalogue see 61-96 with *Addenda* at 96-97.

Alexander Petau has catalogued his own manuscripts (ed. de Meyïer 1947: 172-175). Three Actuarius entries are listed (de Meyïer 1947: 174, no. 151). According to de Meyïer 1947: 174 ad 151, one of them is current manuscript Glasgow, Hunterian Museum, U.5.11 (= [0387]). Another may be the Actuarius copy in the collection of the Queen of Sweden Christina now at the Vatican Library (see [1499]). The Leiden library currently contains one copy of Actuarius: Voss. gr. F. 32 (= [0512]). However, this item does not seem to have been owned by either Alexander Petau or his father Paul (1568-1614). The third copy of Actuarius could be the present item 1191, the current location of which is unknown.

See [1548] and also [1568].

| [1568] | **1194** | II.108. |

This manuscript is listed as a copy of Ioannes Zacharias Actuarius, *Opera varia*. Reference is made to "Costomiris, Rev. des ét. gr. X p. 435".

According to Amati et al. 1800-1834: 225r, it contains Iohannes Chrysostomus, *Epistulae*.

The situation of this item is the same as that of the supposed *Vaticani graeci* 517 and 1191 (= [1548] and [1567], respectively).

[1569]	**1276**	I.40.
		Amati et al. 1800-1834: 301v-305r.
[1570]	**1277**	II.95.
		Amati et al. 1800-1834: 305v-308v.
	1283	Aristoteles, *Problemata*.
		Wartelle 1963: 132, no. 1774.
	1290	(f. 69v) *De duodecim segnis et humana constitutione*.
		CCAG V.1 (Cumont and Boll) 1904: 241-242.
[1571]	**1309**	I.38.
		Amati et al. 1800-1834: 325v-326v.
	1334	Aristoteles, *De insomniis* (cum scholiis).
		Wartelle 1963: 132, no. 1781.

[1572]	**1343**	II.20.
		Amati et al. 1800-1834: 327v-348r.
[1573]	**1347**	II.93.
		Amati et al. 1800-1834: 349v-351r; *CCAG* V.3 (Heeg) 1910: 71.
[1574]	**1354**	I.38.
		Amati et al. 1800-1834: 353r-v.
	1409	(ff. 111v-137v) Gregorius Nyssenus, *De hominis opificio.*
		Uthemann 1983 (especially 643).
	1424	Nicolaus Myrepsus, *Antidotarium.*
		Lucà 2012: 343.
[1575]	**1427**	II.71, 72.
		Lucà 2012: 343.
[1576]	**1444**	I.113, 135; II.44, 76, 101.

This manuscript is listed among the copies of the following works (order of folios in the manuscript; references to Diels' catalogue follow the folio numbers):

- Galenus, *Prognostica de decubitu ex mathematica scientia*, f. 22v (I.113);
- Hermes Trismegistus, *Iatromathematica*, f. 217 (II.44);
- Galenus, *De chirurgorum operationibus et de decubitu infirmorum*, f. 223 (I.135);
- Pancharius, *De decubitu infirmorum*: f. 235v (II.76);
- Theophilus, *De principiis mundi collectanea*: f. 243v (II.101).

Amati et al. 1800-1834: 398v, do not provide a detailed list of content.

Although the codex does not contain the Galenic *Prognostica de decubitu ex mathematica scientia* on f. 22v, it contains the other treatises listed in Diels' catalogue at the folios mentioned in Diels. The reference to f. 22v about the Galenic work might be a confusion with f. 222v where a title "... γαλινοῦ ... περὶ κατακλίσεως νοσούντων" can be read.

CCAG V.1 (Cumont and Boll) 1904: 81-82.

	1456	(ff. 99r-101r) Epiphanius, *De metris et ponderibus*; (ff. 107v-108r) *De hominis aetatibus.*
		Amati et al. 1800-1834: ff. 404v-405v.
[1577]	**1467**	I.38.
		Amati et al. 1800-1834: 408r-v.
[1578]	**1470**	II.25.
		Amati et al. 1800-1834: 408v; *CCAG* V.4 (Weinstock) 1940: 19.
	1538	(f. 14v) *Remedium pro obsessis*; (ff. 65v-71r) *Orationes pro infirmis.*
		Giannelli 1950: 100-109.

	1561	Demetrius Pepagomenus, *De podagra*.
		Giannelli 1950: 152-153.
	1568	(ff. 111r-193v) Gregorius Nyssenus, *De hominis opificio*.
		Giannelli 1950: 161-163.
	1569	(ff. 217v-218) Epiphanius, *De mensuris et ponderibus* (frg.).
		Giannelli 1950: 163-166.
[1579]	**1595**	I.114.
		Giannelli 1950: 226-228.
[1580]	**1614**	I.111; II.9, 22.
		Giannelli 1950: 278-279.
[1581]	**1692 B**	I.113; II.10, 44.

This manuscript is listed as a copy of the following three works (order of the folios in the manuscript; references to Diels' catalogue follow the folio numbers):

- Hermes Trismegistus, *Iatromathematica*, f. 1 (II.44);

- Galenus, *Prognosticon*, f. 7 (I.113);

- Alexander Aphrodisiensis, *Excerpta*, f. 34 v (II.10).

The *Vaticanus graecus* 1692 (with "B" omitted from its shelfmark, whatever "B" means [2nd volume?]) does not contain such texts, but it contains instead the following ones (order of folios):

(ff. 1r-85) *In evangelium secundum Mattheum catena*;

(ff. 88r-144r) Iohannes Chrysostomus, *Interpretatio evangelii secundum Iohannem*;

(ff. 144r-177r) Pseudo-Titus Bostrensis, *Commentarius in Lucam*;

(ff. 177v-196) *Catena in evangelium secundum Marcum*

(Giannelli 1961: 12-14).

The manuscript referred to here is *Vaticanus graecus* 1702 (see p. 302), which containts the texts listed in Diels' catalogue for the *Vaticanus* 1692 (order of the folios):

- (ff. 1r-6v) Hermes Trismegistus;

- (ff. 7r-15r) Pseudo-Galenus, *Prognostica de decubitu ex mathematica scientia*;

- (ff. 34v-36r) Alexander Aphrodisiensis, *Quaestionum et solutionum*, 2. 23 (*De pietra Heraclea*).

According to Giannelli 1961: 51 (last paragraph of the description), a number 1692 followed by the letter B appears on the spine of *Vaticanus* 1702:

... praebet in dorso: notam *1692* ... impressam (littera B paullo inferius plumbo adiecta) ...

On *Vaticanus graecus* 1702, see Giannelli 1961: 45-51.

[1582]	**1695**	II.63.
		Giannelli 1961: 20-21.

[1583]	**1700**	I.125.
		Giannelli 1961: 30-41.
	1702	(ff. 7r-15r) Pseudo-Galenus, *Prognostica de decubitu et mathematica scientia.*
		Giannelli 1961: 45-51.
		Same as [1581].
	1719	(ff. 46v-48r) Epiphanius, *De duodecim gemmis.*
		Giannelli 1961: 90-95.
	1729	(ff. 29v-36r) Gregorius Nyssenus, *De hominis opificio* (frg.).
		Giannelli 1961: 108-111.
	1744	(ff. 148v-149r) Johannes Damascenus, *De medicina*; (f. 149r-v) *De nominibus virtutibusque non nullorum fructuum olerumque*; (f. 149v) *De cerebri cavitatibus* ("ut in cod. Vat. 1700, f. 88").
		Giannelli 1961: 148-153.
	1753	(f. 16v) *Remedia*; (ff. 17r-18v) *De cibis.*
		Canart 1970: 36-47.
[1584]	**1759**	I.28.
		Canart 1970: 66-77.
	1826/I	(ff. 2v-4r) Aetius Amidenus, *Libri medicinales* (frg.).
		Canart 1970: 250-261 (especially 250-251).
	1826/X	(ff. 325r-333r) Nicander, *Theriaca* (frg.); (f. 333r-v) Nicander, *Alexipharmaca* (frg.); (f. 333v) Pseudo-Dioscorides, *Alexipharmaca* (frg.).
		Canart 1970: 250-261 (especially 255-256).
[1585]	**1835**	II.71.
		Canart 1970: 280-282.
[1586]	**1845**	I.61, 68, 73, 81 (2), 82, 96, 100, 101.
		Canart 1970: 314-315.
	1852/XIV	(ff. 458r-465r) *Pharmacopoeia.*
		Canart 1970: 325-341 (especially 339).
	1857	(ff. 111r-139r) Gregorius Nyssenus, *De hominis opificio.*
		Canart 1970: 352-356.
[1587]	**1858**	I.107.
		Canart 1970: 356-368.
	1862/XVI	*Remedia varia.*
		Canart 1970: 383.
	1866	Palimpsest (Canart 2004: 47).
		Scriptio inferior: (ff. 1r-4v) Nicander, *Theriaca*, vv. 1-59.

Scriptio superior: Psalterium.

Canart 1970: 395-403 for the whole manuscript.

1871   Palimpsest (Canart 2004: 47).

Scriptio inferior: unidentified text.

Scriptio superior: (ff. 12r-17r) *Physiologus*.

Canart 1970: 415-422.

1878   (ff. 271-316) Erotianus, *Vocum hippocraticorum collectio*; (ff. 337r-338v) Galenus, *De historia philosopha*.

Canart 1970: 442-449.

[1588]   **1879**   II.93.

Canart 1970: 449-466.

1882   Palimpsest.

Scriptio superior: Varia biblica, liturgica, letteraria, historica et medica.

Scriptio media: Galenus, *De locis affectis*.

Scriptio infima: Hagiographico-homiletica.

Canart 1970: 472-488; Canart 2004: 47; Harlfinger, Brunschön and Vasiloudi 2006: 145, 155.

See also *Vaticanus graecus* 984 (see above, p. 296).

[1589]   **1885**   II.42, 71, 91.

Canart 1970: 490-491.

1891   (ff. 113v-115v) *Medicamenta varia*.

Canart 1970: 520-528.

1896/VII   (f. 256r-v), Alexander Trallianus, *De podagra* (frg.).

Canart 1970: 546-554 (especially 551).

[1590]   **1898**   I.114, 115.

Canart 1970: 558-577.

[1591]   **1902**   II.26.

Canart 1970: 587-615.

[1592]   **1904**   II.6, 28, 33; N.43.

Canart 1970: 616-632.

1907   (ff. 205v-216r) Gregorius Nyssenus, *De hominis opificio*.

Canart 1970: 634-639.

1908/III   (ff. 12-16), Galenus, *De humoribus*.

Canart 1970: 639-645 (especially 640).

[1593]   **1911**   II.6; N.43.

Canart 1970: 650.

	1912/VII	(ff. 111r-133v) Gregorius Nyssenus, *De hominis opificio*.
		Canart 1970: 651-664 (especially 660-661).
		Palimpsest: Canart 2004: 47.
[1594]	**1949**	II.8.
		Canart 1970: 734-762.
	2005	Palimpsest.
		Scriptio superior: Euchologium.
		Scriptio media: Formulae medicinarum.
		Scriptio infima: Psalterium.
		Harlfinger, Brunschön and Vasiloudi 2006: 145, 162-163.
	2066	Gregorius Nyssenus, *De hominis opificio*.
		Canart and Lucà 2000: 43.
		See also Washington D.C., Library of Congress, Rare Book and Manuscripts, Medieval and Renaissance MSS, 37 (see p. 347).
[1595]	**2154**	II.26.
		Duffy 1983: 16; Ihm 2002: 203, 236.
	2163	(ff. 115 et seq.) Michael Ephesius, *Commentarium in librum Aristotelis de insomniis*.
		Lilla 1985: 4-6.
[1596]	**2182**	I.93; II.30, 109, 110.
		Lilla 1985: 75-79.
	2183	(ff. 122r-125r) Aristoteles, *De insomniis*.
		Wartelle 1963: 136, no. 1836; Lilla 1985: 80-83.
[1597]	**2202**	II.6; N.43.
		Lilla 1985: 157-159.
	2217	(ff. 270v-271r) Severianus Gabalensis, *De nomine hominis* (frg.); (f. 271r, ll. 6-21) Splenius, *De origine ac resolutione corporis hominis*.
		Lilla 1985: 205-211.
	2220	(ff. 4r-13v) Epiphanius, *De mensuris et ponderibus*; (f. 32r, ll. 12-21) Nemesius Emesenus, *De natura hominis* (frg.).
		Lilla 1985: 224-257.
	2230	(ff. 168v-169r) Epiphanius, *De duodecim gemmis*.
		Lilla 1985: 315-327.
	2236	(ff. 2r-3r) Diocles, *Ad Antigonum regem epistula de tuenda valetudine*.
		Lilla 1985: 348-359.

| [1598] | **2238** | I.18. |

Lilla 1985: 363-367.

2248/IV *De lapidibus* inter quae (ff. 155v-156v) Epiphanius, *De duodecim gemmis*.

Lilla 1985: 406-416 (especially 407-409).

[1599] **2250** II.58.

Lilla 1985: 419-424.

[1600] **2254** I.5, 93; II.104.

Lilla 1985: 430-432.

[1601] **2256** I.114, 128, 133; II.91.

This manuscript is listed with the following contents (order of folios in the manuscript; references to Diels' catalogue follow the folio numbers):

- Rufus, *Excerpta*, f. 26 (II.91);
- Galenus, *De succedaneis*, f. 33 (I.114);
- Galenus, *De urinis*, f. 78v (I.128);
- Galenus, *Remedia*, f. 79v (I.133).

The identification of the content in Cozza Luzi n.d.: 216v is insufficient to allow for an identification ("ἰατρικὰ διαφορά").

The manuscript contains the following three texts:

- (ff. 33r, l. 10-35v, l. 8) Galenus, *De succedaneis* (frg.);
- (ff. 78v, l. 7-79r, l. 6) *De urinis*;
- (ff. 79r, l. 7-79v, l. 18) *Antidotorum methodus*.

The text identified as Rufus, *Excerpta* at f. 26r-v, is not by Rufus of Ephesus, but is instead a "ἱερὰ τῶν περὶ μελαγχολικῶν ρουφῶν" extracted from the *Efodia*.

[1602] **2259** II.24, 95 (2).

This manuscript is mentioned under the following works (order of folios in the manuscript; references to Diels' catalogue follow folio numbers):

- Stephanus Alexandrinus, *De mundo*, f. 16 (II.95);
- Stephanus Alexandrinus, *Epistula ad Theodorum*, f. 25 (II.95);
- Cleopatra, *De mensuris et ponderibus*, f. 132 (II.24).

Whereas Cozza Luzi n.d.: 217r-v, mentions only the first and third texts, the manuscript does also contain Stephanus, *Epistula ad Theodorum* at ff. 25r-41r.

2291 (ff. 247r et seq.) Nicander, *Theriaca*; (ff. 271v et seq.) Nicander, *Alexipharmaca*.

This manuscript was *Vaticanus Chisianus* R.VIII.59.

Franchi de' Cavalieri 1927: 100-101 (no. 50).

[1603]   **2304 [olim 2217]**   I.18; II.7, 27, 89, 101.

This manuscript appears among the copies of the following works (in the order of Diels' mentions; references to Diels' catalogue follow the folio numbers [according to Diels]):

- Hippocrates, *Iusiurandum*, f. 1 (I.18);
- Aëtius Amidenus, *Excerpta*, ff. 8, 17-19, 9-16v, 19 (II .7);
- Democritus, *Prognosticon*, f. 6 (II.27);
- Rufus, *De corporis humani appellationibus* (frg.), f. 6v (II.89);
- Theophilus, *De pulsibus*, f. 1v (II.101).

Whereas Cozza Luzi n.d.: 231v, mentions only "Σχεδιάσματά τινα, Ὀριβασίου τινα, περὶ τῶν ζῴων διαφορά", the manuscript does contain the works listed in Diels' catalogue.

A number 2217 (deleted) appears on f. Ir. As Cozza Luzi n.d.: 231v mentions, this is the shelfmark of the manuscript when it was in the Colonna collection ("Columnensis olim 2217").

On the provenance of this manuscript (Colonna collection), see Lilla 1985: XXIn36, and XLVII, no. 40.

2644/XXI   *Remedia.*

Lilla 1996: 1-17 (especially 16-17).

2672   Dioscorides, *De materia medica*, and Aetius Amidenus, *Libri medicinales* (frg. extracted from a binding).

Ceresa and Lucà 2008.

[1604]   **3062**   N.43.

This codex is listed as a copy of Aetius Amidenus, *Libri medicinales*.

As Mercati 1917: 53-54 has demonstrated, this is actually a *Parisinus graecus*, which contains a catalogue of the Greek manuscripts in the Biblioteca Vaticana. This catalogue lists a Vatican copy of Aetius Amidenus, *Libri medicinales*.

This information probably comes from Costomiris 1890: 176.

See also [1605].

[1605]   **3073**   N.43.

Same incorrect information as above [1604].

See Mercati 1917: 53-54, and Costomiris 1890: 176.

[1606]   **4423**   I.111.

This item is identified as a copy of Galenus, *Definitiones medicae*.

This is not the Greek text of the treatise, but its early 16th-century Latin translation by Euphronymus Boninus (Frosino Bonino [*fl.* 1497-1525]).

Durling 1993: 299.

[1607]   **7152**   II.65.

This copy of Mercurius monachus, *De pulsibus* is not in Greek, but in Latin.

It is listed in Diels' catalogue with a reference to "Daremberg, Not. et Extr. I p. 143 sq." (= Daremberg 1851-1853: 143), where the manuscript is mentioned on the basis of "cardinal A. Mai (Classici auct. T. IV, p. XIII)", that is, Mai 1831: XII-XIV.

As Mai 1831: XIII explicitly mentioned, this item is not a *Vaticanus graecus*, but a *Vaticanus latinus* ("... 7152, seriei latinae ..."). It contains on ff. 90-91 the text referred to in Diels' catalogue, but in Latin and under the title *Abytiani sive Mercurii Monachi dissertatio De pulsibus*.

See also Masullo 2006: 337.

Vatic. lat. (*Vaticani latini*)

[1608]   **5763**   I.76.

Palimpsest (f. 30).

Scriptio superior: Isidorus Hispalensis, *Etymologiae*.

Scriptio inferior: Galenus, *De alimentorum facultatibus* (frg.).

Schoene 1902. More recently, Harlfinger, Brunschön and Vasiloudi 2006: 145, 146-150, and Wilkins 2013: XXV and XXVI-XXVII.

See also [1853].

Roma (Rome) (IT)

Biblioteca Angelica (Angelica Library)

See above **Rom, Bibl. Angelica** (see above, pp. 270-271).

Biblioteca Casanatense (Casanatense Library)

-

1700   Epiphanius, *Physiologus*.

Bancalari 1894: 198-199.

Biblioteca Corsiniana (Corsiniana Library)

-

43. D. 32   See [1440].

36. E. 26   See [1441].

Biblioteca Vallicelliana (Vallicelliana Library)

-

B 53   (f. 145v) *Physiologia*.

Martini 1902: 21-26.

B 70   See [1445].

B 80   (ff. 151v-152r) *Metrologia*; (ff. 152v-153r) *De corporis humani partibus*; (f. 153r) *Medicina*; (f. 153r) *De mensibus*; (ff. 153r-153v) Theophanes [Chrysobalantes], *Epitome de curatione morborum* (frg.).

Martini 1902: 32-33.

B 93   See [1446].

C 4   (ff. 380r-389r) Nicephorus Blemmydes, *De corpore*.

Martini 1902: 48-54.

C 97²   (ff. IIIr) Basilius Caesariensis, *Anthropologia* (frg.).

Martini 1902: 80-83.

E 37   (ff. 87r-87v) *Lexicon plantarum nominum*; (ff. 87v-88r) *Metrologia*; (ff. 88r-88v) *Plantarum nominum explicatio*.

Martini 1902: 113-116.

E 55   (ff. 130r-131v) *Formulae medicae*.

Martini 1902: 119-125.

F 9   See [1447].

F 33   (ff. 111r-121r) Democritus, *Physica et mystica*; (f. 116r) Synesius Cyrenensis, *Scholia ad Democriti librum* (frg.).

Martini 1902: 157-159.

F 68   (ff. 156r-190v) Epiphanius, *Physiologus*.

Martini 1902: 183-185.

F 83   See [1448].

Collegio inglese (English College)

Z 7   (ff. 56v-58v) Gregorius Nazianzenus, *De humana natura*.

Nikolopoulos 1961: 260-262; Domiter 1999: 8.

Pontificio collegio greco (Pontifical Greek College)

3   (f. 198v) Epiphanius, *De mensuris et ponderibus*.

Lampros 1913: 8-11.

4   (ff. 122r et seq.) *Physiologus*.

Lampros 1913: 11-12.

8   Gregorius Nazianzenus, *De humana natura*.

Lampros 1913: 16-17 (does not specifically identify the text); Domiter 1999: 21.

Rosanbo (FR)

Bibl. de M. le marquis de Ros. (Bibliothèque de Monsieur le marquis de Rosanbo [Marquis of Rosanbo's Library]).

[1609]   **286**   I.98.

Omont 1886-1888: 3.381, no. 102.

Salamanca (SP)

Bibl. Univ. (*Bibliotheca Universitatis* [University Library]), now Universidad de Salamanca, Biblioteca General Histórica (Salamanca University, General Historical Library)

[1610]   **1. 1. 11**   II.71.

Graux, ed. Martin 1892: 151-152.

Current shelfmark: M 567.

Also [1612].

[1611]   **1. 1. 14**   II.78.

Graux, ed. Martin 1892: 153-154.

Current shelfmark: M 7.

[1612]   **(Epistt. septem)**   II. 70.

This manuscript listed without shelfmark under Oribasius, *Opera varia*, seems to be current codex M 567 in the Biblioteca General Histórica of the Universidad de Salamanca.

A note "Oribasius. De medicina epistola VII" appears in this manuscript, f. IIr, although no such text can be found in it (see Tovar 1963: 82 "unde idem auctor [i.e. Diels] hauserit notitiam Salamantini cuiusdam codicis continentis epistulas septem Oribasii nescio"; also Martínez Manzano 2005: 290-291).

The information probably comes from the list of manuscripts at Salamanca, University library, compiled by Volger 1859, where a manuscript identified as follows is listed (see p. 377, *sub* Oribasio):

Oribasio. De medicina epistolae septem. (Un tomo en fol. pasta antigua, en tabla, bien cons. sin foliar, en griego).

Although such text is not present in it, the manuscript referred to here seems to be current M 567. The source of the identification of this manuscript as a copy of Oribasius' supposed *Epistolae septem* is unknown.

Same as [1610].

Universidad de Salamanca, Biblioteca General Histórica (Salamanca University, General Historical Library)

M 7   See [1611].

Tovar 1963: 15-16.

M 232   (ff. 66v et seq.) Synesius Cyrenensis, *De insomniis*.

Tovar 1963: 50-55; Lilao Franca-Castrillo González 1997: 185.

M 365   *De theriaca Andromachi*.

Tovar 1963: 71.

M 560   *Geoponica*.

Tovar 1963: 75-79.

M 567   Formerly [1610].

Tovar 1963: 81-82.

2659   See [0589].

Lilao Franca and Castrillo González 2002: 1053; Touwaide 2003.

2710   See [0588].

Lilao Franca and Castrillo González 2002: 1113.

2713   (ff. 393r et seq.) Symeon Seth, *De humani corporis partium nominibus*; (ff. 394v et seq.) Symeon Seth, *De medicinae partibus*; (ff. 398r-403v) Theophilus Protospatharius, *De urinis*; (ff. 403v-434r) Symeon Seth, *Varia de medicina*; (ff. 434r-436v) Symeon Seth, *De animalibus virus eiaculantibus*.

Graux, ed. Martin 1892: 80-82 (no. 17); Lilao Franca and Castrillo González 2002: 1113.

Saloniki (Θεσσαλονίκη [Thessalonica]) (GR)

Bibl. gymnas. (*Bibliotheca gymnasii*, Γυμνασίου Βιβλιοθήκη [Gymnasium Library])

[1613]   **17**   II.40.

On September 3-4, 1890, a fire ravaged the Gymnasium (Serruys 1903: 73, 77). It did not destroy the holdings of the library (contrary to Congourdeau 1996: 99n1), although it damaged many of them (Serruys 1907: 12-13, 77-78). The manuscripts were catalogued in 1903 by Serruys. Their numbers (from 1 to 79) have been introduced by Serruys.

For the present item, see Serruys 1903: 28-30.

Most of the manuscript of this collection are now in Athens, at the National Library (Olivier 1995: 781 no. 2287).

This item is currently Αθήνα, Εθνική Βιβλιοθήκη της Ελλάδος ΕΒΕ (Athens, National Library of Greece–EBE), 2086 (see above, p. 14).

Санкт-Петербург (Sankt-Petersburg [Saint-Petersburg]) (RU)

Российская национальная библиотека (РНБ) (Rossiiskaia natsional'naia biblioteka [RNB] [National Library of Russia [NLR])

The different collections in the library are numbered. The collection below (Greek manuscripts) is Фонд no. 906. This number duplicates the name of the collection and should not necessarily be mentioned if the name of the collection is cited.

Собрание греческих рукописей (Sobranie grecheskich rukopisei [Collection of Greek manuscripts])

115a   4 folios, palimpsest.

Scriptio superior: Psalterium.

Scriptrio media: Evangelia et liturgica;

Scriptio infima: Aetius Amidenus, *Libri medicinales*.

Granstrem 1956; Harlfinger, Brunschön and Vasiloudi 2006: 145, 156-157.

Muralt 1864: 66-67; Granstrem 1961: 271-272, no. 173.

116   Same as [0944] and [1407].

Granstrem 1967: 275-276, no. 522.

770   Gregorius Nyssenus, *De hominis opificio*.

Granstrem 1961: 261, no. 130.

San Lorenzo de El Escorial (ES)

Biblioteca del Real Monasterio de San Lorenzo del Escorial (Library of the Royal Monastery at San Lorenzo del Escorial)

See **Escurial** (pp. 62-66).

Sáros-Patak (now Sárospatak) (HU)

Bibl. d. reform. Colleg. (Bibliothek des reformierten Collegiums [Library of the Reformed College]), now Sárospatakai Református Kollégium Todományos Gyüjteményei, Nagykönyvtár (Sárospatak Reformed College, Great Library, Scholarly Collection)

[1614]   -   II.43.

This copy of Hermes Trismegistus, *Opera omnia* by Johannes Xylander without shelfmark in Diels' catalogue is listed in the same way in Haenel 1840: 424.

Current shelfmark: Kt 405.

Börzsönyi 1986: 83 (where the manuscript is dated 1599 and not 1591 as in Haenel [above]).

Sens (FR)

- (Bibliothèque municipale [Municipal Library])

[1615]   **nr. 209**   I.38.

This is a copy of Hippocrates, *Epistulae*.

As Diels' catalogue mentions, this is a 17th/18th-century manuscript.

It contains (ff. 107r-138v) Hippocrates, *Epistula ad Damagetem*.

Catalogue général des manuscrits 1887: 187.

It is a French translation of a manuscript owned by the French scholar, numismate, and curator of medals at the king's numismatic cabinet Marc-Antoine Oudinet (1645-1712) (see *ibid.* "traduction d'un manuscrit d'Oudinet, graveur des médailles du Roi").

[1616]   **Miscell. 187** I.5.

The mention "Miscell." does not belong to the shelfmark of this manuscript, which is listed as a copy of Hippocrates, *Prognosticon*.

This is a printed edition (Paris, 1560) of *Methodus sex librorum Galeni in differentiis et causis morborum*, with commentaries by Jacques Dubois (better known as Sylvius) (1478-1555) with 17th-century handwritten notes in Latin, also including the following according to the catalogue (below):

(No. 4) Fol. 328. "Aphorismi ex libro Prognosticorum ... Hippocratis."

The text is contained on ff. 328r-356r.

Catalogue général des manuscrits 1887: 184-185; Alexanderson 1963: 89-90.

Σινά Ὄρος (سيناء, Mount Sinai) (EG)

Ἱερά Μονή Θεοβαδίστου Ὄρους Σινά, Ἁγίας Αἰκατερίνης (دير القدّيسة كاترينا, St. Catherine Monastery of Mount Sinai)

150	(ff. 1r et seq.) Epiphanius, *De duodecim gemmis*.
	Gardthausen 1886: 28; Kamil 1970: 68, no. 175; Weitzmann and Galavaris 1990: 89-91.
328	(ff. 60r-100v) Gregorius Nyssenus, *De hominis opificio*.
	Gardthausen 1886: 68; Kamil 1970: 76, no. 390.
424	(ff. 206r-239v) Gregorius Nyssenus, *De hominis opificio*.
	Gardthausen 1886: 102; Kamil 1970: 88, no. 648.
427	(No. 6) Epiphanius, *De duodecim gemmis*.
	Gardthausen 1886: 103; Kamil 1970: 88, no. 651.
485	(ff. 298r-312v) Epiphanius, *Physiologus*.
	Gardthausen 1886: 117-118; Kamil 1970: 90, no. 708.
1207	*Notulae medicae*.
	Gardthausen 1886: 252-253; Kamil 1970: 137, no. 2107.
1387	Hippocrates, *Capitula medica*; *De infirmis*; *Aphorismi*; Galenus, *De succedaneis*.
	Beneševič 1917: 42; Kamil 1970: 137, no. 2134; Karas 1994: 380.
1660	Hippocrates, *Aphorismi*.
	Beneševič 1917: 130-131; Kamil 1970: 138, no. 2151.
1889	(ff. 310v-312r) Nepualius, *De sympathia et antipathia*.
	Beneševič 1917: 252-261 (especially 261); Kamil 1970: 84, no. 564.
2106	no. 4: Gregorius Nyssenus, *De hominis opificio*.
	Beneševič 1917: 324-327; Kamil 1970: 86, no. 600.

New Finds, Arabic

8   Palimpsest

               Scriptio superior: Gospels (Arabic translation) (Kachouh 2008)

               Stratus inferior: medicinalia inter quae (ff. 16v-17r) *Pictura plantae medicae* (ἀδίαντον) (Dioscorides, *De materia medica*, 4.134).

New Finds, Greek

103   *Physiologus.*

               New Finds 1999: 173.

326   *Astrologia* et *alchimia.*

               New Finds 1999: 235.

375   Meletius, *De natura hominis.*

               New Finds 1999: 240.

Σκιάθος (Skiathos) (GR)

Ιερά Μονή Ευαγγελισμού της Θεοτόκου (Monastery of the Annunciation, also known as Evangelistrias Monastery)

-

23   (f. 15r-v) *Iatrosophica*; (f. 25r-v) *Iatrosophica alia*; (ff. 26r-133r) Artemidorus Dalianus, *Oneirocriticon*; (f. 146r-v) *Phlebotomia.*

               Dimitrakopoulos 2012: 67-70.

28   (ff. 11r-15v) *Iatrosophica*; (ff. 18v-19v) *De lapidibus*; (ff. 20r-24v) *Hippocratis et Galeni philosophia de mundi elementis et de hominibus*; (f. 25r-v) *Iatrosophica*; (ff. 26r-39r) Galenus, *Medica quaedam*; (f. 39v) Galenus, *Prognosticum de homine*; (ff. 40r-78v) *Iatrosofion.*

               Dimitrakopoulos 2012: 75-76.

София (Sofia [BG])

Българска Академия на Науките (БАН), Научен Архив (НА) (Bulgarska Akademiia na Naukite [BAN], Nauchen Arkhiv [Bulgarian Academy of Sciences, Scientific Archives])

BAN гр (BAN gr.)

5   Aetius Amidenus, *Libri medicinales* (frg.).

               Getov 2006: 250, 252-253; Getov 2010: 24-25.

               Fragment of [1396].

Народна Библиотека "Св. Св. Кирил и Методий" (НБКМ) (Narodna Biblioteka "Sv. Sv. Kiril i Metodii" [NBKM], National Library "St. Cyril and Methodius")

Гр (Gr.)

118   *Physiologus.*

               Stojanov 1973: 121.

Софийски Университет "Св. Климент Охридски", Научен център за *славяно-византийски* проучвания "Иван Дуйчев" (Sofiiski Universitet Sv. Kliment Ochridski, Nauchen Centăr za Slaviano-Vizantiiski Prouchvanija "Ivan Dujchev" [Sofia University "St Clement of Ohrid", Centre for Slavo-Byzantine Studies "Prof. Ivan Dujchev")

Д. гр (D. gr.)

156   (ff. 322r-354r) Iohannes Zacharias Actuarius, *De spiritu animali*; (f. 354r) *Iatrosophica*; (ff. 357r-362v) *Medica varia*.

Getov, Katsaros and Papastathis 1994: 52-66.

198   (ff. 104v-110r) *Iatrosophica*; (f. 110r-v) *De urinis*.

Getov, Katsaros and Papastathis 1994: 83-84.

297   (ff. 163r-200v) *Physiologus.*

Džurova et al. 1994: 37; Džurova and Canart 2011: 258.

394   [Hippocrates], *De hominis constitutione.*

Džurova et al. 1994: 42; Roselli 2009: 177-178.

Strasbourg (FR)

Bibliothèque nationale et universitaire (National and University Library)

-

MS 1.900   (f. 1r-v) *Calendarium sanitatis*; (ff. 2r-9v) *Lexicon plantarum*; (ff. 9v-10v) *De urinis*; (ff. 11r-22v) *De pulsibus*; (ff. 24r-30v) Index capitulorum; (ff. 30v-109v) Theophanes [Chrysobalantes], *Epitome de curatione morborum*; (ff. 110r-113v) Diocles, *Ad Antigonum regem epistula de tuenda valetudine.*

Welz 1913: 17-19 (the manuscript is identified as number 6); *Catalogue général des manuscrits* 1923: 389-390 (between parentheses "Grec 6"); Sonderkamp 1987: 213-214.

MS 1.906   (ff. 13v-24r) Nemesius Emesenus, *De natura hominis* (frg.).

Welz 1913: 28-42 (the manuscript is identified as number 12); *Catalogue général des manuscrits* 1923: 392 (between parentheses "Grec 12"; does not list Nemesius' text); Morani 1981: 29 (identifies the manuscript as "12").

Θεσσαλονίκη (Thessalonica) (GR)

Αριστοτέλειο Πανεπιστήμιο Θεσσαλονίκης, Κεντρική βιβλιοθήκη (Aristotle University Thessalonica, Central Library)

-

25   Stephanus, *De febrium differentiis.*

Politis 1991: 26-27; Karas 1994: 405.

95/XXIX   *Nomina humani corporis partium.*

Politis 1991: 87-89.

Ἱερά Μονή Βλατάδων (Vlatadon Monastery)

14   Galenus, *Opera*.

             Pietrobelli 2010.

Toledo (ES)

Bibl. del cabillo [*sic*] **de la iglesia catedral** (Biblioteca del cabildo de la iglesia catedral [Library of the Chapter of the Cathedral Church]), now Biblioteca Capitular, Catedral de Toledo (Chapter Library, Toledo Cathedral)

-

[1617]   **101, 15**   II.6, 41.

                             Graux, ed. Martin 1892: 293-294; *CMAG* V (Zuretti and Severyns) 1928: 94, 111-113.

                             Current shelfmark: Fondo Zelada, BCT 101-15.

Biblioteca Capitular, Catedral de Toledo (Chapter's Library, Toledo Cathedral)

Fondo Zelada

    BCT 101-15   See [1617].

Torino (Turin) (IT)

Biblioteca Nazionale Universitaria (National University Library)

Several manuscripts were destroyed in the fire that ravaged the library in 1904 (see Gorrini 1905 and, more recently, Eleuteri 1990).

-

B. I. 6   See [1623] and [1624].

B. I. 14   (f. 256) *Ex Cleopatrae tractatu de ponderibus et mensuris.*

               Pasini et al. 1749: 176-178 (no. LXXXII with shelfmark c. III. 25); Cosentini 1922: 14-15 (no. 92).

B. III. 1   *Geoponica.*

               Pasini et al. 1749: 141-142 (no. XXXVI with shelfmark *b.* V. 16); Cosentini 1922: 18 (no. 129).

B. III. 37   (ff. 1r-55v) Theophilus, *Commentarium in Hippocratis Aphorismos.*

               Pasini et al. 1749: 228 (no. CXXI with shelfmark *c.* V. 12); Cosentini 1922: 21 (no. 163); Magdelaine 1994: 274n3, 275, 279.

B. V. 16   See [1628].

B. V. 33   See [1629] and [1632].

B. V. 39   Possibly [1622].

B. VI. 8   (f. 23r) Apollonius Citiensis, *De articulis.*

               Zuretti 1896: 207; *CCAG* IV (Bassi et al.) 1903: 3; Cosentini 1922: 28 (no. 229).

B. VI. 21	Galenus, *Definitiones medicae.*
	Pasini et al. 1749: 382 (no. CCLXXIX with shelfmark *c*. I. 34); Cosentini 1922: 30 (no. 241).
B. VII. 18	*Varia continet ad medicinam et historiam naturalem pertinentia.*
	Pasini et al. 1749: 472 (no. CCCXLVII with shelfmark *b*. I. 17); Cosentini 1922: 33 (no. 270).
C. I. 11	(ff. 27r et seq.) Gregorius Nyssenus, *De hominis opificio.*
	Pasini et al. 1749: 168-170 (no. LXXI with shelfmark *c*. III. 14); Cosentini 1922: 35 (no. 289).
C. VI. 3	See [1630] and [1633].
C. VI. 10	See [1627].
C. VI. 21	See [1634].
C. VI. 26	(ff. 26v et seq.) *Ex Hippocrate nonnulla afferuntur de temporis prognosi.*
	Pasini et al. 1749: 363 (no. CCXXVIII with shelfmark *b*. VI. 18); Cosentini 1922: 43 (no. 364).

Tübingen (DE)

Univ.-Bibl. (Universitätsbibliothek [University Library])

-

[1618]	**2**	II.95.
		Schmid 1902: 4-6.
		Current shelfmark: Mb 2.
[1619]	**23**	I.20.
		Schmid 1902: 48.
		Current shelfmark: Mb 23.
[1620]	**37**	I.20.
		Schmid 1902: 70-78.
		Current shelfmark: Mb 37.
		It is a 16th-century collection of antiquities by Martin Crusius (1536-1607).
		See Ihm 2002: 234-235, no. 288 (especially 235).

Universitätsbibliothek (University Library)

See **Univ.-Bibl.** (above).

-

Mb 2	See [1618].
Mb 23	See [1619].

Turin (Torino [Turin]) (IT)

Bibl. Nazionale (Universitaria) (National University Library)

Shelfmark systems changed over time. The first system can be found in the catalogue published in 1749 by Pasini et al. (where the manuscripts also have a sequential number appearing before the shelfmark). The second system (currently used) appears in the catalogue by Cosentini 1922 (in which manuscripts are also numbered sequentially, with their previous shelfmark [= Pasini et al. 1749]. There is no table of concordance between ancient and new shelfmarks). Tables of concordance for all of the library's shelfmark systems can be found in Eleuteri 1990.

Apart from [1621] and [1622], which are not identified by any shelfmark, the manuscripts of Torino are identified in three different ways in Diels' catalogue:

- Items [1623]-[1624] and [1627]-[1631] are identified by their sequential number in Pasini et al. 1749 (this number is written in Arabic numerals in Diels' catalogue, whereas it is in Roman numerals in the 1749 catalogue). This number is followed by the shelfmark of the manuscripts according to Pasini et al. 1749. In [1624], this shelfmark is followed by the recent one;

- Manuscripts [1625] and [1626] are identified by the sequential number as assigned in the catalogue of Zuretti 1896, followed by their new shelfmark;

- Codices [1632]-[1634] are identified by their new shelfmarks. For [1632] and [1633], this shelfmark is followed, between parentheses, by the sequential Arabic number and the shelfmark from Pasini et al. 1749. For [1634] the shelfmark is followed, between parentheses, by the shelfmark in Pasini et al. 1749.

There are 3 pairs of duplicates (manuscripts identified according to two of the systems used in Diels' catalogue as above):

- [1623] is the same as [1624], the latter adding the new shelfmark;

- [1629] identified according to Pasini et al. 1749 is the same as [1632] identified according to its new shelfmark;

- [1630] and [1633], the former identified according to Pasini et al. 1749 and the latter according to its new shelfmark.

Several manuscripts were destroyed in the fire that ravaged the library in 1904 (see Gorrini 1905 and, more recently Eleuteri 1990).

[1621]   ?   II.71.

This manuscript listed without any identifier is supposedly a codex of Oribasius, *Medicae collectiones ad Iulianum*.

According to the index in Cosentini 1922: 199-219, the only *Taurinensis* containing a text by Oribasius is B VII 36 (on which see *ibid*. 34 [no. 278]). This codex does not contain the *Medicae collectiones ad Iulianum*, but a text identified as follows by Cosentini:

Oribasius, Anatomica ex libris Galeni desumta.

This text is not listed in the short description by Pasini et al. 1749: 415-416 (no. CCCXXXIII with shelfmark *b*. I. 1).

Probably same as [1631].

[1622]   - («zitiert bei Montfaucon 1837 'Gal.   I.64.

de IV elementis'; nicht verifiziert»)

This manuscript identified by means of a reference to a not otherwise identified work by Montfaucon and the title of a Galenic work is supposed to be a copy of Galenus, *De elementis secundum Hippocratem*.

The information may come from Ackermann 1821: LXXV, no. 8, where a manuscript "In Taurin." is mentioned (without brackets) without further element of identification.

The reference to Montfaucon in Diels' catalogue is to Montfaucon 1739. However, the number 1837 is incorrect as Montfaucon, *Bibliotheca bibliothecarum* contains only 1669 pages. Nevertheless, a work similar to the one referred to here and described as follows can be found at page 1397:

Ejusd[em] (i.e. Galeni) lib. de quattuor elementis, *in*-4°. graec.

This codex appears in a list published in Montfaucon 1739: 2.1393-1402 under the following title (on this list see Blume 1824-1827: 1.80):

Catalogus Manuscriptorum Serenissimi Principis Sardiniae Regis accepti ab ejus Bibliothecario P. Josepho Roma Ordinis Minimorum, Viro eruditissimo, in Taurinensi Universitate Regio Professore ...

This item might correspond to B. V. 39 (see above, p. 315), in which a text identified as follows can be found according to Pasini et al. 1749: 379-380, no. CCLXXV with shelfmark *c.* I. 29 (reproduced in Cosentini 1922: 27-28 [no. 222]):

Varia primo loco habentur opuscula, seu potius excerpta ab ipso Darmario ad medicinam spectantia, in quibus de natura hominis, de quattuor elementis, de partibus humani corporis, aliisque similibus agitur, parvi tamen momenti.

On this manuscript, see Pasini et al. 1749: 379-380, no. CCLXXV. *c.* I. 29; Cosentini 1922: 27-28 (no. 222).

[1623]   **6 b IV 6**   I.126; II.63.

This item has a sequential number VI in Pasini et al. 1749: 70, with a shelfmark *b.* IV. 6. See also Cosentini 1922: 13-14 (no. 84).

Current shelfmark: B. I. 6.

Also [1624].

[1624]   **6 b IV 6 (B I 6)**   I.76, 134.

Same as [1623].

[1625]   **8 B V 31 (B VI 29)**   I.111.

This codex is sequentially numbered 8 in Zuretti 1896: 205-206, with shelfmark B. V. 31 (B. VI. 29).

Although Diels' catalogue does not mention it, this manuscript (with shelfmark B. V. 31) is no longer available as it was destroyed in the fire that ravaged the library in 1904 (it does not appear in Cosentini 1922; see also Eleuteri 1990: 31).

[1626]   **17 B VII 22 (B I 12)**   I.48, 49, 56, 96, 132, 134, 149; II.41, 58, 64.

This manuscript bears a sequential number 17 in Zuretti 1896: 211-215, with shelfmark B. VII. 22 (B. I. 12).

It was B. VII. 22, but it is no longer available as Diels' catalogue noted (*Verbrannt*) (it is not listed in Cosentini 1922; see also Eleuteri 1990: 32).

[1627]   **156 b II 10**   I.5; II.63, 110.

This item is numbered sequentially CLVI in Pasini et al. 1749: 243-344, with shelfmark *b*. II. 10.

Cosentini 1922: 42 (no. 356).

Current shelfmark: C. VI. 10.

[1628]   **177 b II 31**   I.41.

This manuscript has a sequential number CLXXVII in Pasini et al. 1749: 261-265, with shelfmark *b*. II. 31.

This manuscript has been preserved contrary to Diels' information (*Verbrannt*).

See Cosentini 1922: 25-26 (no. 206); Eleuteri 1990: 31.

Current shelfmark: B. V. 16.

[1629]   **179 b II 33**   I.56.

This manuscript is sequentially numbered CLXXIX in Pasini et al. 1749: 266-269, with shelfmark *b*. II. 33.

Cosentini 1922: 27 (no. 219).

Current shelfmark: B. V. 33.

According to Diels, it was *much damaged by fire* ("Durch Feuer stark beschädigt").

Also [1632].

[1630]   **287 c I 42**   II.28.

This codex is sequentially numbered CCLXXXVII in Pasini et al. 1749: 384-385, with shelfmark *c*. I. 42.

Cosentini 1922: 41 (no. 351).

Current shelfmark: C. VI. 3.

Same as [1633].

[1631]   **333 b I 1**   II.59, 74, 89, 93.

This item is sequentially numbered CCCXXXIII in Pasini et al. 1749: 415-416, with shelfmark *b*. I. 1.

Its shelfmark was B. VII. 36.

Whereas Diels' catalogue mentions that it was *much damaged by fire* ("Durch Feuer stark beschädigt") and Cosentini 1922: 34 (no. 278) marks it with an asterisk (*) indicating that it was heavily damaged by the 1904 fire (see Id.: 5n(8): "I manoscritti preceduti da un asterisco * sono assai danneggiati dall'incendio del 1904"), it is listed between brackets by Eleuteri 1999: 32, meaning that it is currently unavailable (see Id.: 39n10: "Le parentesi quadre stanno ad indicare che il codice non è attualmente presente").

Possibly also [1621].

[1632]   **B V 33 (179 b II 33)**   I.14.

Same as [1629].

[1633]   **C VI 3 (287 c I 42)**   I.40, 47.

Same as [1630].

[1634]   **C VI 21 (b VI 18)**   I.44; II.82, 87; N.53.

This manuscript is *b*. VI. 18 in Pasini et al. 1749: 363 (with sequential number CCXXVIII).

Cosentini 1922: 42 (no. 363).

Current shelfmark: C. VI. 21.

Uppsala (SE)

Uppsala Universitetsbibliotek (Uppsala University Library)

Gr

5   (f. 120v [= 117v in prior foliation]) *De vita et morte*.

Torallas Tovar 1994: 208-215.

8   See [1635].

Nyström 2009.

25   See [1636].

28 A-B   (ff. 129r et seq.) Synesius Cyrenensis, *De insomniis*.

Graux, ed. Martin 1889: 341-343.

30   See [1637].

34   See [1638].

Upsala (Uppsala) (SE)

Upsal. bibl. acad. (*Upsaliensis Bibliotheca Academiae* [Library of Uppsala Academy]), now at Uppsala Universitet (Uppsala University)

-

[1635]   **8 (Sparfwenf. 49)**   I.38, 117; II.28, 78.

The mention "Sparfwenf. 49" does not belong to the shelfmark of the manuscript, but refers to the catalogue of the collection that Johan Gabriel Sparwenfeldt (1655-1727) assembled and donated in 1705 to Uppsala university library (*Catalogus* 1706: 55-61).

Graux, ed. Martin 1889: 322-329; Torallas Tovar 1994: 224-242; Nyström 2009.

Current shelfmark: Gr 8.

[1636]	**nr. 25**	I.73.
		Graux, ed. Martin 1889: 339.
		Current shelfmark: Gr 25.
[1637]	**30**	II.63.
		Graux, ed. Martin 1889: 344.
		Current shelfmark: Gr 30.
[1638]	**34**	II.104.
		Graux, ed. Martin 1889: 346; Ihm 2002: 213-216, no. 257 (especially 215).
		Current shelfmark: Gr 34.

Urbana, IL (US)

The Rare Book & and Manuscript Library, University of Illinois at Urbana-Champaign

Pre-1650 MSS

> 0004   Theophilus Protospatharius, *De excrementis* et *De tumoribus*; Hierophilus, *De nutritione*; Michael Psellus, *Poema de medicina*; *medica varia*.
>
> de Ricci and Wilson 1935: 699 (where the manuscript has a shelfmark x. 612.36 – T. 34 e).

Urbini et Pisauri (Urbino and Pesaro) (IT)

Bibl. Ducis (*Bibliotheca Ducis* [Duke's Library])

[1639]   -   II.40.

According to Diels, this copy of Gregorius Nyssenus, *De conditione hominis* is lost (*Verbleib unbekannt*).

The Duke of Urbino and Pesaro is Francesco Maria II Della Rovere (1549-1631). His collection of manuscripts was assembled by Federico da Montefeltro (1422-1482), and was transferred to the Vatican Library in 1631 (D'Aiuto 2011/2).

No Greek copy of Gregorius Nyssenus, *De conditione hominis* seems to appear among the Greek *Urbinati* manuscripts (see Stornajolo 1895, especially 339, the *Index Auctorum, Operum et Rerum Notabilium, sub nomine* Gregorius).

Similarly, no such copy of the work appears among Federico de Montefeltro's manuscripts listed in the so-called "Inventarium vetus" (or "Indice Vecchio") compiled ca. 1487 and published by Stornajolo 1895: CLX-CLXXV (Greek manuscripts).

However, one item with a similar title appears among the Latin manuscripts listed in the "Inventarium vetus" (Stornajolo 1895: LIX-CXXXIX), *sub* no. 109. Its description reads as follows (Stornajolo 1895: LXXVII):

109 Basilii Hexameron Episcopi neo Caesariensis a Rufino In latinum Conversum. *Gregorii* Niceni De homine sive Conditione hominis. In Purpureo.

This item corresponds to the current *Vaticanus Urbinas latinus* 485 (Stornajolo 1902: 494-495, especially 494 for the correspondence between item 109 of ˋ the "Inventarium vetus" and current shelfmark).

Venedig (Venezia [Venice]) (IT)

?

-

[1640]   **cod. Venetus** I.60.

In the section on the manuscripts of Galenus, *De optima secta ad Thrasybulum liber*, reference is made to a codex *Venetus* considered still unidentified (*bisher nicht identifiziert*).

Information is not sufficient to allow for any identification.

Bibl. Andreae Asulani *(Bibliotheca Andreae Asulani* [Andrea Asulanus' library]).

This is a manuscript owned by Andrea Torresanus (also known as Asulanus, 1451-1529), the heir of the Aldine press in Venice.

[1641]   -   I.59.

This is the manuscript *unicum* that was the source of *Galeni paraphrastae Menodoti suasoria ad artes oratio* in the 1525 Aldine edition of Galen published by Andrea Torresanus (on this edition, see Cataldi Palau 1998: 639-640).

According to Diels' catalogue the location of this manuscript is unknown (*Verbleib unbekannt*). More recently, see Boudon 2002: 46-47.

Bibl. Andreae de Rubeis (gr.?) *(Bibliotheca Andreae de Rubeis* [Andrea de Rubeis' Library])

Diels' catalogue mentions one manuscript owned, according to Tomasini 1650, by an apparently unknown Andrea de Rubeis (de' Rossi [?]), who possessed, according to the same, 10 manuscripts (most of which apparently in Greek).

[1642]   -   I.67.

This item, which Diels listed without knowing whether it was a Greek manuscript, is a copy of Galenus, *De ossibus ad tirones*.

Such a manuscript is listed by Tomasini 1650: 103, among the books "Apud V. Cl. Andream de Rubeis" as "Galenus de ossibus".

According to Garofalo and Debru 2005: 9n28, this manuscript cannot be found ("reste introuvable").

Bibl. Josephi de Aromatariis *(Bibliotheca Josephi de Aromatariis* [Giuseppe degli Aromatari's Library])

Diels' catalogue lists six manuscripts as being owned by Josephus de Aromatariis, who can be identified as the physician Giuseppe degli Aromatari (1587-1660). It does not provide any element of identification other than the texts they contain.

These manuscripts have been listed by Tomasini 1650: 94-95 (Manuscripta Graeca & Latina, quae extant in Bibliotheca Viri celeberrimi D. Iosephi de Aromatariis apud Venetos), which is most likely the source of Diels' information.

On this basis, it is possible to establish a correspondence between Diels' and Tomasini's items.

[1643]   -   I.67 (2), 70 (2), 84, 109, 113.

These references could refer to a unique manuscript containing a corpus of Galenic treatises (the treatises are listed below in the order of Tomasini's catalogue; references to Diels' catalogue follow the titles):

- *De foetus formatione* (I.70);

- *De musculorum dissectione* (I.109);

- *De nervorum dissectione* (I.67);

- *De venarum arteriarumque dissectione* (I.67);

- *De pulsibus ad Antonium* (I.113);

- *De causis respirationis* (I.70);

These titles correspond to the following entry in Tomasini 1650: 94, col. 1, ll. 16-27 (except "De Hominis structura", "De Quinque sensibus", and "De Respiratione difficili"):

- *Galenus de conformatione fetus*;

- *De Hominis structura*;

- *De Musculorum resectione, tyronibus*;

- *De Nervoru[m] dissectione*;

- *De Venarum resectione*;

- *De Pulsibus ad Antonium Philologum, & Philosophum*;

- *De Quinque sensibus*;

- *De Respirationis causis*;

- *De Respiratione difficili.*

According to all citations in Diels' catalogue, the manuscript cannot be located ("Verbleib unbekannt"). See also Formentin 1978: 23-24, 53 (about *De nervorum dissectione*), 54 (on *De causis respirationis*), 57 (on *De difficultate respirationis*), 63 (on *De musculorum dissectione ad tirones*), and 64 (on *De pulsibus ad Antonium*).

[1644]   -   II.17, 18 (2), 19.

This manuscript contains Aretaeus, *De causis et signis acutorum morborum*, *De causis et signis diuturnorum*, *De curatione acutorum morborum* and *De curatione diuturnorum morborum*.

This item corresponds exactly to the description by Tomasini 1650: 94, col. 1, ll. 8-15:

Aretaeus Cappadox de Causis & Signis Acutarum Affectionum. Idem de Causis & Signis Diuturnarum Affectionum. Idem de Acutarum affectionum curatione. Idem de Diuturnarum affectionum curatione.

While this manuscript, according to Diels, cannot be identified (*Verbleib unbekannt*), according to Formentin 1978: 24 and 76, it is now Berlin, SBB-PKB, *Phill. gr.* 1531 (= [0127]), which actually contains the four treatises by Aretaeus. See also Cutolo 2012: 26n19.

[1645]   -   II.49.

This copy of Herophilus, *Definitiones pulsuum* is described by Tomasini 1650: 94, col. 1, ll. 8-7 *ab imo* as follows:

Herophili definitiones Pulsuum. Fragmentum.

According to Formentin 1978: 83, this manuscript cannot be located and is probably incorrectly identified as the work is not known by any other copy. Although Herophilus did write on sphygmology (von Staden 1989: 262-288, T262), no manuscript of the work has been located so far.

[1646]   -   II.96.

This is a copy of Stephanus Alexandrinus, *Scholia in Hippocratis praenotiones*.

It corresponds to the following entry in Tomasini 1650: 94, col. 2, ll. 1-3:

Scholia, cum Deo, in Prognosticum Hippocratis, ex auditione (sive ore) Stephani Atheniensis.

The work or fragments of it are preserved in nine manuscripts (Duffy 1983: 13-19):

- *Florentinus Laurentianus* 59.14 (= [0304]) probably acquired by Janus Lascaris (1445-1534) in 1491-92 for the Medici library (Fryde 1996: 646, 790);
- *Londinensis* Wellcome 354 (see p. 122) attributed to Andreas Darmarios (b. 1540) (Moorat 1962: 225), with the text under Damascius' name;
- *Mediolanensis Ambrosianus* A 27 inf. (= [0662]) from the Pinelli collection (Martini and Bassi 1906: 882);
- *Mediolanensis Ambrosianus* L 30 sup. (= [0637]) owned by Girolamo Mercuriale (1530-1606) and purchased in Pisa, where Mercuriale taught (Martini and Bassi 1906: 566);
- *Mediolanensis Ambrosianus* Trotti 373 (see p. 136), owned by the Trivulzio family (Pasini 1997: 78-79);
- *Parisinus graecus* 2296 (= [1244]) owned by Gian Francesco d'Asola (Asulanus; ca. 1498-1157/58) and transferred to the Bibliothèque royale in Paris sometimes in the 1540s (Cataldi Palau 1998: 385-389);
- *Vindobonensis medicus graecus* 15 (= [1778]) purchased by Augier de Busbecq in Constantinople (Hunger and Kresten 1969: 59);
- *Yalensis Scholae medicae* 50 (see p. 166) attributed to Andreas Darmarios (Escobar Chico 1993: 85), with the text ascribed to Damascius and an ex-libris of *Sra Isabel Reyna Hungria*, dated 1779 on the anterior plate of the binding, internal side.

None of these descriptive elements suggests the identity of the item under discussion here, which remains unknown as Formentin 1978: 91 considered.

[1647]   -   II.101.

This manuscript of Theophilus, *De pulsibus* is described in Tomasini 1650: 94, col. 1, l. 5 *ab imo* as follows:

Theophilus de Pulsibus.

According to Formentin 1978: 24 and 94, it is now Berlin, SBB-PKB, *Phill. gr.* 1531 (= [0127]). See also Cutolo 2012: 26n19.

[1648]   -   I.115, 119, 125, 133.

Diels' catalogue mentions four more Galenic treatises as pertaining to Giuseppe de Aromatari (listed here in alphabetical order by titles; references to Diels' catalogue follow the titles):

- *De consuetudinibus* (I.119);
- *De quinque sensibus* (I.115);
- *De victu mensium* (I.125);
- *Remedia* (I.133).

Only the first title appears in Tomasini 1650: 94, col. 1, l. 28, among the items of de Aromatari's library, under the title that the treatise had in historiography at that time: "Claudius Galenus de Moribus".

It is not known if the other three treatises were either in the same volume but not listed by Tomasini, if each was a volume in its own right and none were catalogued by Tomasini, or if this is a mistake in Diels' catalogue.

Formentin 1978: 65 (on *De quinque sensibus*) and 66 (about *De consuetudinibus*) determines that these volumes cannot be located.

Bibl. Mon. St. Michael. (*Bibliotheca Monasterii Sancti Michaelis* [Library of St. Michael's Monastery])

[1649]   [-]   I.64.

This manuscript listed without shelfmark in Diels' catalogue is supposed to be a copy of Galen, *De elementis secundum Hippocratem*.

It does not appear in Mittarelli 1779. The information comes from Ackermann 1821: LXXV, no. 8 (without brackets), where the manuscript is identified as *mont. S. Mich.* without any other element of identification.

Ackermann's spelling *mont. S. Mich.* instead *of monast. St. Michael.* as in Diels I.14 (= [1650]) or *Monast. St. Michaelis prope Murianum* as in Diels I.92 (= [1651]), seems to refer to the library of the monastery of Mont Saint-Michel (*montis Sancti Michaelis*, abbreviated *mont. S. Mich.*) in France (actually, Avranches), rather than to the monastery of San Michele in Murano, Italy.

The Avranches library owns a copy of *De elementis Hippocratis secundum Hippocratem* (shelfmark: 232), listed in Diels I.64 among the Latin copies of the Hippocratic treatise, under Avranches.

On this manuscript, see *Catalogue général des manuscrits* 1872: 543-545; see 544, no. 9 for the text referred to here. Also Thorndike and Kibre 1963: 1274 (under *Quoniam elementum minima est particula* ...), and Kibre 1985: 135.

Bibl. monast. St. Michael. (*Bibliotheca monasterii Sancti Michaelis* [Library of St. Michael's Monastery]).

Although there is no mention of Murano as in [1651]-[1652], this is a reference to the library of San Michele of Murano, which has been dispersed (Merolla 2010).

[1650]   **104**   I.14.

This is a copy of Hippocrates, *Aphorismi*.

It is listed in Mittarelli 1779: 508:

Hippocrates Chius. "Aphorismata.". *Ext. in Cod.* 104.

Similar information (without the number 104, however) is found in Ackermann 1825: LXV (including the reference to Mittarelli 1779: 508), where it is among additions by K. (= Kühn).

Formentin 1978: 23, conjectures that this item could be the manuscript of Oxford, Bodleian Library, Holkham 106 (p. 181 and also [0406]) which contains indeed Hippocrates, *Aphorismi*. However, since Mittarelli 1779: 508, does not mention that it is in Greek (as he usually does when such is the case), this item seems rather to be a Latin manuscript (as Formentin 1978: 43 mentions; see also Magdelaine 1994: 88n1 and 185n3).

Given the paucity of the information, the present item cannot be identified with any of the Latin manuscripts of the treatise listed by Kibre 1985: 29-90. No identification is provided in Merolla 2010: 98. The manuscript is possibly lost.

Mioni 1958: 319; Merolla 2010: 98.

Bibl. Monast. St. Michaelis prope Murianum (*Bibliotheca Monasterii Sancti Michaelis prope Murianum* [Library of St Michael's Monastery, in Murano]), now San Michele di Murano (St. Michael of Murano).

The manuscripts of this library are no longer at the Monastery.

[1651]   **93**   I.92.

This is a copy of Galenus, *Methodi medendi libri XIV.*

This manuscript is listed in Mittarelli 1779: 424, item 2 *sub nomine* Galenus, where it is described as follows:

Idem [i.e. Galenus]. "Methodus Therapeutice." Codex Graecus chartac. in fol. Sec. XIV. Num. 93. cum notis marginalibus Graecis, aliquibus autem Latinis. Initio Codicis legitur: *Iste liber est mei Jani Podocathari Equitis regii & legum Doctoris, nunc autem mei Francisci Barbari.* Ad calcem bis legitur Graecis vocibus: *Hic liber est Johannis filii domini Manuelis ...*

It is now London, British Library, Add. 6898 (= [0527]).

Richard 1952: 6; Mioni 1958: 334-335; Diller 1963: 259 (no. 1600); Formentin 1978: 22-23, 58; Merolla 2010: 93.

[1652]   **132**   I.74.

This is a copy of Galenus, *De placitis Hippocratis et Platonis libri IX.*

The manuscript is listed twice in Mittarelli 1779: 424, item 1 *sub nomine* Galenus:

Galenus. "De Hippocratis & Platonis dogmatibus libri septem." *Codex Graecus in folio num.* 132. sed initio & fine mutilus, atque desunt primus, & initium secundi libri.

and 508, *sub nomine* Hippocrates:

Hippocrates Chius. ... "Dogmata." *In Codice* 132. *inscripto*: *Galenus de Hippocratis & Platonis dogmatibus libri septem Graece scripti.*

It is now Berlin, SBB-PKB, Ms. Ham. 270 (= [0116]).

Mioni 1958: 335; Formentin 1978: 22; De Lacy 2005: 12-18; Merolla 2010: 108-109.

Bibl. Nazionale Marciana (Biblioteca Nazionale Marciana [Marciana National Library]), now Biblioteca Nazionale San Marco (San Marco National Library)

graeci

Diels' catalogue identifies most of the items of this collection by their sequential number in the catalogue of Zanetti and Bongiovanni 1740. In [1665] and [1667], however, it includes a second number between parentheses, with the precision "jetzt" (= "now"), as if this second number was a new shelfmark. This number is the so-called "collocazione", which is part of the complete identification of the items in the Biblioteca Nazionale Marciana.

The list of all the Marciani of this collection that are mentioned here is given again (together with other *Veneti codices* not mentioned by Diels) under Venezia, Biblioteca Nazionale San Marco, with the so-called Zanetti number followed by the "collocazione" (see below, pp. 338-345).

[1653]   **[Marcian.]**   I.20 (2).

This manuscript listed without shelfmark in Diels' catalogue is Hippocrates, *Coacae praenotiones* and *Praenotiones*, liber I.

Similar vague information appears in Ackermann 1825: LIX (*Praedictiones*), and CXIV, no. 2 ctd. (*Coacae praenotiones*), in both cases without brackets:

in bibl. S. Marci

and

in bibl. D. Marci Ven.

According to Formentin 1978: 43 and 44, this manuscript could be *Marcianus gr.* 269 (= [1662]).

See also [1654] and [1656].

[1654]   **[Marcian.]**   I.124.

According to Diels, this manuscript listed without shelfmark is a copy of Hippocrates, *Praenotiones*, liber II.

This item should probably be grouped with [1653] and could be *Marcianus gr.* 269 (= [1662]), according to Formentin 1978: 46.

See [1653] and also [1656].

[1655]   **[Marcian. ?]**   I.10.

This item listed without shelfmark in Diels' catalogue is a copy of Hippocrates, *De morbis popolaribus*, I et III.

The paucity of the information does not allow for an identification. It may be the same as [1657]. In this case, it is not a copy of the Hippocratic treatise, but of the Galenic commentary on it.

[1656]   **[?]**   I.33.

This manuscript listed without shelfmark in Diels' catalogue is a copy of Hippocrates, *Praenotiones*, Liber II.

According to Formentin 1978: 46, this could be *Marcianus graecus* 269 (= [1662]).

The text is listed in the index of the manuscript, but is no longer present because of the loss of folios after f. 408.

Also [1653] and [1654].

[1657]   **[ap. Montf. I 472]**   I.10.

This manuscript listed without any other element of identifidation than a reference to a work by Montfaucon not otherwise identified, is a copy of Hippocrates, *De morbis popolaribus*, I et III.

The same information is found in Ackermann 1825: XXXIX (without brackets), who mentions "in bibl. D. Marci Ven, teste Montfauc. I. p. 472" with no further element of identification.

The reference is to Montfaucon 1739: 1.472, col. 1, item 5, where the following item can be found:

Galeni expositio in epidemias Hippocratis, in papyro

This is not a copy of the Hippocratic treatise, but of Galen's commentary on it (see also Formentin 1978: 42).

Four *Marciani* contain Galen's commentary on the *Epidemiae*:

- *gr.* 283 (coll. 631) (= [1680]), on paper, from Bessarion's collection;
- *gr.* 285 (coll. 708) (= [1683]), on parchment, from Bessarion's collection;
- *app. gr.* V.5 (coll. 1053) (= [1714]), on parchment, from the library of the San Giovanni e Paolo monastery;
- *app. gr.* V.15 (coll. 1299) (= [1727]), on paper, from the Nani collection.

Based on the medium and the provenance, the item listed by Montfaucon could correspond to *gr.* 283 (coll. 631) (= [1680]), unless it is another copy that is now lost. See, however, [1655].

[1658]   **92**   II.25, 30, 32, 79.

This codex is listed among the copies of the following four works (alphabetical order of author's name; references to Diels' catalogue follow the titles):

- Cratevas, *De herbis* (II.25);
- Dioscorides, *De materia medica* (II.30);
- Pseudo-Dioscorides, *De venenis* (II.35);
- Paulus Aegineta, *De succedaneis ex Galeno* (II.70).

Manuscript *Marcianus graecus* 92 (coll. 425) contains Iohannes Chrysostomus (Mioni 1981: 135-136).

The manuscript referred to here is current *Marcianus appendix graeca* XI, 21 (coll. 453) (see p. 344) (Mioni 1959: 374n70; Formentin 1978: 3, 77, 79; Touwaide 1981: 150-153).

Contrary to the indication in Diels' catalogue ("Venedig Marcian."), this manuscript was not originally among the holdings of the Biblioteca Nazionale Marciana in Venice, but in the collection of Giacomo Nani (1725-1797) catalogued by Mingarelli 1784. However, the manuscript *Nanianus* XCII (= 92) described by Mingarelli 1784: 180-182, contains *Patrum vitae et narrationes*. As Mioni 1967: XXV indicates, it corresponds to current *appendix graeca* II.70 (described in Mioni 1967: 197-204).

From the content in Diels, it appears that the manuscript referred to in Diels' catalogue was Nani CCLII (see Mingarelli 1784: 445-447). It was bequeathed to the Biblioteca Marciana (with Nani's whole collection). Mioni 1967: XXVI establishes the identification with current *appendix graeca* XI.21 (coll. 453) (on which see below, p. 344).

The number 92 in Diels' catalogue may come from Wellmann 1897: 23. It is repeated in much of the subsequent literature (among others Premerstein 1906: 185; Wellmann 1906-1914: 2.XX; Singer 1921: 65; Kourilas 1935: 28-29) until Mioni 1959: 374n70, who established the correspondence with current *Marcianus appendix graeca* XI.21 (coll. 453) (nevertheless, see MacKinney 1965: 180, no. 9, where the manuscript is identified as MS 92).

The source of this number 92 in Wellmann (above) is unknown. It might be significant, however, that the text attributed to Cratevas (instead of Pseudo-Dioscorides) by Wellmann 1897: 23, appears on f. 92.

[1659]   **173**   II.95.

Mioni 1981: 265-270; Mioni 1986: 18.

Current shelfmark: Gr. 173 (coll. 476).

[1660]   **257**   II.9, 10, 22.

Mioni 1981: 371–373; Mioni 1986: 22.

Current shelfmark: Gr. 257 (coll. 622).

[1661]   **266**   II.67.

Mioni 1981: 383-386; Mioni 1986: 23.

Current shelfmark: Gr. 266 (coll. 517).

[1662]   **269**   I.4, 5, 8, 10, 11 (2), 12 (2), 14, 18 (2), 19, 20, 21 (2), 22 (2), 23 (2), 24 (2), 25, 26 (2), 27 (3), 28 (2), 29 (2), 30 (3), 31 (2), 33, 34 (2), 35 (3), 38, 57, 110; II.93.

Mioni 1981: 391-393; Mioni 1986: 23.

Current shelfmark: Gr. 269 (coll. 533).

Also [1653], [1654] and [1656].

[1663]   **270**   II.17, 18 (2), 19.

Mioni 1981: 394.

Current shelfmark: Gr. 270 (coll. 624).

[1664]   **271**   II.25, 30, 32 (2).

Mioni 1981: 394-395.

Current shelfmark: Gr. 271 (coll. 727).

Also [1665].

[1665]   **271 (jetzt 727)**   N.49 (2).

Same as [1664].

[1666]   **272**   II.30, 32 (2).

Mioni 1981: 395-396; Mioni 1986: 23.

Current shelfmark: Gr. 272 (coll. 728).

Also [1667].

[1667]   **272 (jetzt 728)**   N.49 (2).

Same as [1666].

[1668]   **273**   II.30.

Mioni 1981: 396-398.

Current shelfmark: Gr. 273 (coll. 669).

[1669]   **275**   I.61, 64 (2), 65, 78, 79 (2), 80.

Mioni 1981: 399.

Current shelfmark: Gr. 275 (coll. 893).

[1670]   **276**   I.70, 73, 74, 75, 83, 92, 129; N.33.

Mioni 1981: 399-400; Mioni 1986: 24.

Current shelfmark: Gr. 276 (coll. 912).

Also [1671].

[1671]   **[276]**   I.114.

This is a copy of *De melancholia ex Galeno, Rufo, Posidonio et Marcello Sicamii Aetii libellus.*

As Diels' catalogue mentions, the texte referred to here is *De atra bile*, which appears in *Marcianus graecus* 276, ff. 261r-268r (Mioni 1981: 399-400).

Same as [1670].

[1672]   **277**   I.101, 105.

Mioni 1981: 400-401.

Current shelfmark: Gr. 277 (coll. 630).

[1673]   **278**   I.101, 105.

Mioni 1981: 402.

Current shelfmark: Gr. 278 (coll. 873).

[1674]   **279**   I.66, 69, 73, 76, 94, 95, 99, 106, 108 (2), 114; II.7, 86, 91.

Mioni 1981: 402-403.

Current shelfmark: Gr. 279 (coll. 705).

Also [1675].

[1675]   **[279 (?)]**   I.67.

This is supposed to be a copy of Galenus, *De venarum arteriarumque dissectione*. The same information appears in Ackermann 1821: LXXXVII (without brackets or question mark).

The text referred to here is probably one or more of the following three Galenic treatises contained in the manuscript (listed below according to the folio numbers) (Mioni 1981: 402-403):

- (ff. 243v-253r) *De venae sectione adversos Erasistrateos Romae degentes*;
- (ff. 253r-258v) *De venae sectione adversus Erasitratum*;
- (ff. 259r-267v) *De curandi ratione per venae sectionem*.

Same as [1674].

[1676]   **280**   I.85, 93, 98.

Mioni 1981: 403-404.

Current shelfmark: Gr. 280 (coll. 706).

[1677]   **281**   I.70, 72, 73 (2), 81, 83, 86, 99 (3), 100, 102, 103, 112; II.14.

Mioni 1981: 404-405.

Current shelfmark: Gr. 281 (coll. 581).

[1678]   **282**   I.28, 60, 71 (2), 73, 74, 75, 80, 81, 82, 83, 84, 89, 91, 96, 101 (2), 107, 113.

Mioni 1981: 405-406.

Current shelfmark: Gr. 282 (coll. 648).

Also [1679].

[1679]   **[282]**   I.114.

This is supposed to be a copy of *De melancholia ex Galeno, Rufo, Posidonio et Marcello Sicamii Aetii libellus*.

As Diels' catalogue mentions, the text referred to here is *De atra bile*, which appears in *Marcianus graecus* 282, ff. 194r-199v (Mioni 1981: 405-406).

Same as [1678].

[1680]   **283**   I.104.

Mioni 1981: 407; Mioni 1986: 24.

Current shelfmark: Gr. 283 (coll. 631).

See [1657].

[1681]   **284**   I.73, 74 (2), 92; N.33.

Mioni 1981: 407-408.

Current shelfmark: Gr. 284 (coll. 707).

Also [1682].

[1682]   **[284]**   I.114.

This is supposed to be a copy of *De melancholia ex Galeno, Rufo, Posidonio et Marcello Sicamii Aetii libellus.*

As Diels' catalogue mentions, the text referred to here is *De atra bile*, which appears in *Marcianus graecus* 284, ff. 223v-228v (Mioni 1981: 407-408).

Same as [1681].

[1683]   285   I.77, 98, 101, 104, 105.

Mioni 1981: 408-409.

Current shelfmark: Gr. 285 (coll. 708).

[1684]   286   I.96.

Mioni 1981: 409-410.

Current shelfmark: Gr. 286 (coll. 626).

[1685]   287   I.68, 87, 88 (2), 89.

Mioni 1981: 410-411.

Current shelfmark: Gr. 287 (coll. 709).

[1686]   288   I.98, 115; N.34.

Mioni 1981: 411-412; Mioni 1986: 24.

Current shelfmark: Gr. 288 (coll. 913).

[1687]   289   II.6; N.43.

Mioni 1981: 412.

Current shelfmark: Gr. 289 (coll. 627).

[1688]   290   II.6.

Mioni 1981: 412-413.

Current shelfmark: Gr. 290 (coll. 628).

[1689]   291   II.6, 8; N.43.

Mioni 1981: 413-416; Mioni 1986: 24.

Current shelfmark: Gr. 291 (coll. 298).

[1690]   292   II.78; N.62.

Mioni 1981: 416-418; Mioni 1986: 24.

Current shelfmark: Gr. 292 (coll. 914).

[1691]   293   II.74, 78.

Mioni 1981: 418-419.

Current shelfmark: Gr. 293 (coll. 299).

[1692]   294   II.71, 72.

Mioni 1981: 419-420.

Current shelfmark: Gr. 294 (coll. 288).

[1693]	**295**	I.114; II.4, 11, 79; N.37, 42, 61, 62.
		Mioni 1981: 420-423; Mioni 1986: 24.
		Current shelfmark: Gr. 295 (coll. 729).
[1694]	**296**	I.8; N.109.
		Mioni 1981: 423-424; Mioni 1986: 24.
		Current shelfmark: Gr. 296 (coll. 632).
[1695]	**297**	II.63.
		Mioni 1981: 425-426.
		Current shelfmark: Gr. 297 (coll. 633).
[1696]	**298**	II.109, 110.
		Mioni 1981: 426-427.
		Current shelfmark: Gr. 298 (coll. 583).
[1697]	**299**	II.95, 111, 112 (2), 115.

Mioni 1981: 427-433; Mioni 1986: 24; *CMAG* II (Zuretti et al.) 1927: 1-2, 341-358; *CMAG* IV (Goldschmidt) 1932: 399-432.

Current shelfmark: Gr. 299 (coll. 584).

[1698]	**334**	N.52.
		Mioni 1985: 66-71.
		Current shelfmark: Gr. 334 (coll. 553).
[1699]	**335**	II.82; N.53.
		Mioni 1985: 71-77.
		Current shelfmark: Gr. 335 (coll. 645).
[1700]	**336**	I.113; II.44, 82.
		Mioni 1985: 77-83.
		Current shelfmark: Gr. 336 (coll. 646).
[1701]	**480**	II.8.

Formentin 1978: 73-74 identifies this manuscript of Aglaias as *Marcianus graecus* 280, which is incorrect. *Marcianus* 280 (= [1676]) does contain medical texts (Galen), but not Aglaias. This is probably a typographical error in Formentin above (280 instead of 480).

Mioni 1985: 272-276.

Current shelfmark: Gr. 480 (coll. 589).

[1702]	**509**	I.149.
		Mioni 1985: 362-364.
		Current shelfmark: Gr. 509 (coll. 845).
[1703]	**510**	II.109.
		Mioni 1985: 365-367.
		Current shelfmark: Gr. 510 (coll. 769).

[1704]   **529**   II.109.

Mioni 1985: 415-417.

Current shelfmark: Gr. 529 (coll. 847).

[1705]   **596**   II.6; N.43.

Mioni 1985: 517-518.

Current shelfmark: Gr. 596 (coll. 867).

[1706]   **597**   II.30, 32 (2).

Mioni 1985: 518.

Current shelfmark: Gr. 597 (coll. 661).

[1707]   **609**   I.38.

Mioni 1985: 535-536.

Current shelfmark: Gr. 609 (coll. 686).

appendix graeca

Diels' catalogue includes a mention "olim Nanian." in [1709], [1722] and [1724], and "olim Na." in [1726]. This mention is followed by a number in Arabic numerals. This information refers to the collection of Giacomo Nani (1725-1797) catalogued by Mingarelli 1784 and bequeathed to the Biblioteca Marciana. These manuscripts entered the library after Nani's death. A table of concordance can be found in Mioni 1967: XXV-XXVI. This reference to Nani's collection is not part of the current shelfmark of the manuscripts.

[1708]   **II, 171**   I.95, 134; II.15, 91.

Mioni 1967: 97-98.

Current shelfmark: App. Gr. II.171 (coll. 445).

[1709]   **IV, 36 (olim Nanian. 258)**   II.43.

In Mingarelli 1784: 450, this manuscript is described among the *Philosophici* manuscripts of the collection assembled by Giacomo Nani.

Mioni 1967: 225-226.

Current shelfmark: App. Gr. IV.36 (coll. 1425).

[1710]   **V, 1**   II.78.

Mioni 1967: 253; Mioni 1986: 49.

Current shelfmark: App. Gr. V.1 (coll. 834).

Former [0902], and possibly [0903], 2nd part.

[1711]   **V, 2**   II.30.

Mioni 1967: 253.

Current shelfmark: App. Gr. V.2 (coll. 1246).

[1712]   **V, 3**   II.30.

Mioni 1967: 253.

Current shelfmark: App. Gr. V.3 (coll. 1280).

[1713]   **V, 4**   I.59, 64, 66, 68, 70, 71, 74 (2), 78, 79 (2), 80, 89, 91, 92, 93, 95, 102, 106 (2), 110, 111, 115, 121; II.59.

Mioni 1967: 254-255; Mioni 1986: 49.

Current shelfmark: App. Gr. V.4 (coll. 544).

[1714]   **V, 5**   I.61, 68, 69, 70, 73, 78, 80, 81 (2), 82 (2), 84, 85, 95 (2), 96, 102, 103, 104, 105, 107, 109, 112, 113, 128, 130.

Mioni 1967: 255-258; Mioni 1986: 49-50.

Current shelfmark: App. Gr. V.5 (coll. 1053).

[1715]   **V, 6**   I.96.

Mioni 1967: 258.

Current shelfmark: App. Gr. V.6 (coll. 1207).

[1716]   **V, 7**   I.98.

Mioni 1967: 258-261.

Current shelfmark: App. Gr. V.7 (coll. 1054).

[1717]   **V, 8**   I.89, 91; II.22, 100, 102, 110.

Mioni 1967: 262-265.

Current shelfmark: App. Gr. V.8 (coll. 1334).

[1718]   **V, 9**   I.29, 60, 68, 68-69, 73, 81 (2), 82, 96 (2), 101, 102, 105, 120; II.11, 12; N.30, 34, 36, 41.

Mioni 1967: 265-270.

Current shelfmark: App. Gr. V.9 (coll. 1017).

[1719]   **V, 10**   I.101, 105, 149; II.9.

Mioni 1967: 270; Mioni 1986: 50.

Current shelfmark: App. Gr. V.10 (coll. 1444).

[1720]   **V, 11**   I.76.

Mioni 1967: 271; Mioni 1986: 50.

Current shelfmark: App. Gr. V.11 (coll. 1064).

[1721]   **V, 12**   I.69, 79; II.101, 102 (2).

Mioni 1967: 271-273.

Current shelfmark: App. Gr. V.12 (coll. 1317).

Also [1722].

[1722]   **V, 12 (olim Nanian. 246)**   II.101.

In Mingarelli 1784: 437-438, this manuscript is described among the *Medici* manuscripts of the collection assembled by Giacomo Nani.

Same as [1721].

[1723]   **V, 13**   I.49, 149; II.7, 41, 45, 49, 65, 68, 80, 86, 109; N.53.

Mioni 1967: 273-276; Mioni 1986: 50; *CMAG* II (Zuretti et al.) 1927: 263-278.

Current shelfmark: App. Gr. V.13 (coll. 1221).

Also [1724].

[1724]   **V, 13 (olim Nanian. 247)**   II.43.

In Mingarelli 1784: 438-442, this manuscript is described among the *Medici* manuscripts of the collection assembled by Giacomo Nani.

Same as [1723].

[1725]   **V, 14**   I.34.

Mioni 1967: 276.

Current shelfmark: Gr. V.14 (coll. 1408).

Also [1726].

[1726]   **V, 14 (olim Na. 248)**   I.4, 26, 28, 31, 35.

In Mingarelli 1784: 442, this manuscript is described among the *Medici* manuscripts of the collection assembled by Giacomo Nani.

Same as [1725].

[1727]   **V, 15**   I.104; II.37; N.35.

Mioni 1967: 276-277.

Current shelfmark: App. Gr. V.15 (coll. 1299).

[1728]   **V, 16**   I.40 (2); II.7, 9, 28, 34, 80, 96.

Mioni 1967: 277-282; Mioni 1986: 50.

Current shelfmark: App. Gr. V.16 (coll. 1318).

[1729]   **V, 18**   I.149.

This item goes together with the following four (= [1730]-[1733]). These five numbers are not manuscripts but the five volumes of the 1525 printed edition of Galen (Venetiis, apud Aldum Manutium). All but vol. 3 (V.20 [coll. 987] = [1731]) contain handwritten notes attributed to Melchior Guillandini (ca. 1520-1589) by Mioni 1967: 284.

Mioni 1967: 283-284.

Current shelfmark: App. Gr. V.18 (coll. 985).

[1730]   **V, 19**   I.21, 149.

See [1729].

Current shelfmark: App. Gr. V.19 (coll. 986).

[1731]   **V, 20**   I.149.

See [1729].

Current shelfmark: App. Gr. V.20 (coll. 987).

[1732]	**V, 21**	I.149.

See [1729].

Current shelfmark: App. Gr. V.21 (coll. 988).

[1733]	**V, 22**	I.149.

See [1729].

Current shelfmark: App. Gr. V.22 (coll. 989).

[1734]	**XI, 5**	I.91.

Mioni 1973: 84-86; Mioni 1986: 66.

Current shelfmark: App. Gr. XI.5 (coll. 1254).

[Bibl. S. Anton.] (Biblioteca di San Antonio di Castello [San Antonio of Castello Library])

[1735]	[-]	I.14.

According to Diels' catalogue, this manuscript listed without any identifier is a copy of Hippocrates, *Aphorismi*.

The library of San Antonio monastery in Venice held the collection formed by Cardinal Domenico Grimani (1461-1523). Several catalogues and inventories of this collection have been published by Diller et al. 2003. In the first catalogue (probably compiled in 1522 when the cardinal's collection was moved from Rome to Venice), a manuscript of the Hippocratic *Aphorismi* can be found (see p. 157, no. 331). The text is listed in the analytical index of San Antonio library possibly compiled ca. 1545 (Diller et al. 2003: 177 [H27], shelfmark 3.11.331). It is no longer included in the list dating to 1598 (published in Diller et al. 2003: 191-195) or in the library catalogue compiled by Giovanni Filippo Tomasini and published in 1650 (ff. 15v-18v, reproduced in Diller et al. 2003: 197-203).

Whereas this manuscript was considered lost by Formentin 1978: 21-22, according to Diller et al. 2003: 157 (no. 331), it corresponds to current manuscript Vienna, *historicus graecus* 130 (= [1763]). According to Hunger 1961: 133, the manuscript contains a note referring to a 1490 acquisition. See also Magdelaine 1994: 90 and 162-163.

[1736]	[-]	I.20.

This manuscript listed without shelfmark in Diels' catalogue is a copy of Hippocrates, De *humoribus*.

A mention of this manuscript is made in Ackermann 1825: CXVI, no. 3 ctd.: "in bibl. S. Anton. Ven.".

This manuscript was in the collection of Cardinal Domenico Grimani (on which see [1735]). It is listed in the 1522 catalogue (Diller et al. 2003: 120, no. 69, l. 1) and in the 1545 ca. analytical index of San Antonio library (Diller et al. 2003: 177 [H5], shelfmark 3.6.69). It no longer appears in the subsequent catalogues (1598 and 1650).

Considered to be lost by Formentin 1978: 21-22, it corresponds to the current manuscript Paris, *graecus* 2253 (= [1184]) according to Diller et al. 2003: 120, no. 69, and Jackson 2009: 105.

Venezia (Venice) (IT)

Biblioteca Nazionale San Marco (San Marco National Library)

graeci

26 (coll. 340)	(f. 307r) *Praescriptiones medicae.*
	Mioni 1981: 41-44; Mioni 1986: 14.
58 (coll. 499)	(ff. 66v-116r) Gregorius Nyssenus, *De hominis opificio.*
	Mioni 1981: 83-85; Mioni 1986: 15.
66 (coll. 352)	(ff. 2r-55r) Gregorius Nyssenus, *De hominis opificio.*
	Mioni 1981: 91; Mioni 1986: 15.
82 (coll. 373)	(ff. 363v-369r) Gregorius Nazianzenus, *De humana natura.*
	Mioni 1981: 122-125; Mioni 1986: 15; Domiter 1999: 21.
83 (coll. 512)	(ff. 113r-116v) Gregorius Nazianzenus, *De humana natura.*
	Mioni 1981: 125-128; Mioni 1986: 15; Domiter 1999: 21.
130 (coll. 665)	(f. Vv) *De ictero et tabe.*
	Mioni 1981: 181-182.
172 (coll. 574)	(f. 170r) *De hominis aetatibus.*
	Mioni 1981: 261-265; Mioni 1986: 18.
173 (coll. 476)	See [1659].
175 (coll. 575)	(f. 242v) *De generatione hominis.*
	Mioni 1981: 276-277; Mioni 1986: 19.
177 (coll. 347)	(f. 14v) *De hominis aetatibus.*
	Mioni 1981: 278-279; Mioni 1986: 19.
200 (coll. 327)	(ff. 122v-124v) Aristoteles, *De insomniis*; (ff. 289-293v) Aristoteles, *Physiognomonica*; (ff. 317-370) Aristoteles, *Problemata.*
	Wartelle 1963: 155-156, no. 2101; Mioni 1981: 311-313; Mioni 1986: 20.
206 (coll. 747)	(ff. 312r-315v) Aristoteles, *De insomniis.*
	Wartelle 1963: 156, no. 2107; Mioni 1981: 320-321.
209 (coll. 1023)	(ff. 105r-111v) Aristoteles, *De insomniis.*
	Wartelle 1963: 156-157, no. 2120; Mioni 1981: 322-323.
212 (coll. 606)	(ff. 435v-438r) Aristoteles, *De insomniis.*
	Wartelle 1963: 157, no. 2113; Mioni 1981: 326-327.

214 (coll. 479)	(ff. 181r-183r) Aristoteles, *De insomniis.*
	Wartelle 1963: 157, no. 2115; Mioni 1981: 328-329.
215 (coll. 752)	(ff. 185r-193r) Aristoteles, *Physiognomonica*; (ff. 211v-299) Aristoteles, *Problemata.*
	Wartelle 1963: 157, no. 2116; Mioni 1981: 329-330; Mioni 1986: 21.
216 (coll. 404)	(ff. 5r-22r) Aristoteles, *Physiognomonica*; (ff. 150r-347r) Aristoteles, *Problemata.*
	Wartelle 1963: 157-158, no. 2117; Mioni 1981: 330-331.
237 (coll. 755)	(ff. 83r-93r) Michael Ephesius, *In Aristotelis de insomniis.*
	Wartelle 1963: 159, no. 2137; Mioni 1981: 349-350.
238 (coll. 618)	(ff. 84v-94r) Michael Ephesius, *In Aristotelis de insomniis.*
	Wartelle 1963: 159, no. 2138; Mioni 1981: 351.
239 (coll. 911)	(ff. 296r-302r) Theodorus Metochites, *In Aristotelis de insomniis.*
	Wartelle 1963: 159, no. 2139; Mioni 1981: 351-353; Mioni 1986: 22.
257 (coll. 622)	See [1660].
259 (coll. 982)	(ff. 45v-54v) Cassius iatrosophista, *Problemata*; (ff. 54v-141r) Aristoteles, *Problemata.*
	Wartelle 1963: 160, no. 2145; Mioni 1981: 374-375; Mioni 1986: 23.
263 (coll. 1025)	(ff. 130r-139v) Aristoteles, *Physiognomonica* (frg.); (f. 166r-v) Nemesius Emesenus, *De natura hominis* (frg.).
	Wartelle 1963: 160, no. 2147; Mioni 1981: 378-380; Mioni 1986: 23.
264 (coll. 758)	(ff. 340v-357v) Synesius Cyrenensis, *De insomniis.*
	Mioni 1981: 380-381; Mioni 1986: 23.
266 (coll. 517)	See [1661].
269 (coll. 533)	See [1662].
270 (coll. 624)	See [1663].
271 (coll. 727)	See [1664].
272 (coll. 728)	See [1666].
273 (coll. 669)	See [1668].
275 (coll. 893)	See [1669].
276 (coll. 912)	See [1670].

277 (coll. 630)   See [1672].

278 (coll. 873)   See [1673].

279 (coll. 705)   See [1674].

280 (coll. 706)   See [1676].

281 (coll. 581)   See [1677].

282 (coll. 648)   See [1678].

283 (coll. 631)   See [1680].

284 (coll. 707)   See [1681].

285 (coll. 708)   See [1683].

286 (coll. 626)   See [1684].

287 (coll. 709)   See [1685].

288 (coll. 913)   See [1686].

289 (coll. 627)   See [1687].

290 (coll. 628)   See [1688].

291 (coll. 298)   See [1689].

292 (coll. 914)   See [1690].

293 (coll. 299)   See [1691].

294 (coll. 288)   See [1692].

295 (coll. 729)   See [1693].

296 (coll. 632)   See [1694].

297 (coll. 633)   See [1695].

298 (coll. 583)   See [1696].

299 (coll. 584)   See [1697].

308 (coll. 636)   (ff. 48v-49v) Epiphanius, *De duodecim gemmis* (frg.).
                         Mioni 1985: 15-17.

320 (coll. 638)   (f. 14v) *Medicamentum contra pulices.*
                         Mioni 1985: 34-35.

327 (coll. 642)   (f. 21v) *De phlebotomia.*
                         Mioni 1985: 52-54.

333 (coll. 644)   (ff. 23v-25v) Hippocrates, *De natura hominis* (frg.).
                         Mioni 1985: 61-66.

334 (coll. 553)   See [1698].

335 (coll. 645)   See [1699].

336 (coll. 646)   See [1700].

406 (coll. 791)   (f. 93v) Adamantius, *Physiognomica* (frg.).
                         Mioni 1985: 157-159.

422 (coll. 900)   (ff. 119r-133r) Synesius Cyrenensis, *De insomniis*
                         cum Nicephori Gregorae commentario.
                         Mioni 1985: 185-187.

440 (coll. 761)   (f. 125v) *Medicamentum contra λυποϑυμίαν.*

Mioni 1985: 210-211.

477 (coll. 879)   (ff. 1v-43r) Nicander, *Theriaca*; (ff. 43v-74v) Nicander, *Alexipharmaca.*

Mioni 1985: 269.

480 (coll. 589)   See [1701].

494 (coll. 331)   (ff. 206v-207r) Gregorius Nazianzenus, *De humana natura.*

Mioni 1985: 307-318; Mossay and Coulie 1998: 255-256.

497 (coll. 292)   (ff. 184r-227v) Gregorius Nyssenus, *De hominis opificio.*

Mioni 1985: 323-324.

498 (coll. 432)   (ff. 93r-95v) Epiphanius, *De duodecim gemmis* (frg.); (ff. 247v-248v) *Medicamenta varia*; (f. 305r-v) *De hominis septem aetatibus.*

Mioni 1985: 324-335.

500 (coll. 803)   (ff. 147v-148r) Splenius, *De generatione hominis.*

Mioni 1985: 336-337.

501 (coll. 555)   (f. 176v) *Oratio contra capitis dolorem et ophthalmiam.*

Mioni 1985: 338-341.

506 (coll. 768)   (ff. 26r-50r) Hippocrates, *Aphorismi*, cum Theophili Protospatharii scholiis.

Mioni 1985: 354-357.

507 (coll. 293)   (f. 76r) *De homine.*

Mioni 1985: 357-360.

508 (coll. 844)   (ff. 133r-141r) Basilius Caesariensis, *De hominis opificio*; (ff. 148r-154v) Gregorius Nyssenus, *De hominis opificio.*

Mioni 1985: 360-362.

509 (coll. 845)   See [1702].

510 (coll. 769)   See [1703].

512 (coll. 678)   (f. 104v) *Praescriptiones medicae*; (f. 177v) *Praescriptiones medicae in morbos oculorum*; (f. 179v) *De podagra*; (ff. 239v-256v) *Cyranides* (frg.).

Mioni 1985: 369-374.

516 (coll. 904)   (f. Iv) *Medicamenta.*

Mioni 1985: 381-384.

517 (coll. 886)	(ff. 121r-122r) *Medicamenta*; (ff. 124r-125r) Aetius Amidenus, *Libri medicinales*, 13 (frg.); (ff. 126r-128r) Diocles, *Ad Antigonum regem epistula de tuenda valetudine.*
	Mioni 1985: 384-386.
521 (coll. 316)	(ff. 21r-51r) Meletius, *De natura hominis*; (ff. 97r-99v) Cassius iatrosophista, *Problemata* (frg.); (f. 100r-v) Galenus, *Definitiones medicae* (frg.).
	Mioni 1985: 390-393.
523 (coll. 846)	(ff. 40v-42r) Synesius Cyrenensis, *De insomniis* (frg.).
	Mioni 1985: 396-398.
524 (coll. 318)	(ff. 9r-10v) *De dentibus*; (ff. 190r-192r) *Geoponica* (frg.).
	Mioni 1985: 399-407; Mioni 1986: 26.
529 (coll. 847)	See [1704].
589 (coll. 830)	(ff. 108v-109r) *De generatione infantium.*
	Mioni 1985: 508-511.
596 (coll. 867)	See [1705].
597 (coll. 661)	See [1706].
602 (coll. 418)	(ff. 100r-123v) Nemesius Emesenus, *De natura hominis.*
	Mioni 1985: 527-528.
603 (coll. 685)	(ff. 22r-23r) *De cibis qui per singulos menses utiles sunt ad sanitatem tuendam.*
	Mioni 1985: 528-529.
604 (coll. 910)	(ff. 1r-122r) Aristoteles, *Problemata.*
	Wartelle 1963: 161, no. 2156; Mioni 1985: 529-531.
609 (coll. 686)	See [1707].
appendix graeca	
II.53 (coll. 1165)	(ff. 107v-116v) Gregorius Nyssenus, *De hominis opificio* (frg.).
	Mioni 1967: 167-168; Mioni 1986: 33.
II.105 (coll. 563)	(ff. 83r-99r) Manuel Philes, *De animalium proprietate.*
	Mioni 1967: 316-320.
II.123 (coll. 567)	(ff. 146v-161r) *Physiologus* (frg.).
	Mioni 1972: 8-12; Mioni 1986: 41.
II.163 (coll. 444)	(f. 45r) *Medicamentum*; (ff. 100r-107v) *De herba paeonia*; (ff. 112r-113v) *Oneirocriticon.*
	Mioni 1972: 74-76; Mioni 1986: 42.

II.171 (coll. 445)	See [1708].
II.183 (coll. 1000)	(ff. 83r-103v) Basilius Caesariensis, *De hominis opificio*.
	Mioni 1972: 111-112; Mioni 1986: 43.
III.4 (coll. 1076)	(ff. 438v-439r) *De generatione*.
	Mioni 1972: 144-156; Mioni 1986: 44.
IV.28 (coll. 543)	(ff. 7r-11r) Nicephorus Constantinopolitanus Patriarcha, *Oneirocriticon*; (ff. 11v-12v) *Geoponica* (frg.); (ff. 130r-132r) Cleopatra, *De mensuris et ponderibus*.
	Mioni 1972: 214-221; Mioni 1986: 47.
IV.35 (coll. 1383)	*Physiologus*.
	Mioni 1972: 225.
IV.36 (coll. 1425)	See [1709].
IV.46 (coll. 1464)	(f. 15v) *De hominis septem aetatibus*; (f. 38v) *De hominum quinque sensibus*; (f. 39r-v) *De hominis fabrica*; (f. 40r-v) *De urinis*; (f. 40v) *De sanguine*; (f. 41r) *De morte*; (f. 68r) *De generatione*; (f. 70r) *De morbis humanis secundum singulum* ζώδιον; (f. 71r) *Hominis imago cum zodiaci signis quae singulis membris praesident*; (f. 76v) *Hominis figura cum zodiaci signis*; (f. 82r) *De phlebotomia*.
	Mioni 1972: 233-239; Mioni 1986: 48.
IV.55 (coll. 1191)	(f. 297r) *Nomina plantarum medicinalium*.
	Mioni 1972: 244-245; Mioni 1986: 49; Touwaide 1999: 216, 228.
IV.58 (coll. 1206)	(ff. 15r-26r) Aristoteles, *Physiognomica*; (ff. 34v-152v) Aristoteles, *Problemata* (frg.); (ff. 194v-210r) Nemesius Emesenus, *De natura hominis*.
	Wartelle 1963: 161, no. 2165; Mioni 1972: 247; Morani 1981: 56-57; Mioni 1986: 49.
V.1 (coll. 834)	See [1710].
V.2 (coll. 1246)	See [1711].
V.3 (coll. 1280)	See [1712].
V.4 (coll. 544)	See [1713].
V.5 (coll. 1053)	See [1714].
V.6 (coll. 1207)	See [1715].
V.7 (coll. 1054)	See [1716].
V.8 (coll. 1334)	See [1717].
V.9 (coll. 1017)	See [1718].

V.10 (coll. 1444)	See [1719].
V.11 (coll. 1064)	See [1720].
V.12 (coll. 1317)	See [1721].
V.13 (coll. 1221)	See [1723].
V.14 (coll. 1408)	See [1725].
V.15 (coll. 1299)	See [1727].
V.16 (coll. 1318)	See [1728].
V.17 (coll. 1281)	*Iatrosofion* (16th century).
	Mioni 1972: 282-283.
V.18 (coll. 985)	See [1729].
V.19 (coll. 986)	See [1730].
V.20 (coll. 987)	See [1731].
V.21 (coll. 988)	See [1732].
V.22 (coll. 989)	See [1733].
VII.38 (coll. 1385)	(161r-v) *De conceptione, De fetu, De generatione*; (f. 172v) Splenius, *De generatione hominis* (frg.).
	Mioni: 1960: 69-84; Mioni 1986: 56-57.
IX.18 (coll. 1432)	Manuel Philes, *De animalium proprietate*.
	Mioni 1973: 19-20.
XI.5 (coll. 1254)	See [1734].
XI.9 (coll. 1232)	(ff. 2r-38r) Synesius Cyrenensis, *De insomniis* cum Nicephori Gregorae scholiis (ff. 38v-40v) *De nominibus membrorum humani corporis*; (f. 40v) *De victus ratione*.
	Mioni 1973: 89-91; Mioni 1986: 67.
XI.12 (coll. 1084)	(ff. 1r-150v) *Geoponica*.
	Mioni 1973: 95; Mioni 1986: 67.
XI.18 (coll. 1042)	(f. 171r-v) Aetius Amidenus, *Excerpta medica tria*.
	Mioni 1973: 102-106; Mioni 1986: 68.
XI.20 (coll.1475)	(f. 302v) *Exhorcismus contra morsus viperarum et serpentium*; (f. 302v) *Exhorcismus contra astheniam*; (f. 301v) *Quo cibo per totum annum utendum sit*.
	Mioni 1973: 109-112; Mioni 1986: 69.
XI.21 (coll. 453)	Formerly [1658].
	Mioni 1973: 112-115; Mioni 1986: 69.
XI.23 (coll. 1292)	(ff. 178r-182v) *Physiologus* (frg.); (ff. 212v-213r) *Prognostica de vita et morte*.
	Mioni 1973: 131-133; Mioni 1986: 70.

XI.24 (coll.1293)	(ff. 75r-77r) Epiphanius, *De duodecim gemmis* (frg.); (ff. 96v-101v) *Physiologus* (frg.); (f. 157v) *De hominis septem aetatibus et quinque sensibus.*
	Mioni 1973: 133-138; Mioni 1986: 70.
XI.26 (coll. 1322)	(f. 348r) Adamantius sophista ex Aetio Amideno, *Libri medicinales*, 3.163-164.
	Mioni 1973: 141-146; Mioni 1986: 70.
XI.31 (coll. 1354)	(f. 103v) *De sanitate tuenda praecepta*; (f. 103v) Dioscorides, *Praecepta per singulos menses*; (f. 104r) *Alia praecepta*, et *De victu* (f. 168r-v) *Praecepta medica*; (f. 168v) *Dies fasti et nefasti ad usum medicorum.*
	Mioni 1973: 157-165; Mioni 1986: 72.

Verona (IT)

    Bibl. Capitolare (Biblioteca Capitolare [Chapter Library])

[1737]   **CXXIX (118)**   II.63.

           Omont 1891: 6-7; Mioni 1965: 2.498-499; Marchi 1996: 216.

[1738]   **57**   II.108.

This is a copy of Ioannes Zacharias Actuarius, *Opera*.

According to Formentin 1978: 27-28, Diels' catalogue probably reproduced one item taken from Montfaucon 1739: 1.490. There (line E9), Montfaucon mentions the following item:

57. Actuarius

This manuscript appears in a collection identified as follows (Montfaucon 1739: 1.490): *In Museo Joannis Saibante*. According to the same, the information was reproduced from the following source:

In Verona Illustrata V. CL. D. Scipionis Maffei, parte tertia pag. 242.

In Maffei, *Verona Illustrata*, Parte terza, 1732 (in-folio edition), the manuscript referred to here did not belong to the Biblioteca Capitolare of Verona contrary to Diels, but to the 18th-century Veronese book collector Giovanni Saibante (fl. 1732). His collection is catalogued in Maffei 1732: 3.241-244, and the manuscript numbered 57 appears in column 244 (and note 242 as in Montfaucon 1739). This catalogue of Saibante's collection in Maffei 1732 is directly followed by the list of the *Manoscritti Capitolari* (Maffei 1732: 3.244-251), something that may have created confusion in Diels.

Whereas Formentin (above) considers this manuscript lost, it is Oxford, Bodleian Library, Auct. T. 4. 3 (= [0862] and [0863]), as was clear from Coxe 1853: 774-809; more recently, Jeffreys 1977: 258.

Vicenza (IT)

Bibl. Bertoliana (Biblioteca Bertoliana [Bertoliana Library]), now Biblioteca Civica Bertoliana [Bertoliana City Library])

[1739]   **44 (I.6.15)**   II.71, 89.

Mazzatinti 1892: 10.

This is not a Greek copy of Oribasius (II.71) and Rufus (II.89), but a Latin translation of Oribasius, *De cerebro eiusque tunicis* and *De ossibus, de musculis et de nervorum distributione*, and Rufus, *De partium corporis appellationibus*, as Formentin 1978: 28 noticed. Instead of Rufus, however, she mentions Paul of Aegina, whose text is not present in the manuscript according to Mazzatinti's catalogue.

Viterbo (IT)

Biblioteca Capitolare (Chapter Library)

11   *Physiologus.*

Mioni 1965: 2.527-528 (the manuscript is identified as no. 68).

49   Hippocrates, *Aphorismi*, cum Theophili Protospatharii *Commentario.*

Mioni 1965: 2.527 (numbered 8).

Warschau (Warsawa [Warsaw]) (PL)

Bibl. Zamoyski (*Bibliotheca Zamoyski* [Zamoyski Library])

[1740]   **142**   I.61.

According to Diels' catalogue, this is a copy of Galenus, *Ars medica.*

Although most manuscripts of this library were destroyed during World War II, codex 142 has been preserved (Aland 1956: 20). After the war, the remaining items of the Zamoyski library were transferred to the Biblioteka Narodowa (see p. 347).

The codex 142 (Current shelfmark:BN BOZ 142) does not contain Galen's *Ars medica* (Foerster 1900: 444; Aland 1956: 22; Canart 1974: 554-555), but mostly Herennius, *Commentarius in Aristotelis Metaphysicae libros.* Aland 1956: 22. For an analysis of the manuscript, see Foerster 1900: 435-448.

Contrary to Boudon 2002: 197n109 ctd, this manuscript can, in fact, be found.

The information contained in Diels results from an unaccountable mistake.

Warsawa (Warsaw) (PL)

    Biblioteka Narodowa (National Library)

        BOZ

125	(ff. 220r-230v and 234r-236r) Manuel Philes, *De animalium proprietate*.
	Kaliszuk and Szyller 2012: 55.
155	Johannes Zacharias Actuarius; Galenus.
	Description in Turyn 1928: 507-511; Aland 1956: 22-23; Kaliszuk and Szyller 2012: 61.

Washington, D.C. (US)

    Library of Congress

    Rare Book and Manuscripts, Medieval and Renaissance MSS.

        37   Gregorius Nyssenus, *De hominis opificio* (frg.).

A bifolium (actually the first of a quire signed as number 8 on the verso of the current second folio). Black and white reproduction in Jaeger 1947: plates I-IV.

A description (with an incorrect identification of the text) is provided in de Ricci and Wilson 1935: 211.

This bifolium is incorrectly quoted in the literature under the sequential number 60 that it received in de Ricci and Wilson 1935: *ibid.* (see for example Jaeger 1947; Mercati 1956; Olivier 1995: 830; and, more recently Canart and Lucà 2000: 43).

As Jaeger 1947 noticed, this bifolium comes from manuscript *Vaticanus graecus* 2066 (see p. 304).

Weimar (DE)

    Herzogin-Anna-Amalia-Bibliothek (Duchess Anna-Amalia Library)

        Q 733   (pp. 1-55) *Iatrosofion*, 16th century.

                    No published catalographic description is currently available.

Wien (Vienna) (AT)

[1741]   **(bei Berth.-Ruelle, Alchim. gr. I p. 56-69)**   II.100.

This manuscript listed in Diels' catalogue without library name and shelfmark, is vaguely identified in Berthelot and Ruelle 1888 referred to in the catalogue.

In the edition of Synesius Cyrenensis, *Ad Dioscorum, scholia in librum Democriti* (published in Berthelot and Ruelle 1888: 56-69), reference is made (p. 56) to an unidentified Vienna manuscript ("le ms. de Vienne").

In the edition of Pelasgius, *De chrysopoeia* contained in the same work (Berthelot and Ruelle 1888: 253-261), reference is made to the Vienna codices 51 and 52 (*ibid.*: 253).

Also, in the edition of Ostanes, *De chrysopoeia* that follows (Berthelot and Ruelle 1888: 261-262) reference is made (*ibid.*: 261) to one manuscript ("le ms. de Vienne dit Codex medicus gr. 51").

No mention of one or more Vienna manuscript(s) is made in the "Note préliminaire sur les abréviations, les sigles des manuscrits, etc." (Berthelot and Ruelle 1888: 2), which precedes the several editions contained in the same volume.

The Vienna collection owns two manuscripts (twin codices dating back to 1564) that contain Synesius Cyrenensis, Pelasgius, and Ostanes:

- *medicus graecus* 2 (see below, p. 357): (ff. 47v-53r) Synesius Cyrenensis; (ff. 37r-40v) Pelasgius; (ff. 40v-41r) Ostanes;
- *medicus graecus* 3 (= [1767]): (ff. 36v-40r) Pelasgius; (ff. 40v-41r) Ostanes; (ff. 47v-52v), Synesius Cyrenensis.

The reference to "le ms. de Vienne" (singular, in Berthelot and Ruelle 1888: 56) and to the "Codex medicus 51" (*ibid.*: 261) seem to indicate that only the manuscript *medicus graecus* 2 was intended in Diels' catalogue, although *medicus graecus* 2 and 3 are almost identical (on both manuscripts, see Hunger and Kresten 1969: 41-43 and 44-46 respectively).

See below (p. 357) for *medicus graecus* 2 and [1767] for *medicus graecus* 3.

Bibl. Colleg. S. J. Rossia (*Bibliotheca Collegii Societatis Jesu Rossia* [Rossia Library of Jesuit Company College], actually Jesuitenkollegiums [Jesuits' College]; see Gollob 1908)

[1742]   **XI.167**   N.27 (2), 28, 30, 39, 51, 56 (2), 63 (2), 65, 66.

Diels' catalogue confuses two different manuscripts:

- all references (except N.30) are about the item with shelfmark XI.167;
- N.30 is about Galenus, *De usu partium*, which is not in XI.167 (Gollob 1908: 1-12), but in another codex of the same collection: XI.132 (on which Gollob 1908: 12-13).

Both manuscripts are now Città del Vaticano, Biblioteca Apostolica Vaticana (table of concordance of shelfmarks in Canart and Peri 1970: 322-323):

- XI.167 is now *Rossianus* 1018;
- XI.132 is now *Rossianus* 982. On this codex, see also [1442].

On these two manuscripts see pp. 55-56, Città del Vaticano, Biblioteca Apostolica Vaticana.

Gollob Privatbesitz (Private collection Eduard Gollob)

[1743]   -   N.27.

This miscellaneous manuscript contains on ff. 143r-162v Hippocrates, *Epistulae*. When Diels' catalogue was compiled, it belonged to Eduard Gollob (1856-1922), in Krems (Gollob 1903: 29-31).

It is now in Wien, Österreichische Nationalbibliothek, *Supplementum graecum* 179 (Hunger and Hannick 1994: 313-315) (see below, p. 366).

Hofbibliothek (Court Library), now Österreichische Nationalbibliothek (National Library of Austria)

In the list of the manuscripts preserved by that library, Diels' catalogue refers to three different printed catalogues about items [1744]-[1757]:

- in [1744]-[1751], references to **Lambec.** are to Petri Lambecii, *Commentariorum de Augustissima Bibliotheca Caesarea Vindobonensi Liber primus* [*secundus* and *sextus*]. Vindobonae: Typis Matthaei Cosmerovii, 1665, 1669, 1674 respectively;

- in [1752]-[1754], references to **Lambec. ed. Kollar** are to Petri Lambecii Hamburgensis, *Commentariorum de Augustissima Bibliotheca Caesarea Vindobonensis Liber primus* (*secundus, ...* usque ad *octavum*). Editio altera opera et studio Adam Francisci Kollarii ..., 8 vols. Vindobonae: Typis et sumptibus Ioan. Thomae nob. de Trattnern, 1766-1782;

- in [1755]-[1756] (to which [1757] must be added), references to **Nessel** are to D. Danielis de Nessel, *Breviarium & Supplementum Commentariorum Lambecianorum, Sive Catalogus aut Recensio specialis Codicum Mstorum Graecorum, nec non Linguarum Orientalium Augustissimae Bibliothecae Caesareae Vindobonensis* ..., 2 vols. Vindoboneae & Norimbergae: Typis Leopoldi Voigt, & Joachimi Balthasaris Endteri, 1690.

[1744]

    [ap. Lambec. I 181]   I.65, 83, 89.

This manuscript is supposed to contain the following three Galenic treatises (order of Diels' catalogue):

- *De facultatibus naturalibus* (I.65);

- *De marcore* (I.83);

- *De crisibus libri III* (I.89).

The information comes from Ackermann 1821 (where the same reference to Lambecius can be found, without brackets) (same order of texts as above):

- LXXXI, no. 14 ctd.: *De facultatibus naturalibus*;

- CXXXIII, no. 61: *De marcore*;

- CVIII, no. 43: *De crisibus libri III*.

The notice about this manuscript in Lambeck, *Liber primus*, p. 181 (published in 1665) reads as follows (ll. 14-24):

Claudii Galeni Opuscula quaeda[m] Medica; nempe ... *de Marasmo* sive *marcore*, ..., *de Facultatibus naturalibus*, ..., *de Crisibus*, ...; translata ex *Arabica* in *Hebraicam* linguam à R. *Chanim Ben Isaac* ante annos plùs minùs *sexcentos* ... Codex preastantissimus partim in membranâ, partim in chartâ; fol. N. 24.

According to this description, this is a Hebrew manuscript which contains the *Compendium Alexandrinum* of Galen's works translated from Arabic into Hebrew. Ackermann 1821: CXXXIII, no. 61 (who lists the manuscripts under "graeci" with a reference to "Lamb. I. p. 181") includes it in the same paragraph as "*Hebraicus* cod. Ex arabico versus a R. Chanin ben Isaac ... in bibl. Vind. Lamb. Ed. Koll. I, p. 290).

The current shelfmark at the Österreichische Nationalbibliothek is Cod. Hebr. 29.

See Schwarz 1925: 187-191.

[1745]   **[ap. Lamb. II c. 6]**   I.98.

This is supposed to be a copy of Galenus, *De compositione medicamentorum secundum locos libri X.*

The information comes from Ackermann 1821: CXXIV, no. 54 ctd. (without brackets), mentioning that the *Vindobonensis* referred to by Lambecius II. c. 6 contains only books VI-VIII ("Libri VI. VII. VIII. Codex est in bibl. Vindob. Lamb. II. c. 6.")

The reference seems to be to *Liber Secundus*, Chapter 6 in Lambeck 1669 (= p. 465-519). This chapter is entitled "De *Henrici Gundelsingij* Historia Austriaca hactenus inedita, cujus Codex Mstus ... est inter Mstos Codices Historicos Latinos *trecentesimus vigesimus primus*", where there is no mention of any Greek manuscript containing a treatise by Galen.

The only manuscript containing Galenus, *De compositione medicamentorum secundum locos libri X* in the current collections of the Österreichische Nationalbibliothek is *medicus graecus* 15 (= [1778]). However, it contains only fragments of books 1-10 of the work (Hunger and Kresten 1969: 55-59).

No other *Vindobonensis* seems to contain the treatise. See:

- Hunger 1961: 454 for the *Vindobonenses historici* and *philosophici et philologici*;

- Hunger and Kresten 1976: 186 for the *theologici* 1-100;

- Hunger, Kresten and Hannick 1984: 507 for the *theologici* 101-200;

- Hunger, Lackner and Hannick 1992: 496 for the *theologici* 201-337;

- Hunger and Hannick 1994: 379 for the *Supplementum*.

There was a mistake in Ackermann 1821 (above) followed by Diels, in the reference to Lambeck. It should not have been "II c. 6" (seemingly referring to *Liber Secundus, Capitulum* 6), but "Pars Secunda Libri VI" (= Lambeck 1674) where a manuscript identified as XXXIV is described (pp. 141-143). This manuscript contains books VI-VIII (as per Ackermann 1821: CXXIV, no. 54 ctd.) of a treatise on medicines by Galen (see Lambeck p. 142). However, this treatise is not *De compositione medicamentorum secundum locos* but *De simplicium medicamentorum temperamentis et facultatibus.*

The codex identified as XXXIV in Lambeck (above) corresponds to the current *medicus graecus* 48 (= [1811]) (Hunger 1953: 31). This manuscript contains (ff. 46r-60v, 62v-114r, 126v-164r) books VI-VIII of *De simplicium medicamentorum temperamentis et facultatibus* (see Hunger and Kresten 1969: 100; for a description of the whole manuscript, see *ibid.*: 100-101).

Same as [1811].

[1746]

[Lamb. VI 85]   I.8.

This is a copy of Hippocrates, *De diaeta (regimine) acutorum*.

In Lambeck, *Liber sextus*, 1674: 85, there is no mention of this treatise in the description of the codex then identified as *medicus* I. However, *De victus ratione* (and not *de victus ratione acutorum*) is mentioned (p. 86) as being in the same codex, ff. 174v-241r.

The codex *medicus graecus* I of Lambeck 1674 corresponds to the current *medicus graecus* 4 (Hunger 1953: 31) (= [1768]). This codex contains indeed Hippocrates, *De victus ratione* on ff. 174v-233v (and not 174v-241r as in Lambeck 1674: *ibid.*).

Same as [1768].

[1747]

[Lambec. VI p. 93]   I.149.

According to Diels' catalogue, this codex contains *Excerpta* of Galen.

The reference is to Lambeck, *Liber sextus*, 1674: 93, ll. 11-16, in the description of codex *medicus* VIII (*ibid.*: 92-93) which reads as follows:

Tertiò, et quidem à fol. 11 pag. 1 usque ad fol. 121 pag. 1, *Excerpta varia ex Galeno*, inter quae praecipuè est *Epitome alphabetica* (1) *Libri sexti, septimi, octavi et noni* περὶ τῆς τῶν ἁπλῶν φαρμάκων δυνάμεως, sive, *de Simplicium medicamentorum facultatibus*; ...

The manuscript *medicus* VIII in Lambeck 1674 corresponds to the current *medicus* 25 (Hunger 1953: 31) (= [1789]). However, according to Hunger and Kresten 1969: 71-72, *medicus graecus* 25 does not contain any text that can be identified as Galenic *excerpta*. Nevertheless, the identification in Lambeck 1674 (above) may correspond to the following texts (by Galen or incorrectly attributed to Galen) actually contained in the manuscript (order of the folios in the manuscript):

- (f. 11r-v) Galenus, *De theriaca ad Pisonem* (frg.);

- (ff. 12r-103r) Paulus Aegineta, *Epitome medica* (frgs.), inter alia tabula plantarum ex *tractatu De simplicium medicamentorum facultatibus* desumpta;

- (ff. 103r-131r) Aetius Amidenus, *Libri medicinales* (frgs.).

It is possibly the same as [1789].

[1748]

[Lambec. VI p. 100]   I.149.

This codex is supposed to contain Galenus, *Excerpta*.

The reference is to Lambeck, *Liber sextus*, 1674: 100, where four *medici* manuscripts are described: XI (partim), XII, XIII and XIV (partim). The only one for which *Excerpta* of Galen are mentioned is XIII, with the following content:

... Continentur eo *anonymi cuiusdam Autoris Eclogae sive Excerpta ex variis Hippocratis & Galeni Operibus, ut & ex Aristotelis Problematibus Physicis*. Primum inter hasce Eclogas tenent locum *Eclogae ex Galeni Libris de Locis affectis*.

If this is the text identified as "Excerpta" in Diels' catalogue, *medicus* XIII of Lambecius is the manuscript referred to here. It corresponds to current *medicus* 15 (Hunger 1953: 31) (= [1778]).

Also [1755].

[1749]   **[v. Lambec. VI 145]**   I.42.

This manuscript is supposed to contain Hippocrates, *Medendi methodus*.

This text does not appear in Lambeck, *Liber sextus*, 1674: 145, in the description of the manuscript *medicus* XXXV (*ibid.*: 144-152), corresponding to current *medicus* 16 (Hunger 1953: 31) (= [1780]). It does not appear in the index of Lambeck 1674: 205-206 *sub nomine* Hippocratis, either.

The current *Vindobonensis medicus graecus* 16 (= 1780]) does not contain either a text identified (or identifiable) as Hippocrates, *Medendi methodus*, or the treatise with the same title by Galen.

Diels' catalogue might have merged two different items found in Ackermann 1825: CLXXVII:

- *Methodus curandi Hippocratica*, for which Ackermann provides the following reference to a manuscript: "... in bibl. Narcissi, archiep. Dublin, nr. 1709". This manuscript is [0230], and is an Arabic manuscript that, according to *C.M.A.* 1697: 2.2.61, contains a treatise entitled as in Ackermann;

- *Hippocrates therapeutica* (on the same page in Ackermann 1825), with the following reference to a Vienna manuscript: "in biblioth. Vindob. Lambec. VI. p. 145". This is the information that appears in Diels I.42, but for a treatise entitled *Medendi methodus*, that is, a title similar to that above, which is provided by Ackermann 1825 for the Dublin manuscript.

[1750]   **[Lambec. VI p. 151]**   I.149.

This is a copy of Galenus, *Excerpta* (*Anonymus tabula in libros Galeni*).

The reference is to Lambeck, *Liber sextus*, 1674: 151, where *Tabulae Divisionum* related to several of Galen's works are mentioned on ff. 329r-359v, in the description of the manuscript *medicus* XXXV (*ibid.*: 144-152) corresponding to current *medicus* 16 (Hunger 1953: 31).

This is the current *medicus graecus* 16 (= [1780]), where such tables can be found ff. 329r-359v.

[1751]   **[Lambec. VI p. 153]**   I.149.

This manuscript is supposed to contain Galenus, *Excerpta*.

The reference is to Lambeck, *Liber sextus*, 1674: 153, where the description of the manuscript *medicus* XXXVII includes the following mention:

... anonymi cuiusdam Autoris *Eclogae miscellanea ex Hippocratis, Galeni, aliorumque veterum Medicorum et Philosophorum Operibus* ...

The number XXXVII of Lambeck corresponds to the current *medicus* 13 (Hunger 1953: 31) (= [1776]), which contains a compilation of medical extracts, including by Galen.

[1752]   **[Lambec. ed. Kollar I p. 272]**   I.123.

According to Diels' catalogue, this is a copy of Galenus, *Iatrosophia*.

The reference is to the edition of Lambecius by A. F. Kollar, tome 1 (= 1776), col. 272 (and not p. as in Diels), where this item appears among the corrections made by Kollar to the list of manuscripts in the Constantinopolitan collection of an unidentified *Grammaticus* published by du Verdier 1585: 57-59 (see [0440]-[0441]). Kollar 1766-1782: 1.272, ll. 1-4, reads as follows:

Ibidem (i.e., "In Catalogo librorum 174, a Grammatico quodam exhibito [Kollar 1766-1782: 1.269, ll. 1-2]); *Galeni Medicinale ad Hippocratem.* In Codice Caesareo (i.e. in *Vindobonensis historicus graecus* 98) legitur Ἰατροσόφιον Γαληνοῦ καθ᾽ Ἱπποκράτους.

This is a correction of du Verdier 1585: 57, col. 2, l. 35, which reads:

Galeni Medicinale ad Hippocratem.

The first edition of this catalogue is by Hartung 1578: Bii recto, no. 13. Recent editions by Foerster 1877: 20, no. ιδ΄, and Papazoglu 1983: 380.

The title *Galeni Medicinale ad Hippocratem* appears in Ackermann 1821: CLXXXVII, § 6, where a reference to "Verdier II 57" can be found.

Since this catalogue is considered to be a forgery (see above, on [0440]-[0441]), this item probably does not correspond to any preserved manuscript. See Papazoglou 1983: 186, no. 14.

[1753]   **[ap. Lambec.-Kollar I p. 273]**   I.124.

This is supposed to be a copy of Galenus, *Hippocratis liber resolutionis, quem Galenus explicat.*

The reference to "Lambec.-Kollar I p. 273" is to Kollar 1766-1782: 1.273, ll. 12-17 (col. and not p. as in Diels), that is, to Kollar's correction of the description of this item in du Verdier 1585: 59, col. 1, ll. 48-49 (see above, about [0440] and [0441]).

Diels' catalogue mistakenly considered that Kollar's notice refers to a manuscript in the Imperial Library in Vienna, whereas the present item is a correction of the title of item [0440] supposedly in a Constantinopolitan collection.

Since the catalogue in which item [0440] is listed is considered to be a forgery (see above [0440]-[0441]), the item [1753] does not correspond to any extant manuscript.

[1754]   **[Lambec. ed. Kollar I p. 275]**   I.149.

This is supposed to be a copy of Galenus, *Excerpta*, which, according to Diels' catalogue, "seems to have pertained to Michael Cantacuzenus" ("Videtur fuisse Mich. Cantacuzeni").

The reference to "Lambec. ed. Kollar I p. 275" is to Kollar 1766-1782:1.275 (col. and not p. as in Diels), where corrections to the list of manuscripts once owned by Michael Cantacuzenus published by du Verdier 1585 can be found.

No item specifically identified as containing *Excerpta* of Galen appears in Kollar 1766-1782: 1.275, unless this is a reference to the manuscript described *ibid.* as follows (275, l. 41-276, l. 7):

Ibidem (i.e. In Catalogo librorum Michaelis Cantacuzeni ... [275, l. 41-276, l. 7]): *Joannici sacri monachi, itemque Cardani et Protesyngeli Corcyrae Insulae, collecta omnia necessaria a tribus Medicis, Hippocrate, Galeno et Melchio [sic].*

Quae verba sic supplenda et mutanda sunt: Ἰατροσόφιον, Ἰωάννου ἱερομονάχου τοῦ καὶ ἐπίκλην Καρτάνου, καὶ Πρωτοσυγκέλλου γενομένου τῆς τῶν Κερκυραίων νήσου, συναχθὲν καὶ ἐκλεχθὲν ἀπὸ τῶν τριῶν ἰατρῶν Ἱπποκράτους, Γαληνοῦ καὶ Μελετίου.

This notice is about du Verdier 1585: 62, col. 2, ll. 30-34, which reads:

Ioannicis sacri Monachi, itémque Cardani et Prothesingeli Corcyrae Insulae, omnia necessaria à tribus medicies: Hippocrate, Galeno et Melechio: praeterea de astris, Sole et Luna, et de Dieta XII. mensium, et de sectione vena in ipsis (in charta bibacina.)

First edition of this item in Hartung 1578: Eii verso, ll. 12-16. Recent editions by Foerster 1877: 28, cols 1-2, no. μβ´, and Papazoglu 1983: 401.

The current location of this item is unknown. See also Papazoglou 1983: 346, no. 42, and above [0442] and [0443].

[1755]   **[ap. Nessel P. III]**   I.102.

This manuscript is supposed to contain Galenus, *In Hippocratis librum de acutorum victu commentarii V*.

The information comes from Ackermann 1821: CLXXXIV, no. 15 (without brackets).

The reference is to Nessel 1690, part III, entitled as follows:

Catalogi Bibliothecae Caesareae Manuscriptorum Pars III, quae complectitur Manuscriptos Medicos Graecos.

No manuscript containing this text is listed in Nessel 1690, part III. According to the *Index ... alphabeticus* in Id., part VI, pp. 3-119, *sub nomine* Claudius Galenus (= pp. 54-55), there is only one codex containing this treatise (only Book I) in Kollar's catalogue: *philosophicus et philologicus* 208, ff. 123r-134r (described in Id., part IV, p. 114; see no. 7 for this specific text) (on this manuscript, see Hunger 1961: 317-318)

Nevertheless, according to Hunger and Kresten 1969: 55-59, especially 59, the current *medicus graecus* 15 (= [1778]) contains a fragment of Galen's commentary on Hippocrates, *De acutorum victu* (f. 134r-v). However, in Nessel 1690, Part III, p. 26, no. XV, the list of the texts contained in this manuscript does not include any specific mention of this treatise:

... Continentur eo Anonymi *cuiusdam Autoris Eclogae sive Excerpta ex variis Hippocratis & Galeni Operibus, ut & ex Aristotelis Problematibus Physicis.* Primum inter hasce Eclogas tenent locum *Eclogae ex Galeni Libris de Locis affectis.*

This manuscript is described in the same way in [1748], without mention of the text listed here, however.

Same as [1778].

[1756]   **[ap. Nessel III 27 (?) no. 5]**   I.80.

This manuscript is supposed to contain Galenus, *De differentiis febrium libri II*.

The information comes from Ackermann 1821: CI, no. 2 (without brackets or question mark).

The reference to Nessel is to Nessel 1690, part III, page 27, text no. 5, which is contained ff. 49r-55v in the manuscript *medicus* 16 (described *ibid.*, at pp. 26-28).

The manuscript corresponds to the current *medicus graecus* 16 (= [1780]) where the text of Galen appears at ff. 49r-55v (Hunger and Kresten 1969: 60-62 for the manuscript, 60 for the text).

Same as [1780].

[1757]   **[38 (?)]**   I.80.

This codex is supposed to contain Galenus, *De differentiis febrium libri II*.

This information is probably an incorrect reproduction of the item identified as follows in Ackermann 1821: CI, no. 2, ctd. (without brackets or question mark):

Alius cod., isque integer, est no. 28. vid. De Nessel P. III. p. 38.

On this basis, it appears that, contrary to Diels' catalogue, the number 38 is not a shelfmark (supposedly corresponding to *medicus graecus* 38 = [1801]), but a reference to page 38 in Nessel 1690, part III.

Nessel 1690, part III, pp. 38-40 describes the codex *medicus graecus* XXVIII (as correctly noted by Ackermann 1821: CI, ll. 6-7) as containing (ff. 18r-26v) a *Liber de Febrium differentiá*, attributed by Nessel to "Eiusdem", that is, Theophilus.

This codex corresponds to the current *medicus graecus* 28 (= [1792]), on which see Hunger and Kresten 1969: 76-78. In this catalogue, the text of ff. 18r-26v is identified as Anonymus, πόσαι διαφοραὶ τῶν πυρετῶν β΄. The manuscript opens with texts by Theophilus Protospatharius (ff. 2r-17v) and Galenus (f. 17v), the first of which may have induced Nessel to attribute the text of ff. 18r-26v to Theophilus.

[1758]   **69 B 101**   I.3.

This item is a copy of the 1538 Froben (Basel) edition of Hippocrates, *Opera omnia*, with handwritten notes by Janus Cornarius (ca. 1500-ca. 1558) in the margins, particularly in *De regimine* and *De morbo sacro*.

Current shelfmark is *69.B.101.

[1759]   **131**   I.79.

This is a copy of fragments from Galenus, *De morborum causis*.

The number 131 does not seem to correspond to any shelfmark in the present collections of the Österreichische Nationalbibliothek. Among the *medici graeci* manuscripts of the library, Galenus, *De morborum causis* appears in the codex no. 15 (= [1778]) ff. 75r-77r according to Hunger and Kresten 1969: 55-59, especially 56.

The number 131 might be an incorrect transformation of 231 as the codex *medicus graecus* 15 (= [1778]) is described in Lambeck ed. Kollar vol. 6 (1780) on colls. 230-231.

Possibly the same as [1778]. Also [1760].

[1760]   **[131]**   I.126.

The manuscript here is supposed to contain Galenus, *De morbis excerpta*.

This item might be the same as [1759], and the text referred to here might be *De morborum causis*.

Possibly the same as [1759] and [1778].

[1761]   **[179]**   I.44.

This manuscript is supposed to be a copy of Hippocrates, *Prognostica*.

The number 179 does not seem to correspond to any shelfmark in the current collections of the Österreichische Nationalbibliothek. Among the *medici graeci* manuscripts of the library, the Hippocratic *Prognostica* appear in the no. 15 (= [1778]), ff. 169r-174v, according to Hunger and Kresten 1969: 55-59, especially 59.

The number 179 might be an incorrect reproduction of 169, that is, the folio where the text starts in the codex *medicus graecus* 15.

Possibly the same as [1778].

histor. (*historici*)

91   (f. 110r) *Fragmentum medicum*.

             Hunger 1961: 94-102.

[1762]   **94**   II.20.

             Hunger 1961: 103.

95   (f. 327r) *Phlebotomia*.

             Hunger 1961: 103-104.

112   (ff. 38r-80r) Manuel Philes, *De animalium proprietate*.

             Hunger 1961: 115-116.

113   (ff. 169r-172r) *De somniis*.

             Hunger 1961: 116-118.

[1763]   **130**   I.14.

             Hunger 1961: 132-133.

             Formerly [1735].

juridici

1   (ff. 343v-344r) Splenius, *De generatione hominis*.

             Hunger and Kresten 1969: 1-3.

10   (f. 84r) Splenius, *De generatione hominis*.

             Hunger and Kresten 1969: 19-22.

18   Palimpsest.

             Scriptio superior: *Ecloga legum, Appendix Eclogae, Basilika, Prochiron*.

             Scriptio inferior: *Formulae medicamentorum*.

Harlfinger, Brunschön and Vasiloudi 2006: 146, 161-162; Grusková 2010: 130-169, esp. 158-159.

Hunger and Kresten 1969: 33-34.

lat. (*latini*)

[1764]   **16**   II.30.

This manuscript is now Napoli, Biblioteca Nazionale Vittorio Emanuele III, *olim Vindobonensis latinus* 2 (see above, p. 158).

Tabulae codicum 1868: 2-3.

        2277   Iconae plantarum ex *Vindobonensi medico graeco* 1 (= [1766]) desumptae.

Unterkircher 1957: 66.

[1765]   **4772 (tab. cod. III 382)**   I.14, 18.

This is a Latin manuscript. The mention *tab. cod. III 382* is a reference to the catalogue of Latin manuscripts in Vienna, entitled *Tabulae codicum manu scriptorum praeter graecos et orientales in Bibliotheca Palatina Vindobonensi asservatorum* (Vindobonae: Caroli Geroldi Filius, 1869), vol. 3, page 382, where this manuscript is listed (actual reference is pp. 382-383). This codex contains the following texts on ff. 58r-109r:

Collectanea varia ex historia litteraria medica, videlicet: Vita Hippocratis, jusjurandum Hippocratis, graece et latine, Epistola Hippocratis de Microcosmo ad regem Ptolomaeum [*sic*], Epistola eadem ab anonymo metrica redacta, ... omnia a manu ipsius Cuspiniani perscripta.

Johannes Cuspinianus is Johan Spiesshaymer (1473-1529).

Tabulae codicum 1869: 382-383.

med. (*medici*)

[1766]   **1**   I.96, 117; II.25, 30, 38, 39 (3)

Hunger and Kresten 1969: 37-41.

        2   (ff. 84r-85v) Cleopatra, *De mensuris et ponderibus*.

Hunger and Kresten 1969: 41-43.

Possibly also [1741].

[1767]   **3**   II.109.

Hunger and Kresten 1969: 44-46.

Possibly also [1741].

[1768]   **4**   I.23 (2), 24, 25, 26 (2), 27 (2), 30.

Hunger and Kresten 1969: 46-47.

Also [1746].

[1769]   **5**   II.25, 39.

Hunger and Kresten 1969: 47-48.

[1770]   **6**   II.6, 25.

Hunger and Kresten 1969: 48-49.

[1771]   **8**   I.41, 61; II.15, 55, 63, 78, 79 (2), 82, 90, 102 (2).

Hunger and Kresten 1969: 49-51.

Also [1772].

[1772]   **[8]**   I.56.

This manuscript of Hippocrates, *Excerpta varia*, may be the *medicus graecus* 8 (= [1771]), which contains on ff. 282r-283r the *Sententiae de vita et morte* attributed to Hippocrates (see Hunger and Kresten 1969: 49-51).

[1773]   **10**   II.10.

Hunger and Kresten 1969: 52.

[1774]   **11**   II.28, 33.

Hunger and Kresten 1969: 52-53.

[1775]   **12**   II.6; N.43, 62.

Hunger and Kresten 1969: 53-54.

[1776]   **13**   I.28, 42, 43, 93, 149.

Hunger and Kresten 1969: 54.

Also [1751].

[1777]   **14**   I.31, 42; II.30.

Hunger and Kresten 1969: 54-55.

[1778]   **15**   I.119, 149; II.60; N.57.

Hunger and Kresten 1969: 55-59.

Also possibly [1748], [1755], [1759], [1760], [1761], and [1779].

[1779]   **[15]**   I.56; II.10.

This codex, supposedly containing Hippocrates, *Excerpta varia* (I.56) and Galenus, *De febribus* (II.10), may very well be the *medicus graecus* 15 (= [1778]), containing among others (ff. 81v-83r) extracts from Galenus, *De febribus*, and (ff. 139r-182r) excerpts from several Hippocratic treatises (Hunger and Kresten 1969: 55-59).

See [1778].

[1780]   **16**   I.49, 58, 111; II.30, 60, 97, 98, 104, 105; N.57.

Hunger and Kresten 1969: 60-62.

Also [1750], [1756] and [1781], and possibly [1749].

[1781]   **16 (ol. 35)**   I.5; II.71.

This manuscript containing Hippocrates *Prognosticon* (I.5) and Oribasius, *Opera varia* (II.71) is the *medicus graecus* 16 (= [1780]), where the Hippocratic treatise and fragments from Oribasius, *Collectiones medicae*, can be found in the margins of ff. 185v-261v and on ff. 284v-287r, respectively (Hunger and Kresten 1969: 60-62; also Alexanderson 1963: 91 for Hippocrates).

The mention "ol. 35" is not part of its current shelfmark; it is the one attributed to the manuscript in Lambeck 1674: 144-152 (also Hunger 1953: 31, table *Codices medici II, sub numero* 35).

Same as [1780].

	17	Iohannes Zacharias Actuarius, *De methodo medendi*.
		Hunger and Kresten 1969: 62-63.
[1782]	**18**	I.85, 93; II.33, 97.
		Hunger and Kresten 1969: 63-64.
[1783]	**[19 (?)]**	I.128.

Since 1809, this manuscript of Paul of Aegina has been in Paris, Bibliothèque nationale de France, *Supplementum graecum* 446 (= [1351]) (Mencik 1909/1910: XIX; Heiberg 1919: 270; Hunger 1953: 30n5; Hunger and Kresten 1969: 64; Irigoin 1970: 522).

Same as [1351].

[1784]	**20**	I.114, 133.
		Hunger and Kresten 1969: 64-66.
[1785]	**21**	II.79, 109 (2), 110.
		Hunger and Kresten 1969: 66-67.
[1786]	**22**	I.85; II.28, 110.
		Hunger and Kresten 1969: 67.
[1787]	**23**	II.44, 45 (2), 47-48, 48, 79, 110.
		Hunger and Kresten 1969: 67-69.
[1788]	**24**	I.24, 38.
		Hunger and Kresten 1969: 69-71.
[1789]	**25**	I.96; II.20, 79.
		Hunger and Kresten 1969: 71-72.
		Possibly also [1747].
[1790]	**26**	I.114; II.79, 109, 110.
		Hunger and Kresten 1969: 72-74.
[1791]	**27**	II.28, 36, 37, 45, 74, 79, 91.
		Hunger and Kresten 1969: 74-75.
[1792]	**28**	I.14, 89, 92, 134, 136; II.6, 33, 34, 49, 58, 63, 80, 105, 106.
		Hunger and Kresten 1969: 76-78.
		Also [1757] and [1793].

[1793]   **[28 (?)]**   I.20, 114.

This codex is supposed to contain Hippocrates, *De humoribus* (I.20), and Galenus, *De succedaneis* (I.114).

According to Hunger and Kresten 1969: 111, *sub nomine* Galenos, and 112, *sub nomine* Hippokrates, no *Vindobonensis medicus graecus* contains these two treatises.

However, the codex *medicus graecus* 28 (= [1792]) contains Galenus, *De humoribus ex Hippocrate* on ff. 184r-186v.

As for Galenus, *De succedaneis*, it does not seem to be available in any *Vindobonensis medicus* (see Hunger and Kresten 1969: 111, *sub nomine* Galenos). Diels' information may be a transformation of Ackermann 1821: CLXX, no. 138 (where there are no brackets or question mark):

Excerpta ex Pauli Aeginetae libro VII. De medicamentis succedaneis secund. Galen. sunt in bibl. Vind. no. 28 de Ness. III. P. 39.

Ackermann's reference is to Nessel 1690, part III, p. 39, about the codex *medicus* 28 described on pp. 38-40 (corresponding to the *medicus graecus* 28). On p. 39, Nessel lists the following item:

Quinto ... item Excerpta ex (1) Paul Aeginetae Libro septimo de Medicamentis succedaneis secundum Galenum.

The codex *medicus graecus* 28 contains, ff. 138v-139v, a text entitled Γαληνοῦ ἐκ τὰ ἀντίβολα, which corresponds to Paulus Aegineta, *Epitome medica*, 7.25 (*De succedaneis*).

Same as [1792].

[1794]   **29**   I.134; II.30, 35, 36, 79, 80, 102.

Hunger and Kresten 1969: 78-80.

[1795]   **30**   I.78, 129; II.75.

Hunger and Kresten 1969: 80-82.

[1796]   **31**   I.14; II.37, 58, 69, 81; N.39, 51, 56 (2), 63, 66.

Hunger and Kresten 1969: 83.

[1797]   **32**   I.39, 114, 125; II.28, 33, 79.

Hunger and Kresten 1969: 83-86.

                 33   *Iatrosofion* (15th cent.).

Hunger and Kresten 1969: 86-87.

[1798]   **34**   I.101, 105; N.34, 35.

According to N.34 and 35, this manuscript is now Paris, *Supplementum graecum* 447 (Menčik 1909/1910: XIX; Hunger 1953: 30n14; Hunger and Kresten 1969: 87; Irigoin 1970: 522).

Same as [1352].

[1799]   **35**   I.96.

Hunger and Kresten 1969: 87.

                 36   (ff. 71r-118v) Symeon Seth, *De alimentorum facultatibus*; (ff. 119r-130v) Michael Psellus, *De diaeta*.

Hunger and Kresten 1969: 87-88.

[1800]	**37**	I.149; II.48, 102.
		Hunger and Kresten 1969: 89-90.
[1801]	**38ᶜ**	II.37.
		Hunger and Kresten 1969: 91.
[1802]	**39**	II.33, 66.

This manuscript contains Moschion as II.66 rightly states, and not Dioscorides, *Liber agens de experientia medica* as per II.33.

Hunger and Kresten 1969: 91-92.

[1803]	**40**	I.40; II.20, 79.
		Hunger and Kresten 1969: 92-93.
[1804]	**41**	I.46; II.81; N.27 (2), 28, 39, 51, 56 (2), 63, 65, 66.
		Hunger and Kresten 1969: 93-94.
		Possibly also [1805].
[1805]	**[41]**	I.56.

The text identified in Diels' catalogue as Hippocrates, *Excerpta varia*, could very well be the treatise *De quatro elementis et humoribus* attributed to Hippocrates that can be found in *medicus graecus* 41, ff. 81r-83v (Hunger and Kresten 1969: 93).

Possibly same as [1804].

[1806]	**42**	II.71.
		Hunger and Kresten 1969: 94.
[1807]	**43**	II.37, 93.
		Hunger and Kresten 1969: 94-95.
[1808]	**44**	I.5, 107; II.9, 97, 98, 104, 109; N.35.
		Hunger and Kresten 1969: 95-96.
[1809]	**45**	II.63.
		Hunger and Kresten 1969: 96-97.
	46	*Geoponica.*
		Hunger and Kresten 1969: 98.
[1810]	**47**	I.24, 123, 128.
		Hunger and Kresten 1969: 98-99.
[1811]	**48**	I.14, 96, 99; II.78, 88.
		Hunger and Kresten 1969: 100-101.
		Also [1745].
[1812]	**49**	I.14; II.87.
		Hunger and Kresten 1969: 101.
[1813]	**50**	II.43.
		Hunger and Kresten 1969: 102-103.

[1814]	**51**	II.6.

Hunger and Kresten 1969: 103.

[1815]	**52**	I.40, 41, 56, 86; II.6, 33, 49 (2), 105.

Hunger and Kresten 1969: 103-105.

[1816]	**53**	I.39, 42, 125, 149; II.64.

Hunger and Kresten 1969: 105-106.

Possibly also [1817].

[1817]	**[53]**	I.56.

The *Excerpta varia* of Hippocrates could very well be the *Testamentum* contained in the codex *medicus graecus* 53, ff. 8v-11r (Costomiris 1889: 383; Hunger and Kresten 1969: 105).

Possibly same as [1816].

phil.

These items actually are *philosophici et philologi graeci*.

[1818]	**34**	II.67.

Hunger 1961: 160-161.

[1819]	**37**	II.82.

Hunger 1961: 162-163.

[1820]	**74**	II.104.

Hunger 1961: 188-190.

[1821]	**82**	I.38.

Hunger 1961: 194-195.

[1822]	**108**	II.82 (2).

Hunger 1961: 213-217.

[1823]	**178**	I.41, 42, 128; II.20, 79; N.39, 68.

Hunger 1961: 283-286.

[1824]	**179**	I.14.

Hunger 1961: 286-288.

Also [1830].

[1825]	**181**	II.67.

Hunger 1961: 288-290.

[1826]	**192**	I.26.

Hunger 1961: 301-303.

[1827]	**219**	I.18.

Hunger 1961: 326-330.

[1828]	**290**	II.35.

Hunger 1961: 388.

[1829]   **303**   I.72; II.89.

Hunger 1961: 397-398.

philos. et philol. (*philosophici et philologici*)

14   (ff. 9r-11r) Michael Psellus, *Lectiones medicophysicae*.

Hunger 1961: 145-147.

34   See [1818].

37   See [1819].

59   (ff. 114r-115r) Democritus, *Epistula ad Hippocratem*.

Hunger 1961: 177-178.

64   (ff. 180v-184v) Aristoteles, *De insomniis*.

Hunger 1961: 181-182; Wartelle 1963: 163-164, no. 2187.

74   See [1820].

82   See [1821].

108   See [1822].

110   (ff. 406v-415r) Aristoteles, *De insomniis*; (ff. 434r-456r) Gregorius Nyssenus, *De hominis opificio*; (ff. 458r-484v) Nemesius Emesenus, *De natura hominis*.

Hunger 1961: 218-222; Wartelle 1963: 165, no. 2197; Morani 1981: 57.

111   (ff. 1r-42r) Achmet, *Oneirocriticon*.

Hunger 1961: 222.

112   (f. 1r-22v) *Geoponica*.

Hunger 1961: 222-223.

134   (ff. 185r-198r) Aristoteles, *De insomniis*.

Hunger 1961: 241; Wartelle 1963: 165, no. 2200;

149   (f. 274r-v) Splenius, *De generatione hominis*.

Hunger 1961: 250-255.

154   (f. 376r) *De infirmis*.

Hunger 1961: 257-259.

157   (ff. 74r-81v) Aristoteles, *De insomniis*.

Hunger 1961: 260; Wartelle 1963: 166, no. 2207.

162   (ff. 1r-160r) Achmet, *Oneirocriticon*.

Hunger 1961: 265.

166   (ff. 32r-39r) *Lexicon botanicum*; (ff. 39v-40v) *De urinis*.

Hunger 1961: 269-270.

168   (ff. 79r-83r) Synesius Cyrenensis, *De insomniis*.

Hunger 1961: 271-273.

178   See [1823].

[1830]   **179**   II.114.

This item, which is not listed among the copies of *De IV aetatibus praenotio* in Diels' catalogue (I.49), appears in the *Addenda* (= II.114). There, the catalogue specifies that this text is an extract from *De aere, aquis, locis* (Littré 2.42-50).

The text does appear (f. 123v) in the manuscript *Vindobonensis philosophicus et philologicus* 179 (= [1824]). However, it is not a fragment from *De aere, aquis, locis*, but from *Aphorismi* (Littré 4.490-492) on prognosis (Hunger 1961: 288; on the text see Magdelaine 1994: 203n1).

Same as [1824] (see also Magdelaine 1994: 203 and 203n1).

181   See [1825].

187   (ff. 46r-47v) *De plantis.*

             Hunger 1961: 295-296.

190   (ff. 49r-58v) *Quaestiones medicinales.*

             Hunger 1961: 298-300.

192   See [1826].

199   (f. 75r) *De mensuris.*

             Hunger 1961: 311-312.

208   (ff. 123r-134r) Galenus, *In Hippocratis de diaeta acutorum commentarium.*

             Hunger 1961: 317-318.

219   See [1827].

220   (ff. 181r-188v) *Formulae remediorum*; (f. 189v) Galenus, *De humoribus in capite*; (ff. 190v-197v) *Capitula medica.*

             Hunger 1961: 330-332.

222   (f. 1v) *De tempore phlebotomiae.*

             Hunger 1961: 332-333.

224   (ff. 202r-209v) Synesius Cyrenensis, *De insomniis* (frg.).

             Hunger 1961: 334-336.

225   (f. 86r-v) *De humani corporis partibus.*

             Hunger 1961: 336-338.

231   (ff. 1r-23v) Aristoteles, *Physiognomonica* (frg.).

             Hunger 1961: 340-341; Wartelle 1963: 168, no. 2225.

241   (f. 286v) *Somnium.*

             Hunger 1961: 349-351.

254   (f. 113r) Splenius, *De generatione hominis.*

             Hunger 1961: 364-365.

271   (f. 46r-v) Hippocrates, *Epistula ad Ptolemaeum regem de tuenda valetudine.*

             Hunger 1961: 375-377.

273	(ff. 1r-54v) Synesius Cyrenensis, *De insomniis*, et Nicephorus Gregoras, *Commentarium in Synesii De insomniis*.
	Hunger 1961: 377-378.
277	(ff. 1r-12r) *Geoponica* (frg.).
	Hunger 1961: 380.
287	(ff. 1r-37v) Achmet, *Oneirocriticon*.
	Hunger 1961: 386.
290	See [1828].
297	(ff. 1r-78v) Achmet, *Oneirocriticon*.
	Hunger 1961: 392.
301	(ff. 39v-40v) *Praecepta salubria*.
	Hunger 1961: 395-396.
303	See [1829].
309	(ff. 79v-80v) *De mensuris*.
	Hunger 1961: 402.
321	(f. 309r) Splenius, *De generatione hominis*.
	Hunger 1961: 409-418.
333	(f. 188r) Epiphanius, *De duodecim gemmis* (frg.).
	Hunger 1961: 427-430.

suppl. (*Supplementum graecum*)

[1831]	**8**	II.6.
		Hunger and Hannick 1994: 16-18.
	13	(ff. 1v-257v) Hippocrates: (ff. 2r-12v) *Lexicon*; (ff. 13r-17r) *De arte*; (ff. 17v-26r) *De prisca medicina*; (ff. 27r-35v) *Prognostica*; (ff. 39r-62r) *De diaeta acutorum*; (ff. 62v-72r) *Coa praesagia*; (ff. 72v-157v) *De morbis popularibus*; (ff. 159r-228r) *De morbis*; (ff. 229r-241r) *De diaeta*; (ff. 245r-253r) *Praesagia*; (ff. 255r-257v) *De alimento*; (ff. 160r-354r) Galenus: (ff. 260r-288v) *Ars medica*; (ff. 290r-350r) *De antidotis*; (ff. 350r-354r) *De theriaca ad Pisonem*.
		Hunger and Hannick 1994: 25-28.
[1832]	**28 (olim Neapolitan.)** II.30.	
		This manuscript is now Naples, Biblioteca Nazionale Vittorio Emanuele III, *Neapolitanus olim Vindobonensis graecus* 1 (see above, p. 158).
		Originally in Naples, it has been in Vienna, at the Hofbibliothek, during the period 1718-1919 as the mention "Olim Neapolitan[us]" in Diels' catalogue states.
	39	(f. 262r-v) *De gemmis*.
		Hunger and Hannick 1994: 74-77.
	45	(ff. 327r-328v) *De humani corporis partibus*.
		Hunger and Hannick 1994: 85-87.

	71	(f. 214r) *Formula medicamenti.*
		Hunger and Hannick 1994: 119-121.
[1833]	**81**	II.6.
		Hunger and Hannick 1994: 137-138.
	91	(ff. 105v-123v, 147r-152v) *De mensuris et ponderibus.*
		Hunger and Hannick 1994: 154-162.
	125	(f. 12r-v) *Formulae medicae.*
		Hunger and Hannick 1994: 212-214.
	179	(143r-162v), Hippocrates, *Epistulae.*
		Hunger and Hannick 1994: 313-315.
		Formerly [1743].
	198	(ff. 19v-21v, 4r-13r) Epiphanius, *Physiologus.*
		Hunger and Hannick 1994: 355-359.

theol. (*theologici*)

	68	II.67.
[1834]		Hunger and Kresten 1976: 126-127.
	113	(ff. 79r-138r) Gregorius Nyssenus, *De hominis opificio.*
		Hunger, Kresten and Hannick 1984: 36-40.
[1835]	**128**	II.35.
		Hunger, Kresten and Hannick 1984: 98-110.
	134	(ff. 87r-94r) Basilius Caesariensis, *De hominis opificio*; (ff. 95r-150r) Gregorius Nyssenus, *De hominis opificio*; (ff. 212v, 220r-v, 214v-215r) *Medicina varia*, including Galenus, *De locis affectis* (frg.).
		Hunger, Kresten and Hannick 1984: 126-132.
	139	(f. 5r) fragmentum therapeuticum (?).
		Hunger, Kresten and Hannick 1984: 144-147 (especially p. 146).
	160	(ff. 60r-113v) Gregorius Nyssenus, *De hominis opificio.*
		Hunger, Kresten and Hannick 1984: 242-247.
	168	(ff. 73r-120r) Gregorius Nyssenus, *De hominis opificio.*
		Hunger, Kresten and Hannick 1984: 275-279.
	193	(ff. 223r-224v) Epiphanius, *De duodecim gemmis* (frg.).
		Hunger, Kresten and Hannick 1984: 411-417.
[1836]	**199**	II.67.

This manuscript is listed as containing Nemesius Emesenus, *De natura hominis* (frg.) on f. 1, whereas it does not (Hunger, Kresten and Hannick 1984: 428-433). No other *theologicus graecus* seems to contain Nemesius' work on f. 1.

Actually, this manuscript contains Anastasius Sinaites, *Quaestiones et responsiones*, 24-35 that includes fragments from Nemesius (Morani 1981: 122).

200   (ff. 117v-118v) *De dysuria.*

Hunger, Kresten and Hannick 1984: 433-442.

203   (ff. 43v-48v) *Recepta medica.*

Hunger, Lackner and Hannick 1992: 7-16.

[1837]   **207**   II.95.

This manuscript is listed as containing Splenius, *De generatione hominis*, on f. 61v. The current *Vindobonensis theologicus graecus* 207 does not contain such text (see Hunger, Lackner and Hannick 1992: 28-31), which appears, instead, in *theologicus graecus* 315, ff. 61v-62r (see Hunger, Lackner and Hannick 1992: 413-418).

See below (p. 368).

222   (ff. 134r-187v) Gregorius Nyssenus, *De hominis opificio*; (ff. 189r-192v) Nemesius Emesenus, *De natura hominis* (frg.).

Hunger, Lackner and Hannick 1992: 77-82.

231   (ff. 77r-93v) *Iatrosofion* (16th century).

Hunger, Lackner and Hannick 1992: 105-110.

236   (ff. 345r-353r) Germanus Patriarcha Constantinopolitanus, *Oneirocriticon.*

Hunger, Lackner and Hannick 1992: 122-125.

244   (f. 53/1v) *Iatrosophica* (16th century); (f. 154r-v) *De quattuor elementis et humoribus.*

Hunger, Lackner and Hannick 1992: 145-157.

245   (ff. 312r-316r) Nicephorus Blemmydes, *De urinis*; (f. 316r-v) Nicephorus Blemmydes, *De distinctione sanguinis*; (ff. 316v-319r) *Paraphrasis ad Blemmidis de urinis.*

Hunger, Lackner and Hannick 1992: 157-160.

256   (tegumentum, posterius) *Formula medicinae.*

Hunger, Lackner and Hannick 1992: 186-192.

264   (f. 161v) *Geoponica* (frg.); (f. 168v) *De elementis et humoribus.*

Hunger, Lackner and Hannick 1992: 216-220.

278   (ff. 2r-49v) Gregorius Nyssenus, *De hominis opificio.*

Hunger, Lackner and Hannick 1992: 262-263.

287   (f. 44r) *De vermis.*

Hunger, Lackner and Hannick 1992: 298-302.

	288	(f. 21r) Epiphanius, *De mensuris et ponderibus* (frg.).
		Hunger, Lackner and Hannick 1992: 302-304.
[1838]	**293**	I.40.
		Hunger, Lackner and Hannick 1992: 316-321.
	302	(ff. 13r-14r, in marg.) Epiphanius, *De duodecim gemmis* (frg.).
		Hunger, Lackner and Hannick 1992: 345-356.
	304	(f. 258v) Epiphanius, *De mensuris et ponderibus* (frg.).
		Hunger, Lackner and Hannick 1992: 361-366.
	315	See [1837].
		Hunger, Lackner and Hannick 1992: 413-418.
	324	(f. IIv) *Formula medicinae*; (f. 296v) *Formula medicinae*.
		Hunger, Lackner and Hannick 1992: 436-447.
	325	(f. IIIv) *De hominis septem aetatibus*.
		Hunger, Lackner and Hannick 1992: 447-453.

Österreichische Nationalbibliothek (National Library of Austria)

See above **Hofbibliothek** (see above, pp. 349-368).

Wolfenbüttel (DE)

Bibl. Guelf. August. (*Bibliotheca Guelfi Augusti* [August Guelph's Library]), now Herzog August Bibliothek Wolfenbüttel (Herzog August Library Wolfenbüttel)

Of the several collections preserved in Wolfenbüttel library, the following four contain Greek medical manuscripts (listed here in alphabetical order of their usual Latin designation):

- *Augustei* (Augustiani in Diels; see [1839] and [1840]);
- *Gudiani* (see [1481]-[1485]);
- *Helmstadienses* (Helmstatenses in Diels; see [1851] and [1852]);
- *Weissenburgerani* (see [1853] and [1854]).

Diels' catalogue distinguishes them, and also uses the general designation *Guelferbytani* (referring to Wolfenbüttel) with the abbreviation Gud. (= Gudiani) (see [1842]-[1850]).

Diels also refers to the catalogue by Ebert 1827 (explicitly in [1841] and implicitly in [1842]-[1850]), and cites it as if it were a collection within Wolfenbüttel Library.

Diels' catalogue identifies the manuscripts according to three different systems and uses more than one such system for some manuscripts (generating duplicates):

- shelfmark in [1839] and [1853];
- shelfmark followed by the sequential number of the manuscript (between parentheses or not) in a catalogue in [1851];
- sequential number of the manuscript in a catalogue followed by the shelfmark (between parentheses or not) in [1840]-[1850], [1852] and [1854].

Augustiani

[1839]   **[18, 1]**   I.38.

Current shelfmark: 18.1 Aug. 4to.

von Heinemann 1900: 234-236.

Also [1840].

[1840]   **3132 (18.1 Aug. 4°)**   N.27.

The number 3132 is the sequential number of the manuscript in von Heinemann 1900: 234-236.

Same as [1839].

Ebert

[1841]   **364 (7 und 8 Gud. lat.)**N.29.

The mention "Ebert" refers to the catalogue by Ebert 1827. The number 364 is the sequential number of the manuscript in this catalogue (Ebert 1827: 75).

Current shelfmark: 7 and 8 Gud. Lat. 2°.

This is the 1525 edition of Galen, *Opera omnia* (in Greek), Venetiis, in aedibus Aldi, et Andreae Asulani soceri, with marginal notes by Joseph Justus Scaliger (1540-1609).

Köhler and Milchsack 1913: 81.

Also [1844].

Guelferb. (*Guelferbytani*)

Under this designation, Diels' catalogue lists items of the Gudiani collection. Numbers are not shelfmarks, but the sequential numbers in Ebert 1827. Following this number, Diels' catalogue provides between parentheses the shelfmark as in Ebert 1827 (which does not exactly corresponds to current shelfmarks).

[1842]   **2 (47 Gud. gr.)**   N.62.

The number 2 is the sequential number of the manuscript in Ebert 1827: 1.

Current shelfmark: 47 Gud. graec. fol.

Köhler and Milchsack 1913: 34-35, where Köhler hypothesizes that this manuscript might be [0903], 2nd part.

Also [1843].

[1843]   **2 (Gud. 47)**   II.78.

Same as [1842].

[1844]   **364 (Gud. 7 et 18)**   I.58.

The number 364 is a sequential number in Ebert 1827: 75.

Current shelfmark: 7 and 8 Gud. lat. 2° (and not 7 and 18).

Same as [1841].

[1845]   **368 (11 Gud. gr.)**   N.33 (2).

The number 368 is the sequential number of the manuscript in Ebert 1827: 75.

Current shelfmark: 11 Gud. graec. fol.

Köhler and Milchsack 1913: 6.

Also [1846].

[1846]   **368 (Gud. 11)**   I.86, 87.

Same as [1845].

[1847]   **369 (Gud. 69)**   I.92.

The number 369 is the sequential number in Ebert 1827: 76.

Current shelfmark: 69. Gud. graec. 4to.

Köhler and Milchsack 1913: 43-44.

17th-century manuscript, possibly autograph by Friedrich Lindenbrog (1573-1648).

Also [1848]-[1850].

[1848]   **369 (69 Gud. gr.)**   N.33.

Same as [1847].

[1849]   **369. 370 (Gud. 69)**   I.93.

The numbers 369 and 370 are sequential numbers in Ebert 1827: 76, where the same manuscript is dealt with in two different entries.

Same as [1847].

[1850]   **370 (69 Gud. gr.)**   N.34.

The number 370 is a sequential number in Ebert 1827: 76.

Same as [1847].

Helmstatenses

[1851]   **757.837**   I.73.

The number 757 is the shelfmark of the manuscript and the number 837 its sequential number in von Heinemann 1886: 193.

Current shelfmark: 757 Helmst.

von Heinemann 1886: 193.

Also [1852].

[1852]   **837 (757 Helmst.)**   N.31.

The number 837 is the sequential number of the manuscript in von Heinemann 1886: 193, and 757 its shelfmark.

Same as [1851].

Weissenb. (*Weissenburgerani*)

[1853] **64** I.76.

Palimpsest.

Scriptio superior: Isidorus Hispalensis, *Etymologiae.*

Scriptio inferior: Galenus, *De alimentorum facultatibus* (frg.).

von Heinemann 1903: 295-296; more recently: Butzmann 1964: 204-210; Harlfinger, Brunschön and Vasiloudi 2006: 146-150.

For other folios of the same manuscript, see [1608].

Current shelfmark: 64 Weiss.

Also [1854].

[1854] **4148** N.32.

(64 Weissenb.) The number 4148 is the sequential number of the manuscript in von Heinemann 1903: 295-296, and 64 is its shelfmark.

Same as [1853].

Herzog August Bibliothek Wolfenbüttel (Herzog August Library Wolfenbüttel)

Augustei (Aug.)

18.1 Aug. 4to See [1839] and [1840].

Gudiani graeci (Gud. graec.)

11 fol. See [1845]-[1846].

47 fol. See [1842]-[1843].

84 4to Gregorius Nyssenus, *De hominis opificio.*

Köhler and Milchsack 1913: 51.

86 4to Cassianus Bassus, *Geoponica.*

Köhler and Milchsack 1913: 52.

87 4to Gregorius Nyssenus, *De creatione hominis.*

Köhler and Milchsack 1913: 52.

93 4to Symeon Seth, *De ciborum facultatibus.*

Köhler and Milchsack 1913: 55.

Helmstadienses (Helmst.)

757 See [1851]-[1852].

Weissenburgerani (Weiss.)

64 See [1853]-[1854].

Wrocław (PL)

Biblioteka Uniwersytecka we Wrocławiu (University Library Wrocław)

Rehd.

34 See [0171].

Երևան (Yerevan) (AM)

Մատենադարան. Մ. Մաշտոցի անվան հին ձեռագրերի գիտահետազոտական ինստիտուտ (Matenadaran. M. Maštoc`i anvan hin jeřagreri gitahetazotakan institut [Matenadaran. Mesrop Mashtots Institute of Ancient Manuscripts])

-

M 141   Dioscorides, *De materia medica.*

             Chétanian 2008: 69-70.

             See [0233].

Ζάβορδα (Zavorda) (GR)

Ιερά Μονή Οσίου Νικάνορος (St. Nikanor Monastery)

-

95   (ff. 365r-366r) Nicephorus Constantinopolitanus Patriarcha, *Oneirocriticon*; (f. 366r) *Iatrosofion.*

             Politi 2012: 63-67.

123   (ff. 16r et seq.) Symeon Seth, *De alimentorum facultatibus*; (f. 55r) *Lexicon botanicum*; (f. 55v) *Diagnostica.*

             Politi 2012: 105-107.

Zaragoza (ES)

Bibl. d. Cat. d. Pil. (Biblioteca de la Catedral del Pilar [Library of the Cathedral del Pilar]), now Santa Iglesia mayor del Pilar (Basilica of Our Lady of the Pilar)

-

[1855]   **1106 (ol. 562)**   II.89 (2), 90.

             Graux, ed. Martin 1892: 212-213, no. 562.

             The actual shelfmark at the Pilar was 562. When the collection moved to the Archivo-Biblioteca del Cabildo metropolitano (La Seo) in Zaragoza, the shelfmark was 11-35.

             The number 1106 in Diels is of unknown origin (Olivier 1976: 56) and probably comes from an old catalogue. It is still used in Ihm 2002: 81, no. 39.

             This manuscript is now New Haven, Yale University, Harvey Cushing/John Jay Whitney Medical Library, Manuscript 32 vault (see above, p. 165) (Olivier 1976: 53; Escobar Chico 1993: 84).

[1856]   **1115 (olim 1427)**   II.26.

             Graux, ed. Martin 1892: 218, no. 1427.

             The actual shelfmark at the Pilar was 1427. When the collection moved to the Archivo-Biblioteca del Cabildo metropolitano (La Seo), the shelfmark was 5-55.

The shelfmark 1115 in Diels is of unknown origin (Olivier 1976: 56, 57) and probably comes from an old catalogue.

It is now New Haven, Yale University, Harvey Cushing/John Hay Whitney Medical Library, Manuscript 50 vault (see above, p. 166) (Olivier 1976: 53; Escobar Chico 1993: 85).

Zeitz (DE)

Stiftsbibliothek (Abbey Library), now Stiftsbibliothek und Stiftsarchiv Zeitz (Abbey Library and Archive, Zeitz)

-

[1857]   **66**   I.72.

Wendel 1921: 372-373; Eleuteri 1999: 45.

Stiftsbibliothek und Stiftsarchiv Zeitz (Abbey Library and Archive, Zeitz)

See above **Stiftsbibliothek**.

Zürich (CH)

Stadtbibliothek (City Library), now Zentralbibliothek Zürich-Kantons-, Stadt- und Universitätsbibliothek (Zurich Central Library-Cantonal, City and University Library)

-

[1858]   **C 50**   II.97.

Gagliardi and Forrer 1982: 360.

Current shelfmark: Ms. C 50.

[1859]   **C 136**   I.39, 43; II.34.

Mohlberg 1951: 64; Leu et al. 2008: 288-289.

Current shelfmark: Ms. C 136.

Zentralbibliothek Zürich-Kantons-, Stadt- und Universitätsbibliothek (Zurich Central Library-Cantonal, City and University Library)

See above **Stadtbibliothek.**

Bibliography[1]

Abbott 1900: Thomas Kingsmill Abbott, *Catalogue of the manuscripts in the Library of Trinity College, Dublin*. Dublin: Hodges, Figgis, & Co., and London: Longman, Green, & Co., 1900.

Ackermann 1821: Johannes Chr. Ackermann, "Libri Quarti Caput XIX (olim XVIII): Claudius Galenus", in Ioannes Albertus Fabricius, *Bibliotheca Graeca sive Notitia Scriptorum Veterum Graecorum quorumcumque Monumenta Integra aut Fragmenta edita exstant tum plerorumque e MSS. ac deperditis ab auctore recognita*. Editio tertia variorum curis emendatior atque auctior curante Gottlieb Christophoro Harles. Accedunt Christophori Augusti Heumanni Supplementa inedita, Volumen quintum. Hamburgi: apud Carolum Ernestum Bohn; Lipsiae: Ex Officina Breitkopfia et Haertelia, 1796, pp. 377–500 (reproduced as *Historia literaria Claudii Galeni ... ex Jo. Alb. Fabricii Biblioth. Graec. ex ed. Gli. Cph. Harles, vol. V. P. 377–500*, in Carolus Gottlob Kühn [ed.], *Claudii Galeni Opera omnia*, Tomus 1 [Medicorum Graecorum Opera quae exstant 1]. Leipzig: Carl Cnobloch, 1821, pp. XVII-CCLXV).

Ackermann 1825: Johannes Chr. Ackermann, "Libri Secundi Caput XXIII: De Hippocrate, Medicorum Principe, et Polybo eius Discipulo", in Ioannes Albertus Fabricius, *Bibliotheca Graeca sive Notitia Scriptorum Veterum Graecorum quorumcumque Monumenta Integra aut Fragmenta edita exstant tum plerorumque e MSS. ac deperditis ab auctore recognita*. Editio quarta variorum curis emendatior atque auctior curante Gottlieb Christophoro Harles. Accedunt B. I. A. Fabricii et Christoph. Augusti Heumanni Supplementa inedita, Volumen secundum. Hamburgi: apud Carolum Ernestum Bohn; Lipsiae: Ex Officina Breitkopfia, 1791, pp. 506–611 (reproduced as *Historia literaria Hippocratis ... ex Jo. Alb. Fabricii Biblioth. Graec. ex edit. Gli. Cph. Harles, vol. II. P. 506–511. Desunta et hinc inde aucta et emendata*, in Carolus Gottlob Kühn [ed.], *Magni Hippocratis Opera omnia*, Tomus 1 [Medicorum Graecorum Opera quae exstant 21]. Leipzig: Carl Cnobloch, 1825, pp. I-CCVI).

Adrados 2005: Francisco Rodríguez Adrados, *A History of the Greek Language: From its Origins to the Present*. Leiden: Brill, 2005.

Agati 2007: Maria Luisa Agati, *Catalogo dei manoscritti greci della Biblioteca dell'Accademia nazionale dei Lincei e Corsiniana* ("Bollettino dei Classici", Supplemento 24). Roma: Accademia nazionale dei Lincei, 2007.

Aland 1956: Kurt Aland, *Die Handschriftenbestände der polnischen Bibliotheken* (Deutsche Akademie der Wissenschaften zu Berlin, Schriften der Sektion für Altertumswissenschaft 7). Berlin: Akademie Verlag, 1956.

Alexanderson 1963: Bengt Alexanderson, *Die hippokratische Schrift Prognostikon. Überlieferung und Text* (Studia graeca et latina gothoburgensia 17). Göteborg: Acta Universitatis Gothoburgensis, 1963.

Alexanderson 1967: Bengt Alexanderson, *Galenos Περὶ κρίσεων. Überlieferung und Text* (Studia graeca et latina gothoburgensia 23). Göteborg: Acta Universitatis Gothoburgensis, 1967.

---

[1] Titles in Greek respect the exact spelling of the publications (including the poly- or monotonic accentuation). For the transformation of Greek spelling during the 20th century, see Adrados 2005, *passim*.

Alexopoulou 1998: Maria-Parthena Alexopoulou, *Das Iatrosophion des sog. Meletios. Edition mit sprachlichen und sachlichen Kommentar*. Inaugural-Dissertation zu Erlangung des Doktorgrades der Philosophie an der Ludwig-Maximilians-Universität München. München, unpublished thesis, 1998.

Allaci 1614–1630: [Leo Allaci], *Index* (= *Inventarium*) *Graecorum Codicum Manu Scriptorum, Pars Prima, a Laurentio Portio Scriptore Graeco descriptum*. Città del Vaticano, Biblioteca Apostolica Vaticana, Manuscripts *Vaticani graeci* 2668–2669.

Amati et al. 1800–1834: Girolamo Amati et al., *Inventarium codicum Vaticanorum Graecorum 993–2160*. Città del Vaticano, Biblioteca Apostolica Vaticana, Manuscript *Vaticanus graecus* 2664.

Andrist 2007: Patrick Andrist, *Les manuscrits grecs conservés à la Bibliothèque de la Bourgeoisie de Berne - Burgerbibliothek Bern. Catalogue et histoire de la collection*. Dietikon-Zurich: Urs Graf, 2007.

***Aristoteles graecus* 1976**: Paul Moraux, Dieter Harlfinger, Diether Reinsch, and Jürgen Wiesner, *Aristoteles graecus. Die griechischen Manuskripte des Aristoteles*. Erster Band: Alexandrien-London (Peripatoi 8). Berlin and New York: Walter De Gruyter, 1976.

Astruc 1985: Charles Astruc, "Deux fragments anciens (en minuscule de type «Anastase») du *De hominis opificio* de Grégoire de Nysse", *Scriptorium* 39 (1985), pp. 265–269.

Astruc and Concasty 1960: Charles Astruc, and Marie-Louise Concasty, *Bibliothèque nationale, Département des manuscrits, Catalogue des manuscrits grecs*, Troisième partie: Le Supplément grec, Tome III: Nᵒˢ 901–1371. Paris: Bibliothèque nationale, 1960.

Astruc, Concasty et al. 2003: Charles Astruc, Marie-Louise Concasty, Cécile Bellon, Christian Förstel et alii, *Catalogue des manuscrits grecs. Supplément grec, numéros 1 à 150*. Paris: Bibliothèque nationale de France, 2003.

***Badische Landesbibliothek* 1896/1970**: *Die Handschriften der grossherzoglich-badischen Hof- und Landesbibliothek in Karlsruhe*, IV. Die karlsruher Handschriften. Karlsruhe: Ch. Th. Gross, 1896 (reprint: *Die Handschriften der badischen Landesbibliothek in Karlsruhe, IV Die karlsruher Handschriften*, Erster Band: Nr. 1–1299 mit einem Vorwort von Wilhelm Brambach. Neudruck mit bibliographischen Nachträgen. Wiesbaden: Otto Harrassowitz, 1970).

Baffioni 1963: Giovanni Baffioni, "Il *Codex Scorialensis* Y. I. 8", *Bollettino del Comitato per la preparazione della Edizione nazionale dei classici greci e latini* N.S. 11 (1963), pp. 25–32.

Balayé 1988: Simone Balayé, *La Bibliothèque Nationale des origines à 1800* (Histoire des idées et critique littéraire 262). Genève: Droz, 1988.

Bancalari 1894: Francesco Bancalari, "Index codicum graecorum Bibliothecae Casanatensis", *Studi italiani di filologia classica* 2 (1894), pp. 161–207 (reproduced in Christa Samberger [ed.], *Catalogi codicum graecorum qui in minoribus bibliothecis italicis asservantur in duo volumina collati et novissimis additamentis aucti*, 2 volumes [Catalogi codicum graecorum lucis ope reimpressi]. Lipsiae: Zentral Antiquariat der Deutschen Demokratischen Republik, 1965–1968, volume 2, pp. 203–249).

Bandini 1764–1770: Angelo Maria Bandini, *Catalogus codicum manuscriptorum Bibliothecae Mediceae Laurentianae* ..., 3 volumes. Florentiae: Typis Caesareis (volume 1); Typis Regiis (volumes 2–3), 1768-1770 (reprint: Fridolf Kudlien [ed.], *Angelo Maria Bandini, Catalogus codicum manuscriptorum Bibliothecae Mediceae Laurentianae. Accedunt supplementa tria ab E. Rostagno et N. Festa congesta, necnon Additamentum ex inventariis Bibliothecae Laurentianae depromptum*, 2 volumes [Catalogi codicum graecorum lucis ope reimpressi]. Leipzig: Zentral-Antiquariat der Deutschen Demokratischen Republik, 1961).

Bandini 1774: Angelo Maria Bandini, *Catalogus codicum latinorum Bibliothecae Mediceae Laurentianae*, Tomus 1: *In quo Sancti Patres Latini Et Scriptores Ecclesiastici Recensentur, Operum Singulorum Notitia Datur, Plura Nondum Vulgata Indicantur Aut Proferuntur, Edita Supplentur et Emendantur*. Florentiae: s.n., 1774.

Bandini 1776: Angelo Maria Bandini, *Catalogus codicum latinorum Bibliothecae Mediceae Laurentianae*, Tomus 3: *In quo Medici, Chirurgici, Philosophi, Politici, Nomici, Tam Veteris, Quam Recentioris Aetatis Aevi Accuratissime Recensentur, Operum Singulorum Notitia Datur, Plura Nondum Vulgata Indicantur, Aut Proferuntur, Edita Supplentur et Emendantur*. Florentiae: typis Caesareis, 1776.

Barbour 1960: Ruth Barbour, "Summary Description of the Greek Manuscripts from the Library at Holkham Hall", *The Bodleian Library Record* 6 (1960), pp. 591–613.

Beaujouan 1962: Guy Beaujouan, *Manuscrits scientifiques médiévaux de l'Université de Salamanque et de ses "Colegios Mayores"* (Bibliothèque de l'Ecole des hautes études hispaniques, 32). Bordeaux: Féret et Fils, 1962.

Bees 1967: Νίκος Α. Βέης, *Τὰ χειρόγραφα τῶν Μετεώρων. Κατάλογος περιγραφικὸς τῶν χειρογράφων κωδίκων τῶν ὑποκειμένων εἰς τὰς μονὰς τῶν Μετεώρων ...*, Τόμος Α΄. Ἐκδιδόμενος ἐκ τῶν καταλοίπων ... Ἀθῆναι: Ἀκαδημία Ἀθηνῶν, Κέντρον Ἐρεύνης τοῦ Μεσαιωνικοῦ καὶ Νέου Ἑλληνισμοῦ, 1967 — Nikos A. Bees, *Les manuscrits des Météores. Catalogue descriptif des manuscrits conservés dans les monastères des Météores*, volume 1: Les manuscrits du monastère de Transfiguration. Oeuvre posthume ... Athènes: Académie d'Athènes, Centre de recherches médiévales et néo-helléniques, 1967 (2nd edition including: Λεάνδρος Βρανούση — Δημήτριος Ζ. Σοφιανός, *Προλεγόμενα — Προσθῆκαι*; Leandros Vranoussis, and Demetrios Z. Sophianos, *Prolégomènes-Additions*. Ἀθῆναι: Ἀκαδημία Ἀθηνῶν, Κέντρον Ἐρεύνης τοῦ Μεσαιωνικοῦ καὶ Νέου Ἑλληνισμοῦ; Athènes: Académie d'Athènes, Centre de recherches médiévales et néo-helléniques, 1998).

Bees 1984: Νίκος Α. Βέης, *Τὰ χειρόγραφα τῶν Μετεώρων. Κατάλογος περιγραφικὸς τῶν χειρογράφων κωδίκων τῶν ὑποκειμένων εἰς τὰς μονὰς τῶν Μετεώρων ...*, Τόμος Β΄ Τὰ χειρόγραφα τῆς Μονῆς Βαρλαάμ. Ἐκδιδόμενος ἐκ τῶν καταλοίπων ... Ἀθῆναι: Ἀκαδημία Ἀθηνῶν, Κέντρον Ἐρεύνης τοῦ Μεσαιωνικοῦ καὶ Νέου Ἑλληνισμοῦ, 1984 — Nikos A. Bees, *Les manuscrits des Météores. Catalogue descriptif des manuscrits conservés dans les monastères des Météores*, volume 2: Les manuscrits du monastère de Barlaam. Oeuvre posthume. Athènes: Académie d'Athènes, Centre de recherches médiévales et néo-helléniques, 1984.

Beneševič 1917: Vladimir Beneševič, *Catalogus codicum manuscriptorum graecorum qui in monasterio Sanctae Catharinae in Monte Sina asservantur*. Tomi III pars I. Codices numeris 1224–2150 signati. Petropoli: Academiae Scientiarum imperialis, 1917.

Berger 1807: Franz Xavier Berger, "Asclepiadarum praecepta de sanitate conservanda, antiquissimum rei medicae monumentum", *Beytraege zur Geschichte und Literatur vorzüglich aus den Schätzen der königl. Hof- und Centralbibliothek zu München* 9 (1807), pp. 1001–1008.

Berger 2014: Friederike Berger, *Katalog der griechischen Handschriften der Bayerischen Staatsbibliothek München*, Band 9: Codices graeci Monacenses 575–650 (Handschriften des Supplements) (Catalogus codicum manu scriptorum Bibliothecae Monacensis, Tomus II, Pars 9). Wiesbaden: Otto Harrassowitz, 2014.

Bergsträsser 1914: Gotthelf Bergsträsser (ed.), *Pseudogaleni In Hippocratis De septimanis commentarium ab Hunaino q. f. Arabice versum*, edidit et Germanice vertit (Corpus Medicorum Graecorum XI 2, 1). Lipsiae et Berolini: In aedibus B. G. Teubneri, 1914.

Berthelot and Ruelle 1888: Marcelin Berthelot in collaboration with Charles-Emile Ruelle, *Collection des anciens alchimistes grecs. Texte grec avec variantes, notes et index*. Paris: Georges Steinheil, 1888.

Bibliotheca Academiae Lugduno-Batavae 1932: *Bibliotheca Academiae Lugduno-Batavae, Catalogus,* Deel XIV: Inventaris van de handschriften, Eerste afdeeling. Leiden: Universiteits-Bibliotheek, 1932.

Bibliotheca Meermanniana 1824: *Bibliotheca Meermanniana, sive, Catalogus librorum impressorum et codicum manuscriptorum quos maximam partem collegerunt viri nobilissimi Gerardus et Joannes Meerman, morte dereliquit Joannes Meerman, toparcha in Dalem et Vuren, etc. etc. quorum publica fiet auctio die VIII sqq. Junii, anni MDCCCXXIV, Hagae Comitum, in aedibus defuncti (Boschkant, Wijk K. no. 261).* Lugduni Batavorum: S. et J. Luchtmans, and Hagae et Amstellodami: Fratres van Cleeft; Hagae: B. Scheurleer, 1824.

Bibliotheca Regia 1740: *Catalogus Codicum Manuscriptorum Bibliothecae Regiae.* Tomus secundus. Parisiis: E Typographia Regia, 1740.

Bingeli et al. 2014: André Bingeli, Matthieu Cassin, and Vassa Kontouma, "Inventaire des manuscrits de l'Institut français d'études byzantines", *Revue des études byzantines* 72 (2014), pp. 5–128.

Björck 1938: Gudmund Björck, "Remarques sur trois documents médicaux de la Bibliothèque universitaire de Leyde", *Mnemosyne* 3rd series, 6 (1938), pp. 139–150.

Björnbo 1911: Axel Anthon Björnbo, "Nachtrag: Handschriftenbeschreibung", in Axel Anthon Björnbo, and Seb. Vogl, *Alkindi, Tideus und Pseudo-Euklid, Drei optische Werke.* Herausgegeben und erklärt (Abhandlungen zur Geschichte der mathematischen Wissenschaften mit Einschluss ihrer Anwendungen 26.3). Leipzig: B.G. Teubner, 1911, pp. 121–147.

Black 1845: William Henry Black, *Descriptive, Analytical, and Critical Catalogue of the Manuscripts Bequeathed to the University of Oxford by Elias Ashmole..., also of Some Additional MSS. Contributed by Kingsley, Lhuyd, Borlase and Others.* Oxford: University Press, 1845.

Bleskina et al. 2013: Olga N. Bleskina, and Natalia A. Elagina with the collaboration of Krzystoff Kossarzecki, and Sławomir Szyller, *The Inventory of Manuscripts from the Zaluski Library in the Imperial Public Library* (National Library of Russia, Saint Petersburg, National Library of Poland, Warsaw). Warzawa: Biblioteka Narodowa, 2013.

Blume 1824–1827: Friedrich Blume, *Iter italicum,* 2 volumes: 1. *Archive, Bibliotheken und Inschriften in den Sardinischen und Œsterreichischen Provinzen*; 2. *Archive, Bibliotheken und Inschriften in Parma, Modena, Massa, Lucca, Toscana, dem Kirchenstaat und S. Marino.* Berlin und Stetting: In der Nicolaischen Buchhandlung, 1824–1827.

Bodenheimer and Rabinowitz 1949: Friedrich Shimon Bodenheimer, and Alexander Rabinowitz, *Timotheus of Gaza Περὶ ζῴων. Fragments of a Byzantine Paraphrase of an Animal-book of the 5th Century A.D. Translation, Commentary and Introduction* (Collection de travaux de l'Académie internationale d'histoire des sciences 3). Paris: Académie internationale d'histoire des sciences, and Leiden: E. J. Brill, 1949.

Boinet 1908: Amédée Boinet, *Catalogue des manuscrits de la bibliothèque de la Faculté de Médecine.* Paris: Plon-Nourrit, 1908.

Bono et al. 2002: Nicolas Bono, Gábor Görgey, Francesco Sicilia, István Monok, *Nel segno del corvo. Libri e miniature della biblioteca di Mattia Corvino re d'Ungheria (1443–1490).* Modena: Il Bulino, 2002.

Borland 1916: Catherine R. Borland, *A Descriptive Catalogue of the Western Medieval Manuscripts in Edinburgh University Library.* Edinburgh: University of Edinburgh, 1916.

Börzsönyi 1986: József Börzsönyi, *A Tiszáninnemi Református Egyházkerülwt Nagykönyvtáránnak (Sárospatak) kéziratkatalógusa* (Magyaroszági egyházi könyvtárak kéziratkalogúsai - Catalogi manuscriptorum, quae in bibliothecis ecclesiasticis Hungariae asservantur 4). Budapest: Országos Széchényi Könyvtár, 1986.

Bosquillon 1784: Eduardus-Franciscus-Maria Bosquillon, *Hippocratis Aphorismi et Praenotiones Liber*. Recensuit, notasque addidit -. Parisiis: Excudebat J. Fr. Valade, 1784.

Boudon 2002: Véronique Boudon, *Galien*, Tome II: *Exhortation à l'étude de la médecine. Art médical*. Texte établi et traduit (Collection des Universités de France). Paris: Belles Lettres, 2002.

Boudon-Millot 2007: Véronique Boudon-Millot, *Galien*, Tome I: *Introduction générale. Sur l'ordre de ses propres livres. Sur ses propres livres. Que l'excellent médecin est aussi philosophe*. Texte établi, traduit et commenté (Collection des Universités de France). Paris: Belles Lettres, 2007.

Bouras-Vallianatos 2015: Petros Bouras-Vallianatos, "Greek Manuscripts at the Wellcome Library in London: A Descriptive Catalogue", *Medical History* 59 (2015), pp. 275–326.

Browne 1900: Edward G. Browne, *A Hand-list of the Muhammadan Manuscripts, including all those written in the Arabic character, preserved in the Library of the University of Cambridge*. Cambridge: University Press, 1900.

Burgon 1839: John William Burgon, *The Life and Times of Sir Thomas Gresham; compiled chiefly from his correspondence preserved in Her Majesty's State-paper Office, including notices of many of his contemporaries*, 2 volumes. London: Robert Jennings, 1839.

Bussemaker 1862: Ulgo Cats Bussemaker, "Fragmenta poematum rem naturalem vel medicinam spectantium ... Omnia collegit, denuo recognovit; pleraque fragmenta medicinalia cum cod. comparavit; pauca quaedam nunc demum primum edidit", in *Poetae bucolici et didactici*. Parisiis: Ambrosius Firmin Didot, 1862, pars 3, pp. 71–134.

Bussemaker and Daremberg 1851: Ulco Cats Bussemaker, and Charles Daremberg (eds.), *Oeuvres d'Oribase*. Texte grec, en grande partie inédit, collationné sur les manuscrits, traduit pour la première foix en français avec une introduction, des notes, des tables et des planches, Tome premier. Paris: Imprimerie nationale, 1851.

Butzmann 1964: Hans Butzmann, *Die Weissenburger Handschriften neu beschrieben* (Kataloge der Herzog-August-Bibliothek Wolfenbüttel, Neue Reihe, Bd. 10). Frankfurt am Main: Vittorio Klostermann, 1964.

Byl 1977: Simon Byl, "Note sur un recentior hippocratique (*Parisinus gr.* 2145, K)", *Revue d'Histoire des Textes* 7 (1977), pp. 271–280.

Calcoen 1965–1975: Roger Calcoen, *Inventaire des manuscrits scientifiques de la Bibliothèque royale de Belgique*, 3 volumes. Bruxelles: Bibliothèque royale, 1965–1975.

Calcoen 1980: Roger Calcoen, *Inventaire des manuscrits scientifiques de la Bibliothèque royale Albert I*er, tome 4 (Publications du Centre national d'histoire des sciences I, 4). Bruxelles: Centre national d'histoire des sciences, 1980.

Canart 1966: Paul Canart, *Catalogue des manuscrits grecs de l'Archivio di San Pietro* (Studi e Testi 246). Città del Vaticano: Biblioteca Apostolica Vaticana, 1966.

Canart 1970: Paul Canart, *Bibliothecae Apostolicae Vaticanae codices manu scripti recensiti. Codices Vaticani Graeci. Codices 1745–1962*. Volumen I: Codicum enarrationes. [Città del Vaticano]: In Bibliotheca Vaticana, 1970.

Canart 1974: Paul Canart, "Notes sur quelques manuscrits grecs des bibliothèques de Pologne", in John H. Keller (ed.), *Serta Turyniana. Studies in Greek Literature and Palaeography in honor of Alexander Turyn*. Urbana, Chicago and London: University of Illinois Press, 1974, pp. 547–563.

Canart 1977–1979: Paul Canart, "Démétrius Damilas, *alias* le «Librarius Florentinus»", *Rivista di studi bizantini e neo-ellenici* 14–16 (1977–1979), pp. 281–347 (reproduced in Paul Canart, *Etudes de paléographie et de codicologie*. Reproduites avec la collaboration de Maria Luisa Agati, and Marco D'Agostino, 2 volumes [Studi e Testi 450–451]. Città del Vaticano: Biblioteca Apostolica Vaticana, 2008, volume 1, pp. [451]-[522]).

Canart 2004: Paul Canart, "Les palimpsestes des fonds grecs de la Bibliothèque Vaticane. Une liste sommaire et quelques précisions" in Bart Janssens, Bram Roosen, and Peter Van Deun (eds.), *Philomathestatos. Studies in Greek and Byzantine Texts presented to Jacques Noret for his Sixty-fifth Birthday. Etudes de patristique grecque et textes byzantins offerts à Jacques Noret à l'occasion de ses soixante-cinq ans* (Orientalia Lovaniensia Analecta 137). Leuven, Paris and Dudley, MA: Peeters, 2004, pp. 45–55 (reproduced in Paul Canart, *Etudes de paléographie et de codicologie. Reproduites avec la collaboration de Maria Luisa Agati et Marco D'Agostino*, 2 volumes [Studi e Testi 450–451]. Città del Vaticano: Biblioteca Apostolica Vaticana, 2008, volume 2, pp. [1311]-[1321]).

Canart and Lucà 2000: Paul Canart, and Santo Lucà, *Codici greci dell'Italia meridionale. Catalogo della mostra (Grottaferrata-Biblioteca del Monumento Nazionale, 31 marzo-31 maggio 2000)*. Roma: Retablo, 2000.

Canart and Peri 1970: Paul Canart, and Vittorio Peri, *Sussidi bibliografici per i manoscritti greci della Biblioteca Vaticana* (Studi e Testi 261). Città del Vaticano: Biblioteca Apostolica Vaticana, 1970.

Capocci 1958: Valentinus Capocci, *Codices Barberiniani graeci*, Tomus I: Codices 1–163. [Città del Vaticano]: In Bybliotheca Vaticana, 1958.

Carter 1966: Robert E. Carter, "The Greek Manuscripts of Hamburg. Their Present Disposition", *Scriptorium* 20 (1966), pp. 69–70.

Cataldi Palau 1990: Annaclara Cataldi Palau, *Catalogo dei manoscritti greci della Biblioteca Franzoniana (Genova), Urbani 2–20* («Bollettino dei Classici», Accademia nazionale dei Lincei, Supplemento 8). Roma: Accademia nazionale dei Lincei, 1990.

Cataldi Palau 1998: Annaclara Cataldi Palau, *Gian Francesco d'Asola e la tipografia aldina. La vita, le edizioni, la biblioteca dell'Asolano*. Genova: Sagep, 1998.

Catalogue général des manuscrits 1872: *Catalogue général des manuscrits des bibliothèques publiques des départements*, Tome IV: *Arras, Avranches, Boulogne*. Paris: Imprimerie nationale, 1872.

Catalogue général des manuscrits 1879: *Catalogue général des manuscrits des bibliothèques publiques des départements*, Tome V: *Metz, Verdun, Charleville*. Paris: Imprimerie nationale, 1879.

Catalogue général des manuscrits 1887: *Catalogue général des manuscrits des bibliothèques publiques de France*, Départements, Tome VI: *Auxerre ...* Paris: Librairie Plon, 1887.

Catalogue général des manuscrits 1893: *Catalogue général des manuscrits des bibliothèques publiques de France*, Départements, Tome XIX: *Amiens*. Paris: Librairie Plon, 1893.

Catalogue général des manuscrits 1899: *Catalogue général des manuscrits des bibliothèques publiques de France*, Départements, Tome XXXV: *Carpentras*, Tome 2. Paris: Librairie Plon, 1899.

Catalogue général des manuscrits 1900: *Catalogue général des manuscrits des Bibliothèques publiques de France*, Départements, Tome XXX: *Lyon*. Paris: Librairie Plon, 1900.

Catalogue général des manuscrits 1901: *Catalogue général des manuscrits des bibliothèques publiques de France*, Départements, Tome XXXIV: Carpentras, Tome 1. Paris: Librairie Plon, 1901.

Catalogue général des manuscrits 1904: *Catalogue général des manuscrits des bibliothèques publiques de France,* Départements, Tome XLII: Supplément, Tome III: *Lyon, Orléans*. Paris: Librairie Plon, 1904.

Catalogue général des manuscrits 1909: *Catalogue général des manuscrits des bibliothèques publiques de France, Paris*, Tome I. Paris: Librairie Plon, 1909.

Catalogue général des manuscrits 1923: *Catalogue général des manuscrits des bibliothèques publiques de France,* Départements, Tome XLVII: *Strasbourg*. Paris: Librairie Plon, 1923.

Catalogue général des manuscrits 1962: *Catalogue général des manuscrits des bibliothèques publiques de France*, Tome LIII: *Manuscrits des bibliothèques sinistrées de 1940 à 1944*. Paris: Bibliothèque nationale, 1962.

***Catalogue of Additions* 1850**: *Catalogue of Additions to the Manuscripts in the British Museum in the Years 1841–1845.* London: British Museum, 1850.

***Catalogue of Additions* 1864**: *Catalogue of Additions to the Manuscripts in the British Museum in the Years 1846–1847.* London: British Museum, 1864.

***Catalogue ULCambridge* 1856–1867**: *A Catalogue of the Manuscripts preserved in the Library of the University of Cambridge,* 5 volumes. Cambridge: University Press, 1856–1867.

***Catalogus* 1706**: *Catalogus centuriae librorum rarissimorum manuscript[orum] & partim impressorum, Arabicorum, Persicorum, Turcicorum, Graecorum, Latinorum, etc. Qua anno MDCCV Bibliothecam Publicam Academiae Upsalensis auxit et exornavit Vir illustris et generosissimus Ioan. Gabr. Sparvenfeldius* ... Upsaliae: Typis Joh. Henr. Werneri, 1706.

***Catalogus Bibliothecae Monacensis* 1892**: *Catalogus Codicum Latinorum Bibliothecae Regiae Monacensis.* Editio altera emendatior. Tomi I pars I. Codices num. 1–2329 complectens (Catalogus Codicum Manu Scriptorum Bibliothecae Regiae Monacensis. Tomi III Pars 1. Codices latinos continens. Editio altera). Monachii: Sumptibus Bibliothecae Regiae, 1892.

***Catalogus Vratislaviensis* 1889**: *Catalogus codicum graecorum qui in Bibliotheca Urbica Vratislaviensi adservantur a philologis vratislaviensibus compositus. Civitatis vratislaviensis sumptibus impressus. Accedit Appendix qua Gymnasii regii Fridericiani codices graeci describuntur.* Vratislavae: Apud Guilelmum Koebnerum, 1889.

***CCAG* I (Olivieri) 1898**: Alexander Olivieri, *Catalogus Codicum Astrologorum Graecorum,* Tomus I, *Codices Florentinos.* Accedunt fragmenta selecta primum edita ab Francisco Boll, Francisco Cumont, Guilelmo Kroll, Alexandro Olivieri. Bruxellis: In Aedibus Henrici Lamertin, 1898.

***CCAG* IV (Bassi et al.) 1903**: Dominicus Bassi, Franciscus Cumont, Aemygdius Martini, et Alexander Olivieri, *Catalogus Codicum Astrologorum Graecorum,* Tomus IV: *Codices italicos praeter Florentinos, Venetos, Mediolanenses, Romanos descripserunt -.* Bruxellis: In Aedibus Henrici Lamertin, 1903.

***CCAG* V.1 (Cumont and Boll) 1904**: Franciscus Cumont et Franciscus Boll, *Catalogus Codicum Astrologorum Graecorum,* Tomus V, Pars 1: *Codicum romanorum pars prior.* Bruxellis: In Aedibus Henrici Lamertin, 1904.

***CCAG* V.2 (Kroll) 1906**: Guilelmus Kroll, *Catalogus Codicum Astrologorum Graecorum,* Tomus V, Pars 2: *Codicum romanorum pars secunda.* Bruxellis: In Aedibus Henrici Lamertin, 1906.

***CCAG* V.3 (Heeg) 1910**: Iosephus Heeg, *Catalogus Codicum Astrologorum Graecorum, Codicum romanorum pars tertia.* Bruxellis: In Aedibus Henrici Lamertin, 1910.

***CCAG* V.4 (Weinstock) 1940**: Stephanus Weinstock, *Catalogus Codicum Astrologorum Graecorum, Codicum romanorum pars quarta.* Accedit Porphyrii philosophi *Introductio in Tetrabiblum Ptolemaei* ab Aemilia Boer et Stephano Weinstock edita. Bruxellis: In Aedibus Academiae, 1940.

***CCAG* VIII.1 (Cumont) 1929**: Franciscus Cumont, *Catalogus Codicum Astrologorum Graecorum,* Tomus VIII, Pars 1: *Codicum Parisinorum Pars prima.* Bruxellis: In Aedibus Mauricii Lamertin, 1929.

***CCAG* VIII.2 (Ruelle) 1911**: Charles Emile Ruelle, *Catalogus Codicum Astrologorum Graecorum,* Tomus VIII, Pars 2: *Codicum Parisinorum Pars secunda.* Accedunt Hermetica edita ab Iosephus Heeg. Bruxellis: in Aedibus Henrici Lamertin, 1911.

***CCAG* VIII.3 (Boudreaux) 1912**: Petrus Boudreaux, *Catalogus Codicum Astrologorum Graecorum,* Tomus VIII, Pars 3: *Codicum parisinorum pars tertia.* Bruxellis: In Aedibus Henrici Lamertin, 1912.

***CCAG* IX.2 (Weinstock) 1953**: Stephanus Weinstock, *Catalogus Codicum Astrologorum Graecorum,* Tomus IX, Pars 2: *Codices Britannici,* Pars altera *Codices Londinenses, Cantabrigienses, bibliothecarum minorum. Accedunt codices Batavi, Danenses, Sueci.* Bruxellis: In Aedibus Academiae, 1953.

CCAG X (Delatte) 1924: Armandus Delatte, *Catalogus Codicum Astrologorum Graecorum*, Tomus X: *Codices Athenienses*. Bruxellis: In Aedibus Mauritii Lamertin, 1924.

CCAG XI.2 (Zuretti) 1934: Carolus Orestes Zuretti, *Catalogus Codicum Astrologorum Graecorum*, Tomus XI, Pars 2: *Codices Hispanenses, Pars altera: Codices Scorialenses, Matritenses, Caesaraugustani*. Bruxellis: In Aedibus Mauritii Lamertin, 1934.

CCAG XII (Šangin) 1936: Mstislav Antoninus P. Šangin, *Catalogus Codicum Astrologorum Graecorum*, Tomus XII: *Codices rossici*. Bruxellis: In Aedibus Henrici Lamertin, 1936.

Ceresa and Lucà 2008: Massimo Ceresa, and Santo Lucà, "Frammenti greci di Dioscoride Pedanio e Aezio Amideno in una edizione a stampa di Francesco Zanetti (Roma 1576)", *Miscellanea Bibliothecae Vaticanae* 15 (Studi e Testi 453). Città del Vaticano: Biblioteca Apostolica Vaticana, 2008, pp. 191–229.

Chétanian 2008: Rose Varteni Chétanian, *Catalogue des fragments et manuscrits grecs du Matenadaran d'Erevan*. Turnhout: Brepols, 2008.

Choulant 1841: Ludwig Choulant, *Handbuch der Bücherkunde für die ältere Medicin zur Kenntniss der griechischen, lateinischen und arabischen Schriften im ärzlichen Fache und zur bibliographischen Unterscheidung ihrer verschiedener Ausgaben, Übersetzungen und Erläuterungen.* Zweite durchaus umgearbeitete und stark vermehrte Auflage. Leipzig: Leopold Voss, 1841 (reprint: Graz: Akademische Druck- und Verlagsanstalt, 1956).

Christie's 2006: Christie's London. *Valuable Manuscripts and Printed Books, Wednesday 7 June 2006. Auction Wednesday 7 June 2006 ... 8 King Street, St. James's, London ... Auction code and number ... BEHEAD-7233.* London: Christie's, 2006.

Clavis Patrum Graecorum 1974: Mauritii Geerard, *Clavis Patrum Graecorum*. Volumen II: Ab Athanasio ad Chrysostomum (Corpus Christianorum). Turnhout: Brepols, 1974.

Clavis Patrum Graecorum, Supplementum 1998: Maurits Geerard, and Jacques Noret, *Clavis Patrum Graecorum, Supplementum* (Corpus Christianorum). Turnhout: Brepols, 1998.

C.M.A. 1697: Edouard Bernard, *Catalogus codicum manuscriptorum Angliae et Hiberniae in unum collecti, cum indice alphabetico*. Oxoniae: E Theatro Sheldoniano, 1697.

CMAG I (Lebègue) 1924: Henri Lebègue, *Catalogue des manuscrits alchimiques grecs*, Tome I: *Les Parisini*. En appendice: *Les manuscrits des Coeranides* et *Tables générales* par Marie Delcourt. Bruxelles: Maurice Lamertin, 1924.

CMAG II (Zuretti et al.) 1927: Carlo Oreste Zuretti, avec la collaboration de Otto Lagercrantz, Johan Ludvig Heiberg, Ingeborg Hammer-Jensen, Domenico Bassi et Æmidio Martini, *Catalogue des manuscrits alchimiques grecs*, Tome II: *Les manuscrits italiens*. En appendice: *Les Manuscrits des Coeranides* par C. O. Z.; *Excerpta* par J. L. H. et C. O. Z.; *Ueber das Verhältnis des Cod. Paris. 2327 (A) zum Cod. Marc. 299 (M)* von O. L.; *Tables* par Marie Delcourt. Bruxelles: Maurice Lamertin, 1927.

CMAG III (Anderson et al.) 1924: Annie Anderson, William J. Anderson et Otto Lagercrantz, *Catalogue des manuscrits alchimiques grecs*, Tome III: *Les manuscrits des iles britanniques*, décrits par A. A. and W. J. A. En appendice: *Les recettes alchimiques du Codex Holkamicus*, éditées par O. L. Bruxelles: Maurice Lamertin, 1924.

CMAG IV (Goldschmidt) 1932: Günther Goldschmidt, *Catalogue des manuscrits alchimiques grecs*, Tome IV: *Manuscrits d'Allemagne, d'Autriche, de Danemark, de Hollande et de Suisse*. En appendice: *Die Diatribe des Th. Reinesius aus cod. Gothanus A 242*, hrg. von G. G.; *Ueber das Verhältnis des Cod. Paris. 2327 (A) zum Cod. Marc. 299 (M). (Fortsetzung von Catalogue, II, 341–358)*, von O. Lagercrantz. Bruxelles: Secrétariat administratif de l'Union Académique Internationale, 1932.

CMAG V (**Zuretti and Severyns**) **1928**: Carlo Oreste Zuretti et Albert Severyns, *Catalogue des manuscrits alchimiques grecs*, Tome V: *Les manuscrits d'Espagne*, décrits par C. O. Z.; 2. *Les manuscrits d'Athènes*, décrits par A. S. Bruxelles: Maurice Lamertin, 1928.

***Codices D'Orvilliani* 1806**: [Thomas Gaisford], *Codices manuscripti, et impressi cum notis manuscriptis, olim d'Orvilliani, qui in Bibliotheca Bodleiana apud Oxonienses adservantur*. Oxonii: E Typographeo Clarendoniano, 1806.

Condylis-Bassoukos 1997: Hélène Condylis-Bassoukos, *Stéphanitès kai Ichnélatès, traduction grecque (XIᵉ siècle) du livre Kalîla wa-Dimna d'Ibn al-Muqaffaᶜ (VIIIᵉ siècle). Etude lexicologique et littéraire* (Académie royale de Belgique, Classe des lettres, Fonds René Draguet XI). Lovanii: Aedibus Peeters, 1997.

Congourdeau 1996: Marie-Hélène Congourdeau, "Le traducteur grec du traité de Rhazès sur la variole", in Antonio Garzya (ed.), *Storia e ecdotica dei testi medici greci, Atti del II Convegno Internazionale Parigi 24–26 maggio 1994* (Collectanea 10). Napoli: M. D'Auria, 1996, pp. 99–111.

Cosentini 1922: Francesco Cosentini, *Torino [Biblioteca Nazionale]* (Inventari dei manoscritti delle biblioteche d'Italia 28). Torino: Olschki, 1922.

Costomiris 1889: Georges A. Costomiris, "Etudes sur les écrits inédits des anciens médecins grecs et ceux dont le texte original est perdu, mais qui existent en latin ou en arabe. Première série: Hippocrate, Cratevas, Aelius Promotus, Galien", *Revue des études grecques* 2 (1889), pp. 343–383.

Costomiris 1890: Georges A. Costomiris, "Etudes sur les écrits inédits des anciens médecins grecs et ceux dont le texte original est perdu, mais qui existent en latin ou en arabe. Deuxième série: L'Anonyme de Daremberg, Métrodora, Aétius", *Revue des études grecques* 3 (1890), pp. 145–179.

Costomiris 1891: Georges A. Costomiris, "Etudes sur les écrits inédits des anciens médecins grecs et ceux dont le texte original est perdu, mais qui existent en latin ou en arabe. Troisième série: Alexandre (Sophiste et Roi), Timothée, Léon le Sophiste, Théophane Nonnos, les Ephodes", *Revue des études grecques* 4 (1891), pp. 97–110.

Costomiris 1897: Georges A. Costomiris, "Etudes sur les écrits inédits des anciens médecins grecs et ceux dont le texte original est perdu, mais qui existent en latin ou en arabe. Cinquième série: XIIIᵉ-XIVᵉ siècles, Jean Tzetzès, Nicolas Myrepsus, Jean Actuarius", *Revue des études grecques* 10 (1897), pp. 405–445.

Courtonne 1957: Yves Courtonne, *Saint Basile, Lettres*, Tome I. Texte établi et traduit (Collection des Universités de France). Paris: Belles Lettres, 1957.

Courtonne 1961: Yves Courtonne, *Saint Basile, Lettres*, Tome II. Texte établi et traduit (Collection des Universités de France). Paris: Belles Lettres, 1961.

Coxe 1852: Henry O. Coxe, *Catalogus Codicum MSS. qui in Collegiis Aulisque Oxoniensibus hodie adservantur*, 2 volumes. Oxonii: E Typographo Academico, 1852 (reprint of volume 1: *Catalogue of the Manuscripts in the Oxford Colleges by H. O. Coxe*. Volume I. Introduction by Kenneth William Humphreys. Republished 1972 by E. P. Publishing Limited from the edition of 1852 published by the Oxford University Press. Wakefield: E. P. Publishing, 1972).

Coxe 1853: Henry O. Coxe, *Catalogi Codicum Manuscriptorum Bibliothecae Bodleianae Pars Prima Recensionem Codicum Graecorum Continens*. Oxonii: E Typographo Academico, 1853 (reprint: Oxford: Bodleian Library, 1969).

Coxe 1854: Henry O. Coxe, *Catalogi Codicum Manuscriptorum Bibliothecae Bodleianae Pars Tertia Codices Graecos et Latinos Canonicianos Complectens*. Oxonii: E Typographo Academico, 1854.

Coxe 1858: Henry O. Coxe, *Catalogus MSS. Laudianorum. Codices Latini* (Catalogi Codicum Manuscriptorum Bibliothecae Bodleianae Partis Secundae Fasciculus Primus). Oxonii: E Typographo Academico, 1858.

Coxe 1858/2: Henry O. Coxe, *Report to Her Majesty's Government, on the Greek Manuscripts yet Remaining in Libraries of the Levant*. London: George E. Eyre and William Spottiswoode, 1858.

Cozza Luzi n.d.: *Inventarium codicum Graecorum Bibliothecae Vaticanae a 1501 (pro 2001) auspice Leone XIII P.O.M. I.B. Card. Pitra S.R.E. Bibliothecarie confectum a Josepho Cozza Luzi Abate S. Mariae Cryptaeferratae Scriptore Bibl. Vaticanae*. Città del Vaticano, Biblioteca Apostolica Vaticana, Manuscript *Vaticanus graecus* 2670.

Csapodi and Csapodi-Gárdony 1982: Csaba Csapodi, and Klára Csapodi-Gárdony, *Bibliotheca Corviniana. La bibliothèque du roi Mathias Corvin de Hongrie*. Budapest: Corvinia Kiadó-Helikon Kiadó, 1982.

Cutolo 2012: Carmelo Cutolo, "Sulla tradizione manoscritta di Areteo di Cappadocia", *Galenos* 6 (2012), pp. 25–47.

Cyrillus 1832: Salvator Cyrillus, *Codices Graeci MSS. Regiae Bibliothecae Borbonicae descripti, atque illustrati*, Tomus II. Neapoli: Ex Regia Typographia, 1832.

D'Aiuto 2011: Francesco D'Aiuto, "[Barberiniani]", in Francesco D'Aiuto e Paolo Vian (eds.), *Guida ai fondi manoscritti, numismatici, a stampa della Biblioteca Vaticana*, 2 volumes: I. *Dipartimento Manoscritti*; II. *Dipartimento Stampati - Dipartimento del Gabinetto Numismatico - Uffici della Prefettura. Archivio - Addenda, elenchi e prospetti, indici* (Studi e Testi 466–467). Città del Vaticano: Biblioteca Apostolica Vaticana, 2011, volume 1, pp. 336–340.

D'Aiuto 2011/2: Francesco D'Aiuto, "[Urbinati]", in Francesco D'Aiuto e Paolo Vian (eds.), *Guida ai fondi manoscritti, numismatici, a stampa della Biblioteca Vaticana*, 2 volumes: I. *Dipartimento Manoscritti*; II. *Dipartimento Stampati - Dipartimento del Gabinetto Numismatico - Uffici della Prefettura. Archivio - Addenda, elenchi e prospetti, indici* (Studi e Testi 466–467). Città del Vaticano: Biblioteca Apostolica Vaticana, 2011, volume 1, pp. 538–545.

d'Ancora 1794: Caietani de Ancora, *Xenocratis de alimento ex aquatilibus, cum Latina interpretatione Jo. Bapt. Rasarii, Scholiis Conradi Gesneri, et Notis integris Jo. Friderici Franzii. Accedunt Novae variantes Lectiones ex Codd. Mss. depromtae, et Animadversiones Diamantis Coray nunc primum editae; itemque Annotationes in Auctorum, Additamenta in Glossarium Franzii hodiernam Ichthyologiam illustrantia, et Lucubratio de Piscium esu*. Neapoli: Typis regiis, 1794.

d'Ancora 1796: Gaetano d'Ancora, "Codices graeci MSS. qui adservantur Neapoli in Bibliotheca Augustinensium S. Iohannis ad Carbonariam", in Jo. Alberti Fabricii, *Bibliotheca graeca sive notitia scriptorum veterum graecorum quorumcumque monumenta integra aut fragmenta edita exstant tum plerorumque e mss. ac deperditis ab auctore recognita*. Editio tertia variorum curis emendatior atque auctor curante Gottlieb Christophoro Harles. Accedunt Christophori Augusti Heumanni Supplementa inedita, Volumen quintum. Hamburgi: apud Carolum Ernestum Bohn, Lipsiae: Ex Officina Breitkopfia et Haertelia, 1796, pp. 796–800.

Daremberg 1845: Charles Daremberg, "Rapport adressé à M. le Ministre de l'Instruction Publique par ... chargé d'une mission médico-littéraire en Allemagne", *Journal général de l'Instruction publique* 14, nos. 33 (23 avril 1845), pp. 193–196, and 34 (26 avril 1845), pp. 198–202.

Daremberg 1845/2: Charles Daremberg, *Rapport adressé à M. le Ministre de l'Instruction Publique par ... chargé d'une mission médico-littéraire en Allemagne*. Paris: P. Dupont, 1845.

Daremberg 1848: Charles Daremberg, *Résumé d'un voyage médico-littéraire en Anglettere; Lu à l'Académie des inscriptions et belles-lettres, dans la séance du 6 octobre. Extrait de la* Gazette médicale de Paris *du 4 novembre 1848*. [Paris]: [Thunot et Cie], 1848.

Daremberg 1850: Charles Daremberg, "Lettre de M. DAREMBERG, bibliothécaire de l'Académie, en date de Rome, 19 novembre", *Bulletin de l'Académie nationale de médecine* 15 (1849–1850), pp. 228–232.

Daremberg 1850/2: Charles Daremberg, "Post-scriptum à la lettre de M. DAREMBERG, bibliothécaire de l'Académie, en date de Rome, 19 novembre", *Bulletin de l'Académie nationale de médecine* 15 (1849–1850), pp. 264–266.

Daremberg 1851: Charles Daremberg, "Notices et extraits des manuscrits médicaux grecs et latins des principales bibliothèques d'Angleterre", *Archives des missions scientifiques et littéraires*, Ière série, 2e volume (1851), pp. 113–168, 409–434, 470–471 and 484–548;

Daremberg 1852: Charles Daremberg, "Notices et extraits des manuscrits médicaux grecs et latins des principales bibliothèques d'Angleterre", *Archives des missions scientifiques et littéraires. Choix de rapports et instructions publiés sous les auspices du Ministère de l'instruction publique et des cultes*, Ière série, IIIe volume, Ier cahier (1852), pp. 1–76.

Daremberg 1853: Charles Daremberg, *Notices et extraits des manuscrits médicaux grecs, latins et français des principales bibliothèques de l'Europe. Ire partie. Manuscrits grecs d'Angleterre suivis d'un fragment inédit de Gilles de Corbeil et de scolies inédites sur Hippocrate*. Paris: Imprimerie Impériale, 1853.

Daremberg 1879: Charles Daremberg, and Charles Emile Ruelle (eds.), *Oeuvres de Rufus d'Ephèse, texte collationné sur les manuscrits. Traduit pour la première fois en français, avec une introduction* (Collection des médecins grecs et latins). Paris: Baillière, 1879.

Dawson 1932: Warren R. Dawson, *Manuscripta Medica. A Descriptive Catalogue of the Manuscripts in the Library of the Medical Society of London*. London: John Bale, Sons & Danielsson for the Medical Society, 1932.

de Andrés 1965: Gregorio de Andrés, *Catálogo de los códices griegos de la Real Biblioteca de El Escorial*, tomo 2. Madrid: [Real biblioteca de El Escorial], 1965.

de Andrés 1967: Gregorio de Andrés, *Catálogo de los códices griegos de la Real Biblioteca de El Escorial*, tomo 3. Madrid: [Real biblioteca de El Escorial], 1967.

de Andrés 1974: Gregorio de Andrés, "Catálogo de los códices de las colecciones: Complutense, Lázaro Galdiano y March de Madrid", *Cuadernos de filología clásica* 6 (1974), pp. 221–265.

de Andrés 1987: Gregorio de Andrés, *Catálogo de los códices griegos de la Biblioteca nacional*. Madrid: Ministerio de Cultura, Dirección general del libro y bibliotecas, 1987.

de Boor 1897: Carl de Boor, *Verzeichniss der griechischen Handschriften der Königlichen Bibliothek zu Berlin*, II. Berlin: A. Asher & Co, 1897.

De Lacy 1996: Philip De Lacy, *Galen, On the elements according to Hippocrates*. Edition, translation and commentary (Corpus Medicorum Graecorum V 1, 2). Berlin: Akademie Verlag, 1996.

De Lacy 2005: Philip De Lacy, *Galen, On the doctrines of Hippocrates and Plato*. Edition, translation and commentary. First part: Books I-V. Third, unrevised edition (Corpus Medicorum Graecorum V 4, 1, 2). Berlin: Akademie Verlag, 2005.

de Meyïer 1946: Karel Adriaan de Meyïer, *Codices Perizoniani* (Bibliotheca Universitatis Leidensis, Codices manuscripti 4). Lugduni Batavorum: E. J. Brill, 1946.

de Meyïer 1947: Karel Adriaan de Meyïer, *Paul en Alexandre Petau en de geschiedenis van hun hanschriften (voornamelijk op grond van de Petau-handschriften in de Universiteitsbibliotheek te Leiden)*. Proefschrift ter verkrijging van de graad van Doctor in de Letteren en Wijsbegeerte aan de Rijksuniversiteit te Leiden ... Leiden: E.J. Brill, 1947.

de Meyïer 1955: Karel Adriaan de Meyïer, *Codices Vossiani Graeci et Miscellanei* (Bibliotheca Universitatis Leidensis, Codices manuscripti 6). Lugduni Batavorum: In Bibliotheca Universitatis, 1955.

de Meyïer 1975: Karel Adriaan de Meyïer, *Codices Vossiani Latini*, Pars II: Codices in quarto (Bibliotheca Universitatis Leidensis, Codices manuscripti 14: Codices Vossiani latini 2). Leiden: Universitaire Pers Leiden, 1975.

de Meyïer and Hulshoff Pol 1965: Karel Adriaan de Meyïer, and Elfriede Hulshoff Pol, *Codices bibliothecae publicae graeci* (Bibliotheca Universitatis Leidensis, Codices manuscripti 8). Lugduni Batavorum: Bibliotheca Universitatis, 1965.

De Paolis 1996: Paolo De Paolis, "1. Miscellanea grammaticale", in Mariano Dell'Olmo (ed.), *Virgilio e il Chiostro. Manoscritti di autori classici e civiltà monastica. Abbazia di Montecassino, 8 luglio-8 dicembre 1996*. Roma: Fratelli Palombi Editori, 1996, pp. 105–107.

de Ricci 1907: Seymour de Ricci, "Liste sommaire des manuscrits grecs de la Bibliotheca Barberina", *Revue des bibliothèques* 17 (1907), pp. 81–125.

de Ricci and Wilson 1935: Seymour de Ricci, and William Jerome Wilson, *Census of Medieval and Renaissance Manuscripts in the United States and Canada*, volume 1. New York: H. W. Wilson, 1935.

Deissmann 1933: Adolf Deissmann, *Forschungen und Funde im Serai mit einem Verzeichnis der nichtislamischen Handschriften im Topkapu Serai zu Istanbul*. Berlin and Leipzig: Walter de Gruyter, 1933.

Delisle 1861: Léopold Delisle, "Recherches sur l'ancienne bibliothèque de Corbie", *Mémoires de l'Institut impérial de France. Académie des inscriptions et belles-lettres* 24, Première partie (1861), pp. 266–342.

Delisle 1863: Léopold Delisle, *Inventaire des manuscrits latins conservés à la Bibliothèque nationale sous les numéros 8823–18613, et faisant suite à la série dont le catalogue a été publié en 1744*. Paris: Auguste Durand et Pedone-Lauriel, 1863 (reprint: Hildesheim: Olms, 1974).

Denig 1899: Carl Denig, *Mitteilungen aus dem griech. Miscellancodex 2773 der Grossherzoglichen Holfbibliothek zu Darmstadt. Beiträge zur Kritik d. Plato, Marc Aurel, Pseudo-Proclus, Jo. Glykys, Themistius, Pseudo-Dioscorides, Hephaestion; ein Brief eines christlichen Autors und eine Tafel mit Zeitchnungen von Windrosen u.a.* Programm des Grossherzoglichen Gymnasiums zu Mainz. Schuljahr 1898–99. Mainz: Buchdrukerei von H. Prickarts, 1899.

Dermul 1939: Amédée Dermul, *Catalogue des manuscrits de la bibliothèque de la ville d'Anvers* (Catalogue général des manuscrits des bibliothèques de Belgique 5). Gembloux: J. Duculot, and Paris: Belles Lettres, 1939.

Devreesse 1937: Robert Devreesse, *Codices vaticani graeci*. Tomus II: Codices 330–603. [Città del Vaticano]: In Bibliotheca Vaticana, 1937.

Devreesse 1945: Robert Devreesse, *Bibliothèque nationale, Département des manuscrits, Catalogue des manuscrits grecs*, II. Le fonds Coislin. Paris: Imprimerie nationale, 1945.

Devreesse 1950: Robert Devreesse, *Codices vaticani graeci*. Tomus III: Codices 604–866. [Città del Vaticano]: In Bibliotheca Vaticana, 1950.

Devreesse 1965: Robert Devreesse, *Le fonds grec de la Bibliothèque Vaticane des origines à Paul V* (Studi e Testi 244). Città del Vaticano: Biblioteca Apostolica Vaticana, 1965.

Dickson 1990: Keith M. Dickson, "Gadaldini's Hand (Ms. Hauniensis Bibl. Univ. e Donat. var. fol. 29)", *Mnemosyne* 43 (1990), pp. 441–445.

Dictionary of German Biography: Walther Killy, and Rudolf Vierhaus (eds.), *Dictionary of German Biography*, 10 volumes. München: K. G. Saur Verlag, 2001–2006.

Diels 1905: Hermann Diels, *Die Handschriften der antiken Ärzte*. I. Teil. *Hippokrates und Galenos*. Im Auftrage der akademischen Kommission herausgegeben von - (Abhandlungen der Königlich

Preussischen Akademie der Wissenschaften vom Jahre 1905, Philosophisch-historische Klasse, Abhandlung III). Berlin: Königliche Akademie der Wissenschaften, 1905.

Diels 1906: Hermann Diels, *Die Handschriften der antiken Ärzte. II. Teil. Die übrigen griechischen Ärzte ausser Hippokrates und Galenos.* Im Auftrage der akademischen Kommission herausgegeben von - (Abhandlungen der Königlich Preussischen Akademie der Wissenschaften vom Jahre 1906, Philosophisch-historische Klasse, Abhandlung I). Berlin: Königliche Akademie der Wissenschaften, 1906.

Diels 1906/2: Hermann Diels, *Die Handschriften der antiken Ärzte. Griechische Abteilung.* Im Auftrage der akademischen Kommission herausgegeben von - aus den Abhandlungen der Königlich Preussischen Akademie der Wissenschaften der Jahre 1905 und 1906. Berlin: Königliche Akademie der Wissenschaften, 1906.

Diels 1908: Hermann Diels, *Bericht über den Stand des interakademischen Corpus Medicorum Antiquorum und Erster Nachtrag zu den in den Abhandlungen 1905 und 1906 veröffentlichten Katalogen: Die Handschriften der antiken Ärzte. I. und II. Teil.* Zusammengestellt im Namen der Kommission der Königlich Preussischen Akademie der Wissenschaften von - (Abhandlungen der Königlich Preussischen Akademie der Wissenschaften vom Jahre 1907, Philosophisch-historische Klasse, Abhandlung II). Berlin: Königliche Akademie der Wissenschaften, 1908.

Diels et al. 1915: Hermann Diels (ed.), *Galeni, In Hippocratis Prorrheticum I commentaria III*; Johannes Mewaldt (ed.), *Galeni, De comate secundum Hippocratem*; Josef Heeg (ed.), *Galeni, In Hippocratis Prognosticum commentaria III* (Corpus Medicorum Graecorum V 9, 2). Lipsiae et Berolini: In aedibus B. G. Teubneri, 1915.

Dietz 1827: Friedrich Reinhold Dietz (ed.), Ἱπποκράτους, Περὶ ἱερῆς νούσου βίβλιον. Recensuit, novam interpretationem latinam notasque addidit -. Lipsiae: sumptibus Leopoldi Vossii, 1827.

Dietz 1834: Friedrich Reinhold Dietz (ed.), *Apollonii Citiensis, Stephani, Palladii, Theophili, Meletii, Damasci, Ioannis aliorum Scholia in Hippocratem et Galenum e codicibus mss. Vindobonens. Monacens. Florentin. Mediolanens. Escorialens. etc. primum graece edidit*, 2 volumes. Regimontii Prussorum: apud Fratres Borntraeger, 1834 (reprint: Amsterdam: Adolf M. Hakkert, 1966).

Diller 1963: Aubrey Diller, "The Library of Francesco and Ermolao Barbaro", *Italia medioevale e umanistica* 6 (1963), pp. 253–262 (reproduced in Aubrey Diller, *Studies in Greek Manuscript Tradition*. Amsterdam: Hakkert, 1983, pp. 427–437).

Diller 1983: Aubrey Diller, "Greek codices strayed from the Vatican Library", *Italia medioevale e umanistica* 26 (1983), pp. 383–388.

Diller et al. 2003: Aubrey Diller, Henri D. Saffrey, and Leender G. Westerink, *Bibliotheca Graeca Manuscripta Cardinalis Dominici Grimani (1461–1523)* (Biblioteca Nazionale Marciana, Collana di Studi 1). Mariano del Friuli: Edizioni della Laguna, 2003.

Diller 1932: Hans Diller, *Die Überlieferung der hippokratischen Schrift* περὶ ἀέρων ὑδάτων τόπων (Philologus Supplementband XXIII, Heft III). Leipzig: Dieterich'sche Verlagsbuchhandlung, 1932.

Diller 1970: Hans Diller, *Hippokrates, Über die Umwelt*, herausgegeben und überstezt (Corpus Medicorum Graecorum I 1, 2). Berlin: Akademie Verlag, 1970.

Dilts et al. 1998: Mervin R. Dilts, Mark L. Sosower, and Antonio Manfredi, *Librorum Graecorum Bibliothecae Vaticanae Index a Nicolao De Majoranis compositus et Fausto Saboeo collatus, Anno 1533* (Studi e documenti sulla formazione della Biblioteca Apostolica Vaticana 3; Studi e testi 384). Città del Vaticano: Biblioteca Apostolica Vaticana, 1998.

Dimitrakopoulos 2012: Φώτιος Αρ. Δημητρακόπουλος, *Κατάλογος χειρογράφων τῆς ἱερᾶς μονῆς Εὐαγγελισμοῦ Σκιάθου*. Αθήνα: Παρρησία, 2012.

Domiter 1999: Kristian Domiter, *Gregor von Nazianz, De humana natura (c. 1, 2, 14)*. Text, Übersetzung, Kommentar (Patrologia-Beiträge zum Studium der Kirchenväter 6). Frankfurt am Main: Peter Lang, 1999.

du Verdier 1585: Antonius Verderius, *Supplementum Epitomes Bibliothecae Gesnerianae. Quo longè plurimi libri continentur qui Conrad. Gesnerum, Ios. Simlerum, & Io. Iac. Frisium postremum huiusce Bibliothecae locupletatorem latuerunt, vel post eorum editiones typis mandati sunt. Adiecta est ob subiecti similitudinem Bibliotheca Constantinopolitana. Qua antiquitates eiusdem urbis & permulti libri manuscripti in hac extantes recensentur. Accessit & de Calcographia inventione Poëma encomiasticum, olim ab Io. Arnoldo Bergellano conscriptum, núncque suo candori restitutum.* Lugduni: Apud Bartholomeum Honorati, 1585.

Duffy 1983: John M. Duffy, *Stephanus the Philosopher, A Commentary on the Prognosticon of Hippocrates*. Edition and Translation (Corpus Medicorum Graecorum XI 1, 2). Berlin: In Aedibus Academiae Scientiarum-Akademie-Verlag, 1983.

Duminil 1998: Marie-Paule Duminil. *Hippocrate. Oeuvres complètes*, Tome VIII: *Plaies. Nature des os. Coeur. Anatomie*. Texte établi et traduit (Collection des Universités de France). Paris: Belles Lettres, 1998.

Durling 1961: Richard J. Durling, "A Chronological Census of Renaissance Editions and Translations of Galen", *Journal of the Warburg and Courtauld Institutes* 24 (1961), pp. 230–305.

Durling 1967: Richard J. Durling, "Corrigenda and addenda to Diels' Galenica. I. Codices Vaticani". *Traditio* 23 (1967), pp. 461–476.

Durling 1981: Richard J. Durling, "Corrigenda and addenda to Diels' Galenica. II. Codices Miscellanei". *Traditio* 37 (1981), pp. 373–381.

Durling 1993: Richard J. Durling, "A Guide to the Medical Manuscripts Mentioned in Kristeller's *Iter Italicum* V-VI", *Traditio* 48 (1993), pp. 253–316.

Džurova et al. 1994: Axinia Džurova, Vassilis Atsalos, Krassimir Stančev, and Vassilis Katsaros, *"Checklist" de la collection de manuscrits grecs conservée au Centre de recherches slavo-byzantines «Ivan Dujčev» auprès de l'université «St. Clement d'Ohrid» de Sofia* (Ἀριστοτέλειο Πανεπιστήμιο Θεσσαλονίκης, Publications du programme de la coopération entre le Centre «Ivan Dujčev» de l'université «St. Clement d'Ohrid» de Sofia et l'Université Aristote de Thessalonique 3). Thessalonique: [Université Aristote], 1994.

Džurova and Canart 2011: Axinia Džurova, and Paul Canart, *Le Rayonnement de Byzance. Les manuscrits enluminés des Balkans (VIe-XIIIe siècles). Catalogue d'exposition (XXIIe Congrès Internationales* [sic] *d'Etudes Byzantines), Sofia, 22–27 août 2011*. Sofia: Galerie Nationale d'Art Etranger, 2011.

Ebert 1822: Friedrich Adolf Ebert, *Geschichte und Beschreibung der königlichen öffentlichen Bibliothek zu Dresden*. Leipzig: F. A. Brockhaus, 1822.

Ebert 1827: Friedrich Adolf Ebert, *Bibliothecae Guelferbytanae codices graeci et latini classici*. Lipsiae: apud Steinackerum et Harknochium, 1827.

Ehrhard 1893: Albert Ehrhard, "Zur Catalogisirung der kleineren Bestände griechischer Handschriften in Italien (I. Genova]", *Zentralblatt für Bibliothekswesen* 10 (1893), pp. 189–218 (reproduced in Christa Samberger [ed.], *Catalogi codicum graecorum qui in minoribus bibliothecis italicis asservantur in duo volumina collati et novissimis additamentis aucti*, 2 volumes [Catalogi codicum graecorum lucis ope reimpressi]. Lipsiae: Zentral Antiquariat der deutschen demokratischen Republik, 1965–1968, volume 1, pp. 263–292).

Eleuteri 1990: Paolo Eleuteri, "Biblioteca Nazionale Universitaria di Torino. Concordanze delle segnature dei manoscritti greci", *Codices Manuscripti* 15 (1990), pp. 28–39.

Eleuteri 1993: Paolo Eleuteri, *I manoscritti greci della Biblioteca Palatina* (Documenti sulle arti del libro 17). Milano: Il Polifilo, 1993.

Eleuteri 1999: Paolo Eleuteri, "Noterelle sui manoscritti greci di Schleusingen e Zeitz" *Codices Manuscripti* 27/28 (1999), pp. 43–45.

Elsheikh 1990: Mahmoud Salem Elsheikh, *Medicina e farmacologia nei manoscritti della Biblioteca Riccardiana di Firenze*. Roma: Vecchiarelli, 1990.

Escobar Chico 1993: Angel Escobar Chico, *Codices Caesaraugustani graeci. Catálogo de los manuscritos griegos de la Biblioteca Capitular de La Seo (Zaragoza)*. Zaragoza: Institución Fernando El Católico, 1993.

Eustratiades 1918: Σωφρόνιος Εὐστρατιάδης, *Κατάλογος τῶν ἐν τῇ Μονῇ Βλατάδων (Τσαούς-Μοναστήρι) ἀποκειμένων κωδίκων*. Θεσσαλονίκη: Σ. Παντελῆ καὶ Ν. Ξενοφωντίδου, 1918.

Eustratiades and Arcadios 1924: Sophronios Eustratiades, and Arcadios Vatopedinos, *Catalogue of the Greek Manuscripts in the Library of the Monastery of Vatopedi on Mt. Athos* (Harvard Theological Studies 11). Cambridge (MA): Harvard University Press, 1924 (reprint: New York: Kraus reprint, 1969).

Fabricius 1719: Jo. Alberti Fabricii, *Bibliothecae graecae volumen nonum, sive Libri V. Pars V. Et ultima, in qua praeter multos alios traduntur scriptores, qui vitas sanctorum, monachorumque composuere; et de Theodoris, Anastasiis, Joanne Philopono, Photio, Scriptisque censurae ejus subjectis, ac de Suida plenius disseritur. Accedunt nonnulla hactenus inedita, ut Xenocratis de alimento ex aquatilibus, longe quam Gesnerus eum olim vulgaverat, plenior: Himerii oratio qua Athenis Julianum Imp. Excepit; specimen Lexici Photii; nec non Maximi Sophistae De objectionibus insolubilibus eludendis, et Troili Prolegomena rhetorica*. Hamburgi: Sumtu Christiani Liebezeit et Theodori Christophori Felginer, 1719.

Fabricius, ed. Harles 1796: Jo. Alberti Fabricii, *Bibliotheca graeca sive notitia scriptorum veterum graecorum quorumcumque monumenta integra aut fragmenta edita exstant tum plerorumque e mss. ac deperditis ab auctore recognita*. Editio tertia variorum curis emendatior atque auctor curante Gottlieb Christophoro Harles. Accedunt Christophori Augusti Heumanni Supplementa inedita, Volumen quartum. Hamburgi: apud Carolum Ernestum Bohn, et Lipsiae: Ex Officina Breitkopfia et Haertelia, 1796.

Faye and Bond 1962: Christopher Urdahl Faye, and William Henry Bond, *Supplement to the Census of Medieval and Renaissance Manuscripts in the United States and Canada*. New York: Bibliographical Society of America, 1962.

Fedwick 1993: Paul Jonathan Fedwick, *Bibliotheca Basiliana Universalis. A study of the manuscript tradition of the works of Basil of Caesarea*. I. The letters (Corpus Christianorum). Turnhout: Brepols, 1993.

Feron and Battaglini 1893: Ernest Feron, and Fabio Battaglini, *Codices manuscripti graeci Ottoboniani Bibliothecae Vaticanae descripti*. Romae: Ex Typographeo Vaticano, 1893.

Ferrari 1991: Mirella Ferrari, *Medieval and Renaissance Manuscripts at the University of California, Los Angeles*. Edited by Richard H. Rouse (Medieval and Renaissance Manuscripts in California Libraries, II. University of California, Los Angeles; University of California Publications: Catalogs and Bibliographies 7). Berkeley and Los Angeles, CA: University of California Press, 1991.

Fichtner 2012: Gerhard Fichtner, *Corpus Galenicum. Bibliographie der galenischen und pseudogalenischen Werke*. Weitergeführt durch die Arbeitstelle "Galen als Vermittler, Interpret und Vollender der antiken Medizin (Corpus Medicorum Graecorum)" der Berlin-Brandenburgischen Akademie der Wissenschaften. Erweiterte und verbesserte Ausgabe. Berlin: Berlin-Brandenburgische Akademie der Wissenschaften, 2012.

Fischer 1774: Iohannes Fridericus Fischerus, Ἀκτουαρίου περὶ ἐνεργειῶν καὶ παϑῶν τοῦ ψυχικοῦ πνεύματος καὶ τῆς κατ' αὐτὸ διαιτῆς λόγοι B quorum alterum e Paris. exemplo Martini iuvenis, alterum e cod. Monacensi cum varietate lectionis nunc primum in Germania edidit. Lipsiae: sumtu Iohannis Friderici Langenhemii, 1774.

Fink-Errera 1959: Guy Fink-Errera, "A propos des bibliothèques d'Espagne. Tables de concordance", *Scriptorium* 13 (1959), pp. 89–118.

Fleury and Paris 1837: Henri Fleury, and Louis Paris (eds.), *La Chronique de Champagne*. Tome premier (1ère Année). Reims: Bureau, et Paris: Techkner, 1837.

Foerster 1877: Richard Foerster, *De antiquitatibus et libris manuscriptis constantinopolitanis commentatio*. Rostochii: Formis Academicis Adlerianis, 1877.

Foerster 1884: Richard Foerster, "Mittheilungen aus handschriften. 1. Handschriften in Holkham", *Philologus* 42 (1884), pp. 158–167.

Foerster 1900: Richard Foerster, "Zu Handschriftenkunde und Geschichte der Philologie. VI. Handschriften der Zamoyski'schen Bibliothek", *Rheinisches Museum für Philologie* Neue Folge 55 (1900), pp. 435–459.

Fohlen 1979: Jeannine Fohlen, "Recherches sur le manuscrit palimpseste Vatican, Pal. Lat. 24", *Scrittura e Civiltà* 3 (1979), pp. 195–222.

Fohlen et al. 1982: Jeannine Fohlen, Colette Jeudy, Yves-François Riou, *Les manuscrits classiques latins de la Bibliothèque vaticane*, Tome II, 2me partie: Fonds Palatin, Rossi, Ste-Marie Majeure et Urbinate (Documents, Etudes et Répertoires publiés par l'Institut de recherche et d'histoire des textes). Paris: Editions du Centre national de la recherche scientifique, 1982.

Fonkič 2000: Boris L. Fonkič, "Aux origines de la minuscule stoudite (les fragments moscovite et parisien de l'oeuvre de Paul d'Egine)", in Giancarlo Prato (ed.), *I manoscritti greci tra riflessione e dibattito. Atti del V Colloquio Internazionale di Paleografia Greca (Cremona, 4–10 ottobre 1998)*, 4 volumes (Papyrologica florentina 31). Firenze: Gonnelli, 2000, volume 1, pp. 169–186; volume 3, pp. 117–124.

Fonkič 2006: Борис Львович Фонкич, *Греческие рукописи Научной библиотеки Московского государственного университета имени М.В. Ломоносова*. Москва: Московский государственного университет им. М.В. Ломоносова, Научной библиотека, 2006.

Formentin 1978: Mariarosa Formentin, *I codici greci di medicina nelle tre Venezie* (Università di Padova, Studi bizantini e neogreci 10). Padova: Liviana editrice, 1978.

Formentin 1995: Maria Rosa Formentin, *Catalogus codicum graecorum Bibliothecae Nationalis neapolitanae*, volume II (Indici e cataloghi, Nuova serie 8). Roma: Istituto Poligrafico e Zecca dello Stato, Libreria dello Stato, 1995.

Formentin 1997: Maria Rosa Formentin, "Codici greci di medicina nella Biblioteca Nazionale Vittorio Emanuele III di Napoli: le vie di acquisizione", in Sergio Sconocchia and Lucio Toneatto (eds.), in collaboration with Daria Crismani, Michele Faraguna, and Italo Pin, *Lingue tecniche del greco e del latino II. Atti del II Seminario internazionale sulla letteratura scientifica e tecnica greca e latina (Trieste, 4–5 ottobre 1993)*. Bologna: Pàtron, 1997, pp. 208–216.

Fortuna 1997: Stefania Fortuna, *Galeni, De constitutione artis medicae ad Patrophilum*. Edidit et in linguam italicam vertit (Corpus Medicorum Graecorum V 1, 3). Berlin: In Aedibus Academiae Scientiarum-Akademie Verlag, 1997.

Fortuna and Raia 2006: Stefania Fortuna, and Annamaria Raia, "Corrigenda and Addenda to Diels Galenica by Richard J. Durling: III. Manuscripts and Editions", *Traditio* 61 (2006), pp. 1–30.

Foti 1987: Maria Bianca Foti, "Frammenti di Paolo d'Egina in un manoscritto messinese", *Codices manuscripti* 31 (1987), pp. 88–91.

Fraccaroli 1897: Giuseppe Fraccaroli, "Dei codici greci del Monastero del SS. Salvatore che si conservano nella biblioteca universitaria di Messina", *Studi italiani di filologia classica* 5 (1897), pp. 487–514.

Franchi de' Cavalieri 1927: Pius Franchi de' Cavalieri, *Biblioteca Apostolica Vaticana, Codices Graeci Chisiani et Borgiani recensuit*. Romae: Typis Polyglottis Vaticanis, 1927.

Franchi de' Cavalieri and Muccio 1896: Pio Franchi de' Cavalieri, and Giorgio Muccio, "Index codicum graecorum Bibliothecae Angelicae", *Studi italiani di filologia classica* 4 (1896), pp. 33–184 (reproduced in Christa Samberger, *Catalogi codicum graecorum qui in minoribus bibliothecis italicis asservantur in duo volumina collati et novissimis additamentis aucti*, 2 volumes [Catalogi codicum graecorum lucis ope reimpressi]. Lipsiae: Zentral Antiquariat der deutschen demokratischen Republik, 1965–1968, volume 2, pp. 47–199).

Franke 1967: Konrad Franke, "Zacharias Conrad von Uffenbach als Handschriftensammler. Ein Beitrag zur Kulturgeschichte des 18. Jahrhunderts", *Archiv für Geschichte des Buchwesens* 8 (1967), cols. 1–208.

Franz 1774: Ioannes Georgius Fridericus Franzius, Ξενοκράτους περὶ τῆς ἀπὸ ἐνύδρων τροφῆς *cum latina interpretatione Ioh. Bapt. Rasarii et Conradi Gesneri scholiis nunc primum integritati restituit varietate lectionis atque glossarium adiecit*. Francofurti et Lipsiae: Sommer, 1774 (2nd print 1779).

Fryde 1996: Edmund B. Fryde, *Greek Manuscripts in the Private Library of the Medici 1469–1510*, 2 volumes. Aberystwyth: The National Library of Wales, 1996.

Gagliardi and Forrer 1982: Ernst Gagliardi, and Ludwig Forrer, *Katalog der Handschriften der Zentralbibliothek*, II, Neuere Handschriften seit 1500. Zurich: Zentralbibliothek, 1982.

Gardthausen 1886: Victor Gardthausen, *Catalogus codicum Graecorum Sinaiticorum*. Oxonii: E Typographeo Clarendoniano, 1886.

Gardthausen 1898: Viktor Gardthausen, *Katalog der griechischen Handschriften der Universitäts-Bibliothek zu Leipzig*. Leipzig: O. Harrassowitz, 1898.

Garnier 1843: Jacques Garnier, *Catalogue descriptif et raisonné des manuscrits de la bibliothèque communale de la ville d'Amiens*. Amiens: Imprimerie de Duval et Herment, 1843.

Garofalo 1986: Ivan Garofalo, *Galenus, Anatomicarum Administrationum Libri qui supersunt novem. Earundem interpretatio arabica Hunaino Isaaci filio adscripta*. Tomus prior libros I-IV continens. Neapoli: Istituto universitario orientale, 1986.

Garofalo 2010: Ivan Garofalo, "Prolegomena à l'édition du *De pulsibus ad tirones* de Galien", in Véronique Boudon-Millot, Antonio Garzya, Jacques Jouanna, and Amneris Roselli (eds.), *Storia della tradizione e edizione dei medici greci. Atti del VI Colloquio internazionale, Paris 12–14 aprile 2008* (Collectanea 27). Napoli: M. D'Auria, 2010, pp. 89–108.

Garofalo and Debru 2005: Ivan Garofalo, and Armelle Debru, *Galien*, Tome VII: *Les os pour les débutants. L'anatomie des muscles*. Texte établi et annoté par Ivan Garofalo. Traduit par Ivan Garofalo et Armelle Debru (Collection des Universités de France). Paris: Belles Lettres, 2005.

Geel 1852: Jacob Geel, *Catalogus librorum manuscriptorum qui inde ab anno 1741 bibliothecae Lugduno Batavae accesserunt*. Lugduni Batavorum: E.J. Brill, 1852.

Gessner 1545: Conradus Gesnerus, *Bibliotheca universalis, sive Catalogus omnium scriptorum locupletissimus in tribus linguis, Latina, Graeca & Hebraica, extantium & non extantium, veterum & recentiorum in hunc usque diem, doctorum & indoctorum, publicatorum & in bibliothecis latentium. Opus novum, & non Bibliothecis tantum publicis privatisque instituendis necessarium, sed studiosis omnibus cuiuscumque artis aut scientiae ad studia melius formanda utilissimum*. Tigvri: Apvd Christophorvm Froschouerum, 1545.

Gessner 1559: Conradus Gesnerus, *Xenocratis de alimento ex aquatilibus Animantium libellus, Graecè nunc primùm editus, imperfectus. Idem Latinè perfectior, Io. Baptista Rasario medico Novariensi interprete. Accedunt Conradi Gesneri Scholia, in ea Xenocratis que Grece hic damus: et eorundem interpretationem Latinam.* Tiguri: Apud Gesneros Fratres, 1559.

Getov 1997: Dorotei Getov, *A Checklist of the Greek Manuscript Collection at the Ecclesiastical Historical and Archival Institute of the Patriarchate of Bulgaria* ("Ivan Dujčev" Centre for Slavo-Byzantine Studies, University of Sofia "St. Kliment Ochridski", Series catalogorum 5). Sofia: St. Kliment Ochridski University Press, 1997.

Getov 2006: Dorotei Getov, "Fragmenta Serdicensia Lost and Found", *Jahrbuch der Österreichischen Byzantinistik* 56 (2006), pp. 245–260.

Getov 2010: Dorotei Getov, A *Catalogue of Greek Manuscripts in the Scientific Archives of the Bulgarian Academy of Sciences.* Sofia: Bulgarian Academy of Sciences, Institute for Literature, "Boyan Penev" Publishing Centre, 2010.

Getov 2014: Dorotei Getov, *A Catalogue of the Greek Manuscripts at the Ecclesiastical Historical and Archival Institute of the Patriarchate of Bulgaria*, volume 1: Bačkovo Monastery. Turnhout: Brepols, 2014.

Getov, Katsaros and Papastathis 1994: Dorotei Getov, Vassilis Katsaros, and Charalambos Papastathis, *Catalogue des manuscrits grecs juridiques déposés au Centre de Recherches Slavo-Byzantines «Ivan Dujčev» de l'Université «St. Clément d'Ohrid» de Sofia* (Ἀριστοτέλειο Πανεπιστήμιο Θεσσαλονίκης, Publications du programme de coopération entre le Centre «Ivan Dujčev» de l'Université «St. Clément d'Ohrid» de Sofia et l'Université de Thessalonique 2). Thessalonique: [Université Aristote de Thessalonique], 1994.

Geymonat 1974: Mario Geymonat, *Scholia in Nicandri Alexipharmaca cum glossis*, edidit (Testi e documenti per lo studio dell'antichità 48). Milano: Istituto Editoriale Cisalpino-La Goliardica, 1974.

Giannelli 1950: Cyrus Giannelli, *Codices vaticani graeci. Codices 1485–1683.* Città del Vaticano: In Bybliotheca Vaticana, 1950.

Giannelli 1961: Cyrus Giannelli, *Codices vaticani graeci. Codices 1684–1744.* Addenda et indices curavit Paulus Canart. Città del Vaticano: In Bybliotheca Vaticana, 1961.

Giorgianni 2006: Franco Giorgianni, *Hippokrates, Über die Natur des Kindes (De genitura und De natura pueri).* Herausgegeben, ins Deutsche und Italienisch übersetzt und textkritisch kommentiert (Serta Graeca 23). Wiesbaden: Ludwig Reichert, 2006.

Glorieux 1933–1934: Palémon Glorieux, *Répertoire des maîtres en théologie de Paris au XIIIe siècle*, 2 volumes (Etudes de philosophie médiévale 17–18). Paris: Vrin, 1933–1934.

Gkinis 1963: Δημήτριος Γκίνης, "Διορθώσεις, συμπληρώσεις καὶ προσθῆκες στὸ "Répertoire" τοῦ M. Richard", *Ὁ Ἐρανιστής* 1 (1963), pp. 111–116.

Gollob 1903: Eduard Gollob, *Verzeichnis der griechischen Handschriften in Österreich ausserhalb Wiens* (Sitzungsberichte der Kaiserlichen Akademie der Wissenschaften in Wien, Philosophisch-historische Klasse, Band 146, 7. Abhandlung). Wien: Carl Gerold's Sohn, 1903.

Gollob 1908: Eduard Gollob, *Medizinische griechische Handschriften des Jesuitenkollegiums in Wien (XIII. Lainz)* (Sitzungsberichte der Philosophisch-historischen Klasse der Kaiserlichen Akademie der Wissenschaften in Wien, 158. Band, 5. Abhandlung). Wien: Alfred Hölder, 1908.

Gollob 1908/2: Eduard Gollob, *Die griechischen Handschriften der öffentlichen Bibliothek in Besançon* (Sitzungsberichte der philosophisch-historischen Klasse der Kaiserlichen Akademie der Wissenschaften, Band 157, Abhandlung 6). Wien: Alfred Hölder, 1908.

Gollob 1910: Eduard Gollob, *Die griechische Literatur in den Handschriften der Rossiana in Wien*, I. Teil (Sitzungsberichte der Kaiserlichen Akademie der Wissenschaften in Wien, Philosophisch-historische Klasse, 164. Band, 3. Abhandlung). Wien: Alfred Hölder, 1910.

Gorrini 1905: Giovanni Gorrini, *L'incendio della Biblioteca nazionale di Torino*. Torino-Genova: Renzo Streglio, 1905.

Grafinger 1997: Christine Maria Grafinger, "Eine Bibliothek auf der Reise zwischen Rom und Wien-Eine Darstellung der Geschichte der Bibliotheca Rossiana", in Ead., *Beiträge zur Geschichte der Biblioteca Vaticana* (Studi e documenti sulla formazione della Biblioteca Apostolica Vaticana III = Studi e Testi 373). Città del Vaticano: Biblioteca Apostolica Vaticana, 1997, pp. 95–146.

Granstrem 1956: Евгения Эдуардовна Гранстрем, "Отрывок Медицинского Трактата Аэция, из Амиды b Списке X—XI Века", *Византийский Временник* 9 (1956), pp. 159–169.

Granstrem 1961: Евгения Эдуардовна Гранстрем, "Каталог Греческих Рукописей Ленинградских Хранилищ Выпуск. 2. Рукописи X Века ", *Византийский Временник* 18 (1961), pp. 254–274.

Granstrem 1967: Евгения Эдуардовна Гранстрем, "Каталог Греческих Рукописей Ленинградских Хранилищ Выпуск 6. Рукописи XIV Века", *Византийский Временник* 27 (1967), pp. 273–294.

Graux 1879: Charles Graux, "Rapport sur une mission en Espagne", *Archives des Missions scientifiques et littéraires, choix de rapports et instructions...*, 3e série, tome 5 (1879), pp. 111–136.

Graux, ed. Martin 1889: Charles Graux, "Notices sommaires des manuscrits grecs de Suède mises en ordre et complétées par Albert Martin", *Archives des Missions scientifiques et littéraires, choix de rapports et instructions ...*, 3e série, tome 15 (1889), pp. 293–370 (reprint: *Notices sommaires des manuscrits grecs de Suède*. Mises en ordre et complétées par Albert Martin. Extrait des *Archives des Missions*, 3ᵉ série, tome XV, revu et augmenté d'une table analytique. Paris: Ernest Leroux, 1889).

Graux, ed. Martin 1892: Charles Graux, and Albert Martin (ed.), "Rapport sur une mission en Espagne et en Portugal. Notices sommaires des manuscrits grecs d'Espagne et de Portugal", *Nouvelles Archives des Missions scientifiques et littéraires* 2 (1892), pp. 1–322 (reprinted as *Notices sommaires des manuscrits grecs d'Espagne et de Portugal*. Paris: Ernest Leroux, 1892).

Grensemann 1968: Hermann Grensemann, *Hippokrates, Über Achtmonatskinder, Über das Siebenmonatskind (unecht)*. Herausgegeben, übersetzt und erläutert (Corpus Medicorum Graecorum I 2, 1). Berlin: Akademie Verlag, 1968.

Gritsopoulos 1952: Τάσος Αθανάσιος Γριτσόπουλος, "Κατάλογος τῶν χειρογράφων κωδίκων τῆς Βιβλιοθήκης τῆς Σχολῆς Δημητσάνης", Ἐπετηρὶς Ἑταιρείας Βυζαντινῶν Σπουδῶν 22 (1952), pp. 183–226.

Grusková 2010: Jana Grusková, *Untersuchungen zu den griechischen Palimpsesten der Österreichischen Nationalbibliothek. Codices historici, Codices philosophici et philologici, Codices Iuridici* (Veröffentlichungen zur Byzanzforschung 20) (Österreichische Akademie der Wissenschaften, Philosophisch-historische Klasse, Denkschriften 401). Wien: Verlag der Österreichischen Akademie der Wissenschaften, 2010.

Guérin 1856: Victor Guérin, *Description de l'île de Patmos et de l'île de Samos*. Paris: Auguste Durand, 1856.

Gundert 2009: Beate Gundert, *Galen, Über die Verschiedenheit der Symptome*. Herausgegeben, übersetzt und erläutert (Corpus Medicorum Graecorum V 5, 1). Berlin: Akademie Verlag, 2009.

Gutiérrez 1966: David Gutiérrez, "La biblioteca di San Giovanni a Carbonara di Napoli", *Analecta augustiniana* 29 (1966), pp. 59–212.

Hænel 1840: Gustav Hænel, "Ungedruckte Handschriften-Kataloge, II. Manuscripta B. Collegii Ref. S. Patak", *Neue Jahrbücher füf Philologie und Paedagogik oder Kritische Bibliothek für das Schul- und Unterrichtswesen* 6. Supplementband (1840), pp. 423–424.

Hajdú 2003: Kerstin Hajdú, *Katalog der griechischen Handschriften der Bayerischen Staatsbibliothek München*, Band 3: Codices graeci Monacenses 110–180. Neu beschrieben (Catalogus codicum manu scriptorum Bibliothecae Monacensis, Tomus II, Pars 3). Wiesbaden: Otto Harrassowitz, 2003.

Hajdú 2012: Kerstin Hajdú, *Katalog der griechischen Handschriften der Bayerischen Staatsbibliothek München*, Band 4: Codices graeci Monacenses 181–265. Neu beschrieben (Catalogus codicum manu scriptorum Bibliothecae Monacensis, Tomus II, Pars 4). Wiesbaden: Otto Harrassowitz, 2012.

Haller 1771–1772: Albertus von Haller, *Bibliotheca botanica. Qua scripta ad rem herbariam facientia a rerum initiis recensentur*, 2 volumes. Tiguri: apud Orell, Gessner, Fuessli, et Socios, 1771–1772 (reprinted with a preface by Gunter Mann [volume 1, pp. V*-X*], Hildesheim and New York: Georg Olms, 1969).

Haller 1776: Albertus von Haller, *Bibliotheca medicinae practicae qua scripta ad partem medicinae practicam facientia a rerum initiis ad a. MDCCLXXV recensentur*, Tomus I: Ad annum MDXXXIII. Bernae: Apud Em. Haller, Basileae: apud Joh. Schweighauser, 1776.

Hardt 1806–1812: Ignaz Hardt, *Catalogus Codicum Manuscriptorum Graecorum Bibliothecae Regiae Bavaricae*, 5 volumes. Monachii: Typis I. E. Seidelii Solisbacensis, 1806–1812.

Harlfinger, Brunschön and Vasiloudi 2006: Dieter Harlfinger, Carl Wolfram Brunschön, and Maria Vasiloudi, "Die griechischen medizinischen Palimpseste (mit Beispiele ihrer digitalen Lektüre)", in Carl Werner Müller, Christian Brockmann, and Carl Wolfram Brunschön (eds.), *Ärzte und ihre Interpreten. Medizinische Fachtexte der Antike als Forschungsgegenstand der klassischen Philologie. Fachkonferenz zu Ehren von Diethard Nickel* (Beiträge zur Altertumskunde 238). München and Leipzig: K. G. Saur, 2006, pp.143–164.

Hartung 1578: Ioannes Hartung, *Bibliotheca Sive Antiquitates Urbis Constantinopolitanae*. Argentorati: Excudebat Nicolaus Wyriot, 1578.

Heiberg 1919: Johannes L. Heiberg, "De codicibus Pauli Aeginetae observationes", *Revue des études grecques* 32 (1919), pp. 268–277.

Heiberg 1921: Johannes L. Heiberg (ed.), *Paulus Aegineta*, Pars prior: Libri I-IV (Corpus Medicorum Graecorum IX 1). Lipsiae et Berolini: In Aedibus B. G. Teubneri, 1921.

Heiberg 1924: Johan Ludwig Heiberg (ed.), *Paulus Aegineta*, Pars altera: Libri V-VII (Corpus Medicorum Graecorum IX 1). Lipsiae et Berolini: In aedibus B. G. Teubneri, 1924.

Helmreich 1907–1909: Georgius Helmreich, *Galeni De usu partium Libri XVII*. Ad codicum fidem recensuit, 2 volumes. Lipsiae: In Aedibus B. G. Teubneri, 1907–1909.

Hoffmann 1836: Samuel Friedrich Wilhelm Hoffmann, *Lexicon bibliographicum sive Index editionum et interpretationum scriptorum graecorum tum sacrorum tum profanorum*, Tomus tertius: L-Z. Lipsiae: Sumptibus I. A. G. Weigel, 1836.

Hude 1958: Carolus Hude, *Aretaeus*, edidit -. Editio altera lucis ope expressa nonnullis locis correcta indicibus nominum verborumque et addendis et corrigendis aucta (Corpus Medicorum Graecorum II). Berolini: In Aedibus Academiae Scientiarum, 1958.

Hunger 1953: Herbert Hunger, *Codices Vindobonenses Graeci. Signaturkonkordanz der griechischen Handschriften der Österreichischen Nationalbibliothek* (Biblos-Schriften 4). Wien: Brüder Hollinek, 1953.

Hunger 1961: Herbert Hunger, *Katalog der griechischen Handschriften der Österreichischen Nationalbibliothek*, Teil 1: Codices historici, codices philosophici et philologici (Museion, Veröffentlichungen der Österreichischen Nationalbibliothek, Neue Folge, Vierte Reihe:

Veröffentlichungen der Handschriftensammlung, Erster Band: Katalog der griechischen Handschriften der Österreichischen Nationalbibliothek, Teil 1). Wien: Georg Prachner, 1961.

Hunger and Hannick 1994: Herbert Hunger unter Mitarbeit von Christian Hannick, *Katalog der griechischen Handschriften der Österreichischen Nationalbibliothek*, Teil 4: Supplementum graecum (Museion, Veröffentlichungen der Österreichischen Nationalbibliothek, Neue Folge, Vierte Reihe: Veröffentlichungen der Handschriftensammlung, Erster Band: Katalog der griechischen Handschriften der Österreichischen Nationalbibliothek, Teil 4). Wien: Hollinek, 1994.

Hunger and Kresten 1969: Herbert Hunger, and Otto Kresten, *Katalog der griechischen Handschriften der Österreichischen Nationalbibliothek*, Teil 2: Codices juridici, codices medici (Museion, Veröffentlichungen der Österreichischen Nationalbibliothek, Neue Folge, Vierte Reihe: Veröffentlichungen der Handschriftensammlung, Erster Band: Katalog der griechischen Handschriften der Österreichischen Nationalbibliothek, Teil 2). Wien: Georg Prachner, 1969.

Hunger and Kresten 1976: Herbert Hunger, and Otto Kresten, *Katalog der griechischen Handschriften der Österreichischen Nationalbibliothek*, Teil 3/1: Codices theologici 1–100 (Museion, Veröffentlichungen der Österreichischen Nationalbibliothek, Neue Folge, Vierte Reihe: Veröffentlichungen der Handschriftensammlung, Erster Band: Katalog der griechischen Handschriften der Österreichischen Nationalbibliothek, Teil 3/1). Wien: Hollinek, 1976.

Hunger, Kresten, and Hannick 1984: Herbert Hunger, Otto Kresten, and Christian Hannick, *Katalog der griechischen Handschriften der Österreichischen Nationalbibliothek*, Teil 3/2: Codices theologici 101–200 (Museion, Veröffentlichungen der Österreichischen Nationalbibliothek, Neue Folge, Vierte Reihe: Veröffentlichungen der Handschriftensammlung, Erster Band: Katalog der griechischen Handschriften der Österreichischen Nationalbibliothek, Teil 3/2). Wien: Hollinek, 1984.

Hunger, Lackner, and Hannick 1992: Herbert Hunger, and Wolfgang Lackner, in collaboration with Christian Hannick, *Katalog der griechischen Handschriften der Österreichischen Nationalbibliothek*, Teil 3/3: Codices theologici 201–337 (Museion, Veröffentlichungen der Österreichischen Nationalbibliothek, Neue Folge, Vierte Reihe: Veröffentlichungen der Handschriftensammlung, Erster Band: Katalog der griechischen Handschriften der Österreichischen Nationalbibliothek, Teil 3/3). Wien: Hollinek, 1992.

Hunt 1953: Richard William Hunt, *A Summary Catalogue of Western Manuscripts in the Bodleian Library at Oxford*, Volume 1: Historical Introduction and Conspectus of Shelf-marks. Oxford: Clarendon Press, 1953.

Ideler 1841–1842: Julius Ludovicus Ideler, *Physici et medici graeci minores*. Congessit, ad fidem codd. mss. praesertim eorum, quos Beatus Diezius contulerat, veterumque editionum partim emendavit partim nunc prima vice edidit, commentariis criticis indicibusque tan rerum quam verborum instruxit, 2 volumes. Berlin: G. Reimer, 1841–1842 (reprint: Amsterdam: Adolf M. Hakkert, 1963).

Ihm 2002: Sibylle Ihm, *Clavis Commentariorum der antiken medicinischen Texte* (Clavis Commentariorum Antiquitatis et Medii Aevi 1). Leiden, Boston and Köln: Brill, 2002.

Ikonomakou 2002: Κωνσταντῖνος Οἰκονομάκος, *Προλεγόμενα στὴν κριτικὴ ἔκδοση τῶν Ἀλεξιφαρμάκων τοῦ Νικάνδρου* (Πονήματα 4). Ἀθῆναι: Ἀκαδημία Ἀθηνῶν, Κέντρον Ἐκδόσεως Ἔργων Ἑλλήνων Συγγραφέων, 2002.

Ikonomakou 2002/2: Κωνσταντῖνος Οἰκονομάκος, *Νικάνδρου Ἀλεξιφάρμακα* (Ἀκαδημία Ἀθηνῶν, Ἑλληνικὴ Βιβλιοθήκη). Ἀθῆναι: Ἀκαδημία Ἀθηνῶν, Κέντρον Ἐκδόσεως Ἔργων Ἑλλήνων Συγγραφέων, 2002.

Ilberg 1889: Ioannes Ilberg, "Galeniana", *Philologus* 48 (N.F. 2) (1889), pp. 57–66.

Ilberg 1927: Ioannes Ilberg (ed.), *Soranus* (Corpus Medicorum Graecorum 4). Lipsiae et Berolini: In Aedibus B. G. Teubnerii, 1927.

Iriarte 1769: Joannes Iriarte, *Regiae Bibliothecae Matritensis Codices Graeci MSS.* Volumen prius. Matriti: E Typografia Antonii Perez de Soto, 1769.

Irigoin 1970: Jean Irigoin, "Les manuscrits grecs. I. Quelques catalogues récents", *Revue des études grecques* 83 (1970), pp. 500–529.

Jackson 1998: Donald F. Jackson, "Fabio Vigili's Inventory of Medici Greek Manuscripts", *Scriptorium* 52 (1998), pp. 199–204.

Jackson 2009: Donald F. Jackson, "Greek Manuscripts of the de Mesmes Family", *Scriptorium* 63 (2009), pp. 89–121.

Jacques 2002: Jean-Marie Jacques, *Nicandre, Oeuvres*, Tome II: *Les Thériaques. Fragments iologiques antérieurs à Nicandre.* Texte établi et traduit (Collection des Universités de France). Paris: Belles Lettres, 2002.

Jacques 2007: Jean-Marie Jacques, *Nicandre, Oeuvres*, Tome III: *Les Alexipharmaques. Lieux parallèles du livre XIII des Iatrica d'Aétius.* Texte établi et traduit (Collection des Universités de France). Paris: Belles Lettres, 2007.

Jadart 1902: Henri Jadart (ed.), *Journal de Dom Pierre Chastelain, Bénédictin Rémois, 1709–1782. Avec ses Remarques sur la température et la vigne suivies d'un autre Journal et d'Observations analogues jusqu'en 1848.* Publiés sur les documents originaux de la Bibliothèque de Reims avec une introduction et des notes (Documents inédits publiès par l'Académie de Reims). Reims: F. Michaud, 1902.

Jaeger 1947: Werner Jaeger, "Greek uncial fragments in the Library of Congress in Washington", *Traditio* 5 (1947), pp. 79–102.

James 1899: Montague Rhodes James, *A Descriptive Catalogue of the Manuscripts in the Library of Peterhouse*, with an Essay on the History of the Library by John Willis Clark. Cambridge: University Press, 1899 (reprint: Montague Rhodes James, *A Descriptive Catalogue of the Manuscripts in the Library of Peterhouse.* With an Essay on the History of the Library by John Willis Clark [Cambridge Library Collection-History of Printing, Publishing and Libraries]. Cambridge: Cambridge University Press, 2009).

James 1900: Montague Rhodes James, *The Western Manuscripts in the Library of Trinity College Cambridge. A Descriptive Catalogue*, Volume I containing an account of the manuscripts standing in class B. Cambridge: University Press, 1900 (reprint in the Cambridge Library Collection-History of Printing, Publishing and Libraries. Cambridge: Cambridge University Press, 2009).

James 1902: Montague Rhodes James, *The Western Manuscripts in the Library of Trinity College Cambridge. A Descriptive Catalogue*, Volume III containing an account of the manuscripts standing in class O. Cambridge: University Press, 1902 (reprint in the Cambridge Library Collection-History of Printing, Publishing and Libraries. Cambridge: Cambridge University Press, 2009).

James 1905: Montague Rhodes James, *A Descriptive Catalogue of the Manuscripts in the Library of Pembroke College, Cambridge.* Cambridge: University Press, 1905 (reprint: Montague Rhodes James, *A Descriptive Catalogue of the Manuscripts in the Library of Pembroke College, Cambridge with a Hand List of the Printed Books to the Year 1500.* Edited by Ellis H. Minns [Cambridge Library Collection-History of Printing, Publishing and Libraries]. Cambridge: Cambridge University Press, 2009).

James 1907: Montague Rhodes James, *A Descriptive Catalogue of the Manuscripts in the Library of Gonville and Caius College*, Volume I: Nos. 1–354. Cambridge: University Press, 1907 (reprint in the Cambridge Library Collection-History of Printing, Publishing and Libraries. Cambridge: Cambridge University Press, 2009).

James 1908: Montague Rhodes James, *A Descriptive Catalogue of the Manuscripts in the Library of Gonville and Caius College*, Volume II: Nos. 355–721 with Supplements, Corrigenda, and Index. Cambridge: University Press, 1908 (reprint in the Cambridge Library Collection-History of Printing, Publishing and Libraries. Cambridge: Cambridge University Press, 2009).

James 1913: Montague Rhodes James, *A Descriptive Catalogue of the Manuscripts in the Library of St John's College Cambridge*. Cambridge: University Press, 1913 (reprint in the Cambridge Library Collection-History of Printing, Publishing and Libraries. Cambridge: Cambridge University Press, 2009).

Jeffreys 1977: Elizabeth M. Jeffreys, "The Greek Manuscripts of the Saibante Collection", in Kurt Treu, Jürgen Dummer, Johannes Irmscher, and Franz Paschke (eds.), *Studia codicologica* (Texte und Untersuchungen zur Geschichte der altchristlichen Literatur 124). Berlin: Akademie Verlag, 1977, pp. 249–262.

Jørgensen 1926: Ellen Jørgensen, *Catalogus codicum latinorum medii aevi Bibliothecae Regiae Hafniensis*, fasciculus II. Hafniae: In Aedibus Gyldengalianis, 1926.

Joly 1978: Robert Joly, *Hippocrate. Oeuvres complètes*, Tome XIII: *Les lieux dans l'homme. Du système des glandes. Des fistules. Des hémorrhoïdes. De la vision. Des chairs. De la dentition.* Texte établi et traduit (Collection des Universités de France). Paris: Belles Lettres, 1978.

Jouanna 1988: Jacques Jouanna, *Hippocrate*, Tome V: *Des vents, De l'art.* Texte établi et traduit (Collection des Universités de France). Paris: Belles Lettres, 1988.

Jouanna 1996: Jacques Jouanna, *Hippocrate*, Tome II, 2ᵉ partie: *Airs, eaux, lieux.* Texte établi et traduit (Collection des Universités de France). Paris: Belles Lettres, 1996.

Jouanna 2002: Jacques Jouanna, *Hippocrate, La nature de l'homme.* Edité, traduit et commenté. Deuxième édition anastatique augmentée et corrigée (Corpus Medicorum Graecorum I 1,3). Berlin: Akademie Verlag, 2002.

Jouanna 2013: Jacques Jouanna, *Hippocrate*, Tome III, 1ʳᵉ partie: *Pronostic.* Texte établi, traduit et annoté avec la collaboration d'Anargyros Anastasiou et Caroline Magdelaine (Collection des Universités de France). Paris: Belles Lettres, 2013.

Jouanna and Grmek 2000: Jacques Jouanna, and Mirko D. Grmek, *Hippocrate. Oeuvres complètes*, Tome IV, 3ᵉ partie: *Epidémies V et VI.* Texte établi et traduit par J. J. et annoté par J. J. et M. D. G. (Collection des Universités de France). Paris: Belles Lettres, 2000.

Kaliszuk and Szyller 2012: Jerzy Kaliszuk, and Sławomir Szyller, *Inwentarz rękopisów do połowy XVI wieku w zbiorach Biblioteki Narodowej* (Inwentarze rękopisów Biblioteki Narodowej 3). Warszawa: Biblioteka Narodowa, 2012.

Kachouch 2008: Hikmat Kachouch, "Sinai Ar. N. F. Parchment 8 and 28: Its Contribution to Textual Criticism of the Gospel of Luke", *Novum Testamentum* 50 (2008), pp. 28-57.

Kamil 1970: Murad Kamil, *Catalogue of all Manuscripts in the Monastery of St. Catherine on Mount Sinai.* Wiesbaden: O. Harrassowitz, 1970.

Karas 1994: Γιάννης Καράς, *Οι επιστήμες στην Τουρκοκρατία · Χειρόγραφα και έντυπα*, Τόμος Γ΄: Οι επιστήμες της ζωής. Παράρτημα. Έργα γενικόν γνωσέων (Κέντρο Νεοελληνικών Ερευνών, Ἐθνικό Ἵδρυμα Ερευνών 48). Αθήνα: Βιβλιοπωλείον της «Εστίας», 1994.

Kavrus-Hoffmann 2008: Nadezhda Kavrus-Hoffmann, "Catalogue of Greek Medieval and Renaissance Manuscripts in the Collections of the United States of America, Part IV.1: The Morgan Library and Museum", *Manuscripta* 52 (2008), pp. 65–174.

Kavrus-Hoffmann 2008/2: Nadezhda Kavrus-Hoffmann, "Catalogue of Greek Medieval and Renaissance Manuscripts in the Collections of the United States of America, Part IV.2: The Morgan Library and Museum", *Manuscripta* 52 (2008), pp. 207–324.

Kavrus-Hoffmann 2010: Nadezhda Kavrus-Hoffmann, "Catalogue of Greek Medieval and Renaissance Manuscripts in the Collections of the United States of America, Part V.2: Harvard University, The Houghton Library", *Manuscripta* 54 (2010), pp. 207–274.

Kavrus-Hoffmann 2011: Nadezhda Kavrus-Hoffmann, "Catalogue of Greek Medieval and Renaissance Manuscripts in the Collections of the United States of America, Part V.3: Harvard University, The Houghton Library and Andover-Harvard Theological Library", *Manuscripta* 55 (2011), pp. 1–108.

Kavrus-Hoffmann 2012: Nadezhda Kavrus-Hoffmann, "Catalogue of Greek Medieval and Renaissance Manuscripts in the Collections of the United States of America, Part VI: Boston, Massachusetts, Miscellaneous Collections, and Providence, Rhode Island, Brown University", *Manuscripta* 56 (2012), pp. 47–130.

Kibre 1975–1982: Pearl Kibre, "Hippocrates Latinus. Repertorium of Hippocratic Writings in the Latin Middle Ages", *Traditio* 31 (1975), pp. 99–126; 32 (1976), pp. 257–292; 33 (1977), pp. 253–295; 34 (1978), pp. 193–226; 35 (1979), pp. 273–302; 36 (1980), pp. 347–392; 37 (1981), pp. 267–289; 38 (1982), pp. 165–192.

Kibre 1985: Pearl Kibre, *Hippocrates Latinus. Repertorium of Hippocratic Writings in the Latin Middle Ages*. Revised Edition. New York: Fordham University Press, 1985.

Kitchin 1867: George William Kitchin, *Catalogus codicum MSS. qui in Bibliotheca Aedis Christi apud Oxonienses adservantur*. Oxonii: E Typographo Clarendoniano, 1867.

Koch et al. 1923: Konrad Koch (ed.), *Galeni, De sanitate tuenda*; Georg Helmreich (ed.), *Galeni, De alimentorum facultatibus*; Georg Helmreich (ed.), *Galeni, De bonis malisque sucis*; Karl Kalbfleisch (ed.), *Galeni, De victu attenuante*; Otto Hartlich (ed.), *Galeni, De ptisana* (Corpus Medicorum Graecorum V 4, 1). Lipsiae et Berolini: In aedibus B. G. Teubneri, 1923.

Köhler and Milchsack 1913: Franz Köhler, and Gustav Milchsack, *Die Handschriften der Herzoglichen Bibliothek zu Wolfenbüttel*. Vierte Abteilung. Die Gudischen Handschriften. Die griechischen Handschriften bearbeitet von F. K.. Die lateinischen Handschriften bearbeitet von G. M. Wolfenbüttel: Julius Zwissler, 1913 (reprint: Frankfurt am Main: Vittorio Klostermann, 1966).

Kollar 1766–1782: Petri Lambecii Hamburgensis, *Commentariorum de Augustissima Bibliotheca Caesarea Vindobonensis Liber primus* (*secundus*, ... usque ad *octavum*). Editio altera opera et studio Adam Francisci Kollarii ..., 8 volumes. Vindobonae: Typis et sumptibus Ioan. Thomae nob. de Trattnern, 1766–1782.

Kollesch 1973: Jutta Kollesch, "Hermann Diels in seiner Bedeutung für die Geschichte der antiken Medizin", *Philologus* 117 (1973), pp. 278–283.

Kollesch 1989: Jutta Kollesch, "Die Erschliessung der antiken medizinischen Texte und ihre Probleme-das *Corpus Medicorum Graecorum* et *Latinorum*", *Gesnerus* 46 (1989), pp. 195–210.

Kollesch 1999: "Die Organisation und Herausgabe des *Corpus Medicorum Graecorum*: ergänzenden Details aus der Korrespondenz zwischen Hermann Diels und Johannes Mewaldt", in William M. Calder III, and Jaap Mansfeld (eds.), with the participation of Alex Leukart, François Paschould, and Olivier Reverdin, *Hermann Diels (1848–1922) et la science de l'Antiquité. Huit exposés suivis de discussion ... Vandoeuvres-Genève, 17–21 août 1998* (Entretiens sur l'Antiquité classique 45). Genève: Fondation Hardt, 1999, pp. 207–223.

Kollesch, Kudlien, and Nickel 1965: Jutta Kollesch, and Friedolf Kudlien, *Apollonios von Kition, Kommentar zu Hippokrates Über das Einrenken der Gelenke*. Herausgegeben von -. Übersetzt von J. K., Diethard Nickel (Corpus Medicorum Graecorum XI 1,1). Berlin: Akademie Verlag, 1965.

Kominis 1988: Αθανάσιος Δ. Κομίνης, *Πατμιακὴ βιβλιοθήκη ἤτοι Νέος κατάλογος τῶν χειρογράφων κωδίκων τῆς Ἱερᾶς Μονῆς Ἁγίου Ἰωάννου τοῦ Θεολόγου Πάτμου. Τόμος Α΄. Κώδικες 1–101*. Ἀθῆναι: Εκδοτική Ελλάδος, 1988.

Kougeas n. d.: Σωκράτης Κουγέας, "Κώδ. 2786", in *Περιγραφικὸς κατάλογος χειρογράφων κωδίκων Ἀρ. 2731–2840*. [Ἀθῆναι]: Ἐθνικὴ Βιβλιοθήκη Ἑλλάδος, Τμῆμα Χειρογράφων καὶ Ἐντύπων, n. d.: f. 75.

Kourilas 1935: Εὐλόγιος Κουρίλας Λαυριώτης, *Διοσκορίδειοι Μελέται καὶ ὁ Λαυριωτικός Διοσκορίδης*. Ἀθῆναι: Ι. Λ. Αλευρόπουλου, 1935.

Kournoutou n. d.: Γεώργιος Π. Κουρνούτου, *Περιγραφικὸς κατάλογος χειρογράφων κωδίκων Ἀρ. 2981–3121*. [Ἀθῆναι]: Ἐθνικὴ Βιβλιοθήκη Ἑλλάδος, Τμῆμα Χειρογράφων καὶ Ἐντύπων, n. d.

Kouroupou and Géhin 2008: Matoula Kouroupou, and Paul Géhin, *Catalogue des manuscrits conservés dans la Bibliothèque du Patriarcat Oecuménique. Les manuscrits du monastère de la Panaghia de Chalki*, 2 volumes. Turnhout: Brepols, 2008.

Kraus 1978: Hans P. Kraus, *Greek Manuscripts from the Library of Sir Thomas Phillipps*. New York: H. P. Kraus, 1978 (typewritten catalogue).

Kraus 1979: Hans P. Kraus, *Bibliotheca Phillippica. Manuscripts on vellum and paper from the 9th to the 18th centuries From the Celebrated Collection formed by Sir Thomas Phillipps. The Final Section* (Catalogue 153). New York: H. P. Kraus, 1979.

Kristeller 1963: Paul Oskar Kristeller, *Iter Italicum. A Finding List of Uncatalogued or Incompletely Catalogued Humanistic Manuscripts of the Renaissance in Italian and Other Libraries*, volume 1: Italy, Agrigento to Novara. London: Warburg Institute, and Leiden: E.J. Brill, 1963.

Kristeller 1983: Paul Oskar Kristeller, *Iter Italicum accedunt alia itinera. A Finding List of Uncatalogued or Incompletely Catalogued Humanistic Manuscripts of the Renaissance in Italian and Other Libraries*, volume 3: Alia itinera I: Australia to Germany. London: Warburg Institute, and Leiden: E.J. Brill, 1983.

Kristeller 1991: Paul Oskar Kristeller, *Iter Italicum*, volume 6: Italy III and alia itinera IV. Supplement to Italy (C-G), Supplement to Vatican and Austria to Spain. Leiden: E. J. Brill, 1991.

Krumbacher 1897: Karl Krumbacher, *Geschichte der byzantinischen Litteratur von Justinian bis zum Ende des oströmischen Reiches (527–1453)*, 2. Auflage, bearbeitet unter Mitwirkung von Albert Ehrhard und Heinrich Gelzer. München: C. H. Beck'sche Verlagsbuchhandlung, 1897.

Kubinyi 1956: Maria Kubinyi, *Libri manuscripti graeci in bibliothecis budapestinensibus asservati*. Budapestini: In Aedibus Academiae Scientiarum Hungaricae, 1956.

Kühn 1821–1833: Carl Gottlob Kühn (ed.), *Claudii Galeni Opera Omnia*, 20 tomes in 22 volumes (Medicorum Graecorum Opera quae exstant 1–20). Leipzig: Carl Cnobloch, 1821–1833.

Kühn 1825–1827: Carl Gottlob Kühn (ed.), *Magni Hippocratis Opera Omnia*, 3 volumes (Medicorum Graecorum Opera quae exstant 21–23). Leipzig: Carl Cnobloch, 1825–1827.

Kühn 1828: Carl Gottlob Kühn (ed.), *Aretaei Cappadocis Opera Omnia* (Medicorum Graecorum Opera quae exstant 24). Leipzig: Carl Cnobloch, 1828.

Labbé 1653: Philippi Labbei ..., *Nova bibliotheca MSS. Librorum, sive specimen antiquarum lectionum latinarum et graecarum in quattuor partes tributarum, cum coronide duplici, poetica et libraria. Ac Supplementis decem*. Parisiis: Apud Ioannem Henault, 1653.

Lambeck 1665: Petri Lambecii, *Commentariorum de Augustissima Bibliotheca Caesarea Vindobonensi Liber primus*. Vindobonae: Typis Matthaei Cosmerovii, 1665.

Lambeck 1669: Petri Lambecii, *Commentariorum de Augustissima Bibliotheca Caesarea Vindobonensi Liber secundus*. Vindobonae: Typis Matthaei Cosmerovii, 1669.

Lambeck 1674: Petri Lambecii, *Commentariorum de Augustissima Bibliotheca Caesarea Vindobonensi Liber sextus*. Vindobonae: Typis Matthaei Cosmerovii, 1674.

Lambert 1862: Charles-Godefroy-Alphonse Lambert, *Catalogue descriptif et raisonné des manuscrits de la bibliothèque de Carpentras*, 3 volumes. Carpentras: E. Rolland, 1862.

Lamberz 2006: Erich Lamberz, *Katalog der griechischen Handschriften des Athosklosters Vatopedi*, Band I: Codices 1–102 (Κατάλογοι Ελληνικών Χειρογράφων Αγίου Όρους 2). Θεσσαλονίκη: Πατριαρχικόν Ἵδρυμα Πατερικῶν Μελετῶν, 2006.

Lamberz and Litsas 1978: Erich Lamberz, Εὐθύμιος Κ. Λίτσας, *Κατάλογος Χειρογράφων τῆς Βατοπεδινῆς Σκήτης Ἁγίου Δημητρίου* (Κατάλογοι Ελληνικῶν Χειρογράφων Αγίου Ορους 1). Θεσσαλονίκη: Πατριαρχικὸν Ἱδρυμα Πατερικῶν Μελετῶν, 1978.

Lami 1756: Johannes Lamius, *Catalogus codicum manuscriptorum qui in Bibliotheca Riccardiana Florentiae adservantur in quo multa opuscula anecdota in lucem passim proferuntur et plura Ad Historiam litterariam locuplentandam inlustrandamque idonea, antea ignota exhibentur*. Liburni: Ex Typographio Antonii Sanctinii et Sociorum, 1756.

Lampros 1895–1900: Spyridon P. Lampros, *Catalogue of the Greek Manuscripts on Mount Athos*, 2 volumes. Cambridge: University Press, 1895–1900.

Lampros 1898: Σπυρίδων Π. Λάμπρος, *Κατάλογος τῶν ἐν τῇ κατὰ τὴν Ἄνδρον μονῇ τῆς Ἁγίας κωδίκων*. Ἀθῆναι: Ἑστία, 1898.

Lampros 1905: Σπυρίδων Π. Λάμπρος, "Κατάλογος τῶν κωδίκων τῶν ἐν Ἀθήναις βιβλιοθηκῶν πλὴν τῆς Ἐθνικῆς. Α΄. Κώδικες τῆς Βιβλιοθήκης τῆς Βουλῆς", *Νέος Ἑλληνομνήμων* 2 (1905), pp. 226–235, 357–364, 490–500 (reproduced in José Declerck, Jacques Nore, and Constant De Vocht [eds.], *Catalogi Manuscriptorum Graecorum qui, in periodico «Νέος Ἑλληνομνήμων» olim publici iuris facti, adhuc usui sunt*, Volumen primum (Publicaties van de Redactie van het Corpus Christianorum, Series Graeca). Leuven: Redactie van het Corpus Christianorum, Series Graeca, and Bruxelles: Editions Culture et civilisation, 1981).

Lampros 1906: Σπυρίδων Π. Λάμπρος, "Κατάλογος τῶν κωδίκων τῶν ἐν Ἀθήναις βιβλιοθηκῶν πλὴν τῆς Ἐθνικῆς. Α΄. Κώδικες τῆς Βιβλιοθήκης τῆς Βουλῆς", *Νέος Ἑλληνομνήμων* 3 (1906), pp. 113–121, 243–248, 447–473 (reproduced in José Declerck, Jacques Noret, and Constant De Vocht [eds.], *Catalogi Manuscriptorum Graecorum qui, in periodico «Νέος Ἑλληνομνήμων» olim publicati iuris facti, adhuc usui sunt*, Volumen primum (Publicaties van de Redactie van het Corpus Christianorum, Series Graeca). Leuven: Redactie van het Corpus Christianorum, Series Graeca, and Bruxelles: Editions Culture et civilisation, 1981).

Lampros 1907: Σπυρίδων Π. Λάμπρος, "Κατάλογος τῶν κωδίκων τῶν ἐν Ἀθήναις βιβλιοθηκῶν πλὴν τῆς Ἐθνικῆς. Α΄. Κώδικες τῆς Βιβλιοθήκης τῆς Βουλῆς", *Νέος Ἑλληνομνήμων* 4 (1907), pp. 105–112, 225–236, 368–374, 476–483 (reproduced in José Declerck, Jacques Noret, and Constant De Vocht [eds.], *Catalogi Manuscriptorum Graecorum qui, in periodico «Νέος Ἑλληνομνήμων» olim publicati iuris facti, adhuc usui sunt*, Volumen primum (Publicaties van de Redactie van het Corpus Christianorum, Series Graeca). Leuven: Redactie van het Corpus Christianorum, Series Graeca, and Bruxelles: Editions Culture et civilisation, 1981).

Lampros 1913: Σπυρίδων Π. Λάμπρος, "Τὸ ἐν Ῥώμῃ Ἑλληνικὸν Γυμνάσιον καὶ οἱ ἐν τῷ ἀρχείῳ αὐτοῦ ἑλληνικοὶ κώδικες", *Νέος Ἑλληνομνήμων* 10 (1913), pp. 3–32 (reproduced in Christa Samberger [ed.], *Catalogi codicum graecorum qui in minoribus bibliothecis italicis asservantur in duo volumina* *collati et novissimis additamentis aucti*, 2 volumes [Catalogi codicum graecorum lucis ope reimpressi]. Lipsiae: Zentral Antiquariat der deutschen demokratischen Republik, 1965–1968, volume 2, pp. 253–284).

Lappa-Zizica and Rizou-Kouroupou 1991: Ευρυδίκη Λάππα-Ζιζήκα και Ματούλα Ρίζου-Κουρουπού, *Κατάλογος Ελληνικών χειρογράφων του Μουσείου Μπενάκη (10ος- 16ος αι.) - Catalogue des Manuscrits grecs du Musée Benaki (10e - 16e s.)*. Αθήνα: Μουσείο Μπενάκη, 1991.

Lauxtermann 2013: Marc D. Lauxtermann, "And many, many more. A Sixteenth-Century Description of Private Libraries in Constantinople, and the Authority of Books", in Pamela Armstrong (ed.), *Authority in Byzantium* (Publications of the Centre for Hellenic Studies, King's College London 14). Farnham and Burlington, VT: Ashgate, 2013, pp. 269–282.

Lejeune 1956: Albert Lejeune, *L'optique de Claude Ptolémée, dans la version latine d'après l'arabe de l'émir Eugène de Sicile*. Edition critique et exégétique augmentée d'une traduction française et de compléments (Université catholique de Louvain, Bibliothèque de l'Université, Bureau du recueil, 1956; Recueil de travaux d'histoire et de philologie, 4e série, fascicule 8). Louvain: Université catholique de Louvain, 1956 (reprint under the same title as Collection de travaux de l'Académie internationale d'histoire des sciences 31. Leiden: E.J. Brill, 1989).

Leu et al. 2008: Urs B. Leu, Raffael Keller, and Sandra Weidmann, *Conrad Gessner's Private Library* (History of Science and Medicine Library 5). Leiden and Boston: Brill, 2008.

Lilao Franca and Castrillo González 1997: Óscar Lilao Franca, and Carmen Castrillo González (eds.), *Catálogo de manuscritos de la Biblioteca universitaria de Salamanca*. I. Manuscritos 1–1679bis. Salamanca: Ediciones Universidad de Salamanca, 1997.

Lilao Franca and Castrillo González 2002: Óscar Lilao Franca, and Carmen Castrillo González (eds.), *Catálogo de manuscritos de la Biblioteca universitaria de Salamanca*. II Manuscritos 1680–2777. Salamanca: Ediciones Universidad de Salamanca, 2002.

Lilla 1985: Salvator Lilla, *Codices vaticani graeci*. Codices 2162–2254 (Codices columnenses). [Città del Vaticano]: In Biblioteca Vaticana, 1985.

Lilla 1996: Salvator Lilla, *Codices vaticani graeci*. Codices 2644–2663. Città del Vaticano: In Biblioteca Vaticana, 1996.

Lilla 2011: Salvatore Lilla, "Vaticani greci", in Francesco D'Aiuto, and Paolo Vian (eds.), *Guida ai fondi manoscritti, numismatici, a stampa della Biblioteca Vaticana*, 2 volumes: I. Dipartimento Manoscritti; II. Dipartimento Stampati - Dipartimento del Gabinetto Numismatico - Uffici della Prefettura. Archivio - *Addenda*, elenchi e prospetti, indici. (Studi e Testi 466–467). Città del Vaticano: Bibliotheca Apostolica Vaticana, 2011, volume 1, pp. 584–615.

Littré 1839–1861: Emile Littré, *Oeuvres complètes d'Hippocrate*. Traduction nouvelle avec le texte grec en regard, collationné sur les manuscrits et toutes les éditions; accompagnée d'une introduction, de commentaires médicaux, de variantes et de notes philologiques; Suivie d'une table générale des matières, 10 volumes. Paris: J.-B.Baillière, 1839–1861.

Litzica 1909: Constantin Litzica, *Catalogul manuscriptelor greceşti*. Bucureşti: Institutul de Arte Grafice "Carol Göbl", 1909.

Lo Monaco 2007: Francesco Lo Monaco, "Fra Oriente e Occidente passando per la Lombardia. Vicende di un palinsesto degli *Aforismi* d'Ippocrate con commento", in Antonio Manfredi, and Carla Maria Monti (eds.), *L'antiche e le moderne carte. Studi in memoria di Giuseppe Billanovich* (Medioevo e Umanesimo 112). Roma and Padova: Antenore, 2007, pp. 331–360.

Lo Monaco 2008: Francesco Lo Monaco, "Il codice Cassaforte 1.8 della Civica Biblioteca «Angelo Mai» di Bergamo: un palinsesto degli *Aforismi* d'Ippocrate con commento", in Santo Lucà (eds.), *Libri palinsesti greci: conservazione, restauro digitale, studio. Atti del Convegno internazionale, Villa*

Mondragone-Monte Porzio Catone-Università di Roma «Tor Vergata»-Biblioteca del Monumento Nazionale di Grottaferrata, 21–24 aprile 2004. Indici a cura di Alessia Adriana Aletta e Maria Teresa Rodriquez. Roma: Comitato nazionale per la celebrazione del millenario della fondazione dell'Abbazia di S. Nilo a Grottaferrata, 2008, pp. 59–69.

Lucà 2003: Santo Lucà, "Su origine e datazione del Crypt. B. β. VI (ff. 1–9). Appunti sulla collezione manoscritta greca di Grottaferrata", in Lidia Perria (ed.), *Tra Oriente e Occidente. Scritture e libri greci fra le regioni orientali di Bisanzio e l'Italia* (Testi e Studi bizantino-neoellenici, 14). Roma: Università di Roma «La Sapienza», Dipartimento di filologia greca e latina, Sezione bizantino-neoellenica, 2003, pp. 145–224.

Lucà 2012: Santo Lucà, "La silloge manoscritta greca di Guglielmo Sirleto. Un primo saggio di ricostruzione", *Miscellanea Bibliothecae Apostolicae Vaticanae* 19 (Studi e Testi 474). Città del Vaticano: Biblioteca Apostolica Vaticana, 2012, pp. 317–355.

Maas 1938: Paul Maas, "Review of G. Przychocki, *De Menandri comici codice in Patriarchali bibliotheca Constantinopolitana olim asservato ...*, Krakau, 1938", *Byzantinische Zeitschrift* 38 (1938), pp. 409–412.

MacKinney 1965: Loren MacKinney, *Medical Illustrations in Medieval Manuscripts* (Publications of the Wellcome Historical Medical Library, New Series, V). London: Wellcome Historical Medical Library, 1965.

Madan 1897: Falconer Madan, *A Summary Catalogue of Western Manuscripts in the Bodleian Library at Oxford which have not hitherto been catalogued in the quarto series with references to the Oriental and other manuscripts*, volume 4, Collections received during the first half of the 19th Century, Nos. 16670–24330. Oxford: Clarendon Press, 1897.

Madan and Craster 1922: Falconer Madan, and Herbert Henry Edmund Craster, *A Summary Catalogue of Western Manuscripts in the Bodleian Library at Oxford which have not hitherto been catalogued in the quarto series with references to the Oriental and other manuscripts*, volume 2, Part 1: Collections received before 1660 and miscellaneous MSS. Acquired during the first half of the 17th Century, Nos. 1–3490. Oxford: Clarendon Press, 1922.

Madan and Craster 1924: Falconer Madan, and Herbert Henry Edmund Craster, *A Summary Catalogue of Western Manuscripts in the Bodleian Library at Oxford with references to the Oriental manuscripts and papyri*, Volume 6: Accessions, 1890–1915, Nos. 31001–37299. Oxford: Clarendon Press, 1924.

Madan, Craster and Denholm-Young 1937: Falconer Madan, Herbert Henry Edmund Craster, and Noël Denholm-Young, *A Summary Catalogue of Western Manuscripts in the Bodleian Library at Oxford which have not hitherto been catalogued in the quarto series with references to the Oriental and other manuscripts*, Volume 2, Part 2: Collections and miscellaneous MSS. acquired during the second half of the 17th century. Oxford: Clarendon Press, 1937.

Maffei 1732: Scipione Maffei, *Verona illustrata, Parte Terza. Contiene la notizia delle cose in questa città più osservabili.* Verona: Per Jacopo Vallarsi e Pierantonio Berno, 1732.

Magdelaine 1994: Caroline Magdelaine, *Histoire du texte et édition critique, traduite et commentée des Aphorismes d'Hippocrate*, Tome I: *Introduction.* Université de Paris-Sorbonne-Paris IV, Unpublished PhD thesis, 1994.

Mai 1831: Angelo Mai, *Classicorum auctorum e vaticanis codicibus editorum Tomus IV. Complectens scripta aliquot Oribasii, Procopii, Isaei, Themistii, Porphyrii, Philonis, Aristidis, et alia quaedam.* Romae: Typis Vaticanis, 1831.

Mai 1853: Angelo Mai, *Novae patrum Bibliothecae, Tomus sextus continens in parte I. Sancti Athanasi Epistolas festales syriace et latine cum chronico et fragmentis aliis. In parte II. Leonis Allatii tres* *grandes dissertationes De Nicetis, De Philonibus et de Theodoris cum ipsius Allatii vita et plurimis aliorum opusculis ac tabulis XI.* Romae: Typis Sacri Consilii Propagando Christiano Nomini, 1853.

Majus 1720: Iohannes Henricus Maius, *Bibliotheca Uffenbachiana MSSTA seu catalogus et recensio Msstorum codicum qui in bibliotheca Zachariae Conradi ab Uffenbach Traiecti ad Moenum adservantur et in varias classes distinguuntur quarum priores ... recensuit.* Reliquas possessor ipse digessit qui omnem etiam hanc supellectilem literariam suam ad usus publicos offert. Halae Hermundorum: Impensis Novi Bibliopoli, 1720.

Mancini 1907: Augusto Mancini, *Codices graeci monasterii Messanensis S. Salvatoris.* Descripsit – (Atti della Reale Accademia Peloritana, tome 22.2 [Anno Accademico 179–180]). Messanae: Typis d'Amico, 1907.

Mandarini 1897: Enrico Mandarini, *I codici manoscritti della Biblioteca Oratoriana di Napoli illustrati.* Napoli and Roma: Andrea e Salvatore Festa, 1897.

Marchetti 2010: Francesca Marchetti, "Le illustrazioni dei testi *Sulle Articolazioni* (Περὶ ἄρθρων πραγματεία) di Apollonio di Cizio e *Sulle fasciature* (Περὶ ἐπιδέσμων) di Sorano di Efeso", in Massimo Bernabò (ed.), *La collezione di testi chirurgici di Niceta. Firenze, Biblioteca Medicea Laurenziana, plut. 74.7. Tradizione medica classica a Bisanzio* (Folia Picta. Manoscritti miniati medievali 2). Roma: Storia e Letteratura, 2010, pp. 55-90.

Marchi 1996: Silvia Marchi (ed.), *I manoscritti della Biblioteca Capitolare di Verona.* Catalogo descrittivo. Redatto da don Antonio Spagnolo. Verona: Casa Editrice Mazziana, 1996.

Marganne 1981: Marie-Hélène Marganne, *Inventaire analytique des papyrus grecs de médecine* (Centre de recherches d'histoire et de philologie de la IVᵉ Section de l'Ecole pratique des Hautes Etudes, III Hautes études du monde gréco-romain 12). Genève: Librairie Droz, 1981.

Martelli 2011: Matteo Martelli, *Pseudo-Democrito, Scritti alchemici con il commentario di Sinesio.* Edizione critica del testo greco, traduzione e commento (Textes et Travaux de Chrysopoeia 12). Paris: S.É.H.A, and Milano: Archè, 2011.

Martínez-Manzano 2005: Teresa Martínez-Manzano, "Tres copistas griegos del s. XVI en el fondo antiguo de la biblioteca universitaria de Salamanca", *Studi medievali e umanistici* 3 (2005), pp. 285–309.

Martini 1893: Emidio Martini, *Catalogo di manoscritti greci esistenti nelle biblioteche italiane*, volume 1, Parte 1. Milano: Ulrico Hoepli, 1893 (reprinted under the same title, as: Indici e cataloghi 19, 1. [Roma]: Istituto Poligrafico dello Stato-Libreria dello Stato, 1967).

Martini 1896: Emidio Martini, *Catalogo di manoscritti greci esistenti nelle biblioteche italiane*, volume 1, Parte 2. Milano: Ulrico Hoepli, 1896 (reprinted under the same title, as: Indici e cataloghi 19, 1. [Roma]: Istituto Poligrafico dello Stato-Libreria dello Stato, 1967).

Martini 1902: Emidio Martini, *Catalogo di manoscritti greci esistenti nelle biblioteche italiane*, volume 2: Catalogus codicum Graecorum qui in Bibliotheca Vallicellana Romae adservantur. Milano: Ulrico Hoepli, 1902 (reprinted under the same title, as: Indici e cataloghi 19, 2. [Roma]: Istituto Poligrafico dello Stato-Libreria dello Stato, 1967).

Martini and Bassi 1906: Aemidius Martini, and Dominicus Bassi, *Catalogus codicum graecorum Bibliothecae Ambrosianae.* Digesserunt -, 2 volumes. Mediolani: Impensis U. Hoepli, 1906 (reprint: Hildesheim and New York: Georg Olms, 1978).

Marx 1915: Fridericus Marx, *A. Cornelii Celsi quae supersunt.* Edidit - (Corpus Medicorum Latinorum I). Lipsiae et Berolini: In aedibus B. G. Teubneri, 1915.

Masullo 2006: Rita Masullo, "Sul ΠΕΡΙ ΣΦΥΓΜΩΝ attribuito a Mercurio Monaco", in Véronique Boudon-Millot, Antonio Garzya, Jacques Jouanna, and Amneris Roselli (eds.), *Ecdotica e ricezione* *dei testi medici greci. Atti del V Convegno Internazionale Napoli, 1–2 ottobre 2004* (Collectanea 24). Napoli: M. D'Auria, 2006, pp. 335–346.

Matthaei 1805: Christian Friderich de Matthaei, *Accurata codicum graecorum MSS. bibliothecarum mosquensium Sanctissimae Synodi notitia et recensio ...*, Tomus secundus. Lipsiae: Ex Libraria Joachimica, 1805.

Mavroudis and Sakellaridou-Sotiroudi 1987: Αἰμίλιος Δημ. Μαυρούδης καί Ἀλεξάνδρα Σακελλαρίδου-Σώτηρούδη, ""Ἕνα χειρόγραφο του γιατρού Αετίου του Ἀμιδηνού (Κώδικας Αθων. Λαύρα 630 Ε 168)", *Ἑλληνικά* 38 (1987), pp. 318–341.

Mazzatinti 1892: Giuseppe Mazzatinti, "Vicenza", in Giuseppe Mazzatinti, *Inventari dei manoscritti delle biblioteche d'Italia*, volume 2. Forlì: Luigi Bordandini, 1892, pp. 1–103.

Mazzini 1999: Innocenzo Mazzini, *A. Cornelio Celso, La chirurgia (Libri VII e VIII del De medicina)*. Testo, traduzione, commento (Università degli Studi di Macerata, Facoltà di Lettere e Filosofia, Testi e Documenti 5). Pisa and Roma: Istituti Editoriali e Poligrafici Internazionali, 1999.

McKendrick 1999: Scot McKendrick, *The British Library. A Summary Catalogue of Greek Manuscripts*, volume 1. London: British Library, 1999.

Menčik 1909/1910: F. Menčik, "Die Wegführung der Handschriften aus der Hofbibliothek durch die Franzosen im Jahre 1809" *Jahrbuch der kunsthistorischen Sammlungen des Allerhöchsten Kaiserhauses* 28 (1909/1910), Teil II, pp. IV-XXVIII.

Mercati 1916: Giovanni Mercati, "Minuzie – 5. Per la Vita Porphyrii di Marco diacono. – 6–8. Pretesi scritti di Paolo d'Egina e di Galeno. – 9–11. Pretesi scritti di medicina greca. – 12. Ancora Callisto Angelicude", *Bessarione* 32 (1916), pp. 207–211 (reprinted in Giovanni Mercati, *Opere minori raccolte in occasione del settantesimo natalizio*, volume 3 [1907–1916] [Studi e Testi 78]. Città del Vaticano: Biblioteca Apostolica Vaticana, 1937, pp. 520–524).

Mercati 1917: Giovanni Mercati, "Minuzie.– 13–17. Altre correzioni ed aggiunte all'op. *Die Handschriften der antiken Aerzte*. – 18. Per Aezio. – 19–20. Appunti al Νέος Ἑλληνομνήμων, XIII.", *Bessarione* 38 (1917), pp. 50–55 (reprinted in Giovanni Mercati, *Opere minori raccolte in occasione del settantesimo natalizio*, volume 4 [1917–1936] [Studi e Testi 79]. Città del Vaticano: Biblioteca Apostolica Vaticana, 1937, pp. 16–21).

Mercati 1956: Giovanni Mercati, "Nota su W. Jäger, «Greek Uncial Fragment in the Library of Congress (Ms. 60)»", *Bollettino della Badia Greca di Grottaferrata* N.S. 10 (1956), pp. 131–134.

Mercati and Franchi de' Cavalieri 1923: Giovanni Mercati, and Pio Franchi de' Cavalieri, *Bibliothecae Apostolicae Vaticanae codices manu scripti recensiti, Codices Vaticani graeci*, Tomus I: Codices 1–329. Romae: Typis Polyglottis Vaticanis, 1923.

Merolla 2010: Lucia Merolla, *La biblioteca di San Michele di Murano all'epoca dell'Abate Giovanni Benedetto Mittarelli. I codici ritrovati*. Roma: Vecchiarelli, 2010.

Meyer 1893: Wilhelm Meyer, *Die Handschriften in Göttingen*, 2 volumes (Verzeichniss der Handschriften in Preussischen Staate, I Hannover, 1 Göttingen 1–2). Berlin: A. Bath, 1893.

Mewaldt 1914: Johannes Mewaldt, "I. In Galeni *in Hippocratis De natura hominis commentaria* Praefatio", in Johannes Mewaldt (ed.), *Galeni, In Hippocratis De natura hominis commentaria III*; Georg Helmreich (ed.), *Galeni, In Hippocratis De victu acutorum commentaria IV*; Johann Westenberger (ed.), *Galeni, De diaeta Hippocratis in morbis acutis* (Corpus Medicorum Graecorum V 9, 1). Lipsiae et Berolini: In aedibus B. G. Teubneri, 1914, pp. IX-XXV.

Mewaldt et al. 1914: Johannes Mewaldt (ed.), *Galeni, In Hippocratis De natura hominis commentaria III*; Georg Helmreich (ed.), *Galeni, In Hippocratis De victu acutorum commentaria IV*; Johann Westenberger (ed.), *Galeni, De diaeta Hippocratis in morbis acutis* (Corpus Medicorum Graecorum V 9, 1). Lipsiae et Berolini: In aedibus B. G. Teubneri, 1914.

Migne 1857: Jacques Paul Migne, *Patrologiae cursus completus, seu bibliotheca universalis, integra, uniformis, commoda, oeconomica, omnium SS. Patrum, Doctorum Scriptorumque Ecclesiasticorum, sive latinorum, sive graecorum* ... Series graeca posterior ... Patrologiae graecae tomus 32: S. Basilius Caesariensis episcopus. [Parisii]: apud J.-P. Migne 1857.

Migne 1865: Jacques Paul Migne, *Patrologiae cursus completus, seu bibliotheca universalis, integra, uniformis, commoda, oeconomica, omnium SS. Patrum, Doctorum Scriptorumque Ecclesiasticorum, sive latinorum, sive graecorum* ... Series graeca posterior ... Patrologiae graecae tomus 149: Nicephorus Gregoras, Georgius Lapitha, Theodorus Meliteniota. [Parisiis]: apud J.-P. Migne, 1865.

Miller 1848: Emmanuel Miller, *Catalogue des manuscrits grecs de la bibliothèque de l'Escurial.* Paris: Imprimerie nationale, 1848.

Miller 1886: Emmanuel Miller, "Bibliothèque royale de Madrid. Catalogue des manuscrits grecs (Supplément au catalogue d'Iriarte)", *Notices et extraits des manuscrits de la Bibliothèque nationale et autres bibliothèques* 31.2 (1886), pp. 1–116.

Mingarelli 1784: Giovanni Luigi Mingarelli, *Graeci codices manu scripti apud Nanios patricios Venetos asservati.* Bologna: Typis Laeilli a Vulpe, 1784.

Mioni 1958: Elpidio Mioni, "I manoscritti greci di S. Michele di Murano", *Italia medioevale e umanistica* 1 (1958), pp. 317–343.

Mioni 1959: Elpidio Mioni, "Un ignoto Dioscoride Miniato (Il codice greco 194 del Seminario di Padova)", in Antonio Barzon (ed.), *Libri e stampatori in Padova. Miscellanea di studi storici in onore di Mons. G. Bellini, tipografo, editore, librario.* Padova: Antenore, 1959, pp. 345–376.

Mioni 1960: Elpidio Mioni, *Bibliothecae Divi Marci Venetiarum, Codices graeci manuscripti,* Volumen II: Codices qui in sextam, septimam atque octavam classem includuntur continens (Indici e cataloghi, Nuova serie 6). Roma: Istituto Poligrafico dello Stato-Libreria dello Stato, 1960.

Mioni 1965: Elpidio Mioni, *Catalogo di manoscritti greci esistenti nelle biblioteche italiane,* 2 volumes. (Indici e cataloghi 10). Roma: Istituto Poligrafico dello Stato-Libreria dello Stato, 1965.

Mioni 1967: Elpidio Mioni, *Bibliothecae Divi Marci Venetiarum, Codices graeci manuscripti,* Volumen I: Codices in classes a prima usque ad quintam inclusi, Pars prior: Classis I- Classis II, Codd. 1–120 (Indici e cataloghi, Nuova serie 6). Roma: Istituto Poligrafio dello Stato-Libreria dello Stato, 1967.

Mioni 1972: Elpidio Mioni, *Bibliothecae Divi Marci Venetiarum, Codices graeci manuscripti,* Volumen I: Codices in classes a prima usque ad quintam inclusi, Pars altera: Classis II, Codd. 121–198 - Classis III, IV, V, Indices (Indici e cataloghi, Nuova serie 6). Roma: Istituto Poligrafico dello Stato-Libreria dello Stato, 1972.

Mioni 1973: Elpidio Mioni, *Bibliothecae Divi Marci Venetiarum, Codices graeci manuscripti,* Volumen III: Codices in classes a prima nonam, decimam, undeciman inclusos et Supplementa duo continens (Indici e cataloghi, Nuova serie 6). Roma: Istituto Poligrafico dello Stato-Libreria dello Stato, 1973.

Mioni 1981: Elpidio Mioni, *Bibliothecae Divi Marci Venetiarum, Codices graeci manuscripti,* volumen I, Thesaurus antiquus 1–299 (Indici e cataloghi, Nuova serie 6). Roma: Istituto Poligrafico e Zecca dello Stato, Libreria dello Stato, 1981.

Mioni 1985: Elpidio Mioni, *Bibliothecae Divi Marci Venetiarum, Codices graeci manuscripti,* volumen II, Thesaurus antiquus 300–625 (Indici e cataloghi, Nuova serie 6). Roma: Istituto Poligrafico e Zecca dello Stato, Libreria dello Stato, 1985.

Mioni 1986: Elpidio Mioni, *Bibliothecae Divi Marci Venetiarum, Codices graeci manuscripti. Indices omnium codicum graecorum. Praefatio, supplementa, addenda* (Indici e cataloghi, Nuova serie 6). Roma: Istituto Poligrafico e Zecca dello Stato, Libreria dello Stato, 1986.

Mioni 1992: Elpidio Mioni, *Catalogus codicum graecorum Bibliothecae Nationalis neapolitanae*, volumen I, 1 (Indici e cataloghi, Nuova serie 8). Roma: Istituto Poligrafico e Zecca dello Stato, Libreria dello Stato, 1992.

Mittarelli 1779: Johannis-Benedicti Mittarelli, *Bibliotheca codicum manuscriptorum Monasterii S. Michaelis Venetiarum prope Murianum una cum Appendice librorum impressorum seculi XV. Opus posthumum.* Venetiis: Ex Typographia Fentiana, Sumptibus Praefati Monasterii, 1779.

Mogenet 1989: Joseph Mogenet, *Codices Barberiniani Graeci*, Tomus 2: Codices 164–281. Enarrationes complevit Julien Leroy, Addenda et indices curavit Paul Canart. [Città del Vaticano]: In Bibliotheca Vaticana, 1989.

Mohlberg 1932: Leo Cunibert Mohlberg, *Katalog der Handschriften der Zentralbibliothek Zürich* I. Mittelalterliche Handschriften. Zürich: [Zentralbibliothek Zürich], 1932.

Molhuysen 1910: Philipp Christiaan Molhuysen, *Codices Scaligerani (prater Orientales)* (Bibliotheca Universitatis Leidensis, Codices manuscripti 2). Lugduni-Batavorum: E. J. Brill, 1910.

Molin Pradel 2001: Marina Molin Pradel, "Note su alcuni manoscritti greci della Staats- und Universitätsbibliothek di Amburgo", *Codices manuscripti* 34/35 (2001), pp. 15–21.

Molin Pradel 2002: Marina Molin Pradel, *Katalog der griechischen Handschriften der Staats- und Universitätsbibliothek Hamburg* (Serta graeca 14). Wiesbaden: Ludwig Reichert, 2002.

Molin Pradel 2013: Marina Molin Pradel, *Katalog der griechischen Handschriften der Bayerischen Staatsbibliothek München*, Band 2: Codices graeci Monacenses 56–109. Neu beschrieben (Catalogus codicum manu scriptorum Bibliothecae Monacensis, Tomus II, Pars 2). Wiesbaden: Harrassowitz, 2013.

Molinier 1890: Auguste Molinier, *Catalogue des manuscrits de la Bibliothèque Mazarine*, Tome troisième. Paris: Plon, 1890.

Montfaucon 1715: Bernardus De Montfaucon, *Bibliotheca Coisliniana, olim Segueriana; Sive Manuscriptorum omnium Graecorum, quae in ea continentur, accurata descriptio, ubi operum singulorum notitia datur, aetas cujusque manuscripti indicatur, vetustiorum specimina exhibentur, aliaque multa annotantur, quae ad Palaeographiam Graecam pertinent. Accedunt Anecdota bene multa ex eadem Bibliotheca desunta cum Interpretatione Latina.* Parisiis: Apud Ludovicum Guerin, sub signo S. Thomae Aquinatis; Carolum Robustel, sub signo Arboris Palmae, viâ Jacobaeâ, 1715.

Montfaucon 1739: Bernardus De Montfaucon, *Bibliotheca Bibliothecarum Manuscriptorum Nova, Ubi, quae innumeris pene manuscriptorum bibliothecis continentur, ad quodvis litteraturae genus spectantia et notatu digna, describuntur et indicantur ...*, 2 tomi, Parisiis: Apud Briasson, 1739.

Moody and Clagett 1952: Ernest Addison Moody, and Marshall Clagett, *The Medieval Science of Weights (Scientia de Ponderibus). Treatises ascribed to Euclid, Archimedes, Thabit ibn Qurra, Jordanus de Nemore and Blasius of Parma.* Edited with introductions, English translations and notes. Madison: University of Wisconsin Press, 1952.

Moorat 1962: Samuel Arthur Joseph Moorat, *Catalogue of Western Manuscripts on Medicine and Science in the Wellcome Historical Medical Library*, volume 1: MSS. Written before 1630 AD (Publications of the Wellcome Historical Medical Library, Catalogue Series, MS 1). London: Wellcome Historical Medical Library, 1962.

Morani 1981: Moreno Morani, *La tradizione manoscritta del "De natura hominis" di Nemesio* (Scienze filologiche e letteratura 18). Milano: Vita e pensiero, 1981.

Moraux 1964: Paul Moraux, *Bibliothèque de la Société turque d'histoire, Catalogue des manuscrits grecs (Fonds du Syllogos)* (Türk Tarih Kurumu Yayilarindan, XI. Seri, no. 4). Ankara: Türk Tarih Kurumu Basimevi, 1964.

Morgan 1973: Paul Morgan, *Oxford Libraries outside the Bodleian. A Guide*. Oxford: Oxford Bibliographical Society and Bodleian Library, 1973.

Moschonas 1945: Θεόδωρος Δ. Μοσχονᾶς, *Κατάλογοι τῆς Πατριαρχικῆς Βιβλιοθήκης. Τόμος Α΄. Χειρόγραφα*. Ἀλεξάνδρεια: Πατριαρχεῖον Ἀλεξανδρείας, 1945 (reprint: *Catalogue of MSS of the Patriarchal Library of Alexandria* [Studies and documents 26]. Salt Lake City: University of Utah Press, 1965).

Mošin 1961: Vladimir Mošin, "Les manuscrits du Musée national d'Ochrida", in *Musée national d'Ohrid, Recueil de travaux. Edition spéciale publiée à l'occasion du Xe anniversaire de la fondation du Musée et dédiée au XIIe Congrès international des études byzantines*. Ohrid: Musée national, 1961, pp. 163–243.

Mossay 1981: Justin Mossay, *Repertorium Nazianzenum, Orationes, Textus Grecus,* 1. Codices Galliae (Studien zur Geschichte und Kultur des Altertums, Neue Folge, 2. Reihe: Forschungen zu Gregor von Nazianz, 1). Paderborn: Ferdinand Schöningh, 1981.

Mossay and Coulie 1998: Justin Mossay, and Bernard Coulie, *Repertorium Nazianzenum, Orationes, Textus Grecus,* 6. Codices Aegypti, Bohemiae, Hispaniae, Italiae, Serbiae. Addenda et corrigenda (Studien zur Geschichte und Kultur des Altertums, Neue Folge, 2. Reihe: Forschungen zu Gregor von Nazianz, 14). Paderborn: Ferdinand Schöningh, 1998.

Mueller 1958: Fridericus Mueller (ed.), *Gregorii Nysseni Opera Dogmatica Minora*, Pars I (Gregorii Nysseni Opera, Volumen III, Pars I). Leiden: E. J. Brill, 1958.

Müller 1891: Iwan Müller (ed.), *Claudii Galeni Pergameni Scripta minora*, volume II. Lipsiae: In Aedibus B. G. Teubneri, 1891.

Munby 1960: Alan Noel Latimer Munby, *The Dispersal of the Phillipps Library* (Phillipps studies 5). Cambridge: University Press, 1960.

Münzel 1905: Robert Münzel (ed.), *Philologica Hamburgensia für die Mitglieder der 48. Versammlung deutscher Philologen und Schulmänner ausgestellt von der Stadtbibliothek zu Hamburg*. Hamburg: Lütcke und Wulff, 1905.

Muralt 1864: Eduard von Muralt, *Catalogue des manuscrits grecs de la Bibliothèque impériale publique*, volume 1. St.-Pétersbourg: Imprimerie de l'Académie impériale des sciences, 1864.

Mutschmann 1909: Hermann Mutschmann, "Die Überlieferung der Schriften des Sextus Empiricus", *Rheinisches Museum für Philologie* NF 64 (1909), pp. 244–283.

Napolitano, Nardelli, and Tartaglia 1977: Felicia Napolitano, Maria Luisa Nardelli, and Luigi Tartaglia, *Manoscritti greci non compresi in cataloghi a stampa* (I Quaderni della Biblioteca Nazionale di Napoli, Serie IV, no. 8). Napoli: Biblioteca Nazionale di Napoli, 1977.

Naumann 1838: Aemilius Guilelmus Robertus Naumann, *Catalogus librorum manuscriptorum qui in Bibliotheca senatoria Civitatis Lipsiensis asservantur* ... Grimae: sumptus fecit Julius Mauritius Gebhardt, 1838.

Nessel 1690: Danielis de Nessel, *Breviarium & Supplementum Commentariorum Lambecianorum, Sive Catalogus aut Recensio specialis Codicum Mstorum Graecorum, nec non Linguarum Orientalium Augustissimae Bibliothecae Caesareae Vindobonensis* ..., 2 volumes. Vindoboneae et Norimbergae: Typis Leopoldi Voigt, & Joachimi Balthasaris Endteri, 1690.

New Finds 1999: *The New Finds of Sinai Holy Monastery and Archdiocese of Sinai*. Athens: Ministry of Culture-Mount Sinai Foundation, 1999.

Nikolopoulos 1961: Panagiotis G. Nikolopulos, "Codici greci del Collegio Inglese di Roma", *Rivista di Cultura Classica e Medioevale* 3 (1961), pp. 256–265 (reproduced in Christa Samberger [ed.], *Catalogi codicum graecorum qui in minoribus bibliothecis italicis asservantur in duo volumina collati et novissimis additamentis aucti*, 2 volumes [Catalogi codicum graecorum lucis ope reimpressi]. Lipsiae: Zentral Antiquariat der deutschen demokratischen Republik, 1965–1968, volume 2, pp. 287–296).

Noret 1979: Jacques Noret, "Trente-six grands folios onciaux palimpsestes (avec un fragment inédit de Paul d'Egine)", *Byzantion* 49 (1979), pp. 307–313.

Nutton 1999: Vivian Nutton, *Galen, On my own opinions*. Edition, translation and commentary (Corpus Medicorum Graecorum V 3, 2). Berlin: Akademie Verlag, 1999.

Nutton 2008: Vivian Nutton, "Medicine, Historiography of", in Manfred Landfester, and Hubert Cancik (eds.), *Brill's New Pauly. Encyclopaedia of the Ancient World, Classical Tradition*, volume 3. Leiden and Boston: Brill, 2008, cols. 482–486.

Nyström 2009: Eva Nyström, *Containing multitudes. Codex Upsaliensis Graecus 8 in Perspective* (Acta Universitatis Upsaliensis, Studia Byzantina Upsaliensia 11). Uppsala: Uppsala Universitet, 2009.

Olivier 1976: Jean-Marie Olivier, "Les manuscrits grecs de l'Archivo-Biblioteca del Cabildo metropolitano (La Seo) de Saragosse (ancienne collection du Cabildo de la Santa Iglesia mayor del Pilar)", *Scriptorium* 30 (1976), pp. 52–57.

Olivier 1995: Jean-Marie Olivier, *Répertoire des bibliothèques et des catalogues de manuscrits grecs de Marcel Richard*. Troisième édition entièrement refondue (Corpus Christianorum). Turnhout: Brepols, 1995.

Olivier and Monégier du Sorbier 1983: Jean-Marie Olivier, and Marie-Aude Monégier du Sorbier, *Catalogue des manuscrits grecs de Tchécoslovaquie* (Documents, études et répertoires publiés par l'Institut de recherche et d'histoire des textes). Paris: Editions du Centre national de la recherche scientifique, 1983.

Olivieri 1897: Alessandro Olivieri, "Indicis codicum graecorum Magliabechianorum supplementum", *Studi italiani di filologia classica* 5 (1897), pp. 401–424 (reproduced in Christa Samberger [ed.], *Catalogi codicum graecorum qui in minoribus bibliothecis italicis asservantur in duo volumina collati et novissimis additamentis aucti*, 2 volumes [Catalogi codicum graecorum lucis ope reimpressi]. Lipsiae: Zentral Antiquariat der deutschen demokratischen Republik, 1965–1968, volume 1, pp. 235–258).

Olivieri and Festa 1895: Alessandro Olivieri, and Nicola Festa, "Indice dei codici greci delle biblioteche Universitaria e Comunale di Bologna", *Studi italiani di filologia classica* 3 (1895), pp. 385–495 (reproduced in Christa Samberger [ed.], *Catalogi codicum graecorum qui in minoribus bibliothecis italicis asservantur in duo volumina collati et novissimis additamentis aucti*, 2 volumes [Catalogi codicum graecorum lucis ope reimpressi]. Lipsiae: Zentral Antiquariat der deutschen demokratischen Republik, 1965–1968, volume 1, pp. 1–113).

Olivieri 1935: Alexander Olivieri (ed.), *Aetius of Amida, Libri medicinales I-IV* (Corpus Medicorum Graecorum VIII.1). Lipsiae et Berolini: In aedibus B. G. Teubneri, 1935.

O'Malley and Gnudi 1968: Charles Donald O'Malley, and Martha Teach Gnudi, *The John A. Benjamin Collection of Medical History. Catalogue and First Supplement. Reprinted on the Occasion of the International Conference on the History of Medical Education Sponsored by the Department of Medical History and Supported by the Josiah Macy, Jr. Foundation UCLA, February 5–9, 1968.* Los Angeles: University of California-Los Angeles, 1968.

Omont 1883: Henri Auguste Omont, "Inventaire sommaire des manuscrits grecs conservés dans les bibliothèques de Paris autres que la Bibliothèque nationale", *Bulletin de la Société de l'Histoire de Paris et de l'Île-de-France* 10 (1883), pp. 118–125.

Omont 1884: Henri Omont, "Inventaire sommaire des manuscrits grecs des bibliothèques Mazarine, de l'Arsenal et de Sainte-Geneviève", in *Mélanges Graux. Recueil de travaux d'érudition classique dédié à la mémoire de Charles Graux* ... Paris: Ernest Thorin, 1884, pp. 305–320.

Omont 1885: Henri Auguste Omont, *Catalogue des manuscrits grecs de la Bibliothèque royale de Bruxelles et des autres bibliothèques publiques de Belgique.* Gand: Imprimerie Eug. Vanderhaeghen, and Paris: Alph. Picard, 1885.

Omont 1886: Henri Auguste Omont, "Catalogue des manuscrits grecs des Bibliothèques de Suisse: Bâle, Einsiedeln, Genève, St Gall, Schaffouse et Zürich", *Centralblatt für Bibliothekswesen* 3 (1886), pp. 385–452.

Omont 1886/2: Henri Auguste Omont, *Catalogue des manuscrits grecs des départements.* Paris: Librairie Plon, 1886.

Omont 1886–1888: Henri Auguste Omont, *Inventaire sommaire des manuscrits grecs de la Bibliothèque nationale et des autres bibliothèques de Paris et des Départements*, 3 volumes. Paris: Ernest Leroux, 1886–1888.

Omont 1891: Henri Auguste Omont, "Les manuscrits grecs de la Bibliothèque Capitulaire et de la Bibliothèque Communale de Vérone", *Centralblatt für Bibliothekswesen* 8 (1891), pp. 489–497.

Omont 1897: Henri Auguste Omont, *Catalogue des manuscrits grecs, latins, français et espagnols et des portulans recueillis par feu Emmanuel Miller.* Paris: Ernest Leroux, 1897.

Omont 1898: Henri Auguste Omont, *Inventaire sommaire des manuscrits grecs de la Bibliothèque nationale et des autres bibliothèques de Paris et des Départements. Table alphabétique.* Paris: Ernest Leroux, 1898.

Omont 1909: Henri Auguste Omont, *Anciens inventaires et catalogues de la Bibliothèque nationale*, Tome II: La Librairie royale à Paris au XVIIe siècle. Paris: Ernest Leroux, 1909.

Omont 1910: Henri Auguste Omont, *Anciens inventaires et catalogues de la Bibliothèque nationale*, Tome III: La Librairie royale à Paris au XVIIIe siècle. Paris: Ernest Leroux, 1910.

Omont 1921: Henri Auguste Omont, *Anciens inventaires et catalogues de la Bibliothèque nationale*, Tome V: Introduction et concordances. Paris: Ernest Leroux, 1921.

Pagel 1906: Julius Pagel, "Geschichte der Medicin und der Krankheiten", *Jahresbericht über die Leistungen und Fortschritte in der gesammten Medicin* 41.1 (1906), pp. 416–492.

Papadopoulos-Kerameus 1884-1888 and **1888**: Ἀθανάσιος Παπαδόπουλος Κεραμεύς, "Κατάλογος τῶν ἐν ταῖς βιβλιοθήκαις τῆς νήσου Λέσβου ἑλληνικῶν χειρογράφων", *Σύγγραμμα Περιοδικόν - Ὁ ἐν Κωνσταντινουπόλει Ἑλληνικὸς Φιλολογικὸς Σύλλογος, Παράρτημα τοῦ ΙΕ΄ τόμου*, 1884, pp. α΄-κ΄ and 1–44; *Παράρτημα τοῦ ΙΣΤ΄ τόμου*, 1885, pp. 45–84; *Παράρτημα τοῦ ΙΖ΄ τόμου*, 1886, pp. 85–140; *Παράρτημα τοῦ ΙΗ΄ τόμου*, 1888, pp. 141–212. Reprinted in 1888 as a volume under the same title as Μαυρογορδάτειος Βιβλιοθήκη ἤτοι γενικὸς περιγραφικὸς κατάλογος τῶν ἐν ταῖς ἀνὰ τὴν Ἀνατολὴν βιβλιοθήκαις εὑρισκομένων ἑλληνικῶν χειρογράφων καταρτισθεῖσα καὶ συναχθεῖσα κατ᾽ ἐντολὴν τοῦ ἐν Κωνσταντινουπόλει Ἑλληνικοῦ Φιλολογικοῦ Συλλόγου - Ὁ ἐν Κωνσταντινουπόλει Ἑλληνικὸς Φιλολογικὸς Σύλλογος, Τόμος Α΄. Κωνσταντινουπόλει: Ε.Φ.Σ.-Τύποις Σ. Ι. Βουτυρά. Reprint 1970 of the part devoted to the collection of the Μονή Ἁγίου Ἰωάννου τοῦ Θεολόγου in Ἄντισσα (= pp. 146–161) in Ἰάκωβος Γ. Κλεόμβροτος, *Mytilena Sacra*, Τόμος Α΄: Η Ἱερὰ Μονή Ὑψηλοῦ. Ἱστορία, τέχνη. Ἀθῆναι: s.n., 1970, pp. 133–162.

Papadopoulos-Kerameus 1887: Ἀθανάσιος Παπαδόπουλος Κεραμεύς, "Ἔκθεσις παλαιογραφικῶν καὶ φιλολογικῶν ἐρευνῶν ἐν Θράκῃ καὶ Μακεδονίᾳ κατὰ τὸ ἔτος διὰ τὴν «Μαυρογορδάτειον Βιβλιοθήκην»", *Ἀρχαιολογικὴ Ἐπιτροπή* (*Σύγγραμμα Περιοδικόν - Ὁ ἐν Κωνσταντινουπόλει Ἑλληνικὸς Φιλολογικὸς Σύλλογος, Παράρτημα τοῦ ΙΖ΄*). Κωνσταντινουπόλει: Ε.Φ.Σ.-Τύποις Σ. Ι. Βουτυρά

1887, pp. 3–64 (the *Supplement* [Παράρτημα] contains two title pages; both are exactly identical, except the year of publication: one [the second] is dated to 1886 and the other [the first] to 1887).

Papadopoulos-Kerameus 1891–1915: Ἀθανάσιος Παπαδόπουλος Κεραμεύς, Ἱεροσολυμιτικὴ βιβλιοθήκη ἤτοι Κατάλογος τῶν ἐν ταῖς βιβλιοθήκαις τοῦ ἁγιωτάτου ἀποστολικοῦ τε καὶ ὀρθοδόξου πατριαρχικοῦ θρόνου τῶν Ἱεροσολύμων καὶ πάσης Παλαιστίνης ἀποκειμένων κωδίκων συνταχθεῖσα μὲν καὶ φωτοτυπικοῖς κοσμηθεῖσα πίναξιν, 5 τόμοι. Πετρουπόλει: Β. Κιρσπάουμ, 1891–1915 (reprint: Bruxelles: Culture et Civilisation, 1963).

Papadopoulos-Kerameus 1901: Ἀθανάσιος Παπαδόπουλος Κεραμεύς, "Κατάλογος τῶν ἑλληνικῶν κωδίκων τῆς ἐν Μηλέαις βιβλιοθήκης", Ἐπετηρὶς τοῦ Φιλολογικοῦ Συλλόγου Παρνασσοῦ 5 (1901), pp. 20–74.

Papageorgios 1887: Πέτρος Ν. Παπαγεώργιος, "Παλαιογραφικὴ ἐκδρομὴ εἰς τὴν μονὴν Μπατσκόβου", in Athanasios Palaiologos (ed.), Ἡμερολόγιον τῆς Ἀνατολῆς Φιλολογικὸν καὶ Ἐπιστημονικὸν τοῦ ἔτους 1887. Ἔτος ἕκτον. Κωνσταντινουπόλει: Τύποις Ι. Παλλαραμη, 1887, pp. 115–120.

Papazoglou 1983: Γεώργιος Κ. Παπάζογλου, Βιβλιοθῆκες στην Κωνσταντινουπόλη του ΙΖ αἰώνα (κωδ. Vind. hist. gr. 98). Θεσσαλονίκη: [χ. ὁ.],1983.

Papazoglou 1988: Georges K. Papazoglou, "Le Michel Cantacuzène du codex Mavrocordatianus et le possesseur homonyme du Psautier de Harvard", *Revue des études byzantines* 46 (1988), pp. 161–165.

Papazoglou 1990: Γεώργιος Κ. Παπάζογλου, "Συμπληρωματικὸς κατάλογος χειρογράφων Μονῆς Διονυσίου Ἁγίου Ὄρους (Συνοπτικὴ ἀναγραφή, χφφ. ἀρ. 805–1064", Θεολογία 61 (1990), pp. 443–505.

Pasini 1997: Cesare Pasini, *Codici e frammenti greci dell'Ambrosiana* (Testi e studi bizantino-neoellenici IX). Roma: Dipartimenti di filologia greca e latina, Sezione bizantino-neoellenica, Università di Roma «La Sapienza», 1997.

Pasini et al. 1749: Iosephus Pasinus, Antonius Rivautella, and Franciscus Berta, *Codices manuscripti Bibliothecae Regii Taurinensis Athenaei Per Linguas digesti, & binas in partes distributi, in quarum Prima Hebraei, & Graeci, in altera Latini, Italici, & Gallici*. Recensuerunt, & animadversionibus illustrarunt. Taurini: Ex Typographia Regia, 1749.

Päsler 2007: Ralf G. Päsler, "Zum Handschriftenbestand der ehemaligen Staats- und Universitätsbibliothek Königsberg. Quellenrepertorium und neues Standortverzeichnis", *Scriptorium* 61 (2007), pp. 198–217.

Passow 1825: Franciscus Passow, *Dionysii orbis terrarum descriptio*. Recensuit et adnotatione critica instruxit. Lipsiae: Sumptibus et typis B. G. Teubneri, 1825.

Penny Cyclopedia 1843: *The Penny Cyclopedia of The Society for the Diffusion of Useful Knowledge*, volume 27: *Wales-Zygophyllaceae*. London: Charles Knight, 1843.

Pérez-Martin 2008: Inmaculada Pérez-Martin, "El Escorialensis X.IV.6: un *iatrosophion* palimpsesto en el círculo mesinés de Constantino Láscaris", in Santo Lucà (ed.), *Libri palinsesti greci: conservazione, restauro digitale, studio. Atti del Convegno internazionale, Villa Mondragone-Monte Porzio Catone-Università di Roma «Tor Vergata»-Biblioteca del Monumento Nazionale di Grottaferrata, 21–24 aprile 2004*. Indici a cura di Alessia Adriana Aletta e Maria Teresa Rodriquez. Roma: Comitato Nazionale per le Celebrazioni del Millenario della Fondazione dell'Abbazia di S. Nilo a Grottaferrata, 2008, pp. 279–294.

Perilli 1999: Lorenzo Perilli, "La tradizione manoscritta del Glossario Ippocratico di Galeno (e l'ordinamento alfabetico delle glosse)", in Antonio Garzya, and Jacques Jouanna (eds.), *I testi medici greci. Tradizione e ecdotica. Atti del III Convegno Internazionale, Napoli 15–18 ottobre 1997* (Collectanea 17). Napoli: M. D'Auria, 1999, pp. 429–456.

Perilli 2000: Lorenzo Perilli, "L'ordinamento alfabetico di lessici e glossari: il caso del Glossario Ippocratico di Galeno", *Bollettino della Badia Greca di Grottaferrata* 54 (2000), pp. 27–52.

Perilli 2011: Lorenzo Perilli, "Nuovi manoscritti del Glossario Ippocratico di Galeno e considerazioni stemmatiche. *Codex olim Mosquensis, codex Bodleianus Holkhamensis 92*", in Lorenzo Perilli, Christian Brockmann, Klaus-Dietrich Fischer, and Amneris Roselli (eds.), *Officina Hippocratica. Beiträge zu Ehren von Anargyros Anastassiou und Dieter Irmer* (Beiträge zur Altertumskunde 289). Berlin and Boston: Walter de Gruyter, 2011, pp. 177–201.

Pernot 1979: Laurent Pernot, "La collection de manuscrits grecs de la maison Farnèse", *Mélanges de l'Ecole française de Rome, Moyen Age–Temps Modernes* 91 (1979), pp. 457–506.

Petit 2006: Caroline Petit, "Les manuscrits de Modène et la tradition de l'*Introductio sive medicus* du Pseudo-Galien", in Véronique Boudon-Millot, Antonio Garzya, Jacques Jouanna, and Amneris Roselli (eds.), *Ecdotica e ricezione dei testi medici greci. Atti del V Convegno Internazionale, Napoli, 1–2 ottobre 2004* (Collectanea 24). Napoli: M. D'Auria, 2006, pp. 167–185.

Petit 2009: Caroline Petit, *Galien*, Tome III: *Le médecin. Introduction*. Texte établi et traduit (Collection des Universités de France). Paris: Belles Lettres, 2009.

Petit 2010: Caroline Petit, "La tradition manuscrite du traité des *Simples* de Galien. *Editio princeps* et tradution annotée des chapitres 1 à 3 du livre I", in Véronique Boudon-Millot, Antonio Garzya, Jacques Jouanna, and Amneris Roselli (eds.), *Storia della tradizione e edizione dei medici greci. Atti del VI Colloquio Internazionale Paris 12–14 aprile 2008* (Collectanea 27). Napoli: M. D'Auria, 2010, pp. 143–165.

***Phillipps manuscripts* 1837–1871**: *Catalogus librorum manuscriptorum in bibliotheca D. Thomae Phillipps Bart. A.D. 1837–1871*, 4 parts. [Middle Hill]: Impressus typis Medio-Montanis, 1837–1871 (reprint: *The Phillipps Manuscripts: Catalogus librorum manuscriptorum in bibliotheca D. Thomae Phillipps, BT: impressum typis Medio-Montanis, 1837–1871*, with an introduction by Alan Noel Latimer Munby. [London]: Orskey-Johnson, [2001]).

Piccolomini 1896: Aeneas Piccolomini, "Index codicum graecorum Bibliothecae Angelicae. Praefatio", *Studi italiani di filologia classica* 4 (1896), pp. 7–32 (reproduced in Christa Samberger [ed.], *Catalogi codicum graecorum qui in minoribus bibliothecis italicis asservantur in duo volumina collati et novissimis additamentis aucti*, 2 volumes [Catalogi codicum graecorum lucis ope reimpressi]. Lipsiae: Zentral Antiquariat der deutschen demokratischen Republik, 1965–1968, volume 2, pp. 3–28).

Piccolomini 1898: Aeneas Piccolomini, "Index codicum graecorum Bibliothecae Angelicae ad praefationem additamenta", *Studi italiani di filologia classica* 6 (1898), pp. 167–184 (reproduced in Christa Samberger [ed.], *Catalogi codicum graecorum qui in minoribus bibliothecis italicis asservantur in duo volumina collati et novissimis additamentis aucti*, 2 volumes [Catalogi codicum graecorum lucis ope reimpressi]. Lipsiae: Zentral Antiquariat der deutschen demokratischen Republik, 1965–1968, volume 2, pp. 29–46).

Pierleoni 1901: Gino Pierleoni, "Index codicum graecorum qui Romae in Bybliotheca Corsiniana nunc Lynceorum adservantur", *Studi italiani di filologia classica* 9 (1901), pp. 467–478 (reproduced in Christa Samberger [ed.], *Catalogi codicum graecorum qui in minoribus bibliothecis italicis asservantur in duo volumina collati et novissimis additamentis aucti*, 2 volumes [Catalogi codicum graecorum lucis ope reimpressi]. Lipsiae: Zentral Antiquariat der deutschen demokratischen Republik, 1965–1968, volume 2, pp. 307–320).

Pieralisi n.d.: Sante Pieralisi, *Index codicum manuscriptorum Graecorum et Orientalium Bibliothecae Barberinae*, redactus et digestus cura et studio ... Biblioteca Apostolica Vaticana, Sala Consultazione, Ms. 169-173.

Pietrobelli 2010: Antoine Pietrobelli, "Variation autour du Thessalonicensis Vlatadon 14: un manuscrit copié au Xénon du Kral, peu avant la chute de Constantinople", *Revue des études byzantines* 68 (2010), pp. 95–126.

Politi 2012: Μαρία Α. Πολίτη, *Κατάλογος χειρογράφων Ἱερᾶς Μονῆς Ζάβορδας* (Ἑλληνικὴ Παλαιογραφικὴ Ἑταιρεία). Θεσσαλονίκη: Ἑλληνικὴ Παλαιογραφικὴ Ἑταιρεία, 2012.

Politis n. d./1: Λίνος Πολίτης, *Περιγραφικὸς κατάλογος χειρογράφων κωδίκων Ἀρ. 2571–2730*. [Ἀθήναι]: Ἐθνικὴ Βιβλιοθήκη Ἑλλάδος, Τμῆμα Χειρογράφων καὶ Ἐντύπων, n. d.

Politis n. d./2: Λίνος Πολίτης, "Κώδ. 2922", in *Περιγραφικὸς κατάλογος χειρογράφων κωδίκων Ἀρ. 2841–2980*. [Ἀθήναι]: Ἐθνικὴ Βιβλιοθήκη Ἑλλάδος, Τμῆμα Χειρογράφων καὶ Ἐντύπων, n. d.: ff. 85–87.

Politis 1976: Λίνος Πολίτης, *Συνοπτικὴ ἀναγραφὴ χειρογράφων ἑλληνικῶν συλλόγων* (Ἑλληνικά, Παράρτημα 25). Θεσσαλονίκη: Ἑταιρεία Μακεδονικῶν Σπουδῶν, 1976.

Politis 1991: Λίνος Πολίτης, *Κατάλογος χειρογράφων τοῦ Πανεπιστημίου Θεσσαλονίκης*. Ἐπιμελεία-συμπλήρωσις Παναγιώτης Σωτηρούδης, Ἀλεξάνδρα Σακελλαρίου-Σωτηρούδη. Θεσσαλονίκη: Ἀριστοτέλειο Πανεπιστήμιο Θεσσαλονίκης, Κεντρικὴ Βιβλιοθήκη, 1991.

Politis and Manousakas 1973: Λίνος Πολίτης καὶ Μανοῦσος Ι. Μανούσακας, *Συμπληρωματικοὶ κατάλογοι χειρογράφων Ἁγίου Ὄρους* (Ἑλληνικά, Παράρτημα 24). Θεσσαλονίκη: Ἑταιρεία Μακεδονικῶν Σπουδῶν, 1973.

Politis and Politi 1991: Λίνος Πολίτης, με τη συνεργασία Μαρία Λ. Πολίτη-Σακελλαριάδη, *Κατάλογος τῶν χειρογράφων τῆς Ἐθνικῆς Βιβλιοθήκης τῆς Ἑλλάδος ἀρ. 1857- 2500* (Πραγματείαι τῆς Ἀκαδημίας Ἀθηνῶν 54). Ἀθήναι: Γραφεῖον Δημοσιευμάτων τῆς Ἀκαδημίας Ἀθηνῶν, 1991.

Poussin 1857: Clovis Poussin, *Monographie de l'abbaye et de l'église de St-Rémi de Reims. Précédée d'une Notice sur le saint Apôtre des Francs*. Reims: Lemoine-Canart, 1857.

Premerstein 1906: Antonius de Premerstein, "De Codicis Dioscuridei Aniciae Iulianae, nunc Vindobonensis Med. Gr. I Historia, Forma Argumento", in Iosephus de Karabacek (ed.), *De Codicis Dioscuridei Aniciae Iulianae, nunc Vindobonensis Med. Gr. I Historia, Forma, Scriptura, Picturis*. Lugduni Batavorum: A. W. Sijthoff, 1906, pp. 1–228.

Przychocki 1938: Gustavus Przychocki, *De Menandri comici codice in patriarchali bibliotheca constantinopolitana olim asservato. Accedunt Tabulae II et catalogus bibliothecae patriarchalis constantinopolitanae* (Polska Akademia Umiejętności, Archiwum filologiczne 13). Cracoviae: Sumptibus Academiae Polonae Literarum, 1938.

Puliatti 1965: Pietro Puliatti, "Sigla novissima codicum graecorum Bibliothecae Estensis", in Christa Samberger (ed.), *Catalogi codicum graecorum qui in minoribus bibliothecis italicis asservantur in duo volumina collati et novissimis additamentis aucti*, 2 volumes (Catalogi codicum graecorum lucis ope reimpressi). Lipsiae: Zentral Antiquariat der deutschen demokratischen Republik, 1965–1968, volume 1, pp. 456–459.

Puntoni 1889: Vittorio Puntoni, Στεφανίτης καὶ Ἰχνηλάτης. *Quattro recensioni della versione greca del Kitâb Kalîla wa Dimna* (Pubblicazioni della Società asiatica italiana 2). Firenze: Successori Le Monnier, 1889.

Puntoni 1896: Vittorio Puntoni, "Indice dei codici greci della Biblioteca Estense di Modena", *Studi italiani di filologia classica* 4 (1896), pp. 379–536 (reproduced in Christa Samberger [ed.], *Catalogi codicum graecorum qui in minoribus bibliothecis italicis asservantur in duo volumina collati et novissimis additamentis aucti*, 2 volumes [Catalogi codicum graecorum lucis ope reimpressi]. Lipsiae: Zentral Antiquariat der deutschen demokratischen Republik, 1965–1968, volume 1, pp. 293–452).

Puntoni 1896/2: Vittorio Puntoni, "Indicis codicum graecorum Bononiensium ab Al. Oliverio compositi supplementum", *Studi italiani di filologia classica* 4 (1896), pp. 365–378 (reproduced in Christa Samberger [ed.], *Catalogi codicum graecorum qui in minoribus bibliothecis italicis asservantur in duo volumina collati et novissimis additamentis aucti*, 2 volumes [Catalogi codicum graecorum lucis ope reimpressi]. Lipsiae: Zentral Antiquariat der deutschen demokratischen Republik, 1965–1968, volume 1, pp. 114–127).

Puschmann 1878–1879: Theodor Puschmann, *Alexander von Tralles. Original-text und Übersetzung nebst einer einleitenden Abhandlung. Ein Beitrag zur Geschichte der Medizin*, 2 volumes. Wien: Braumüller, 1878–1879.

***Quinze années* 1969**: *Quinze années d'acquisitions de la pose de la première pierre à l'inauguration officielle de la Bibliothèque* (Exposition, 18 février - 30 mars 1969, Catalogue, 34). Bruxelles: Bibliothèque Royale Albert Iᵉʳ, 1969.

Revilla 1936: Alejo Revilla, *Catálogo de los códices Griegos de la Biblioteca de El Escorial*, tomo I. Madrid: Imprenta Helénica, 1936.

Rice 1980: Eugene F. Rice, "Paulus Aegineta", in F. Edward Cranz, and Paul Oskar Kristeller (eds.), *Catalogus Translationum et Commentariorum: Medieval and Renaissance Latin Translations and Commentaries*, volume 4. Washington, D.C.: Catholic University of America Press, 1980, pp. 145–191.

Richard 1952: Marcel Richard, *Inventaire des manuscrits grecs du British Museum* (Centre National de la Recherche Scientifique, Publications de l'Institut de recherche et d'histoire des textes 3). Paris: Editions du Centre national de la recherche scientifique, 1952.

Richard 1958: Marcel Richard, *Répertoire des bibliothèques et des catalogues de manuscrits grecs*. Deuxième édition (Centre national de la recherche scientifique, Publications de l'Institut de recherche et d'histoire des textes 1). Paris: Centre national de la recherche scientifique, 1958.

Riddle 1980: John Marion Riddle, "Dioscorides", in F. Edward Cranz, and Paul Oskar Kristeller (eds.), *Catalogus Translationum et Commentariorum: Medieval and Renaissance Latin Translations and Commentaries*, volume 4. Washington, D.C.: Catholic University of America Press, 1980, pp. 1–143.

Rivier 1962: André Rivier, *Recherches sur la tradition manuscrite du traité hippocratique "De morbo sacro"* (Travaux publiés sous les auspices de la Société suisse des sciences morales 3). Berne: Francke, 1962.

Robinson and James 1909: J. Armitage Robinson, and Montague Rhodes James, *The Manuscripts of Westminster Abbey*. (Notes and documents relating to Westminster Abbey 1). Cambridge: University Press, 1909.

Rocchi 1883: Antonius Rocchi, *Codices cryptenses seu Abbatiae Cryptae Ferratae in Tusculano digesti et illustrati*. Romae: Ex Typographia Pacis, Philippi Cuggiani, 1883.

Rocchi 1893: Antonius Rocchi, *De coenobio cryptoferratensi eiusque bibliotheca et codicibus praesertim graecis commentarii*. Tusculi: Ex Typographia Tusculana, 1893.

Rodriquez 2008: Maria Teresa Rodriquez, "I palinsesti di Messina: indagine preliminare", in Santo Lucà (ed.), *Libri palinsesti greci: conservazione, restauro digitale, studio. Atti del Convegno internazionale, Villa Mondragone-Monte Porzio Catone-Università di Roma «Tor Vergata»- Biblioteca del Monumento Nazionale di Grottaferrata, 21–24 aprile 2004*. Indici a cura di Alessia Adriana Aletta e Maria Teresa Rodriquez. Roma: Comitato Nazionale per le Celebrazioni del Millenario della Fondazione dell'Abbazia di S. Nilo a Grottaferrata, 2008, pp. 201–213.

Roselli 2009: Amneris Roselli, "Due manoscritti medici greci nelle biblioteche di Sofia", *Galenos* 3 (2009), pp.177–180.

Rosenfeld and Grigorian 1976: Boris A. Rosenfeld, and Ashot Tigranovich Grigorian, "Thâbit ibn Qurra", in Charles Coulston Gillispie (ed.), *Dictionary of Scientific Biography*, volume 13. New York: Charles Scribners' Sons, 1976, pp. 288–295.

Rostagno and Festa 1893: Enrico Rostagno, and Nicola Festa, "Indice dei codici greci Laurenziani non compresi nel catalogo del Bandini", *Studi italiani di filologia classica* 1 (1893), pp. 129–232 (reprinted in Fridolf Kudlien [ed.], *Angelo Maria Bandini, Catalogus codicum manuscriptorum Bibliothecae Mediceae Laurentianae. Accedunt supplementa tria ab E. Rostagno et N. Festa congesta, necnon Additamentum ex inventariis Bibliothecae Laurentianae depromptum*, 2 volumes [Catalogi codicum graecorum lucis ope reimpressi]. Leipzig: Zentral-Antiquariat der Deutschen Demokratischen Republik, 1961, volume 2, pp. 3*-62*).

Sakkelion 1890: Ἰωάννης Σακκελίων, *Πατμιακὴ βιβλιοθήκη ἤτοι ἀναγραφὴ τῶν ἐν τῇ βιβλιοθήκῃ τῆς κατὰ τὴν νῆσον Πάτμον γεραρᾶς καὶ βασιλικῆς μονῆς τοῦ Ἁγίου Ἀποστόλου καὶ Εὐαγγελιστοῦ Ἰωάννου τεθησαυρισμένων χειρογράφων τευχῶν πάλαι μὲν ἐκπονηθεῖσα ... νῦν δὲ φιλοτίμῳ προνοίᾳ καὶ ἀναλώμασι τοῦ Φιλολογικοῦ Συλλόγου Παρνασσοῦ ἐκδιδομένη ἧς ἐν τέλει προσετέθησαν καὶ ἑπτὰ πίνακες πανομοιότυπα περιέχοντες τῆς τῶν διαφόρων ἑκατονταετηρίδων γραφῆς*. Ἀθῆναι: Α. Παπαγεώργιος, 1890.

Sakkelion and Sakkelion 1892: Ἰωάννης Σακκελίων καὶ Ἀλκιβιάδης Σακκελίων, *Κατάλογος τῶν χειρογράφων τῆς Ἐθνικῆς Βιβλιοθήκης τῆς Ἑλλάδος*. Ἀθῆναι: Ἐκ τοῦ Ἐθνικοῦ Τυπογραφείου καὶ Λιθογραφείου, 1892.

Santoro 1965: Caterina Santoro, *I codici medioevali della Biblioteca Trivulziana*. Milano: Biblioteca Trivulziana, 1965.

Savage-Smith 2011: Emilie Savage-Smith, *A New Catalogue of Arabic Manuscripts in the Bodleian Library, University of Oxford*, Volume I: Medicine. Oxford: University Press, 2011.

Savva 1858: Архимандрит Савва, *Указатель для обозрения Московской Патриаршей (ныне Синодальной) библиотеки*. Москва: Въ Университетской Типография,1858.

Savvinidou 2006: Ioanna Savvinidou, "Quelques aspects de l'histoire du texte des Empirica du Ps.-Dioscorides", in Véronique Boudon-Millot, Antonio Garzya, Jacques Jouanna, Amneris Roselli (eds.), *Ecdotica e ricezione dei testi medici greci. Atti del V Convegno Internazionale, Napoli, 1–2 ottobre 2004* (Collectanea 24). Napoli: M. D'Auria, 2006, pp. 347–355.

Scarborough 1981: John Scarborough, "The Galenic Question", *Sudhoffs Archiv* 65 (1981), pp. 1–31.

Schartau 1994: Bjarne Schartau, *Codices Graeci Haunienses: ein deskriptiver Katalog des griechischen Handschriftenbestandes der Königlichen Bibliothek Kopenhagen* (Danish humanist texts and studies 9). Copenhagen: Museum Tusculanum Press, and The Royal Library, 1994.

Schmid 1902: Wilhelm Schmid, *Verzeichnis der griechischen Handschriften der königlichen Universitätsbibliothek zu Tübingen*. Tübingen: Buchdruckerei von G. Schnürlen, 1902.

Schnorr von Carolsfeld 1882: Franz Schnorr von Carolsfeld, *Katalog der Handschriften der Königl. öffentlichen Bibliothek zu Dresden*. Im Auftrage der Generaldirection der königlichen Sammlungen für Kunst und Wissenschaft bearbeitet von -. Erster Band (enthaltend die Abteilungen A-D und F-H). Leipzig: Druck und Verlag von B. G. Teubner, 1882.

Schnorr von Carolsfeld 1979: *Katalog der Handschriften der Sächsischen Landesbibliothek zu Desden, Band 1. Korrigierte und verbesserte, nach dem Exemplar des Landesbibliothek photomechanisch hergestellte Ausgabe des Kataloges der Königlichen Öffentlichen Bibliothek zu Dresden, Band 1. Bearbeitet von Franz Schnorr v, Carolsfeld, Leipzig: Teubner, 1882*. Dresden: Sächsische Landesbibliothek, 1979.

Schoene 1902: Hermann Schoene, "Ein Palimpsestblatt des Galen aus Bobbio", *Sitzungsberichte der königlich preussischen Akademie der Wissenschaften zu Berlin* 21 (1902), pp. 442–447.

Schreiner 1988: Petrus Schreiner, *Codices vaticani graeci*, Codices 867–932. [Città del Vaticano]: In Bibliotheca Vaticana, 1988.

Schwarz 1925: Arthur Zacharias Schwarz, *Die Hebräischen Handschriften der Nationalbibliothek in Wien* (Museion-Veröffentlichungen aus der Nationalbibliothek in Wien, Abhandlungen 2). Wien, Prag und Leipzig: Ed. Strache, 1925.

Sciarra 2009: Elisabetta Sciarra, "Breve storia del fondo manoscritto della Biblioteca Angelica", *La Bibliofilia* 111 (2009), pp. 251–281.

Senguerdii et al. 1716: Wolferdius Senguerdius, Jacobus Gronovius, and Johannes Heyman, *Catalogus librorum tam impressorum quam manuscriptorum bibliothecae publicae universitatis lugduno-batavae ...* Lugduni apud Batavos: Sumptibus Petri van der Aa, 1716.

Seraphim 1909: August Seraphim, *Handschriften-Katalog der Stadtbibliothek Königsberg i. Pr.* Unter Mitwirkung von Dr. Paul Rhode bearbeitet (Mitteilungen aus der Stadtbibliothek zu Königsberg i. Pr. 1). Königsberg in Preußen: Kommissions-Verlag der Fr. Beyerschen Buchhandlung, 1909.

Serbat 1995: Guy Serbat, *Celse, De la médecine*, Tome I. Texte établi, traduit et commenté (Collection des Universités de France). Paris: Belles Lettres, 1995.

Serrai 2004: Alfredo Serrai, *Domenico Passionei e la sua biblioteca*. Milano: Sylvestre Bonnard, 2004.

Serrai 2008: Alfredo Serrai, *La biblioteca Altempsiana ovvero Le raccolte librarie di Marco Sittico III e del nipote Giovanni Angelo Altemps* (Il bibliotecario 22; Le biblioteche private in Italia 6). Roma: Bulzoni, 2008.

Serruys 1903: Daniel Serruys, "Catalogue des manuscrits conservés au Gymnase grec de Salonique", *Revue des bibliothèques* 13 (1903), pp. 12–89.

Sezgin 1970: Fuat Sezgin, *Geschichte des arabischen Schrifttums*, Band 3: Medizin, Pharmazie, Zoologie, Tierheilkunde bis ca. 430 H. Leiden: E.J. Brill, 1970.

Sezgin 1971: Fuat Sezgin, *Geschichte des arabischen Schrifttums*, Band 4: Alchimie, Chemie, Botanik, Agrikultur bis ca. 430 H. Leiden: E.J. Brill, 1971.

Shailor 1984: Barbara Shailor, *Catalogue of Medieval and Renaissance manuscripts in the Beinecke Rare Book and Manuscript Library, Yale University*, volume 1: MSS 1–250. Binghamton, N.Y.: Medieval & Renaissance Texts & Studies, 1984.

Sharpe 1997: Richard Sharpe, *A Handlist of the Latin Writers of Great Britain and Ireland before 1540* (Publications of the Journal of Medieval Latin 1). Turnhout: Brepols, 1997.

Sideras 1977: Alexander Sideras, *Rufus von Ephesos, Über die Nieren- und Blasenleiden*. Herausgegeben und übersetzt (Corpus Medicorum Graecorum 3.1). Berlin: Akademie-Verlag, 1977.

Singer 1921: Charles Singer, "Greek Biology and its Relation to the Rise of Modern Biology", in Charles Singer (ed.), *Studies in the History and Method of Science*, volume 2. Oxford: Clarendon Press, 1921, pp. 1–101.

Sjöberg 1962: Lars-Olof Sjöberg, *Stephanites und Ichnelates. Überlieferungsgeschichte und Text* (Acta Universitatis Upsaliensis, Studia Graeca Upsaliensia 2). Stockholm: Almquist & Wiksell, 1962.

Skouvaras 1967: Εὐάγγελος Σκουβαράς, Ὀλυμπιωτίσσα. Περιγραφὴ καὶ ἱστορία τῆς μονῆς. Κατάλογος τῶν χειρογραφων. Χρονικὰ σημειώματα. Ἀκολουθία Παναγίας τῆς Ὀλυμπιωτίσσης. Ἔγγραφα ἐκ ἀρχείου τῆς μονῆς (1336–1900). Ἀθῆναι: Ἀκαδημία Ἀθηνῶν, Κέντρον Ἐρεύνης τοῦ Μεσαιωνικοῦ καὶ Νέου Ἑλληνισμοῦ, 1967 — Evangelos A. Skouvaras, *Olympiotissa. Description et histoire du monastère. Catalogue des manuscrits. Notices historiques. L'Acolouthie de la Vierge Olympiotissa. Documents tirés des archives du monastère (1336–1900)* (Académie d'Athènes, Centre de recherches médiévales et néo-helléniques). Athènes: Centre de recherches médiévales et néo-helléniques, 1967.

Smets and Van Esbroeck 1970: Alexis Smets, and Michel Van Esbroeck, *Basile de Césarée, Sur l'origine de l'homme. Homélies X et XI de l'Hexaéméron*. Introduction, texte critique, traduction, et notes (Sources chrétiennes 160). Paris: Éditions du Cerf, 1970.

Sofianos 1986: Δημήτριος Ζ. Σοφιανός, *Τὰ χειρόγραφα τῶν Μετεώρων. Κατάλογος περιγραφικὸς τῶν χειρογράφων κωδίκων τῶν ὑποκειμένων εἰς τὰς μονὰς τῶν Μετεώρων ...*, Τόμος Γ´ Τὰ χειρόγραφα τῆς Μονῆς Ἁγίου Στεφάνου. Ἀθῆναι: Ἀκαδημία Ἀθηνῶν, Κέντρον Ἐρεύνης τοῦ Μεσαιωνικοῦ καὶ Νέου Ἑλληνισμοῦ, 1986 — Demetrios Z. Sofianos, *Les manuscrits des Météores. Catalogue descriptif des manuscrits conservés dans les monastères des Météores*, volume 3: Les manuscrits du monastère de Saint Etienne (Hagios Stefanos). Athènes: Centre de recherches médiévales et néo-helléniques, 1986.

Sonderkamp 1987: Joseph A. M. Sonderkamp, *Untersuchung zur Überlieferung der Schriften des Theophanes Chrysobalantes (sog. Theophanes Nonnus)* (Freie Universität Berlin, Byzantinisch-Neogriechisches Seminar, ΠΟΙΚΙΛΑ ΒΥΖΑΝΤΙΝΑ 7). Bonn: Dr. Rudolf Habelt, 1987.

Sotheby 1971: Sotheby & Co., *Bibliotheca Phillippica, Medieval Manuscripts,* New Series: Part VI: *Catalogue of Manuscripts on Papyrus, Vellum and Paper of the 7th Century to the 18th Century. Day of Sale: Tuesday 30th November 1971*. London: Sotheby & Co, 1971.

Sotheby's 1977: Sotheby's, *Bibliotheca Phillippica*, New Series, Nineteenth Part: *Catalogue of English, French, Greek & Icelandic Manuscripts From the Celebrated Collection formed by Sir Thomas Phillipps, Bt. (1792–1872), The Property of the Trustees of the Robinson Trust. Days of Sale: Monday, 17th June, 1977, Lots 4817–4980; Tuesday, 28th June 1977, Lots 4981–5144*. London: Sotheby Parke Bernet & Co., 1977.

Sotheby's 1990: Sotheby's, *Western Manuscripts and Miniatures. London, Tuesday 19th June 1990*. London: Sotheby's, 1990.

Sotiroudis 1998: Παναγιώτης Π. Σωτηρούδης, *Ιερά μονή Ιβήρων. Κατάλογος ελληνικών χειρογράφων.* Τόμος Α´ (1–100). Ἅγιο Ὄρος: Ιερά Μονή Ιβήρων, 1998.

Spyridon and Eustratiades 1925: Spyridon Lauriotes, and Sophronios Eustratiades, *Catalogue of the Greek Manuscripts in the Library of the Laura on Mount Athos, with Notices from other Libraries* (Harvard Theological Studies 12). Cambridge, MA: Harvard University Press, 1925.

Stahl 2004: Irene Stahl (ed.), *Katalog der mittelalterlichen Handschriften der Staats- und Universitätsbibliothek Bremen* (Die Handschriften der Staats- und Universitätsbibliothek 1). Wiesbaden: Harrassowitz, 2004.

Stark 1697: Sebastianus Gottofredus Stark, *Specimen Sapientiae Indorum veterum, id est, liber ethico-politicus pervetustus, dictus arabice Kalîla wa Dimna, graece Stefanîtês kai Ichnêlatês nunc primum Graece ex MSS. Cod. Holsteiniano proditi, cum versione nova Latina*. Berolini: Sumtibus Joh. Michael Rüdigeri. Stanno Ulrici Liebperti, Ypt. Elect., 1697.

Stefou 2011: Loukia Stefou, *Die neugriechische Metaphrase von Stephanites und Ichnelates durch Theodosios Zygomalas*. Inauguraldissertation zur Erlangung des Grades einer Doktorin der Philosophie am Fachbereich Philosophie und Geisteswissenschaften der Freien Universität Berlin, 2011.

Stevenson 1885: Henry Stevenson, *Codices manuscripti Palatini graeci Bibliothecae Vaticanae descripti*. Romae: Ex Typographeo Vaticano, 1885.

Stevenson 1888: Henry Stevenson, *Bibliothecae Apostolicae Vaticanae ... Codices Reginae Suecorum et Pii PP. II graeci*. Romae: Ex Typographeo Vaticano, 1888.

Stockhausen 2001: Annette von Stockhausen, "Katalog der griechischen Handschriften im Besitz der Thüringer Universitäts- und Landesbibliothek Jena", *Byzantinische Zeitschrift* 94 (2001), pp. 684–701.

Stojanov 1973: Маньо Стоянов, *Опис ha Гръцките и Други Чуждоезични Ръкописи b Народна Библиотека Кирил и Методий*. София: Наука и изкуство, 1973 - Manjo Stojanov, *Codices graeci manuscripti bibliothecae "Cyrilli et Methodii" Serdicensis*. Sofia: Nauka i izkustvo, 1973.

Stornajolo 1895: Cosimo Stornajolo, *Codices urbinates graeci Bibliothecae Vaticanae descripti ...* Accedit Index vetus Bibliothecae urbinatis nunc primum editus. Romae: Ex Typographeo Vaticano, 1895.

Stornajolo 1902: Cosimo Stornajolo, *Codices urbinates latini recensuit ...* Tomus I. Codices 1–500. Accessit appendix ad descriptionem picturarum. Romae: Typis Vaticanis, 1902.

Studemund and Cohn 1890: Wilhelm Studemund, and Leopold Cohn, *Codices ex Bibliotheca Meermanniana Phillippici Graeci nunc Berolinenses* (Verzeichniss der griechischen Handschriften der königlichen Bibliothek zu Berlin 1). Berolini: A. Asher & Co, 1890.

***Tabulae codicum* 1868**: *Tabulae codicum manu scriptorum praeter graecos et orientales in Bibliotheca Palatina Vindobonensi asservatorum*. Edidit Academia Caesarea Vindobonensis, volume I. Vindobonae: Venum dat Caroli Geroldi Filius, 1868 (reprint: Nova editio photomechanice impressa, notulis marginalibus aucta. Graz: Akademische Druck- und Verlagsanstalt, 1965*).

***Tabulae codicum* 1869**: *Tabulae codicum manu scriptorum praeter graecos et orientales in Bibliotheca Palatina Vindobonensi asservatorum*. Edidit Academia Caesarea Vindobonensis, volume III: *Codices 3501–5000*. Vindobonae: Venum dat Caroli Geroldi Filius, 1869 (reprint: Nova editio photomechanice impressa, notulis marginalibus aucta. Graz: Akademische Druck- und Verlagsanstalt, 1965*).

Tanner 2008: Marcus Tanner, *The Raven King. Matthias Corvinus and the Fate of his Lost Library*. New Haven, CT, and London: Yale University Press, 2008.

Thomson 2001: Rodney M. Thomson, *A Descriptive Catalogue of the Medieval Manuscripts in Worcester Cathedral Library*. Woodbridge: D. S. Brewer, 2001.

Thomson 2009: Rodney M. Thomson, *A Descriptive Catalogue of the Medieval Manuscripts of Merton College, Oxford*. Woodbridge: D. S. Brewer, 2009.

Thorndike and Kibre 1963: Lynn Thorndike, and Pearl Kibre, *A Catalogue of Incipits of Mediaeval Scientific Writings in Latin*. Revised and augmented edition (Mediaeval Academy of America, Publication 29). Cambridge, MA: Mediaeval Academy of America, 1963.

Thurn 1980: Hans Thurn, *Die griechischen Handschriften der Universitätsbibliothek Erlangen*. Auf der Grundlage des Manuskriptes von Otto Stählin beschrieben (Universitätsbibliothek Erlangen-Nürnberg, Katalog der Handschriften der Universitätsbibliothek Erlangen-Nürnberg 3,2). Wiesbaden: Harrassowitz, 1980.

Tiftixoglu 2004: Viktor Tiftixoglu, *Katalog der griechischen Handschriften der Bayerischen Staatsbibliothek München*. Band 1: Codices graeci Monacenses 1–55. Neu beschrieben, revidiert sowie mit Einleitung und Registern versehen von Kerstin Hajdú und Gerard Duursma (Catalogus codicum manu scriptorum Bibliothecae Monacensis, Tomus II, Pars 1). Wiesbaden: Otto Harrassowitz, 2004.

Tihon 1992: Anne Tihon, "Les *Tables Faciles* de Ptolémée dans les manuscrits en onciale (IXe-Xe siècles)", *Revue d'histoire des textes* 22 (1992), pp. 47–87.

Tinnefeld 1988: Franz Tinnefeld, "Zur Geschichte der Sammlung griechischer Handschriften in der bayerischen Staatsbibliothek München", in Marcel Restle (ed.), *Festschrift für Klaus Wesel in memoriam* (Münchener Arbeiten zur Kunstgeschichte und Archäologie 2). München: Editio Maris, 1988, pp. 303–342.

Tomasini 1639: Iacobus Philippus Tomasini, *Bibliothecae patavinae manuscriptae publicae et privatae*. Utini: Typis Nicolai Schiratti, 1639.

Tomasini 1650: Iacobus Philippus Tomasini, *Bibliothecae venetae manuscriptae publicae et privatae*. Utini: Typis Nicolai Schiratti, 1650.

Torallas Tovar 1994: Sofia Torallas Tovar, "De codicibus graecis Upsaliensibus olim Escurialensibus" *Erytheia* 15 (1994), pp. 191–258.

Touwaide 1981: Alain Touwaide, *Les deux traités de toxicologie attribués à Dioscoride, La tradition manuscrite du texte grec, édition critique et index*, 5 volumes. Louvain-la-Neuve: Université catholique de Louvain, Unpublished PhD thesis, 1981.

Touwaide 1999: Alain Touwaide, "*Lexica medico-botanica byzantina*. Prolégomènes à une étude", in Τῆς φιλίης τάδε δῶρα - *Miscelánea léxica en memoria de Conchita Serrano* (Manuales y Anejos de «Emerita» 41). Madrid: Consejo Superior de Investigaciones Científicas, Centro de Humanidades, 1999, pp. 211–228.

Touwaide 2003: Alain Touwaide, "The Salamanca Dioscorides (Salamanca, University Library. 2659), *Erytheia* 24 (2003), pp. 125–158.

Touwaide 2006: Alain Touwaide, "Latin Crusaders, Greek Herbals", in Jean Givens, Karen M. Reeds, and Alain Touwaide (eds.), *Visualizing Medieval Medicine and Natural History 1200–1550* (AVISTA Studies in the History of Medieval Technology, Science and Art 5). Aldershot and Burlington, VT: Ashgate, 2006, pp. 25–50.

Touwaide 2009: Alain Touwaide, "Byzantine Medical Manuscripts. Towards a New Catalogue, with a Specimen for an Annotated Checklist of Manuscripts based on an Index of Diels' Catalogue", *Byzantion* 79 (2009), pp. 453–595.

Tovar 1963: Antonio Tovar, *Catalogus codicum graecorum Universitatis Salamantinae*. I. Collectio Universitatis Antiqua (Acta Salmanticensia Iussu Senatus Universitatis edita, Filosofia y Letras, Tomo XV, núm. 4). Salamanca: Secretariado de Publicaciones e Intercambio Científico de la Universidad de Salamanca, 1963.

Treu 1973: Kurt Treu, "Griechische Handschriften in Weimar", *Philologus* 17 (1973), pp. 113–123.

Tsakona nd: Kalliopi Tsakonas-Hilas, *ΣΥΛΛΟΓΗ ΤΑΜΕΙΟΥ ΑΝΤΑΛΛΑΞΙΜΩΝ - Musée Benaki, Echangeables*. [Athens: Benaki Museum], n.d. (unpublished list of manuscript).

Tsakopoulos 1956: Αἰμιλιανός Τσακόπουλος, *Περιγραφικός κατάλογος τῶν χειρογράφων τῆς βιβλιοθήκης τοῦ Οἰκουμενικοῦ Πατριαρχείου*, Β΄ Αγ. Τριάδος Χάλκης. Ἰστανμπούλ: Πατριαρχικὸν Τυπογραφεῖον, 1956.

Tselikas 1977: Ἀγαμέμνων Τσελίκας, *Δέκα αἰῶνες ἑλληνικῆς γραφῆς (9ος - 19ος αἰ.)*. Ἀθήναι: Μουσεῖο Μπενάκη, Συλλόγη Χειρογράφων, 1977.

Tsernoglou 1991: Ἀθανάσιος Γ. Τσερνόγλου, "Συμπληρωματικός κατάλογος χειρογράφων τῆς παλαίας Γυμνασιακῆς Βιβλιοθήκης Μυτιλήνης νύν τοῦ Α΄ Λύκειον Μυτιλήνης", *Λεσβιακά* 13 (1991), pp. 347–388.

Tunis 1989: Elizabeth Tunis, *Early Western Manuscripts in the National Library of Medicine. A Short-Title List*. Bethesda, MD: History of Medicine Division, National Library of Medicine, 1989.

Turyn 1928: Alexander Turyn, "Studia Byzantina 1. De Homeri et Ioannis Actuarii codicibus Varsoviensibus", *Eos* 31 (1928), pp. 505–518.

Turyn 1964: Alexander Turyn, *Codices Graeci Vaticani saeculis XIII et XIV scripti annorumque notis instructi* (Codices e Vaticanis selecti quam simillime expressi 28). In Civitate Vaticana: ex Bybliotheca Apostolica Vaticana, 1964.

Tyurina 2012: Галина Тюрина, *Из истории изучения греческих рукописей в Европе в XVIII - начале XIX в. Христиан Фридрих Маттеи (1744–1811)* (Монфокон Вып. 2). Москва: Языки славянской культуры, 2012.

Uffenbach 1720: Zacharius Conradus ab Uffenbach, *Bibliothecae Uffenbachianae Mstae partes septem posteriores, quibus coeteri codices msti diversarum linguarum et argumentorum ... comprehenduntur*, in Iohannes Henricus Maius, *Bibliotheca Uffenbachiana MSSTA seu catalogus et recensio Msstorum codicum qui in bibliotheca Zachariae Conradi ab Uffenbach Traiecti ad Moenum adservantur et in varias classes distinguuntur quarum priores ... recensuit. Reliquas possessor ipse digessit qui omnem etiam hanc supellectilem literariam suam ad usus publicos offert*. Halae Hermundorum: Impensis Novi Bibliopoli, 1720, parts 4–10 of the volume, with separate numbering of columns (1–1364 + index).

Ullmann 1970: Manfred Ullmann, *Die Medizin im Islam* (Handbuch der Orientalistik, Erste Abteilung: Der nahe und der mittlere Osten, Ergänzungsband VI, 1. Abschnitt). Leiden and Köln: Brill, 1970.

Unterkircher 1957: Franz Unterkircher, *Inventar der illuminierten Handschriften, Inkunabeln und Frühdrucke der Österreichischen Nationalbibliothek* (Museion, Neue Folge, Zweiter Reihe, Zweiter Band, Teil 1). Wien: Georg Prachner, 1957.

Uthemann 1983: Karl-Heinz Uthemann, "Der *Codex Vaticanus* 1409. Eine Beschreibung der Handschrift", *Byzantion* 53 (1983), pp. 639–653.

Van de Vorst 1906: Charles Van de Vorst, "Verzeichnis der griechischen Handschriften der Bibliotheca Rossiana", *Zentralblatt für Bibliothekswesen* 23 (1906), pp. 492–508 and 537–550.

Van Der Heide 1977: Albert Van Der Heide, *Hebrew Manuscripts of Leiden University Library* (Codices manuscripti 18). Leiden: Universitaire Pres Leiden, 1977.

Vattasso and Franchi de' Cavalieri 1902: Marcus Vattasso, and Pius Franchi de' Cavalieri, *Codices vaticani latini*, Tomus I: Codices 1–678. Romae: Typis Vaticanis, 1902.

Vieillefond 1935: Jean-René Vieillefond, "Complemento al catálogo de manuscritos griegos de la Biblioteca Nacional de Madrid", *Emerita* 3 (1935), pp. 193–213.

Villa-Amil y Castro 1878: José Villa-Amil y Castro, *Catálogo de los manuscritos existentes en la Biblioteca del Noviciado de la Universidad Central (procedentes de la antigua de Alcalá)*. Parte I: Códices. Madrid: Aribau y Ca, 1878.

Vitelli 1894: Girolamo Vitelli, "Indice de' codici greci Riccardiani, Magliabechiani e Marucelliani", *Studi italiani di filologia classica* 2 (1894), pp. 471–570 (reproduced in Christa Samberger [ed.], *Catalogi codicum graecorum qui in minoribus bibliothecis italicis asservantur in duo volumina collati et novissimis additamentis aucti*, 2 volumes [Catalogi codicum graecorum lucis ope reimpressi]. Lipsiae: Zentral Antiquariat der deutschen demokratischen Republik, 1965–1968, volume 1, pp. 135–234).

Vladimir 1894: Архимандрит Владимир, *Систематическое описаніе рукописей Московской синодальной (патріаршей) библіотеки: Рукописи греческія*. Москва: Синодальная Типографія. 1894.

Volger 1859: Ernst Volger, "Mittheilungen aus Spanien. 23. Verzeichniss der classischen HSS. der Universitätsbibliothek von Salamanca", *Philologus* 14 (1859), pp. 373–379.

Vollmer 1916: Fridericus Vollmer, *Quinti Sereni Libri medicinales*. Edidit - (Corpus Medicorum Latinorum II 3). Lipsiae et Berolini: In aedibus B. G. Teubneri, 1916.

Voltz and Crönert 1897: Ludwig Voltz, and Wilhelm Crönert, "Der Codex 2773 miscellaneus Graecus der Grossherzoglichen Hofbibliothek zu Darmstadt. Ein Beitrag zur griechischen Excerpten-Literatur", *Centralblatt für Bibliothekswesen* 14 (1897), pp. 537–571.

von Euw and Plotzek 1985: Anton von Euw, and Joachim M. Plotzek, *Die Handschriften der Sammlung Ludwig*, Band 4, mit einem Register von Gisela Plotzek-Wederhake. Köln: Schnügen-Museum der Stadt Köln, 1985.

von Gebhardt 1898: Oscar von Gebhardt, "Christian Friedrich Matthaei und seine Sammlung griechischer Handschriften", *Centralblatt für Bibliothekswesen* 15 (1898), pp. 345–357, 393–420, 441–482, 537–566.

von Heinemann 1886: Otto von Heinemann, *Die Handschriften der Herzoglichen Bibliothek zu Wolfenbüttel*. Erste Abteilung. Die Helmstedter Handschriften. II. Wolfenbüttel: Druck und Verlag Julius Zwissler, 1886 (reprint: Frankfurt am Main: Vittorio Klostermann, 1965).

von Heinemann 1900: Otto von Heinemann, *Die Handschriften der Herzoglichen Bibliothek zu Wolfenbüttel*. Zweite Abteilung. Die Augusteischen Handschriften. IV. Wolfenbüttel: Julius Zwissler, 1900 (reprint: Frankfurt am Main: Vittorio Klostermann, 1966).

von Heinemann 1903: Otto von Heinemann, *Die Handschriften der Herzoglichen Bibliothek zu Wolfenbüttel*. Zweite Abteilung. Die Augusteischen Handschriften. V. Dritte Abteilung. *Die Weissenburger Handschriften*. Wolfenbüttel: Julius Zwissler, 1903.

von Staden 1989: Heinrich von Staden, *Herophilus. The Art of Medicine in Early Alexandria*. Edition, translation and essay. Cambridge: Cambridge University Press, 1989.

Waddingus 1650: Lucas Waddingus, *Scriptores Ordinis Minorum quibus accessit Syllabus Illorum qui ex eodem Ordine pro fide Christi forsiter occubuerunt. Priores atramento, posteriores sanguine christianam religionem asseruerunt*. Romae: Ex Typographia Francisci Alberti Tani, 1650.

Warner and Gilson 1921: George F. Warner, and Julius P. Gilson, *British Museum. Catalogue of Western Manuscripts in the Old Royal and King's Collections*, 4 volumes. London: Printed for the Trustees, and Oxford: University Press, 1921.

Wartelle 1963: André Wartelle, *Inventaire des manuscrits grecs d'Aristote et de ses commentateurs* (Collection d'études anciennes). Paris: Belles Lettres, 1963.

Weitzmann and Galavaris 1990: Kurt Weitzmann, and George Galavaris, *The Monastery of Saint Catherine at Mount Sinai. The Illuminated Greek Manuscripts*, 1: From the Ninth to the Twelfth Century. Princeton, NJ: Princeton University Press, 1990.

Wellisch 1975: Hans Wellisch, "Conrad Gessner: a bio-bibliography", *Journal of the Society for the Bibliography of Natural History* 7 (1975), pp. 151–247.

Wellisch 1984: Hans H. Wellisch, *Conrad Gessner. A Bio-Bibliography*. Zug: IDC, 1984.

Wellmann 1897: Max Wellmann, *Kratevas* (Abhandlungen der königlichen Gesellschaft der Wissenschaften zu Göttingen, Philologisch-historische Klasse, Neue Folge, Band 2, Nro. 1). Berlin: Weidmannsche Buchhandlung, 1897.

Wellmann 1906–1914: Max Wellmann, *Pedanii Dioscuridis Anazarbei, De materia medica libri quinque*. Edidit -, 3 volumes. Berlin: Weidmann, 1906–1914 (reprint: 1958).

Wellmann 1908: Max Wellmann, *Philumeni de venenatis animalibus eorumque remediis ex codice vaticano primum edidit* (Corpus Medicorum Graecorum X 1, 1). Lipsiae et Berolini: In Aedibus B. G. Teubneri, 1908.

Wellmann 1914: Max Wellmann, *Die Schrift des Dioskurides περὶ ἁπλῶν φαρμάκων. Ein Beitrag zur Geschichte der Medizin*. Berlin: Weidmannsche Buchhandlung, 1914.

Welz 1913: Karl Welz, *Descriptio codicum graecorum* (Katalog der kaiserlichen Universitäts- und Landesbibliothek in Strassburg). Strassburg: Karl J. Trübner, 1913.

Wendel 1921: Carl Wendel, "Die griechischen Handschriften der Provinz Sachsen", in Georg Leyh (ed.), *Aufsaetze Fritz Milkau gewidmet*. Leipzig: Karl W. Hiersemann, 1921, pp. 354–378.

Wilkins 2013: John Wilkins, *Galien*, Tome V: *Sur les facultés des aliments*. Texte établi et traduit (Collection des Universités de France). Paris: Belles Lettres, 2013.

Wittek 1975: Martin Wittek, "Les manuscrits grecs de la Bibliothèque royale Albert Ier: vingt années d'acquisitions (1954–1973)", in Jean Bingen, Guy Cambier, and Georges Nachtergael (eds.), *Le monde grec. Pensée, littérature, histoire, documents. Hommages á Claire Préaux* (Université Libre de Bruxelles, Faculté de Philosophie et Lettres, 52). Bruxelles: Editions de l'Université Libre de Bruxelles, 1975, pp. 245–253.

Xiropotaminos and Sotiroudis 2012: Ζαχαρία Ξηροποταμινό και Παναγιώτη Σωτηρούδη, *Συμπληρωματικός κατάλογος ελληνικών χειρογράφων Ιεράς Μονής Ξηροποτάμου Αγίου Όρους (426–557)*. Θεσσαλονίκη: Αριστοτελείο Πανεπιστήμιο Θεσσαλονίκης, Κέντρο Βυζαντινών Ερευνών, 2012.

Young 1908: John Young, *A Catalogue of the Manuscripts in the Library of the Hunterian Museum in the University of Glasgow*. Continued and Completed under the Direction of the Young Memorial Committee by Patrick Henderson Aitken. Glasgow: James Maclehose and Sons, 1908.

Zacour and Hirsch 1970: Norman P. Zacour, and Rudolf Hirsch, "Catalogue of Manuscripts in the Libraries of the University of Pennsylvania to 1800: Supplement A (3)", *Library Chronicle* 36 (1970), pp. 79–104.

Zanelli 1890: Agostino Zanelli, "Pistoia, Biblioteca Fabroniana", in Giuseppe Mazzatinti, *Inventari dei manoscritti delle biblioteche d'Italia*, 1. Forlì: Luigi Bordandini, 1890, pp. 268–277.

Zanetti and Bongiovanni 1740: Anton Maria Zanetti, and Antonio Bongiovanni, *Graeca D. Marci Bibliotheca codicum manuscriptorum per titulos digesta* ... Venetiis: apud Simonem Occhi, 1740.

Zervos 1905: Σκεύος Ζερβός, "Ἀετίου Ἀμιδηνοῦ, Περὶ δακνόντων ζῴων καὶ ἰοβόλων ἤτοι Λόγος δέκατος τρίτος", Ἀθηνᾶ 18 (1905), pp. 241–302.

Zipser 2004: Barbara Zipser, "Überlegungen zum Text der *Sunopsis iatrikê* des Leo medicus", in Angela Hornung, Christian Jägel and Werner Schubert (eds.), *Studia Humanitatis ac Litterarum Trifolio Heidelbergensi dedicata. Festschrift für Eckhard Christmann, Wilfried Edelmaier und Rudolf Kettemann* (Studien zur klassischen Philologie 144). Frankfurt am Main: Peter Lang, 2004, pp. 393–399.

Zoras and Bouboulidis 1964: Γεώργιος Θ. Ζώρας καὶ Φαίδων Κ. Μπουμπουλίδης, *Κατάλογος χειρογράφων κωδίκων Σπουδαστηρίου Βυζαντινῆς καὶ Νεοελληνικῆς Φιλολογίας τοῦ Πανεπιστημίου Ἀθηνῶν* (Βιβλιοθήκη Βυζαντινῆς καὶ Νεοελληνικῆς Φιλολογίας 40). Ἀθῆναι: Ἐθνικὸν καὶ Καποδιστριακὸν Πανεπιστήμιον Ἀθηνῶν, Σπουδαστήριον Βυζαντινῆς καὶ Νεοελληνικῆς Φιλολογίας, 1964.

Zuretti 1896: Carlo Oreste Zuretti, "Indice de' mss. greci torinesi non contenuti nel catalogo del Pasini", *Studi italiani di filologia classica* 4 (1896), pp. 201–223.

Index

The index references the library names as in Diels' catalogue and the census. The names cited in Diels, including some owners of manuscripts and collections that no longer exist, exactly reproduce Diels' usage (German, Latin, and transcription into Latin alphabet for Greek names). Library names in the census appear in their original language and alphabet (Armenian, Cyrillic, Greek, Latin). All library names are followed by a city name, unless the name of the library includes the name of the place (e.g. Uppsala Universitetsbibliotek). City names exactly reproduce the information provided in Diels (most often in German) or in the census (in the original language). As a consequence library names may be followed by a city name that does not correspond to current usage (e.g. Venedig as in Diels for Venezia [Venice]) and some library names may be followed by two different appellations of the same location (e.g. the libraries of the monasteries on Mount Athos, followed by Ἅγιον Ὄρος [Holy Mountain] as per the census and by Ἄθως [Athos] as per Diels). The English translation provided for all names in the present volume (place and library names) are included here.

Abbey Library/Abbey Library and Archive, Zeitz: 373

Accademia dei Lincei, Rom: 274

Aedes Christi Library, Oxford: 168

Agios Savva Collection, Patriarchate, Jerusalem: 93

Agiou Panteleimonos Monastery, Holy Mountain: 3; Athos: 25

Alberto Bombace Biblioteca Centrale della Regione Sicilia, Palermo: 194

Ambrosian Library, Mailand: 128

Amstellodamensis: 9

Andrea Asulanus' Library, Venedig: 322

Andrea de Rubeis' Library, Venedig: 322

Angelica Library, Rom: 270; Roma: 307

Antverpensis: 10

Archiepiscopal Library, Lambeth Palace, London: 120

Archiginnasio/Archiginnasio Municipal Library, Bologna: 34

Archives of the Metropolitan Chapter/ Archivio del Capitolo Metropolitano, Mailand: 128

Archivio di San Pietro, Biblioteca Apostolica Vaticana, Città del Vaticano: 53; Rom: 275

Archivio Storico Civico e Biblioteca Trivulziana, Mailand: 136

Ariostea Municipal Library, Ferrara: 66

Ashmolean Museum, Oxford: 39, 167

Asulanus, Andrea, Venedig: 322

August Guelph's Library, Wolfenbüttel: 368

Augustean Library, München: 151

Baden State Library Karlsruhe/Badische Landesbibliothek Karlsruhe: 95

Barberini Library, Rom: 271

Basilica of Our Lady of the Pillar, Zaragoza: 372

Batskobou Monastery, Rhodope: 267

Bavarian State Library, Munich/Bayerische Staatsbibliothek (BSB), München: 151

Beinecke Rare Book and Manuscript Library, Yale University. New Haven, CT: 165

Benaki Museum, Athens: 15

Berlin State Library-Prussian Cultural Heritage: 27

Bertoliana City Library/Bertoliana Library, Vicenza: 346

Biblioteca Academiei Române, București: 37

Biblioteca Ambrosiana, Mailand: 128

Biblioteca Angelica, Rom: 270

Biblioteca Apostolica Vaticana, Città del Vaticano: 53; Rom: 276

Biblioteca Barberina/Biblioteca Barberiniana, Rom: 271

Biblioteca Bertoliana, Vicenza: 346

Biblioteca Borbonica, Neapel: 161

Biblioteca Capitolare Fabroniana, Pitoia: 265; Pistoja: 266

Biblioteca Capitolare, Verona: 345; Viterbo: 346

Biblioteca Capitular, Catedral de Toledo: 315

Biblioteca Casanatense, Roma: 307

Biblioteca civica, Bergamo: 27; Padova: 187

Biblioteca civica Bertoliana, Vicenza: 346

Biblioteca Classense, Ravenna: 267

Biblioteca comunale Ariostea, Ferrara: 66

Biblioteca comunale/Biblioteca comunale dell'Archiginnasio, Bologna: 34

Biblioteca Corsiniana, Rom: 274; Roma: 307

Biblioteca de la Catedral del Pilar, Zaragoza: 372

Biblioteca de la Universidad Complutense, Madrid: 124

Biblioteca dei Gerolamini, Napoli: 158; Neapel: 163, 164

Biblioteca del cabillo de la iglesia catedral, Toledo: 315

Biblioteca del Monumento nazionale di Grottaferrata: 86

Biblioteca del Palacio, Madrid: 127

Biblioteca del Real Monasterio de San Lorenzo del Escorial, Escurial: 62; San Lorenzo de El Escorial: 311

Biblioteca del Seminario Vescovile, Padova: 187

Biblioteca della Missione urbana, Genua: 84

Biblioteca di S. Antonio di Castello, Venedig: 337

Biblioteca di S. Giovanni di Carbonara, Neapel: 163

Biblioteca e Archivio del Capitolo Metropolitano, Mailand: 128

Biblioteca Estense, Modena: 140

Biblioteca Fabroniana, Pitoia: 265; Pistoja: 266

Biblioteca Franzoniana, Genova: 83; Genua: 84

Biblioteca General Histórica, Salamanca: 309

Biblioteca Jagiellońska, Uniwersytet Jagiellońska w Krakowie, Kraków: 103

Biblioteca Labronica, Livorno: 116

Biblioteca Magliabecchiana, Florenz: 80n1

Biblioteca Marucelliana, Florenz: 67

Biblioteca Medicea Laurenziana/Mediceo Laurentiana, Firenze/Florenz: 67

Biblioteca Nacional, Madrid: 124

Biblioteca Nazionale, Firenze: 67; Florenz: 80; Palermo: 194

Biblioteca Nazionale Marciana/San Maro, Venedig: 327; Venezia: 338

Biblioteca Nazionale Universitaria, Torino: 315; Turin: 317

Biblioteca Nazionale Vittorio Emanuele III, Napoli: 158

Biblioteca Oratoriana, Neapel: 164

Biblioteca Palatina, Parma: 262

Biblioteca Reale Borbonica, Neapel: 161

Biblioteca Regionale Universitaria Giacomo Longo, Messina: 137

Biblioteca Riccardiana, Firenze: 67; Florenz: 80

Biblioteca Sanctissimi Salvatoris, Messina: 137

Biblioteca statale oratoriana del Monumento nazionale dei Gerolamini, Neapel: 163

Biblioteca Trivulziana, Mailand: 136

Biblioteca Universitaria, Bologna: 34; Genova: 83; Madrid: 124

Biblioteca Universitaria e Estense, Modena: 140, 143

Biblioteca Vallicellana/Vallicelliana, Rom: 275; Roma: 307

Biblioteca Vaticana, Rom: 276

Biblioteka Narodowa, Warsawa: 347

Biblioteka Uniwersytecka we Wrocławiu, Wrocław: 371

Bibliotheca Aedis Christi, Oxford: 168

Bibliotheca Andreae Asulani, Venedig: 322

Bibliotheca Andreae de Rubeis, Venedig: 322

Bibliotheca Augustea, München: 151

Bibliotheca Bodleiana, Oxford: 168

Bibliotheca Canonicorum Lateranensium, Padua: 187

Bibliotheca Cathedralis, Padua: 188

Bibliotheca Collegii S.J. Rossia, Wien: 348

Bibliotheca Ducis Lobcovic, Raudnitz: 266

Bibliotheca Ducis Urbini et Pisauri: 321

Bibliotheca ecclesiae Westmonasteriensis, London: 116

Bibliotheca Ephesiana, Nea-Ephesos: 164

Bibliotheca Guelfi Augusti, Wolfenbüttel: 368

Bibliotheca gymnasii, Mitylene: 140; Saloniki: 310

Bibliotheca Hunteriana, Glasgow: 84

Bibliotheca Joannis Rhodii, Padua: 189

Bibliotheca Josephi de Aromatariis, Venedig: 322

Bibliotheca Marci Mantuae, Padua: 192

Bibliotheca Mediceo Laurentiana, Florenz: 67
Bibliotheca Mileensis, Mileae: 140
Bibliotheca Monasterii Mpatskobou, Rhodope: 267
Bibliotheca Monasterii S. Johannis Evangelisti, Patmos: 262
Bibliotheca Monasterii S. Michaelis, Venedig: 325, 326
Bibliotheca Narcissi, Dublin: 59
Bibliotheca Norfolciana, Norfolk: 166
Bibliotheca Passinoneiana, Rom: 274
Bibliotheca Philosophica Hermetica, Amsterdam 52
Bibliotheca Regia, Budapest: 38; Paris: 194
Bibliotheca S. Antoni, Venedig: 337
Bibliotheca S. Joannis in Viridario, Padua: 192
Bibliotheca S. Michaelis prope Murianum, Venedig: 326
Bibliotheca S. Petri, Rom: 275
Bibliotheca S. Petri Corbeiensis, Corbie: 56
Bibliotheca S. Remigi, Reims: 267
Bibliotheca S. Salvatoris, Messina: 137
Bibliotheca senatus, Leipzig: 108
Bibliotheca Tomasini, Padua: 194
Bibliotheca Universitatis, Basel: 27; Heidelberg: 88; Kopenhagen: 102; Salamanca: 309
Bibliotheca Universitatis Jagiellonensis, Krakau: 103
Bibliotheca Urbana [Vratislaviensis], Breslau: 36
Bibliotheca Urbis, Königsberg Pr.: 96
Bibliotheca Zamoyski, Warschau: 346
Bibliothek der Serail, Konstantinopel: 100
Bibliothek des Greifes Leicester, Holkham: 89
Bibliothek des heiligen Grabes, Jerusalem: 92
Bibliothek des heiligen Kreuzes, Jerusalem: 93
Bibliothek des Patriarchates, Jerusalem: 94
Bibliothek des reformierten Collegiums, Sáros-Patak: 311
Bibliothek Mar-Saba, Jerusalem: 90
Βιβλιοθήκη Γυμνασίου, Θεσσαλονίκη: 310; Μυτιλήνη: 140
Βιβλιοθήκη Ἐπισκόπου, Rodosto/ Ῥαιδεστός: 268
Βιβλιοθήκη Μαρ-Σάββα: Jerusalem: 93
Βιβλιοθήκη Μηλεῶν, Milies/Μηλεαί: 140
Βιβλιοθήκη Μονῆς Βατοπεδίου, Athos/Ἄθως: 16
Βιβλιοθήκη Μονῆς Διονυσίου, Athos/Ἄθως: 16
Βιβλιοθήκη Μονῆς Δοχειαρίου, Athos/Ἄθως: 17

Βιβλιοθήκη Μονῆς Ἐσφιγμένου, Athos/Ἄθως: 17
Βιβλιοθήκη Μονῆς Θεοτόκου, Chalke/Χάλκη: 50
Βιβλιοθήκη Μονῆς Ἰβήρων, Athos/Ἄθως: 18
Βιβλιοθήκη Μονῆς Κουτλουμουσίου, Athos/Ἄθως: 22
Βιβλιοθήκη Μονῆς Μεγίστης Λαύρας, Athos/Ἄθως: 23
Βιβλιοθήκη Μονῆς Μπατσκόβου, Rhodope/Ροδόπη: 267
Βιβλιοθήκη Μονῆς Ξηροποτάμου, Athos/Ἄθως: 26
Βιβλιοθήκη Μονῆς Παντελεήμονος, Athos/Ἄθως: 25
Βιβλιοθήκη τῆς Ἀστικῆς Σχολῆς, Nea-Ephesos/Νέα Ἔφεσος: 164
Βιβλιοθήκη τῆς Βουλῆς, Ἀθῆναι/Βιβλιοθήκη της Βουλῆς των Ἑλλήνων, Athen/Ἀθῆναι: 10
Βιβλιοθήκη τῆς Μονῆς τοῦ Ἁγίου Ἀποστόλου καὶ Εὐαγγελίστου Ἰωάννου, Patmos/Πάτμος: 262
Βιβλιοθήκη τῆς τοῦ Λειμῶνος Μονῆς, Καλλονὴ Λέσβου, Lesbos: 108
Βιβλιοθήκη τοῦ Παναγίου Τάφου, Ἱερουσαλήμ: 90
Βιβλιοθήκη τοῦ Πατριαρχείου, Jerusalem: 94
Βιβλιοθήκη τοῦ Τιμίου Σταυροῦ, Jerusalem: 93
Βιβλιοθήκη, Πρότυπο Πειραματικό Γενικό Λύκειο Μυτιλήνης του Πανεπιστημίου Αιγαίου, Μυτιλήνη Λέσβου: 157
Bibliothêkê Episkopou, Rodosto: 268
Bibliothêkê Monês Batopediou, Athos: 16
Bibliothêkê Monês Dionysiou, Athos: 16
Bibliothêkê Monês Docheiariou, Athos: 17
Bibliothêkê Monês Esfigmenou, Athos: 17
Bibliothêkê Monês Ibêrôn, Athos: 18
Bibliothêkê Monês Koutloumousiou, Athos: 22
Bibliothêkê Monês Lauras, Athos: 23
Bibliothêkê Monês Panteleêmonos, Athos: 25
Bibliothêkê Monês Theotokou, Chalke: 50
Bibliothêkê tês Boulês, Athen: 10
Bibliothêkê tês tou Leimônos monês, Lesbos: 108
Bibliothèque communale, Orléans: 167
Bibliothèque de Genève: 83
Bibliothèque de l'école [de médecine], Montpellier: 144
Bibliothèque de la Bourgeoisie de Berne: 33
Bibliothèque de la Faculté de Médecine, Paris: 198

Bibliothèque de la ville, Lyon: 123; Paris: 196
Bibliothèque de Monsieur le marquis de
    Rosanbo: 308
Bibliothèque de Paris: 197
Bibliothèque du monastère de Saint-Rémy,
    Reims: 267
Bibliothèque Inguimbertine, Carpentras: 49
Bibliothèque Interuniversitaire de Santé-BIU
    Santé, Paris: 198
Bibliothèque Mazarine, Paris: 200
Bibliothèque municipale Inguimbertine,
    Carpentras: 49
Bibliothèque municipale, Besançon: 34; Lyon:
    123; Sens: 311
Bibliothèque nationale/Bibliothèque nationale
    de France, Paris: 200
Bibliothèque nationale et universitaire,
    Strasbourg: 314
Bibliothèque royale de Belgique, Bruxelles: 36
Bibliothèque Sainte-Geneviève, Paris: 262
Bodleian Library, Oxford: 168
Borbonica Library, Neapel: 161
British Library/British Museum, London: 116,
    117
Българска Академия на Науките (БАН),
    Научен Архив (НА), София: 313
Bulgarian Academy of Sciences, Scientific
    Archives, Sofia: 313
Burgerbibliothek Bern: 33

Caius College, Cambridge: 40
Cambridge University Library: 44, 45
Cantabrigensis Bibliotheca Universitatis: 45
Cantacuzenus, Michael, Konstantinopel: 99
Casanatense Library, Rome: 307
Cathedral Library, Padua: 188
Cathedralis Metensis, Cambridge: 45
Cattaui, Ad., Cairo: 38
Central Library, Aristotle University
    Thessalonica: 314
Centre for Slavo-Byzantine Studies "Prof. Ivan
    Dujčev", Sofia University "St Clement of
    Ohrid": 314
Chapter Library, Toledo Cathedral: 315;
    Verona: 345; Viterbo: 346
Christ Church Library, Oxford: 168
City Library, Antwerp: 10; Bergamo: 27; Bern:
    33; Hamburg: 87; Königsberg Pr.: 96;
    Lyon: 123; Padua: 187; Zürich: 373

Classense Library, Ravenna: 267
Collection of the Holy Sepulchre, Patriarchate,
    Jerusalem: 94
Collection of the Metochion of the Holy
    Sepulchre, Patriarchate, Jerusalem: 92
Collegii Novi, Oxford: 184
Collegio inglese, Roma: 308
Collegium Mertonense, Oxford: 183
Collegium Pembrochianum, Cambridge: 47
Collegium Sanctae Trinitatis, Dublin: 60
Collegium Sancti Johannis, Cambridge: 46
Collegium Sancti Petri, Cambridge: 48
Colonna Collection, Rom: 269
Convent Library, Grottaferrata: 86
Corpus Christi College, Oxford: 185
Corsiniana Library, Rom: 274; Roma: 307
Court and State Library, München: 151
Court Library, Wien: 349

de Rubeis, Andrea, Venedig: 322
Δημόσια Βιβλιοθήκη, Mileae/Μηλεών: 140
Δημόσια Ιστορική Βιβλιοθήκη και Μουσείο της
    Ελληνικής Σχολής Δημητσάνας: 57
Dimantaras, Ach. L., Castellorizo (Megistê): 50
Dionysiou Monastery, Holy Mountain: 4;
    Athos: 16
Duchess Anna-Amalia Library, Weimar: 347
Duke's Library, Urbini et Pisauri: 321
Duke Lobkowicz's Library, Raudnitz: 266

Earl of Leicester's Library, Holkham: 89
Ecclesia Wigornensis, Oxford: 185
Ἐκκλησία Ἁγίου Νικολάου, Gallipoli/Καλλίπολη:
    82
Ekklêsia Agiou Nikolaou, Gallipoli: 82
English College, Rome: 308
Ephesian Library, Nea-Ephesos: 164
Episcopal Library, Rodosto: 268
Episcopal Seminary Library, Padua: 187
Erfgoedbibliotheek Hendrik Conscience,
    Antwerpen: 10
Esfigmenou Monastery, Holy Mountain: 4;
    Athos: 17
Estense Library, Modena: 140
Εθνική Βιβλιοθήκη της Ελλάδος ΕΒΕ, Athen/
    Αθήναι: 11

Fabroniana Library/Fabroniana Capitular
    Library, Pistoia: 265; Pistoja: 266

Fondo Colonna/Fonds Colonna, Rom: 269

Francis A. Countway Library, Medical School, Harvard University, Boston, MA: 35

Franzoniana Library, Genoa: 83

French Institute of Byzantine Studies, Paris: 262

General Historical Library, Salamanca: 309

Geneva Library/Geneva City Library: 83

Genevensis Bibliotheca Urbis, Genf: 83

Gerolamini Library, Neapel: 163

Giacomo Longo Regional University Library, Messina: 137

Giuseppe degli Aromatari's Library, Venedig: 322

Glasgow University Library: 84

Gollob Privatbesitz, Wien: 348

Gonville and Caius College, Cambridge: 40, 47

Государственный Исторический Музей (ГИМ), Синодальная библиотека Московского Патриархата, Moskau: 145; Москва: 148

Great Lavra Monastery, Holy Mountain: 7; Athos, 23

Great Meteora Monastery: 138

Greek Parliament Library, Athens: 10

Gresham College, London: 166

Grossherzogliche Hof- und Landesbibliothek, Karlsruhe: 95

Γυμνασίου Βιβλιοθήκη, Mitylene/Μυτιλήνη Λέσβου: 140; Saloniki/Θεσσαλονίκη: 310

Gymnasium Library, Mytiline, Lesvos: 140; Thessalonica: 310

Hamburg "Carl von Ossietzky" State and University Library: 87

Harvard University, Cambridge MA: 35, 48

Harvey Cushing/John Hay Whitney Medical Library, Yale University, New Haven, CT: 165

Hendrik Conscience Heritage Library, Antwerp: 10

Herzog August Bibliothek/Herzog August Library Wolfenbüttel: 368, 371

Herzogin-Anna-Amalia-Bibliothek, Weimar: 347

Hessische Landes- und Hochschulebibliothek, Darmstadt: 57

Historical Archives and Trivulziana Library, Mailand: 136

Hof- und Staatsbibliothek, München: 151

Hofbibliothek, Wien: 349

Holy Cross Collection, Patriarchate, Jerusalem: 93

Houghton Library, Harvard University, Cambridge, MA: 49

Hunterian Museum, Glasgow: 84

Ιερά Βατοπεδινή Σκήτη Αγίου Δημητρίου, Άγιον Όρος: 3

Ιερά Μονή Αγίου Ιωάννου του Θεολόγου, Patmos: 262; Πάτμος: 264

Ιερά Μονή Αγίου Παντελεήμονος, Άγιον Όρος/ Holy Mountain: 3; Athos/Άθως: 25

Ιερά Μονή Αγίου Σάββα, Jerusalem: 93

Ιερά Μονή Αγίου Στεφάνου, Μετέωρα: 138

Ιερά Μονή Βαρλαάμ, Μετέωρα: 138

Ιερά Μονή Βατοπεδίου, Άγιον Όρος/Holy Mountain: 3; Athos/Άθως: 16

Ιερά Μονή Βλατάδων, Θεσσαλονίκη: 315

Ιερά Μονή Διονυσίου, Άγιον Όρος /Holy Mountain: 4; Athos/Άθως: 16

Ιερά Μονή Εσφιγμένου, Άγιον Όρος /Holy Mountain: 4; Athos/Άθως: 17

Ιερά Μονή Ευαγγελισμού της Θεοτόκου, Σκιάθος: 313

Ιερά Μονή Ζωοδόχου Πηγής ή της Αγίας, Ανδρος: 10

Ιερά Μονή Θεοβαδίστου Όρους Σινά, Αγίας Αικατερίνης Σινά Όρος: 312

Ιερά Μονή Ιβήρων, Άγιον Όρος/Holy Mountain: 4; Athos/Άθως: 18

Ιερά Μονή Κουτλουμουσίου, Άγιον Όρος/Holy Mountain: 6; Athos/Άθως: 22

Ιερά Μονή Λειμώνος Lesbos/Καλλονή Λέσβου: 108

Ιερά Μονή Μεγάλου Μετεώρου, Μετέωρα: 138

Ιερά Μονή Μεγίστης Λαύρας, Άγιον Όρος/Holy Mountain: 7; Athos/Άθως: 23

Ιερά Μονή Μεταμορφώσεως του Σωτήρος, Μετέωρα: 138

Ιερά Μονή Ξηροποτάμου, Άγιον Όρος/Holy Mountain: 8; Athos/Άθως: 26

Ιερά Μονή Οσίου Νικάνορος, Ζάβορδα: 372

Ιερά Μονή Παντοκράτορος, Άγιον Όρος/Holy Mountain: 8; Athos/Άθως: 26

Ιερά Μονή Σταυρονικήτα, Άγιον Όρος/Holy Mountain: 8; Athos/Άθως: 26

Ιερά Μονή Τιμίου Σταυρού, Jerusalem: 93

Inguimbertine Library, Carpentras: 49

Institut français d'études byzantines, Paris: 262

Institut für Geschichte der Medizin, Leipzig: 106

Institute for the History of Medicine, Leipzig: 106

Interuniversity Health Library-BIU Santé, Paris: 198

Iviron Monastery, Holy Mountain: 4; Athos: 18

J. Paul Getty Museum, Los Angeles, CA: 123

Jagiellonian Library, Jagiellonian University/ Jagiellonian University Library, Kraków: 103

Johann Rhodius' Library, Padua: 189

Josephi de Aromatariis Bibliotheca, Venedig: 323

Kaiserliche öffentliche Bibliothek, Petersbourg: 265

Κεντρική βιβλιοθήκη, Αριστοτέλειο Πανεπιστήμιο Θεσσαλονίκης: 314

Klosterbibliothek, Grottaferrata: 86

Kongelige Bibliotek, København : 101; Kopenhagen: 102

Königlich- und Universitätsbibliothek, Königsberg Pr.: 96

Königliche Bibliothek, Berlin: 27; Brüssel: 36; Dresden: 57; Kopenhagen: 102

Koronis Monastery, Karditsa: 95

Koutloumousiou Monastery, Holy Mountain: 6; Athos: 22

Labronica Library, Livorno: 116

Lambeth Palace, Archiepiscopal Library, London: 120

Lee Library, L. Tom Perry Special Collections, Brigham Young University, Provo, UT: 266

Les Enluminures, Paris, Chicago, New York: 52

Library, Model experimental high school of Mytiline of the University of Aegean, Mitylene: 140; Μυτιλήνη/Mytilene: 157

Library of Batskobou Monastery, Rodopi: 267

Library of Canons Regular of the Lateran, Padua: 187

Library of Complutense University, Madrid: 124

Library of Congress, Rare Book and Manuscripts, Medieval and Renaissance MS., Washington, D.C.: 347

Library of Dionysiou Monastery, Athos: 16

Library of Dochiariou Monastery, Athos: 17

Library of Esfigmenou Monastery, Athos: 17

Library of Grottaferrata National Monument: 86

Library of Iviron Monastery, Athos: 18

Library of Koutloumousiou Monastery, Athos: 22

Library of Panteleimonos Monastery, Athos: 25

Library of St. Michael's Monastery, Venedig: 325, 326; in Murano, Venedig: 326

Library of St. Peter at Corbie: 56

Library of the Cathedral del Pilar, Zaragoza: 372

Library of the Chapter of the Cathedral Church, Toledo: 315

Library of the city of Paris: 196

Library of the City School, Nea-Ephesos: 164

Library of the Earl of Leicester, Holkham: 89

Library of the Great Lavra Monastery, Athos: 23

Library of the Holy Cross, Patriarchate, Jerusalem: 93

Library of the Holy Sepulchre, Patriarchate, Jerusalem: 92

Library of the Limonos Monastery, Lesbos: 108

Library of the Monastery of St. John the Evangelist, Patmos: 262

Library of the Reformed College, Sáros-Patak: 311

Library of the Royal Monastery at San Lorenzo del Escorial, Escurial: 62

Library of the Theotokou Monastery, Chalke: 50

Library of Upsala Academy: 320

Library of Vatopedi Monastery, Athos: 16

Library of Westminster Church, London: 116

Library of Xiropotamou Monastery, Athos: 26

Limonos Monastery, Kalloni, Lesvos: 95

Lincei Academy, Rom: 274

Lobkowicz Library/Lobkowiczká Knihovna, Nelahozeves: 164; Raudnitz: 266

Louis M. Darling Biomedical Library,
    University of California Los Angeles: 123
Lower Saxony State and University Library,
    Göttingen: 84

Mantua, Marcus, Padua: 192
Marciana National Library, Venedig: 327
Marco Mantua's Library, Padua: 192
Marquis of Rosanbo's Library: 308
Mar-Saba Library, Patriarchate, Jerusalem: 93
Marsh Library, Dublin: 59
Marucelliana Library, Florenz: 67
Մատենադարան․Մ․ Մաշտոցի
    անվան հին ձեռագրերի
    գիտահետազոտական
    ինստիտուտ, Երևան: 372
Matenadaran. Mesrop Mashtots Institute of
    Ancient Manuscripts, Yerevan: 372
Mazarine Library, Paris: 200
Media Center/Médiathèque, Orléans: 167
Medical School Library, Montpellier: 144;
    Paris: 198
Medical Society, London: 121
Medicea Laurenziana Library, Firenze/
    Florence: 67
Mediomontani, Cheltenham: 50
Merton College, Oxford: 183
Μετόχιον Παναγίου Τάφου, Jerusalem: 92
Μετόχιον Παναγίου Τάφου-ΜΠΤ, Αθήνα: 15
Metochion of the Holy Sepulchre, MPT,
    Αθήνα: 15
Monastery of Panagia Olympiotissa, Ελασσόνα/
    Elassona: 61
Monastery of St. John the Theologian, Patmos:
    262; Πάτμος: 264
Monastery of the Annunciation, also known
    as Evangelistrias Monastery, Σκιάθος/
    Skiathos: 313
Monastery of the Panagia Kamariotissa,
    Chalke/Χάλκη: 50
Monastery of the Transfiguration of the Savior,
    Μετέωρα/Meteora: 138
Monastery of the Zoodochou Pigis or Agias,
    Άνδρος/Andros: 10
Μονή Αγίου Ιωάννου του Θεολόγου, Patmos/
    Πάτμος: 262
Μονή Αγίου Ιωάννου Υψηλού, Άντισσα: 10
Μονή Αγίου Στεφάνου, Μετέωρα: 138
Μονή Βαρλαάμ, Μετέωρα: 138
Μονή Βλατάδων, Θεσσαλονίκη: 315

Μονή Ευαγγελισμού της Θεοτόκου, Σκιάθος: 313
Μονή Θεοσεβαδίστου Όρους Σινά, Αγίας
    Αικατερίνης, Σινά Όρος: 312
Μονή Θεοτόκου, Chalke/Χάλκη: 50
Μονή Κορώνης, Καρδίτσα: 95
Μονή Λειμώνος, Καλλονή Λέσβου: 95
Μονή Μεγάλου Μετεώρου, Μετέωρα: 138
Μονή Μεταμορφώσεως του Σωτήρος, Μετέωρα:
    138
Μονή Μπατσκόβου, Rhodope/Ροδόπη: 267
Μονή Οσίου Νικάνορος, Ζάβορδα: 372
Μονή Παναγίας Καμαριωτίσσης, Chalke/Χάλκη:
    50
Μονή Παναγίας Ολυμπιώτισσας, Ελασσόνα: 61
Morgan Library, New York, NY: 166
Μουσείο Μπενάκη, Αθήνα: 15
Municipal Inguimbertine Library, Carpentras:
    49
Municipal Library, Besançon: 34; Bologna: 34;
    Lyon: 123; Orléans: 167; Sens: 311
Museum nationale Hungaricum, Budapest: 38

Narcissus Library, Dublin: 59
Народна Библиотека "Св. Св. Кирил и
    Методий" (НБКМ), София: 313
National Library, Athens: 11: Florenz: 80;
    Madrid: 124; Paris: 200; Petersburg: 265;
    Санкт-Петербург (Sankt-Petersburg
    [Saint-Petersburg]): 310; Warsawa: 347;
    Wien: 368
National and University Library, Strasbourg:
    314
National Library "St. Cyril and Methodius",
    Sofia: 313
National Library of Medicine, History of
    Medicine Division, U.S. National
    Institutes of Health, Bethesda, MD: 34
National Museum, Ohrid: 167
Националниот музеј, Охрид: 167
National Museum of Hungary, Budapest: 38
National Széchényi Library, Budapest: 38
National University Library, Torino: 315;
    Turin: 317
Nationalbibliothek, Athen: 11
Natsionalnoï Muzeyi, Ohrid: 167
Natural History Museum, London: 122
Научная Библиотека, Московского
    Государственного Университета Имени
    М. В. Ломоносова (МГУ), Москва: 150
New College Library, Oxford: 184, 187

Newberry Library, Chicago, IL: 53
Niedersachsische Staats- und
    Universitätsbibliothek, Göttingen: 84

Öffentliche Bibliothek der Universität Basel: 27
Oratorian Library, Neapel: 164
Országos Széchényi Könyvtár, Budapest: 38
Österreichische Nationalbibliothek, Wien:
    349, 368

Palace Library, Madrid: 127
Palatine Library, Parma: 262
Πανάγιος Τάφος, Jeruslaem/Ιερουσαλήμ: 94
Παντοκράτορος, Athos/Άθως: 26
Pantokrator/Pantokratoros Monastery, Άγιον
    Όρος/Holy Mountain: 8; Athos/Άθως 26
Parliament Library, Athens: 10
Passionei Library, Rom: 274
Patriarchal Collection, Jerusalem: 94
Patriarchal Library, Jerusalem: 94
Patriarchal Library of Alexandria, Αλεξάνδρεια/
    Alexandria: 9; Cairo: 39
Patriarchal Library, Ecumenical Patriarchate of
    Constantinople: 50, 90, 92
Patriarchatus Alexandrinus, Cairo: 39
Πατριαρχική Βιβλιοθήκη, Οικουμενικό
    Πατριαρχείο Κωνσταντινουπόλεως,
    Istanbul: 90
Πατριαρχείο, Jerusalem/Ιερουσαλήμ: 94
Πατριαρχική Βιβλιοθήκη Αλεξανδρείας: 9;
    Πατριαρχείο, Cairo [Αλεξάνδρεια]: 39
Πατριαρχική Βιβλιοθήκη, Πατριαρχείο,
    Ιερουσαλήμ: 90
Pembroke College, Cambridge: 47
Peterhouse, Cambridge: 48
Phillipps, Cheltenham: 50
Pontifical Greek College/Pontificio collegio
    greco, Roma: 308
Privatbibliothek des Königs, Madrid: 127
Public Historical Library and Museum of the
    Hellenic School of Dimitsana: 57
Public Imperial Library, Petersbourg: 265
Public Library of Basel University: 27
Public Library of Milies: 140

Rare Book and Manuscript Library, University
    of Illinois at Urbana-Champaign, Pre-
    1650 MSS: 321
Real Biblioteca, Madrid: 127; Napoli: 161
Reformiertes Collegium, Sáros-Patak: 311

Regimontani, Königsberg Pr.: 95
Research Library, M.V. Lomonosov Moscow
    State University (MSU): 150
Riccardiana Library, Florenz: 80
Romanian Academy Library, Bucureşti/
    Bucharest: 37
Rossia Library of Jesuit Company College,
    Wien/Vienna: 348
Российский государственный архив древних
    актов (ргада), Москва/Moskva: 150
Российская национальная библиотека
    (РНБ), Petersbourg/Санкт-Петербург:
    265; Санкт-Петербург/Saint-Petersburg:
    310
Royal and University Library, Königsberg Pr.:
    96
Royal Bourbon Library, Neapel: 161
Royal Library, Berlin: 27; Brussels: 36;
    Budapest: 38; Copenhagen: 101, 102;
    Dresden: 57; Madrid: 127; Neapel: 161;
    Paris: 194
Russian State Archive of Ancient Documents
    (RGADA), Москва/Moscow: 150

Sächsische Landesbibliothek–Staats- und
    Universitätsbibliothek, Dresden: 57
San Antonio of Castello Library, Venedig: 337
San Marco National Library, Venezia: 338
San Salvatore, Messina: 137
Santa Iglesia mayor del Pilar, Zaragoza: 372
Sárospatak Reformed College, Great Library,
    Scholarly Collection/Sárospataki
    Református Kollégium Todományos
    Gyüjteményei, Nagykönyvtár, Sáros-
    Patak: 311
Saxe State Library–Dresden State and
    University Library: 57
Scaliger, Joseph Justus: 110
Seminary of Byzantine and Neo-Hellenic
    Philology, Department of Philology,
    National and Kapodistrian University of
    Athens, Athens: 16
Senate Library, Leipzig: 108
Serail Library, Constantinople: 100
Σκήτη Αγίου Δημητρίου, Άγιον Όρος/Holy
    Mountain: 3
Skiti Agiou Dimitriou, Άγιον Όρος/Holy
    Mountain: 3
Софийски Универсиетет "Св. Климент
    Охридски", Научен център за *славяно-*

византийски проучвания "*Иван Дуйчев*", София/Sofia: 314
Σπουδαστήριο Βυζαντινής και Νεοελληνικής Φιλολογίας, Τμήμα Φιλολογίας, Εθνικό και Καποδιστριακό Πανεπιστήμιο Αθηνών, Athen: 16
St. Catherine Monastery of Mount Sinai: 312
St. Geneviève Library, Paris: 262
St. John in Viridario Library, Padua: 192
St. John Library at Carbonara, Neapel: 163
St. John's College/Library, Cambridge: 46
St. Nicolas Church, Gallipoli: 82
St. Nikanor Monastery, Ζάβορδα/Zavorda: 372
St. Peter's College, Cambridge: 48
St. Peter's Library, Rom: 275
St. Remy Library/Monastery Library, Reims: 267
St. Salvatore Library/Monastery, Messina: 137
St. Stephen's Monastery, Μετέωρα/Meteora: 138
Staats- und Universitätsbibliothek Bremen, Bremen: 35
Staats- und Universitätsbibliothek Hamburg "Carl von Ossietzky": 87, 88
Staatsbibliothek zu Berlin-Preussischer Kulturbesitz SBB-PKB, Berlin: 27, 33
Stadsbibliotheek/Stadtbibliothek, Antwerpen: 10
Stadtbibliothek, Bern: 33; Hamburg: 87; Zürich: 373
State and University Library, Bremen: 35
State and University Library of Hesse, Darmstadt: 57
State Oratorian Library of Gerolamini's National Monument, Neapel: 163
Stavronikita Monastery, Άγιον Όρος/Holy Mountain: 8; Athos/Άθως 26
Stiftsbibliothek/Stiftsbibliothek und Stiftsarchiv Zeitz: 373
Synodal Library, Moscow/Synodialbibliothek, Moskau: 145
Synodal Library of Moscow Patriarchate, State Historical Museum (GIM), Moskau: 145; Москва/Moscow: 148

Thüringer Universitäts- und Landesbibliothek/ Thuringia University and State Library, Jena: 91
Tomasini, Filippo/Tomasini's Library, Padua: 194

Topkapı Sarayı Kütüphanesi/Topkapi Sarayi Library, Istanbul: 91; Konstantinopel: 100
Trinity College, Cambridge: 48; Dublin: 60
Trivulziana Library, Mailand/Milano: 136
Turk Tarih Kurumu/Turkish Historical Society, Ankara: 10

Uffenbachianus, Hamburg: 87
Università/Universität, Messina: 138
Universitätsbibliothek "Bibliotheca Albertina", Leipzig: 106
Universitätsbibliothek Erlangen-Nürnberg, Erlangen: 61
Universitätsbibliothek, Göttingen: 84; Heidelberg: 88; Leipzig: 106; Leyden: 109; Tübingen: 316
Universitäts-Bibliothek/ Universiteitsbibliotheek, Amsterdam: 9
Universiteitsbibliotheek Leiden: 103; Leyden: 109
University and Estense Library, Modena: 140, 143
University Library, Amsterdam: 9; Basel: 27; Bologna: 34; Copenhagen/Kopenhagen: 102; Edinburgh: 60; Erlangen: 61; Genoa: 83; Glasgow: 84; Göttingen: 84; Heidelberg: 88; Leiden/Leyden: 103, 109; Leipzig: 106; Madrid: 124; Salamanca: 309; Tübingen: 316; Wrocław: 371
University Library "Albertina Library", Leipzig: 106
University Library of Erlangen-Nuremberg: 61
Uppsala Universitetsbibliotek/Uppsala University Library: 320
Upsaliensis Bibliotheca Academiae, Upsala: 320
Urban Mission Library, Genoa: 84
Urbini et Pisauri, Bibliotheca Ducis: 321

Vallicellana/Vallicelliana Library, Rom: 275; Roma: 307
Van Pelt-Dietrich Library, Kislak Center for Special Collections, Rare Books and Manuscripts, Medieval & Renaissance Manuscripts Collection, University of Pennsylvania, Philadelphia, PA: 265
Varllam Monastery, Μετέωρα/Meteora: 138

Vatican Apostolic Library, Rom, 276; Vatican City: 53

Vatopedi Monastery, Ἅγιον Ὄρος/Holy Mountain: 3; Athos/Ἄθως 16

Vlatadon Monastery, Θεσσαλονίκη/ Thessalonica: 314

Vratislava City Library, Breslau: 36

Wellcome Library, London: 122

Westminster Abbey Library, London: 116

Worcester Cathedral, Worcester: 185

Worcester Church, Oxford: 185

Wrocław University Library, Breslau/Wroclaw: 36

Ξενοφώτνος, Ἄθως/Xenophontos Monastery, Athos: 26

Xiropotamou Monastery, Ἅγιον Ὄρος/Holy Mountain: 8; Athos/Ἄθως, 26

Ypsilou Monastery of St. John, Ἄντισσα/ Antissa: 10

Załuski Library, Warsaw: 265

Zamoyski Library, Warschau: 346

Zentralbibliothek Zürich-Kantons-, Stadt- und Universitätsbibliothek/Zurich Central Library-Cantonal, City and University Library: 373